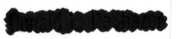

8427/8   1   3   8/11/80

```
 2 215   1475       1    18.40 MDS
11 117     35     1  1      .75 MDS
11 149     41       1      .65 MDS
11 111    835     1  1    13.95 MDS
                         33.75 STL
                          1.01 TAX
                         40.76 ATD
                          6.00 CDU

1 CSH                    34.76 TTL
```

HELMINTHS, ARTHROPODS & PROTOZOA
OF DOMESTICATED ANIMALS

E. J. L. SOULSBY
MA, PhD, MRCVS, DVSM

Chairman, Department of Pathobiology, and Professor of Parasitology, University of Pennsylvania; Chairman, Graduate Department of Parasitology, Graduate School of Arts and Sciences, University of Pennsylvania, Philadelphia. Formerly University Lecturer, Department of Animal Pathology, University of Cambridge

HELMINTHS, ARTHROPODS
& PROTOZOA
OF DOMESTICATED ANIMALS

(Sixth Edition of Mönnig's Veterinary Helminthology & Entomology)

E. J. L. SOULSBY

LEA & FEBIGER   PHILADELPHIA

First edition   1934
Reprinted   1936

Second edition 1938
Reprinted   1941, 1943   By H. O. Mönnig

Third edition   1947
Reprinted   1948, 1950

Fourth edition 1956
Reprinted   1959   Revised by
                                 Geoffrey Lapage
Fifth edition   1962
Reprinted   1965

Sixth edition   1968
Reprinted   1969
Reprinted   1971   Revised by E. J. L. Soulsby
Reprinted   1975
Reprinted   1977

(Helminths, Arthropods & Protozoa of Domesticated Animals)

7020-0237-2

© 1968 Baillière, Tindall and Cassell Ltd
7–8 Henrietta Street
London WC 2

Published in the United States by Lea & Febiger
Philadelphia

Printed at Waverly Press, Inc., Baltimore, Md. 21202 U.S.A.

CONTENTS

LIST OF PLATES

PREFACE TO THE SIXTH EDITION

DESPITE the relatively short time since the fifth edition (6 years) there have been so many advances in the field of parasitology that a new edition of 'Mönnig' has become essential. These advances are such that it becomes increasingly difficult to preserve Professor Mönnig's original intention of a practical manual for veterinarians without losing sight of the basic concepts which permit a full appraisal of the biology of parasites. An attempt has therefore been made to incorporate as much as possible of this basic molecular biology. In addition to this, several other departures have occurred, the major one being the introduction of an entirely new section on the protozoa of veterinary importance. The sixth edition is now, within limits, a text of all the parasites of importance in veterinary medicine. A further departure has been a widening of the geographical scope of the book with an attempt to include important parasitic entities of both developed and developing countries. Other alterations include the placing of references, with title citations, at the end of each major section, the introduction of information on immunity to a parasite in the appropriate part of the text, and a reduction in the amount of detail presented about anthelmintics, insecticides, etc. The latter has been done because the field of therapy of parasitic diseases is moving so rapidly that the time lapse between writing and publication must, inevitably, lead to omission of newer compounds. In any case, it is felt that the main emphasis should be on the parasite, its biology and its pathogenic effects on the host.

Further changes from the fifth edition are an adoption of the Chitwood classification for the nematodes and a reorganisation of the presentation of the arthropods of veterinary importance. No changes have been made in the illustrations for the section of helminthology, but those in the entomology section have been somewhat reorganised so that they are more closely related in the text to the subject matter. The illustrations in the protozoology section have been largely drawn from Wenyon's 'Protozoology' or Hoare's 'Handbook of Medical Protozoology', some are original, two (Plates XXIV and XXV, coccidia of sheep, and of cattle) have been redrawn by the author with the kind permission of Dr J. F. Christensen, University of California, Davis, California and the *Journal of Parasitology*, and one (coccidia of swine, Plate XXVI) is used with the kind permission of Dr John M. Vetterling, Beltsville Parasitological Laboratory, Beltsville, Maryland, the University of Illinois and the *Journal of Parasitology*. To these gentlemen, I offer my grateful thanks.

My thanks also are extended to the many research workers in the field of parasitology. They have contributed with distinction to this exciting age of scientific discovery and I hope the bibliographic citations pay tribute to their efforts. The task of typing, retyping and further re-typing the manuscript and the checking of references has fallen on my secretarial staff Mrs Nancy Barrett, Mrs Helen Roberts, Mrs Nancy Jingozian and Miss Linda Sturgess. To these ladies I owe a debt of gratitude as I do also to Mr Robert Hughes for his expertise in photography. Mr Derek Muncey has now seen four editions of 'Mönnig' prepared; his assistance in the sixth is acknowledged with salutations.

To the publishers I offer my thanks for their co-operation and patience and for the care they have taken in the production of this much revised edition.

Finally, and with the deepest gratitude, I thank my wife for her encouragement, patience and tolerance.

E. J. L. Soulsby

Department of Pathobiology   1968
University of Pennsylvania
Philadelphia

FROM THE PREFACE TO THE FIRST EDITION

SINCE the publication of Neumann's 'Parasites and Parasitic Diseases of Domesticated Animals' in 1892 no textbook that deals adequately with the helminth and arthropod diseases of domesticated animals has appeared, although great progress in this subject can be recorded. Several very useful books have been written on the morphology of helminth and arthropod parasites, but the parasitic diseases with which the veterinarian is primarily concerned, and of which the parasites are only the aetiological factors, have received very little consideration.

During several years of teaching in these subjects the author has felt the great need of a suitable book for veterinary students and practitioners, and the present volume represents an attempt to supply that need. At the same time he hopes that this compilation of practical facts will serve to bring about a realisation of the importance of veterinary parasitology, which is still underrated in many quarters, and that the veterinary student should receive a more adequate training in it.

It has not been the intention to present a complete manual, in which the information required by the veterinarian is buried in a mass of detail, but to give in a scientific way the most important practical facts of the subject. Many known parasites of domesticated animals are not mentioned because they are rarely seen or because little is known about their pathogenicity. It has naturally been difficult to draw the line here, as well as between the hosts themselves. On the whole an attempt has been made to include the important parasites of all the important domesticated animals of all countries. The parasitic diseases of the fur-bearing animals have also been included, because this branch of livestock farming has assumed an importance that deserves the full attention of the veterinarian. If any important parasites of these animals have been omitted, it is only because discrimination on the subject is difficult at the present stage of our knowledge.

H. O. MÖNNIG

INTRODUCTION

PARASITOLOGY is now a multi-disciplinary subject which embraces the fields of biochemistry, physiology, cell biology, immunology and pharmacology, to mention only a few. Rather than attempt an extensive general introduction as has been done in the past, as much basic biological data as space would allow have been introduced into the text, emphasis being placed on those facts which provide a better understanding of the biology of the parasite, its pathogenic effects and control measures against it.

DEFINITIONS

Parasitology is a study of the phenomenon of parasitism—but immediately upon saying this one is faced with the necessity to define parasitism. Until very recently there has been a desire on the part of authors to separate animal associations into parasitism, commensalism and mutualism (or symbiosis). By these definitions it has been implied that commensalism and mutualism are associations of mutual benefit to both partners; in the former the partners retain their physiological independence, while in the latter they are more interdependent. Parasitism, on the other hand, has implied a harmful association; the parasite living at the expense of the host.

Such definitions have invariably led to further qualifying definitions (e.g., temporary parasite, obligatory parasite, periodic parasite), and also to debate as to what is to be regarded as a harmful effect. There are numerous species of organisms which cannot, by any stretch of the imagination, be regarded as pathogens and yet, because they are parasites, it has been assumed *a priori* that they must produce some harmful effect.

With the growth of molecular biological studies of 'parasites' it is clear that there is no longer any justification for retaining strict definitions of animal associations, and certainly none for retaining the idea that a parasite is a form that causes harm to its host. It would seem much more satisfactory to define parasitism as a state in which an organism (the parasite) is metabolically dependent to a greater or lesser extent on another (the host). Within this framework, it would then be useful to designate those forms which are harmful and those which are harmless, or even beneficial, to the host. Two extreme examples might serve to illustrate this: the ciliates of the rumen of the ruminant or the caecum of the horse are metabolically dependent on the host, yet they are far from pathogenic and there is much to indicate that they are beneficial parasites; on the other hand the abomasal worm of sheep, *Haemonchus contortus*, is also metabolically dependent on the host but it is a serious pathogen.

FORMS WHICH ARE PARASITIC

This book deals only with the helminths, arthropods and protozoa which are parasites of domestic animals. It omits the vast assemblage of other parasitic species which also belong to the three groups mentioned above, and the great number of forms which are spread throughout practically every major phylum of the animal kingdom.

The early beginnings of parasitic life must remain obscure since, being invertebrates without exo- or endo-skeletons, they have left no clue to their ancestry. Nevertheless, since they must have evolved with their hosts, the palaeontological history of the host may shed some light on the evolution of parasites. It is probable that early parasitic forms showed little host specificity, but as they became adapted to the host, and evolved with it, the parasites no doubt became increasingly committed to that host.

A more recent consideration of the evolution of host-parasite relationships is based on immunological phenomena. This suggests that the older and better adapted (i.e. non-pathogenic) parasites have increasingly eliminated antigens (? recognition factors) that were foreign to the host. Ultimately, such parasites became forms that shared a number of common antigens with the host, and the degree of antigenic disparity between the host and the parasite determined the success or otherwise of the parasitic organism.

Such a hypothesis could fit into the concept that the pathogenic species of parasites are those which have been parasites for the shortest period of evolutionary time, since they have yet to evolve to the stage where they incite little or no response on the part of the host.

During the evolution of the host-parasite partnership, it is likely that many biological and morphological characters were lost and also that many were gained. The degree to which these took place would depend, amongst other things, on the host parasitized, the site in the host and the environment of the host. Parasites of hosts that are, today, obviously related and which evolved from a common ancestor, probably underwent similar physiological adaptations as these hosts evolved. It is also likely that the physiological changes were expressed as similar changes in morphology, and today, therefore, one would expect a similar series of species in the same habitat in related hosts.

BIOCHEMISTRY AND PHYSIOLOGY

To attempt any broad statement on these subjects would be foolhardy, even if such remarks were restricted to the parasites of domestic animals. Though there are many aspects of the chemical physiology of parasites which are common to many groups, there are also major differences between the members of a family or a genus and it is likely that these differences will become more apparent as knowledge increases. The student is urged to consult Rogers (1962), Read (1966), Read, Rothman and Simmons (1963), von Brand (1966) and others, on this most important aspect of parasitology.

EFFECT OF PARASITES ON THEIR HOSTS

Though there are many species of parasites which are harmless, there are also many forms which produce pathological changes which may lead to severe ill health or death of the host.

As might be expected, the effects are very varied and in many cases represent a combination of several entities. The parasite may compete with the host for food, and where this is a specific effect (e.g., competition for vitamin B_{12} by *Diphyllobothrium latum*) the host may suffer a specific deficiency syndrome (e.g. anaemia in the case of *D. latum* infection). More generally, however, the competition for food is much less well defined. The parasite may indirectly be the cause of decreased food utilisation by the host, it may cause a reduced appetite with a concomitant reduction of food intake, or an increased passage of food through the digestive tract. Changes in the absorptive surface of the intestine may result in marked alterations in the efflux and influx of water and sodium and chloride ions into the bowel and in morphological and biochemical changes in epithelial cells and their microvilli.

The removal of the host's tissues and fluids by parasites is best illustrated by the blood-sucking activities of certain nematodes (e.g. hookworms, *Haemonchus*) and arthropods (e.g. ticks, blood-sucking flies) and in some cases death of the host is directly attributable to excessive loss of blood.

One of the most common effects of parasitism is destruction of the host's tissues. This may be by a mechanical action when, for example, parasites or their larval stages migrate through or multiply in tissues or organs, or when various organs of attachment (e.g. head-spines or teeth, claws, suckers, etc.) are inserted into the tissues as anchors. Destruction may be by pressure as a parasite grows larger (e.g. hyatid, coenurus), or by blockage of ducts such as blood vessels to produce infarction (*Strongylus*), or of lymph vessels to produce oedema and elephantiasis (filariasis) or the intestinal canal to produce necrosis and rupture (ascarids).

Often the destruction of tissues is a secondary effect. It may arise from bacterial infection of lesions caused by a parasite (e.g. bowel ulcers) or by the reaction of the host to the parasite. The latter effect may be due to fibrosis of a lesion (e.g. cirrhosis due to *Fasciola hepatica*), excessive proliferation of epithelium (e.g. *Eimeria stiedae* in the bile ducts of the rabbit), endothelium (e.g. aneurysm caused by *Strongylus*), lymphoid tissue (e.g. leishmaniasis) or the initiation of malignant propensities (e.g. *Spirocerca lupi* in the dog). Tissue damage may also be caused by the immunological response of the host, resulting in necrosis, dermatitis (cercarial dermatitis), oedema (ascariasis and dictyocauliasis of the lung) or excessive cell invasion (scabies, ascariasis of the liver).

These are but a few examples of how pathogenic parasites cause their ill effects; many other examples could be quoted but a comparable list could also be given of those forms for which no adequate explanation can be given of the pathogenic effects. Even with the forms where there is an apparently clear end-result of the parasitism (e.g. anaemia, emaciation or paralysis), often little is known about the chemical pathology and the chronology of the disease process. Anaemia, for example, is a common feature of parasitism and where this is associated with blood sucking parasites the cause and effect may appear relatively clear. Even in these circumstances, however, it is not as simple as has been supposed, and in other parasitic diseases a complex series of nutritional, biochemical and pathological conditions inter-react to manifest themselves as 'anaemia'.

It is clear that a vast amount of investigational work remains to be done on the genesis of the pathology of parasitism.

IMMUNOLOGY

Much evidence has accumulated in the last few decades to indicate that the immune response to parasites is an important phenomenon in the pathology of infection and in the control of parasite populations. Practical uses of the immune response have been the development of immuno-diagnostic tests and the production of vaccines.

The subject of immunology in parasitic infections has now become so immense that, like the biochemistry and physiology of them, it would be unwise to attempt to give a proportionate impression of the vast amount of facts in the limited space of this introduction. This would, inevitably, result in abbreviated treatment of major concepts and in any case, it becomes more and more difficult to present any unified hypothesis, if one exists, of the immunology of parasitism. Consequently, the pertinent facts about immunity to the various species of parasites are presented in the appropriate parts of the text. This aspect of parasitology is very important and the student is urged to consult Sprent (1963), Soulsby (1966, 1962), Garnham, Pierce and Roitt (1963), Kagan (1966), Weinmann (1966), Urquhart, Jarrett and Mulligan (1962), World Health Organisation (1965), International Atomic Energy Agency (1964).

REFERENCES

GARNHAM, P. C. C., PIERCE, A. E. & ROITT, I. (1963). Ed. *Immunity to Protozoa.* Oxford: Blackwell Scientific Publications

INTERNATIONAL ATOMIC ENERGY AGENCY (1964). Production and utilisation of radiation vaccines against helminth diseases. *Technical Reports Series No. 30, International Atomic Energy Agency.* Vienna

KAGAN, I. G. (1966). Mechanisms of immunity in trematode infection. In *Biology of Parasites,* Ed. E. J. L. Soulsby, New York and London: Academic Press

READ, C. P. (1966). Nutrition of intestinal helminths. In *Biology of Parasites,* Ed. E. J. L. Soulsby, New York and London: Academic Press

READ, C. P., ROTHMAN, A. H. & SIMMONS, J. E. (1963). Studies on membrane transport, with special reference to parasite-host integration. *Ann. N.Y. Acad. Sci.,* **113**, 154–205

ROGERS, W. P. (1962). *The Nature of Parasitism.* New York and London: Academic Press

SOULSBY, E. J. L. (1966). The mechanisms of immunity to gastrointestinal nematodes. In *Biology of Parasites,* Ed. Soulsby. New York and London: Academic Press

SOULSBY, E. J. L. (1962). Antigen-antibody reactions in helminth infections. In *Advances in Immunology.* Vol. 2. New York and London: Academic Press

SPRENT, J. F. A. (1962). *Parasitism.* St. Lucia, Queensland: University of Queensland Press

URQUHART, G. M., JARRETT, W. F. H. & MULLIGAN, W. (1962). Helminth immunity. *Adv. Vet. Sci.*, **7**, 87–129

WEINMANN, C. J. (1966). Immunity mechanisms in cestode infections. In *Biology of Parasites*, Ed. E. J. L. Soulsby. New York and London: Academic Press

World Health Organisation (1965). *Immunology and Parasitic Diseases*, Report of a WHO Expert Committee. Technical Report Series No. 315 World Health Organisation, Geneva

In addition to the references above, more information on the biology of parasites may be obtained from a number of other texts, a selection of which is given below.

GENERAL PARASITOLOGY

LAPAGE, G. (1958). *Parasitic Animals*, 2nd Ed. Cambridge: Heffer

BAER, J. G. (1951). *Ecology of Animal Parasites*. Ill.: University of Illinois Press

DOGIEL, V. A. (1962). *General Parasitology*, 3rd Ed. Leningrad University Press. Eng. trans.: Edinburgh and London (1964) Oliver and Boyd, New York (1966) Academic Press

NOBLE, E. R. & NOBLE, G. A. (1966). *Parasitology: The Biology of Animal Parasites*, 2nd Ed. Philadelphia: Lea and Febiger, and London, Kimpton.

CHENG, T. C. (1964). *The Biology of Animal Parasites*. Philadelphia: Saunders

CHANDLER, A. C. & READ, C. P. (1961). *Introduction to Parasitology*. 10th Ed. New York: John Wiley

BIOCHEMISTRY AND PHYSIOLOGY

VON BRAND, T. (1966). *Biochemistry of Parasites*. New York and London: Academic Press

ROGERS, W. P. (1962). *The Nature of Parasitism*. New York and London: Academic Press

SMYTH, J. D. (1962). *Introduction to Animal Parasitology*. London: English Universities Press

STAUBER, L. A. (1960). *Host Influence on Parasite Physiology*. New Brunswick, New Jersey: Rutgers University Press

COLE, W. H. (1955). *Some Physiological Aspects and Consequences of Parasitism*. New Brunswick, New Jersey: Rutgers University Press

LEE, D. L. (1965). *The Physiology of Nematodes*. Edinburgh and London: Oliver and Boyd

SOULSBY, E. J. L. (1966). *Biology of Parasites: Emphasis on Veterinary Parasites*. New York and London: Academic Press

IMMUNOLOGY

TALIAFERRO, W. H. (1929). *Immunology of Parasitic Infections*. New York: Century

SPRENT, J. F. A. (1963). *Parasitism*. St. Lucia, Queensland: University of Queensland Press

SOULSBY, E. J. L. (1966). *Biology of Parasites: Emphasis on Veterinary Parasites*. New York and London: Academic Press

GARNHAM, P. C. C., PIERCE, A. E. & ROITT, I. (1963). *Immunity to Protozoa*. Oxford: Blackwell Scientific Publications

In addition to the titles listed above, review articles on various aspects of parasitology have been published in the series *Advances in Parasitology* (Ed. Ben Dawes. New York and London: Academic Press), in the 'Parasitological Reviews' section of the journal *Experimental Parasitology* (Ed. David R. Lincicome. New York and London: Academic Press) and in the *Annals of the New York Academy of Sciences*, Volume 113, Article 1, pages 1–510, 'Some Biochemical and Immunological Aspects of Host-Parasite Relationship' (Consulting Editor, Thomas C. Cheng).

HELMINTH PARASITES

Helminth Parasites

THE name helminth, which is derived from the Greek words *helmins* or *helminthos*, a worm, is nowadays usually applied only to the parasitic and non-parasitic species belonging to the phyla Platyhelminthes (flukes, tapeworms and other flatworms) and Nemathelminthes (roundworms and their relatives), but it is sometimes still also applied, as it formerly was, to species of the phylum Annelida (earthworms, leeches and other ringed worms). The Annelida are, however, fundamentally different from both the Platyhelminthes and the Nemathelminthes and it is better not to apply the term helminth to them. The only species of the phylum Annelida considered in this book are the relatively few species of leeches that may be parasitic on man and domesticated animals and the earthworms that may be intermediate hosts of Platyhelminthes and Nematoda.

PHYLUM: PLATYHELMINTHES

Dorso-ventrally flattened and usually hermaphrodite worms with solid bodies without a body cavity, all of which, except most of the species of the Class Turbellaria, are parasitic. The organs are embedded in tissue called the parenchyma and the excretory organs are the flame-cells described below. Respiratory and blood-vascular systems are absent. Like the Nemathelminthes, but unlike the Annelida, the Platyhelminthes are not metamerically segmented. The life history is usually indirect.

CLASS: TURBELLARIA (Eddyworms)

A class comprised chiefly of non-parasitic species living in fresh water, the sea or on land, the body having a ciliated covering. The parasitic species are not parasitic in domesticated animals.

CLASS: TREMATODA (Flukes)

Species have an alimentary canal.

CLASS: CESTODA

Species have no alimentary canal (cf. Acanthocephala), food being absorbed through the soft cuticle. The Cestodaria, which are parasitic in fishes and are in some respects intermediate between the Trematoda and the Cestoda, are not considered in this book. Some authorities include them with the Cestoda in a Class called the Cestoidea.

3

PHYLUM NEMATHELMINTHES

CLASS: NEMATODA (Roundworms)

Cylindrical worms, both ends being usually somewhat pointed. The body is not metamerically segmented. The cuticle, which usually looks smooth to the unaided eye and glistens when it is wet, may show various cuticular structures visible under magnification, but the metameric rings visible in annelid worms are not present. Beneath the cuticle there is a hypodermis and beneath this a layer of muscle-cells of a type not found in any other animals. Down the centre of the cylindrical body runs the alimentary canal, which is a tube usually consisting of a mouth at the anterior end of the worm, a muscular oesophagus and an intestine leading to an anus which, unlike that of annelid worms, is not terminal, so that a short tail is present. Between the muscle-cells and the alimentary canal there is a perienteric space filled with fluid under pressure. In the body wall there are organs called lateral canals and other glands associated with them that are regarded as being excretory organs. Flame cells are not present and cilia are absent from the body. The sexes are in separate individuals. The life histories are either direct or indirect.

CLASS: NEMATOMORPHA (Hair worms, Gordiacea)

The adults are non-parasitic, long, threadlike worms living in the water or moist soil. The sexes are in separate individuals. The larvae are parasitic in insects, centipedes and millipedes. Neither the adults nor the larvae are parasitic in domesticated animals, but they may be mistaken for parasitic species.

CLASS: ACANTHOCEPHALA (Thornyheaded worms)

Cylindrical worms with a thick cuticle and a retractable proboscis provided with spines or hooks. There is no alimentary canal (cf. Cestoda). The excretory organs contain bunches of flame-cells. The sexes are in separate individuals and the life-histories are indirect.

Trematodes
(Phylum: Platyhelminthes)

CLASS: TREMATODA

THE bodies of trematodes or flukes are dorso-ventrally flattened and, unlike those of tapeworms, they consist of one piece only. All the organs are embedded in a parenchyma, no body cavity being present. Suckers, hooks or clamps attach these species to the exterior or the internal organs of their hosts. A mouth and an alimentary canal are present, but usually there is no anus. The mouth leads into a muscular pharynx, succeeding which is an intestine, and this divides into two branches, which may themselves branch. The branched excretory system has flame cells and it discharges into an excretory bladder which usually has a posterior opening. The reproductive system is hermaphrodite, except in the family Schistosomatidae, the species of which are unisexual. The life histories are direct (Monogenea) or indirect (Digenea). There are three orders.

ORDER: MONOGENEA

Species of this order are parasitic chiefly on cold-blooded aquatic vertebrates (fishes, amphibia and reptiles), and most of them are ecto-parasitic. None of them attack domesticated animals. The life-histories are, so far as is known, direct.

ORDER: ASPIDOGASTREA

This order contains only one family, the Aspidogastridae, the species of which are parasitic in, or on, fishes, turtles, Mollusca or Crustacea, none being parasitic on domesticated animals.

ORDER: DIGENEA

To this order belong all the species parasitic in domesticated animals. The life-histories require one, two, or more than two, intermediate hosts.

5

ORDER: DIGENEA

In general outline the digenetic trematodes are dorso-ventrally flat-tened, some being long and narrow, some leaf-shaped while a few, the amphistomes, have thick fleshy bodies and the schistosomes are long and worm-like.

The cuticle, or tegument, may be smooth or spiny but as well as serving as an outer covering it is also a physiologically dynamic structure respon-sible for the transport of nutrients (Björkman & Thorsell, 1964). The outer layer is a plasma membrane, the inner layer contains numerous mitochondria and is connected by protoplasmic strands to subcellular cells. With the exception of microvilli the tegument (e.g. of *Fasciola hepatica*) is similar to that of cestodes (see p. 89).

The organs of attachment consist of an anterior sucker (oral sucker) placed at the anterior end of the body and a ventral sucker usually in the anterior third of the ventral surface, but the position varies and in some forms the ventral sucker may be missing.

The digestive system opens at the mouth which is surrounded by the anterior sucker. Posteriorly there is a muscular pharynx then an oeso-phagus, this leading into the intestine which usually divides into two blind caeca. A few species of trematodes have an anus. Secondary branching of the caeca may occur. Electronmicroscopy of the gut epi-thelium (of *F. hepatica*) reveals looped and branching projections, de-limited by a triple membrane and having a dense core (Thorsell & Björkman, 1965). Their function has occasioned debate, some workers considering them active in absorption others in a secretory mechanism. Incorporation of radioactive amino-acids occurs at a high rate in caecal epithelium.

The excretory system consists of a bladder which is sac-like in its simplest form, but may have various shapes, and usually opens at the posterior extremity of the body. From this central collecting organ branched tubes run out into the parenchyma, ending in terminal organs, flame-cells, which are characteristic of the flatworms. These cells have a basal cytoplasmic portion which contains the nucleus and bears a number of long cilia that lie in the proximal wide part of the tube which is attached to the cell. The flame-cell is the excretory cell, collecting from its sur-roundings the waste products to be excreted, while its cilia produce a current in the tubes and so propel these substances to the bladder. The latter gradually fills and ejects the contents at intervals. The flame-cells can best be seen in live cercariae placed under a cover-slip to which slight pressure is applied.

The nervous system is composed of a circum-oesophageal ring of fibres and ganglia, from which a number of nerves run forwards and backwards to all parts of the body. Sense organs as such are not present in the adult, although the free-living larval forms (miracidium and cercaria) may be provided with patches of pigment called 'eye-spots'.

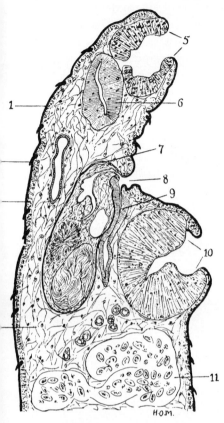

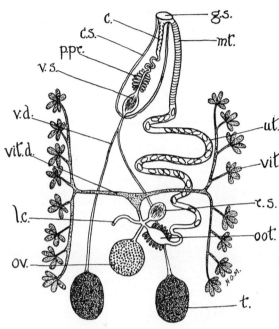

FIG. 2. Reproductive Organs of a Trematode: Diagrammatic (Original)

c.	Cirrus
c.s.	Cirrus-sac
g.s.	Genital sinus
l.c.	Laurer's canal
mt.	Metraterm
oot.	Oötype surrounded by Mehlis's glands
ov.	Ovary
p.pr.	Pars prostatica
r.s.	Receptaculum seminis
t.	Testis
ut.	Uterus
v.d.	Vas deferens
v.s.	Vesicula seminalis
vit.	Vitellaria
vit.d.	Vitelline duct

FIG. 1. Longitudinal Section through *Fasciola hepatica* (after Mönnig)

1. Cuticle
2. Cuticular spine
3. Subcuticular cells
4. Parenchyma
5. Oral sucker
6. Pharynx
7. Cirrus sac
8. Genital sinus
9. Metraterm
10. Ventral sucker
11. Uterus with eggs

With the exception of the *Schistosomatidae* the trematodes are hermaphrodite (Fig. 2). The male organs consist as a rule of two testes which may be spherical, lobed, branched or divided into a number of smaller bodies. The vasa efferentia unite to form the vas deferens, which usually widens distally and forms a vesiculum seminalis surrounded by the prostate gland, and then ends in the cirrus, a protrusible portion which may be armed with spines. There may be a cirrus-sac enclosing these terminal organs. The genital pore is usually anterior and ventral, but may be posterior or lateral. It is surrounded by a genital sinus or atrium, which is in some species (e.g of the family Heterophyidae) developed into a sucker and in which the female pore is also situated. Self-fertilisation usually takes place; the cirrus is evaginated and enters the uterus, or the genital sinus is closed and communication is established in this way.

The female organs (Fig. 2) consist of an ovary which is usually slightly

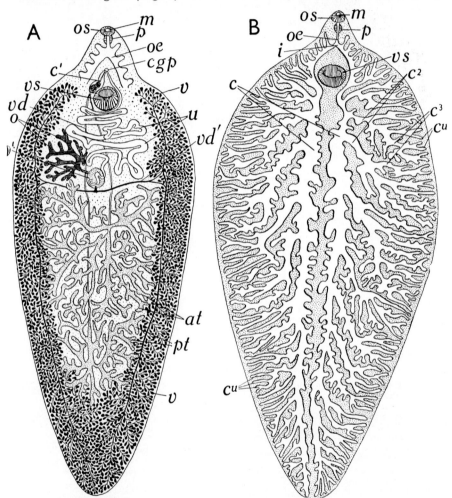

FIG. 3. *Fasciola hepatica*. A, the reproductive system; B, the alimentary canal. (Original by Dawes, B. (1946) *The Trematoda*. Cambridge University Press)

os.	Oral sucker	*c¹.*	Cirrus
vs.	Ventral sucker	*v.*	Vitellaria
m.	Mouth	*vd.*	Vas deferens
p.	Pharynx	*vd¹.*	Duct of the vitelline gland
oe.	Oesophagus	*u.*	Uterus
c.	Intestinal caecum	*o.*	Ovary
c²,c³, cu.	Secondary, tertiary and ultimate branches of the intestinal caeca	*o¹.*	Oötype
		at.	Anterior testis
cgp.	Common genital pore	*pt.*	Posterior testis

lobed and discharges the ova into the oviduct. The latter frequently bears a receptaculum seminis and a narrow canal opening on the dorsal surface of the body, known as Laurer's canal, the function of which is obscure. The insertion of the penis of another fluke into Laurer's canal has been directly observed, but it is not likely that copulation normally occurs in this way. It has been suggested that the function of Laurer's canal is to let out possibly injurious accumulations of material used for making the shells of the eggs (Dawes, 1946). In ectoparasitic (Monogenea) forms a vagino-intestinal canal is present. There is a paired vitelline or yolk gland, consisting usually of a number of follicles situated laterally in the body and discharging into the yolk duct, which joins the oviduct in a special wide portion, the oötype, in which the eggs are formed. The oötype is surrounded by numerous unicellular glands, called Mehlis's glands, which are sometimes collectively called the shell-gland. Recent work has shown that the shells of the eggs are formed from material contributed by both Mehlis's glands and the vitelline glands. For a discussion of the formation of the egg-shell in trematodes and cestodes, see Smyth & Clegg (1959). On leaving the oötype the eggs enter the uterus, which may be short or much convoluted and opens at the genital pore. In some species the distal part of the uterus forms a wide and sometimes muscular portion or metraterm. The eggs usually have an operculum, and those of many species develop in the uterus, so that they are ready to hatch when they are laid.

Life-cycle. The eggs of the *Digenea* are usually passed in the faeces of the host and under suitable conditions of moisture and warmth a larva, *miracidium*, hatches out. The miracidium is roughly triangular in shape, the anterior end being broader and it is usually covered with a ciliated ectoderm, and may have an anterior spine for boring into the intermediate host. The intermediate host is a snail though second intermediate hosts such as other snails or a wide range of other invertebrates, or even vertebrates, may occur in the life-cycle. The miracidium is usually provided with excretory and nervous systems and may have a sac-like gut and an eye-spot. A number of germinal cells are attached to the walls of the body cavity. This larval stage does not feed and further development occurs after it penetrates into a snail. Following penetration the ciliated coat is lost and the form becomes a *sporocyst*—an undifferentiated mass of cells. In due course *rediae* may develop from the germinal cells of the sporocyst. This is not necessarily a feature of all digenetic trematodes. The final stage, the *cercaria* is produced by the sporocyst or the redia. The redia has an oral sucker, a pharynx, a sac-like intestine, an excretory system and a birth-pore, through which cercariae produced inside it escape. The cercaria has suckers and an intestine like that of the adult, excretory and nervous systems, special glands and sometimes an anterior spine. It is frequently also provided with a tail, by means of which it propels itself through the water after escaping from the snail.

The cercaria is the final larval stage and the infective stage and has to reach the definitive host in order to complete its life-cycle. When there is only one intermediate host the cercaria directly enters the definitive host. It may enter this host *passively* when the definitive host drinks water

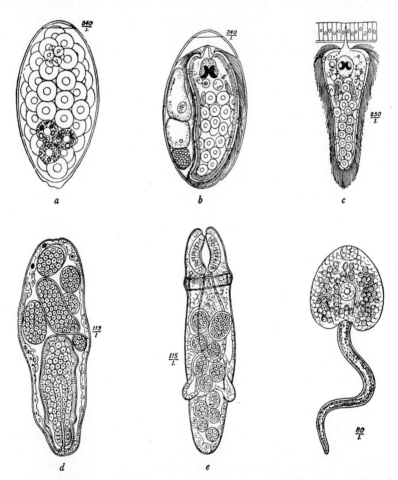

FIG. 4. *Fasciola hepatica*, Development (from Baylis, after Thomas). *a*, egg; *b*, egg containing miracidium; *c*, miracidium; *d*, sporocyst; *e*, redia; *f*, cercaria.

in which the cercaria is swimming, or the cercaria may first enclose itself in a protective cyst on the herbage and this cyst may be eaten with the herbage by the definitive host. The cercariae of some species of flukes, however, such as those belonging to the family Schistosomatidae, can *actively* penetrate the skin of the definitive host. When there is more than one intermediate host, the cercaria, after leaving the first intermediate host, enters the second intermediate host and encysts inside it. There it must wait passively until the second intermediate host is eaten by the definitive host. The term *metacercaria* is given to the cercaria after it has encysted either inside the second intermediate host or on herbage or elsewhere.

When the encysted metacercaria is swallowed by the final host excystation occurs in the intestinal tract and the immature stage migrates to its predilection site. The structure of cercariae varies and they have been given names that refer to details of their anatomical structure. They are discussed by Dawes (1946) and other authors.

Classification of Cercariae according to Lühe (1909)

A. Body of cercaria with a dorsal, longitudinal undulating fin-fold along the body . . . . *Lophocercaria*
B. Body without longitudinal membrane.
   I. Tail with two symmetrical, slender caudal appendages which arise separately and are several times longer than the body. Oral aperture at middle of ventral surface. Intestine simple, sac-like . . . . *Gasterostome cercaria*
   II. Caudal appendage variable, absent or distally forked, but never split to the base. Oral aperture anterior. Intestine bifurcate.
     (a) Ventral sucker absent . . . . . . *Monostome cercaria*
     (b) Ventral sucker present.
       1. Ventral sucker posterior, immediately anterior to base of slender tail . . . . *Amphistome cercaria*
       2. Ventral sucker anterior to hind end of body and well separated from base of tail if latter is present
                       Distome cercaria

Distome Cercariae are further classified as follows:

A. Cercariae single.
   I. Tail well developed.
     (a) Body retractile into a chamber formed by base of tail
                     Cystocercous cercaria
     (b) Body not retractile into tail.
       1. Tail not bifurcate.
         (a) Tail with bristles.
           (i) Tail contractile to equal or exceed width of body
                  Rhopalocercous cercaria
           (ii) Tail always distinctly narrower than body
                  Leptocercous cercaria
        (b) Tail with bristles (marine) . . *Trichocercous cercaria*
       2. Tail distally bifurcate . . . . . *Furcocercous cercaria*
   II. Tail stumpy or absent.
     (a) Tail stumpy . . . . *Microcercous cercaria*
     (b) Tail absent . . . . *Cercariaeum*
B. Cercariae joined into a colony by their tapering tail ends (marine)
                         Rat-king cercariae

A more detailed account of the systematics of the Trematoda may be obtained from Dawes (1946). Silverman (1965) has given a review of the *in vitro* cultivation studies on trematodes, Read (1966) has summarised the mechanism of nutrition and Kagan (1966) has reviewed the mechanisms of immunity in trematode infection.

FAMILY: DICROCOELIIDAE

Species of this family are small or medium-sized flukes parasitic in the biliary and pancreatic ducts of amphibia, reptiles, birds and mammals. The body is flattened and elongate, with weak musculature and loose parenchyma through which the internal organs are easily seen. The cuticle often lacks spines. The suckers are not far apart. A pharynx and an oesophagus are present and the intestinal caeca are simple, not quite reaching the posterior end of the body. The excretory bladder is simple and tubular. The testes are situated not far behind the ventral sucker and the ovary is usually behind them. The genital pore opens in the middle line in front of the ventral sucker. The cirrus is small. A Laurer's canal and a small receptaculum seminis are present. The well-developed vitelline glands lie chiefly in the lateral regions of the body. Most of the space behind the genital glands is filled by the many folds of the uterus. The numerous small eggs are deep brown in colour.

Genus: Dicrocoelium Dujardin, 1845

D. dendriticum (Rudolphi, 1819) Looss, 1899 (syn. *D. lanceolatum*), occurs in the bile ducts of the sheep, goat, ox, deer, pig, dog, donkey, hare, rabbit, elk, coypu and rarely man. Hamsters, cotton rats, white rats and guinea-pigs are also susceptible and the Syrian hamster is the most satisfactory laboratory host. It occurs in Europe, Asia and North America but has not been reported from Central and South Africa or Australia. The fluke is 6–10 mm. long and 1·5–2·5 mm. wide. The body is elongate, narrow anteriorly and widest behind the middle. The cuticle is smooth. The oral sucker is smaller than the ventral. The testes are slightly lobed and lie almost tandem, immediately posterior to the ventral sucker, with the ovary directly behind them. The vitelline glands occupy the middle third of the lateral fields. Behind the gonads the central field is occupied by the transverse coils of the uterus, filled with brown eggs (Fig. 5). The latter measure 36–45 by 22–30 μ and are operculate.

Life History. Two intermediate hosts, a snail and an ant, are required. The two principal snail hosts are *Zebrina detrita* in Europe and *Cionella lubrica* in North America but some twenty-nine other species have been reported to serve as first intermediate hosts (Soulsby, 1965). These include the species *Abida frumentum, Ena obscura, Theba carthusiana, Theba fruticicola, Helicella ericetorum, H. italia* and *Xerophila candidula* but there is no information on the relative roles of these under natural conditions.

The miracidia do not hatch out of the eggs until the eggs have been swallowed by the intermediate host. They hatch in the snail's gut and migrate to the mesenteric gland, where they grow to polymorphous sporocysts lacking a distinct cuticle. These produce a second generation of sporocysts, provided with a cuticle and a birth pore, which in turn produce cercariae, known as *Cercaria vitrina*. Rediae are not formed. The rate of development is slow; 3 months or more being required to produce

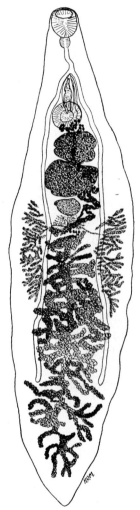

FIG. 5. *Dicrocoelium dendriticum*, Ventral View (Original)

cercariae. The cercariae emerge from the sporocysts only in damp weather following a dry spell and, in the pulmonary chamber of the snail, they clump together in masses called *slime-balls*, in each of which there may be 200–400 cercariae, held together by a sticky, gelatinous substance. These slime-balls are expelled from the snail when a drop in temperature occurs, and adhere to vegetation. The slime-balls are eaten by ants of the genus *Formica*. In the U.S.A., *F. fusca* is concerned (Krull & Mapes, 1953) in Europe *F. fusca*, *F. cunicularia*, *F. gagatis* and *F. rufibarbis* (Hohorst & Graefe, 1961) and in the U.S.S.R., *F. fusca*, *F. rufibarbis* and *Proformica nasuta* (Svadzhian, 1954). Metacercariae are produced in the abdominal cavity, as many as 128 per ant, the time required varying from 26 to 62 days, depending on the environmental temperature. The definitive hosts are infected by swallowing infected ants. It has been generally accepted that the cercariae penetrate into the intestinal wall of the final host; pass by the portal circulation to the liver, and eventually enter the bile ducts. Krull (1958), however, using experimental infections of hamsters and white mice, actually observed the metacercariae entering the intestinal opening of the common bile duct and he states that they enter the liver by this route rather than by penetration of the host's tissues. He found that the metacercariae may, in these hosts, reach all parts of the biliary system within an hour after their entry through the common bile duct. The young flukes develop in the smaller bile ducts, the older ones go to the larger bile ducts. They are full grown after 7 weeks and the first eggs are laid 4 weeks later.

Pathogenesis and Symptoms. These small flukes penetrate into the fine branches of the bile ducts, in which they lie greatly extended and attached by means of their suckers.

Several thousand flukes may occur in field cases, but even with such numbers the pathological changes are of a much lower order than with *Fasciola hepatica*. In advanced infection there is extensive cirrhosis and scarring of the liver surface and the bile ducts are markedly distended with large numbers of flukes. Early fibrosis occurs in the portal triads and this later extends in an interlobular and perilobular manner, ultimately producing a condition resembling portal cirrhosis. Marked proliferation of the bile duct glandular epithelium occurs.

The clinical picture in severe cases consists of anaemia, oedema and emaciation.

Treatment. Hexachloroethane and fouadin, previously recommended treatments, have been shown to inhibit egg production only. Hetolin [$\beta\beta\beta$-tris-4-chlorophenyl propionic acid-4-methylpiperazine hydrochloride] was found by Lämmler (1963) and Enigk & Düwel (1963) to be effective against *D. dendriticum*, doses of 19–22 mg. per kg. being 90 per cent effective. The drug is well tolerated, even by pregnant sheep. Thiabendazole at high dose rates (200–300 mg. per kg.) has been found 96 per cent effective by Šibalić *et al.* (1963).

Control measures rely on treatment of infected animals and the control of snails and ants. However, several factors operate to make control difficult. The eggs of *D. dendriticum* may remain viable for months in soil or faeces and they also withstand sub-zero temperatures. The intermediate hosts live in dry areas and, being scattered over the pasture, are less vulnerable than amphibious or aquatic snails to molluscicide treatment. Wild animals are commonly infected: in the U.S.A. the woodchuck serves as a reservoir host for domestic stock and in Europe the rabbit may maintain infection in an area for considerable periods.

Cultivation of pasture to improve soil texture and disrupt ant nests has been suggested and biological control of snails with domestic poultry has been practised.

Dicrocoelium hospes Looss, 1907, is a closely related species found in the gall-bladder of the ox in the Sudan, Nigeria and Ghana.

Genus: Platynosomum Looss, 1907

P. fastosum (Kossack, 1910) (syn. *P. concinnum*) occurs in the liver of cats in Malaysia, British Guiana, Brazil, Bahamas, Puerto Rico, Florida and other southern states of the U.S.A. It has also been found in a wild cat. It measures 4–8 by 1·5–2·5 mm. It differs from *Dicrocoelium* mainly in being less lanceolate, the testes are horizontal in position and the eggs measure 34–50 by 20–35 μ.

Life-history. Miracidia are present in the eggs when these are passed in the faeces. These are ingested by the snail *Sublina octona*. Cercariae encyst in lizards, *Anolis cristatellus* being important in Puerto Rico (Maldonado, 1945).

Pathogenicity. Leam & Walker (1963) consider the parasite to be the cause of 'lizard poisoning' in cats. A marked dilation of bile ducts occurs with desquamation of bile duct epithelium. The liver may be markedly enlarged. Clinical signs are diarrhoea, vomiting and a progressive icterus. In the terminal stages, diarrhoea and vomiting may be continuous. *Treatment*—unknown.

Platynosomum ariestis Travassos 1918, occurs in the intestine of sheep in Brazil. It is nonpathogenic.

Genus: Eurytrema Looss, 1907

E. pancreaticum (Janson, 1889) is found in the pancreatic ducts and more rarely in the bile ducts and the duodenum of sheep, goat, cattle and buffalo in eastern Asia and Brazil and humans in China. It measures 8–16 by 5–8·5 mm. The body is thick and armed with spines, which are often lost in the adult stage. The suckers are large, the oral being the larger of the two. The pharynx is small and the oesopaghus short. The testes are horizontal, slightly posterior to the level of the ventral sucker. The genital pore opens just behind the bifurcation of the intestine. The cirrus sac is tubular and reaches back past the anterior margin of the ventral sucker. The ovary is situated near the median line, behind the testes, and the uterus fills the posterior part of the body. The vitelline glands are follicular and are laterally situated (Fig. 7). The eggs measure 40–50 by 23–34 μ.

Life-cycle. Tang (1950) found that the two land-snails, *Bradybaena similaris* and *Cathaica ravida sieboldtiana*, belonging to the family Fruiti-coidolidae, serve as first intermediate hosts of this species. Two generations of sporocysts occur in the snails, the second producing cercariae about 5 months after infection. Cercariae are extruded onto herbage and are eaten by grasshoppers, *Conocephalus maculatus* serving as a secondary inter-

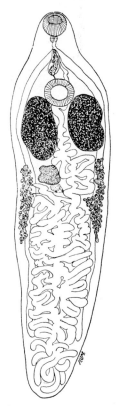

Fig. 6. *Platynosomum fastosum,* Ventral View (Original)

mediate host in Malaysia (Basch, 1966). Metacercariae occur in the haemocoele becoming infective 3 weeks after infection of the grasshopper. Sheep and goats are infected by inadvertently eating infected grass-hoppers, the immature flukes migrating via the pancreatic duct. In goats the prepatent period is 7 weeks.

Several other species of this genus have been described from domestic and other ruminants, but it is not clear whether these are all distinct species. *E. ovis,* described by Tubangui in 1925 from sheep in the Philip-pines, occurs in the peri-rectal fat of that host. *E. coelomaticum* is common in the pancreatic ducts of Brazilian cattle.

Pathogenesis. Basch (1966) has described the pathological lesions in cattle. A few flukes may elicit little change but usually there is catarrhal inflammation with destruction of duct epithelium. Eggs may penetrate into the walls of ducts causing inflammatory foci and granulomata in which plasma cells and eosinophils predominate. The granulomata are confined to the walls of the ducts and the parenchyma is not affected.

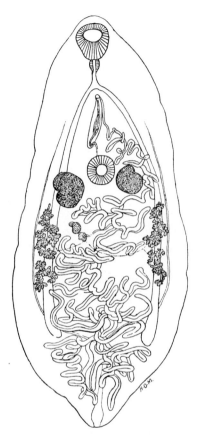 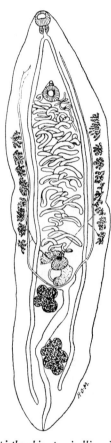

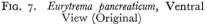

FIG. 7. *Eurytrema pancreaticum*, Ventral FIG. 8. *Opisthorchis tenuicollis*, Ventral
 View (Original) View (Original)

Occasionally severe fibrosis may occur producing atrophy of the pancreas but the remaining parenchyma is normal. Severely infected animals may be poor in condition, but no other clinical signs have been definitely ascribed to these parasites.

Treatment and Prophylaxis—unknown.

E. procyonis Denton, 1942. This species has been reported from the pancreatic ducts, gall bladder and bile ducts of cats, red and grey foxes and racoons in the U.S.A. (New York, Connecticut, Maryland, Kentucky). The snail *Mesodon thyroidus* has been infected experimentally and Denton (1944) suggested animals may be infected by ingestion of the snail.

Generally this parasite causes no apparent ill health. Parasites are found in the medium sized pancreatic ducts. Periductal fibrosis may produce cord-like ducts and there may be atrophy of glandular acini due to duct fibrosis, otherwise the parenchyma is normal (Sheldon, 1966).

E. brumpti Railliet, Henry & Joyeux, 1912, has been recorded from the liver and pancreas of African anthropoid apes.

FAMILY: OPISTHORCHIIDAE

Small to medium-sized flukes, parasitic in the gall-bladder and bile ducts of reptiles, birds and mammals. Usually much flattened with translucent body which is narrow anteriorly. The suckers are weak and not far apart. A pharynx and an oesophagus are present and the intestinal caeca reach near to the posterior extremity. The excretory bladder has a long stem and short branches. The genital pore opens in the middle line just anterior to the ventral sucker. A cirrus-sac is absent, and the tubular seminal vesicle is coiled. The testes lie in the posterior part of the body; they are situated diagonally and are spherical or lobed. The ovary is not far anterior to the testes. The vitelline glands are moderately developed and lie in the lateral fields. The uterine coils usually do not extend behind the ovary. Eggs numerous and light brown.

Genus: Opisthorchis R. Blanchard, 1895

O. tenuicollis (Rud., 1819). This species, which is probably synonymous with *O. felineus*, occurs in the bile ducts, and more rarely in the intestine and the pancreatic ducts of the dog, cat, fox, pig, Cetacea and man. It has been found in southern Asia, Europe and Canada. It measures 7–12 by 1·5–2·5 mm. and has a reddish colour when it is fresh. The cuticle is smooth. The oesophagus is short and the intestinal caeca extend almost to the posterior end. The testes are lobed and the excretory bladder passes between them. The prostate gland and cirrus are absent and there is a weak ejaculatory duct. The ovary is small and lies in the mid-line at the beginning of the posterior third of the body. The vitellaria occupy the middle thirds of the lateral fields; they consist of a series of transversely arranged follicles. The transverse uterine coils do not extend behind the ovary. The eggs measure about 26–30 by 11–15 μ. They have an operculum which fits into a thickened rim of the shell and, when they are laid, they contain a miracidium, the internal structure of which is asymmetrical.

Life-cycle. The first intermediate host is the snail *Bithynia leachi*, according to Vogel (1932), and the metacercariae are found in several fish (*Leuciscus rutilus*, *Blicca björkna*, *Tinca tinca*, *Idus melanotis*, *Barbus barbus*, *Abramis brama* etc.), into which the cercariae penetrate through the skin and encyst in the subcutaneous tissues, especially at the bases of the fins. Infection of the final host occurs through eating raw infected fish, young flukes migrating via the bile duct to the smaller bile ducts.

Pathogenicity, Symptoms and Diagnosis. These are comparable to those seen in *O. sinensis* infection (see below). Dilation of bile ducts with adenomatous thickening of the epithelium is common, marked fibrosis occurring in advanced cases. Several cases of carcinoma of the liver or pancreas of cats and man have been ascribed to *O. tenuicollis.*

Treatment. Erhardt (1932) reported that fouadin at a dose of 0·4 ml. per kg. in cats, given subcutaneously, was effective as a single treatment. More recently, Lienert (1962) reported that hexachlorophene given orally to dogs or cats in gelatine capsules at the rate of 20 mg. per kg. was effective.

O. sinensis (Cobbold, 1875) (syn. *Clonorchis sinensis*). This species, which is often called the Oriental or Chinese liver fluke, occurs in the bile ducts and sometimes in the pancreatic ducts and the duodenum of man and the dog, cat, pig, weasel, mink, badger. It is common in the south-eastern parts of Asia and Japan. Stoll (1947) has estimated the world incidence to be 11 million infected persons. It may reach a size of 25 by 5 mm. It is flat, transparent, wide posteriorly and tapering anteriorly (Fig. 9). The testes are much branched, the cuticle is spiny in the young fluke but smooth in the adult. The eggs measure 27–35 by 12–20 μ; they have a thick light brown wall and contain, when they are laid, a miracidium the internal structure of which is asymmetrical. The operculum of the egg fits into a prominent rim of the shell, while the opposite pole frequently bears a small hook-like structure.

Life-cycle. The eggs normally hatch only after they have been swallowed by the first intermediate host, which may be one of various species of operculated snails, among which are species of the genera *Parafossalurus, Bithynia, Melania* and *Vivipara*. In the snails the miracidium develops into a sporocyst which produces rediae and these in turn produce cercariae which have fairly long tails and elongate bodies with pigmented eye-spots. The second intermediate hosts are fishes belonging to several genera of the family *Cyprinidae*; more than forty have been reported naturally infected. After breaking out of the snail the cercaria swims about, and on meeting a suitable fish it penetrates partly or completely into the tissues of the fish and, losing its tail, becomes encysted in the fish. Infection of the final host occurs through eating raw, infected fish. In some fish the metacercariae are found only under the scales and animals which are fed with the scales and offal of such fish become infected, while humans who eat the rest of the fish do not. The metacercariae are liberated in the duodenum of the final host and reach the liver by way of the bile duct. Eggs of the fluke are passed out of the final host from the sixteenth day after infection.

Pathogenesis. The worms live in the narrow proximal parts of the bile ducts. They cause a catarrhal cholecystitis with desquamation of the epithelium, and may in rare cases bring about bile stasis by blocking up the passages, resulting in jaundice. Papillomatous or even adenomatous proliferation of the epithelium of the bile ducts takes place, together with cirrhosis of the surrounding liver tissue, and this frequently leads to the formation of pockets or cysts enclosing eggs and even worms.

Symptoms are not seen except in fairly heavy infections. The symptoms in man include diarrhoea, followed in severer cases by icterus, ascites and other symptoms, resulting from cirrhosis of the liver and derangement of the portal circulation.

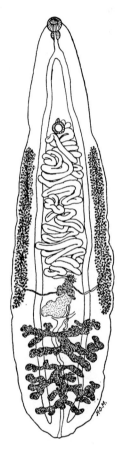

FIG. 9. *Opisthorchis sinensis*, Ventral View (Original)

Diagnosis is confirmed by finding the eggs in the faeces. The eggs must be differentiated from those of other flukes, especially those of species of the family *Heterophyidae*. The latter, however, contain a symmetrically arranged embryo. Serological tests have been used by several workers (Phillipson & McFadzean, 1962; Sadun *et al.*, 1959), and Sawada *et al.* (1964) have produced a potent skin test antigen which is reactive with as little as 0·3 μg. of protein. Cross-reactions with other helminths were minimal.

Treatment. No completely satisfactory treatment is available. Sodium antimony tartrate and chloroquin diphosphate reduce egg output temporarily. Dithiazanine iodine has been used with success in light infections (Yamaguchi *et al.*, 1962).

Prophylaxis. Thorough cooking of all fish used as food. This should stop the infection to a great extent, but further measures to eradicate the snail intermediate hosts (which are operculate) and to prevent their infection from human excreta ought also to be considered. Treatment of night-soil with ammonium sulphate to kill the fluke eggs has been recommended.

Genus: Pseudamphistomum Lühe, 1908

P. truncatum (Rudolphi, 1819) occurs in the bile ducts of the dog, cat, fox, glutton, seal and sometimes man in Europe and India. It measures 2–2·25 by 0·6–0·8 mm. The body is truncate posteriorly, and the cuticle is spiny. The posterior ends of the intestinal caeca bend inwards around the testes, which are spherical and almost horizontal. The uterus extends mainly between the testes and the ventral sucker, which is situated near to the middle of the body (Fig. 10). The eggs measure 29 by 11 μ.

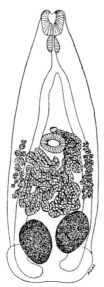

FIG. 10. *Pseudamphistomum truncatum,* Ventral View (Original)

Life-cycle. The first intermediate host snail is unknown. Schuurmans Stekhoven (1931) found the metacercariae in the fresh-water fish *Leuciscus rutilus, Scardinius erythrophthalmus, Abramis brama* and *Blicca björkna.*

Pathogenicity. Not well known. Apparently the fluke is not very pathogenic though liver enlargement and bile duct fibrosis have been described in the silver fox.

Genus: Metorchis Looss, 1899

M. albidus (Braun, 1893) occurs in the gall bladder and bile ducts of dog, cat, fox and grey seal in Europe and North America. It measures 2·5–3·5 mm. by 1·0–1·6 mm., the cuticle is spiny, testes lobed and diagonally placed in the posterior part of the body. The ovary is rounded and just in front of the interior tests. The genital pore opens in front of the ventral sucker. The vitellaria are restricted in the lateral field between the genital pore and the ovary. Egg small, 24–30 μ by 13–16 μ.

Intermediate hosts are fresh water snails and the fish *Blicca björkna*. Pathogenic effects are similar to *Opisthorchis* spp.

M. conjunctus is a similar species in North America occurring in the bile ducts of cat, dog, fox, mink and racoon. It is up to 6 mm. in length and the eggs measure 22–32 μ by 11–18 μ. *Amnicola limosa porosa* serves as first intermediate host and cercariae encyst in the muscles of the common Sucker *Catostomus commersoni*.

Genus: Parametorchis Skrjabin, 1913

Parametorchis complexus (Stiles & Hassall, 1894) has been found in the bile ducts of cats and dogs in Maryland and New York, U.S.A. In this species the uterus forms a rosette around the ventral sucker, the vitelline glands are confined to the anterior third of the body, and the testes are lobed and lie in tandem in the posterior part of the body. The parasite is 5–10 mm. by 1·5–2 mm. and the eggs measure 24 by 12 μ.

The pathogenic effects of the above two liver flukes are similar to the Opisthorchiidae.

FAMILY: FASCIOLIDAE

These are large flukes parasitic in the bile ducts and intestines of mammals, especially ungulates, with a broad, leaf-shaped body and usually a spiny cuticle. The anterior and ventral suckers are close together. A pharynx and a short oesophagus are present and the intestinal caeca are commonly much branched, especially laterally. The excretory bladder is also much branched. The genital pore is median, directly anterior to the ventral sucker. Testes tandem, lobed or branched. Vitellaria strongly developed, filling the lateral fields and extending medially as well. Receptaculum seminis absent. The eggs have thin shells and are operculate.

Genus: Fasciola Linnaeus, 1758

Speciation of genus Fasciola. Several attempts have been made in the past to create new species in this genus. The two principal (and probably only) species are *F. hepatica* and *F. gigantica* which represent the two opposite ends of a range of forms. The new species which have been created at various times include *F. indica* in the Indian subcontinent and *F. halli* and *F. californica* in the U.S.A. The criteria on which these were based most probably represent variations of the two major species and also variations in techniques of fixation and mounting.

F. hepatica Linnaeus, 1758, occurs in the bile ducts of the sheep, goat, ox and other ruminants, pig, hare, rabbit, beaver, coypu, elephant, horse, dog, cat, kangaroo and man. In the unusual hosts, such as man and the horse, the fluke may be found in the lungs, under the skin or in other situations. The fluke is cosmopolitan in its distribution, and is the cause of fascioliasis (liver fluke disease, liver rot), especially in sheep and cattle.

F. hepatica may reach a size of 30 by 13 mm. It is leaf-shaped, broader anteriorly than posteriorly, with an anterior cone-shaped projection which is followed by a pair of broad 'shoulders'. It is greyish-brown in colour, changing to grey when preserved. The ventral sucker is situated at the level of the shoulders, and is about as large as the oral. The cuticle is armed with sharp spines. The intestinal caeca have numerous branches and extend far back. The testes are much branched, filling the median field in about the second and third quarters of the body. There is a well-developed cirrus, and the cirrus-sac also encloses the prostate and seminal vesicle. The ovary is situated to the right of the middle, anterior to the testes, and is branched. The vitelline glands consist of fine follicles filling the lateral fields and the ducts of the follicles unite to form two transverse ducts, which pass inwards to open into a median yolk reservoir, from which a duct passes to the oötype. The uterus lies anterior to the testes. The eggs measure 130–150 by 63–90 μ; and the miracidium develops only after the eggs have been laid.

Life-cycle. The eggs enter the duodenum with the bile and leave the host in the faeces. The rate of development and the hatching of *F. hepatica* eggs depends on temperature (see below) but at 26°C eggs hatch in about 10–12 days producing the first larval stage, the miracidium (see p. 10). The miracidium is broad anteriorly with a small papilliform protrusion, the cuticle is ciliated and the organism has a pair of eye spots. For further development a snail of the genus *Lymnaea* is required. Throughout the years an increasing number of molluscan intermediate hosts of *F. hepatica* have been reported: these are tabulated by Soulsby (1965) but recent considerations of the family Lymnaeidae by Hubendick (1951) and of the species of snails which act as intermediate hosts for *F. hepatica* and *F. gigantica* by Kendall (1954, 1965) indicate that the extensive list of intermediate hosts can be very much reduced. Kendall (1965) suggests that throughout the greater part of the world *F. hepatica* is transmitted by *Lymnaea truncatula* or by snails not readily distinguishable from it on grounds of morphology or ecological requirements. Similarly, for *F. gigantica*, Kendall proposes that it is transmitted by varieties of the super species *Lymnaea auricularia*. *L. truncatula* has a wide range throughout

Europe and North Asia. In North America the principal species incriminated as an intermediate host of *F. hepatica* is *Lymnaea bulimoides techella* and in Australia it is *Lymnaea tomentosa*. Both these show more major differences from *L. truncatula* than many others of the supposedly intermediate hosts, however, Kendall maintains they have many characters in common with *L. truncatula*. At the present state of knowledge, it would seem justified to state that *F. hepatica* is transmitted by the super species *L. truncatula*, or by varieties of it, in the major part of the world: the position with regard to the vector in North America, *L. bulimoides techella*, and in Australia, *L. tomentosa*, requiring further evaluation.

Experimental infection of several other species of snails has been attempted and achieved though this does not necessarily imply that the snail will play a major part in the transmission of the infection under natural conditions. Kendall (1949a), demonstrated that *L. palustris*, *L. pereger*, *L. glabra* and *L. stagnalis* may be infected within the first few days of hatching but there is no evidence that these species in their mature form play any substantial part in the natural incidence of the disease. Berghen (1964) successfully infected *L. stagnalis* and *L. palustris* but was unable to obtain free emergence of cercariae from the snails.

The miracidium penetrates actively into the snail, casting off its ciliate covering, and develops into the sporocyst, which reaches a length of over 1 mm. Dawes (1960) has, however, shown that the final stage of penetration into the snail is performed, not by the miracidium, but by the young sporocyst. Studying the penetration of *Fasciola hepatica* into *Limnaea truncatula* and *F. gigantica* into *L. auricularia*, he found that the miracidium adheres by suction to the epithelial cells of the snail and breaks these down, probably by means of enzymes secreted by the apical organ of the gut, and then casts off, as it enters the snail, its ciliated epithelium, so that the final swift thrust into the snail is effected by the unciliated young sporocyst. Dawes suggests that all the digenetic trematodes enter their intermediate hosts in this manner. Each sporocyst gives rise to five to eight rediae which, when fully developed, are 1–3 mm. long. They are characterised by a circular thickening behind the level of the pharynx and a pair of blunt processes at the beginning of the posterior quarter. Daughter rediae may develop under unfavourable conditions, but the next normal generation is one of cercariae (see Fig. 4). These leave the snail in $4\frac{1}{2}$–7 weeks from the time of infection. They have a body 0·25–0·35 mm. long, a tail of twice that length, no eye-spots, and the dark, granular, cystogenous glands are conspicuous in the lateral parts of the body. Within a few minutes to 2 hours the cercariae settle on blades of grass or other plants just below water-level and, after casting off the tail, secrete a covering from the cystogenous glands forming cysts about 0·2 mm. in diameter. A small number may encyst at the surface of the water and sink to the bottom. The cercariae are now infective. They are swallowed by the final host with the plants on which they are encysted, or animals, like cattle that walk into the water to drink, may stir up the cercariae lying at the bottom and swallow them.

Development in the vertebrate host. Following ingestion of the metacercariae excystation occurs in the duodenum. Factors concerned with this have been studied by Wikerhauser (1960) and Hughes (1963). The former found that excystation could be induced by treating metacercarial cysts with acid pepsin followed by treatment with trypsin and bile. Hughes confirmed the necessity for pre-treatment with acid pepsin and obtained excystation in an artificial intestinal juice composed of trypsin, pancreatin, sodium taurocholate and cholesterol. Hughes found that excystation could occur with cysts no more than 2 days of age. In these *in vitro* experiments, several hours were required for excystation whereas in *in vivo* work, immature trematodes are found in the peritoneal cavity within 2 hours of infection. It is likely that under natural conditions some intrinsic factor, comparable to that responsible for the hatching of *Ascaris* eggs and the exsheathment of strongyle larvae, is operative.

Within 24 hours of infection the majority of immature trematodes occur in the abdominal cavity and by 4–6 days after infection the majority have penetrated the liver capsule and are found migrating in the liver parenchyma. Some young flukes may reach the liver by way of the blood stream but the usual route is via the peritoneal cavity. Migration in the liver occurs for 5–6 weeks and about 7 weeks after infection they begin to enter the main bile ducts and from this time onwards, an increasing number arrive there and reach sexual maturity. For 8 weeks onwards, eggs are found in the bile and subsequently in the faeces, however, there is no synchrony in the behaviour of an infection and even though the infection may be patent, a proportion of developmental stages attain maturity later so that over a period of 2 months a succession of developmental stages reach maturity. Occasionally especially in cattle, immature flukes may be carried to other organs such as the lungs and in pregnant animals, occasionally parasites may be found in the foetus.

Factors affecting development of the egg. At temperatures below 10°C no development occurs in the egg, but from 10° to 26°C there is an increasing rate of development. At 12°C, 60 days or more are required, at 15°C about 40 days and at 26°C about 12 days. Under field conditions in Great Britain, eggs are unlikely to hatch in less than 3 weeks (Rowcliffe & Ollerenshaw, 1960) and in Australia, the incubation period is 21 days in summer and 90 days in winter (Boray, 1963). Eggs may survive for some time at low temperatures and under field conditions accumulation of unhatched eggs may occur over winter leading to mass-hatching and liberation of miracidia in the spring time. Hatching does not occur below 10°C.

Factors affecting the development of the parasite in the snail. Little development occurs in the snail below 10°C, but above this the rate of development increases to about 28°C. The minimum period for completion of the life cycle is about 21 days at 27°C. Boray (1963) found that at temperatures above 20°C there was an increase in mortality of infected snails and also the infectivity of metacercariae fell markedly above this temperature. From extensive studies, Boray concluded that in Australia the contamination of pasture was evenly distributed throughout the year. In warm weather many cercariae of the parasite may be produced but this is offset by an increased mortality of snails and reduced infectivity of metacercariae.

A relationship between the size of the snail and the number of developing parthenitae was observed by Kendall (1949b), larger snails having almost ten times the number of developmental stages than smaller snails, this being a reflection of the amount of food which the snail received. Detailed studies of the effect of population, density, food and other factors which affect snails and the production of cercariae are given by Boray (1963). In field studies, Kendall & Ollerenshaw (1963) confirm that the size of snails and not their numbers appears to be the major factor influencing the number of parasites present.

The ability of the snail hosts of *F. hepatica* (*L. truncatula*, *L. tomentosa*, *L. bulimoides techella*) to undergo aestivation is important in the epidemiology of *F. hepatica* infection. Under field conditions, some snails may survive for several months in dry mud and Taylor (1949) has stated that three out of ten snails may be alive after aestivating under artificial drought conditions for 12 months. Though aestivation of the snail retards the development of *F. hepatica*, the parthenitae of the fluke can survive for at least 10 months in aestivating snails. On the return of moist conditions for the snail it grows to maturity very rapidly and similarly the developmental stages of *F. hepatica* undergo rapid development so that within a short time large numbers of cercariae may accumulate on herbage when moist conditions return to the snail habitat.

Ecology of Lymnaea truncatula. This snail is commonly seen in poorly drained land, drainage ditches, areas of seepages of springs or broken drains, muddy gateways, vehicle-wheel ruts, wet and muddy places near drinking troughs and hoof prints of animals on clay soil. Taylor (1949) in confirming the wide distribution of the snail in Great Britain and probably in Europe, noted that concentrated populations generally occurred in places which became dry for periods of weeks or even months. A return to wetness of these habitats provided optimum conditions for the multiplication of snails. The American species, *L. bulimoides techella*, inhabits similar terrain as *L. truncatula* however, *L. tomentosa* is an amphibious snail and well adapted for aquatic life. It is found in and around ditches, field dams and similar places. The chances of extension of the area of colonisation are greater than with *L. truncatula* and *L. tomentosa* may migrate against the water current at an average speed of migration of 50 cm. per hour against a water velocity of 15 cm. per second. Snails may float or drift with water current for long distances.

Under field conditions in Great Britain, where detailed consideration has been given to the ecology of *L. truncatula*, adult snails commence egg laying in spring and continue to do so throughout the summer. Snails of this population gradually die off so that by October few are left. The daughter generation hatching from such eggs grow and produce eggs throughout the summer. However, this population is inhibited during the winter but forms a nucleus of a parent generation for the following year. Many factors affect this basic ecology, the most important one being moisture. When moisture conditions are optimum during spring and summer, a marked increase in snail numbers may occur and a second generation of snails may be produced in the autumn, this adding to the basic population the following year. On the other hand, when the weather is dry until mid or late summer, breeding is delayed until then. Under ideal conditions, dense populations of snails may develop and Ollerenshaw (1959) has observed up to 3300 snails per square meter.

Longevity of metacercariae. Metacercariae have been shown to survive for more than 1 year under laboratory conditions but under pasture conditions, it is likely that a dangerous level infection does not persist for such a long period. Taylor (1949) indicated that a large proportion of metacercariae fell off certain types of herbage within 4–6 weeks and though such forms may remain viable for some time they are generally unavailable to the grazing animal. In laboratory studies Boray (1963) found that at temperatures of 12–14°C 100 per cent of metacercariae could survive for 6 months and 5 per cent for 10 months. Kendall (1965) reports experiments in which herbage remained infected for periods of between 270 and 340 days. A relative humidity of 70 was necessary for prolonged survival of the metacercariae. Survival of metacercariae below freezing temperatures has been reported. Cercariae may survive on moist hay for 8 months. On the other hand, in normal hay making, it is unlikely that metacercariae will survive the desiccation for an extended period. Failure of metacercariae to survive in silage for more than 35 or 57 days has been demonstrated and in Gulf Coast regions of the United States, Olsen (1947) showed that metacercariae were destroyed by heat and drought during the four summer months. On such pastures, sheep did not become infected until the early winter.

More detailed consideration of the relationship between *F. hepatica* and the snail host may be found in Kendall (1965) and Soulsby (1965).

Pathogenesis. The pathological manifestations depend on the number of metacercariae ingested. Since, under natural conditions, there is little evidence of immunity, additional infections are additive and at autopsy, a succession of developmental stages may be found in an animal. No appreciable damage is done during passage through the intestinal wall or the peritoneal cavity, the principal lesions occurring in the liver, either in the parenchyma or the bile ducts. Essentially the disease entity can be divided into an acute form and a chronic form.

Acute Fascioliasis. This is less common than the chronic entity and is almost invariably seen in sheep. It is essentially a traumatic hepatitis produced by the simultaneous migration of large numbers of immature trematodes and is seen mainly towards the end of summer when large numbers of cercariae are shed onto the herbage. Taylor (1951) estimated that 10,000 cysts must be given to produce the syndrome in sheep. The most damaging stages are those 6–8 weeks of age, these causing extensive destruction of liver parenchyma and marked haemorrhage. In excessive numbers, rupture of the liver capsule may occur with haemorrhage into the peritoneal cavity. Animals may die within a few days of the onset of clinical signs and in these the liver is enlarged, pale and friable, it shows numerous haemorrhagic tracts on the surface and throughout the substance, and fibrinous clots on the liver surface and also throughout the peritoneal cavity. At the proximal part of the tract, an immature parasite may be seen, distal to which is a zone of haemorrhage and then a posterior zone of reddish grey material consisting of infiltrated cells. Small flukes 0·7–2 mm. can be squeezed from the cut surface or obtained from the excess of peritoneal fluid.

In less acute forms of disease, the liver is covered with migratory tracts but an infiltration of white cells is more in evidence and early fibrosis may be seen. This subacute type may be superimposed on an existing chronic infection and then a more marked cellular response may be seen, possibly indicating a form of immune response to the second infection.

The clinical entity of the acute and subacute forms is seen in animals of all ages and states of nutrition. Death may occur rapidly or after several days. Animals are disinclined to move, are anorexic and show a distended abdomen which is painful to the touch.

A complication of the acute condition is 'Black Disease' caused by *Clostridium oedematiens (novyi)*. This is an anaerobe which proliferates in the anaerobic necrotic lesions produced by the immature trematodes. The organism apparently occurs in normal sheep, the clinical entity occurring only after liver damage has been produced by some other agent. Black Disease is common in Australia but is also seen in Europe and the U.S.A. Sheep aged 2–4 years are usually affected. A vaccine is available for the condition.

Chronic Fascioliasis. This is the most common form of the infection in sheep, cattle and other animals (including man). The essential lesion is a progressive biliary cirrhosis which ultimately produces a hard fibrotic liver in which the bile ducts are prominent, thickened, fibrous and, in cattle, often calcified. Histologically the fibrosis is produced by repair to the migratory tracts and a cholangitis. The bile duct walls are markedly thickened and the bile ducts are dilated containing flukes, numerous eggs, white and red blood cells and epithelial debris. Hyperplasia of bile duct epithelium frequently occurs, the cuticular spines of the fluke being embedded in the epithelium which may be extensively damaged by them. The movements of the flukes also aid this action. Ultimately the epithelium may become completely denuded leaving the bile duct as a fibrous tube. In cattle encrustations of calcium are frequently seen, at times these forming complete casts of the bile duct and blocking it. The walls of the ducts are commonly calcified in cattle, they protrude markedly from the surface and are difficult to cut with a knife. They resemble the stem of a clay pipe, giving the common name of 'pipe-stem liver' to the infection.

In cattle, too, parasites are often found in other organs, especially the lungs. Here they occur in hazel-nut sized cysts containing a brownish purulent gelatinous material in which a living, but more frequently a dead and calcified, parasite may be found.

Chemical pathology of Fascioliasis. A profound anaemia and changes in the serum proteins are seen in sheep. These are much less marked in cattle.

The onset of anaemia is associated with the arrival of flukes in the bile ducts and concomitantly there is a fall in serum magnesium and a progressive hypoalbuminaemia. The genesis of the anaemia has aroused much discussion. Dawes (1963) ascribes the blood loss to mechanisms other than the blood sucking activities of the flukes, which he maintains are tissue feeders. However, studies with ^{14}P labelled red cells by Jennings *et al.* (1956) indicated that 0·2 ml. of blood may be lost per fluke per day. More recent work by Sinclair (1964) has indicated that haemorrhage is not the main factor in the anaemia but rather some disturbance of erythropoiesis is a more important cause. In further studies with ^{59}Fe, Sinclair (1965) concluded that the anaemia of fascioliasis is secondary to a disordered reticuloendothelial function with decreased erythrocyte production and probably increased erythrocyte destruction.

Clinical signs. In acute cases, in sheep, the animal dies suddenly; blood-stained froth appears at the nostrils and blood is discharged from the anus, as in a case of anthrax. In the chronic cases the first signs are seen at a time when the young worms, burrowing through the liver parenchyma, have reached a fair size. The sheep is off colour and this is followed by an increasing anaemia. There is an increasing lack of vigour which is observed when the animals are caught or driven. Soon the appetite diminishes, the mucous membranes become pale and oedemas develop. Oedema is more conspicuous in some breeds than in others and it may appear especially in the intermandibular space, the name 'bottle-jaw' being then given to it. The skin becomes dry and doughy to the touch. The wool is dry and brittle, falling out in patches. The debility, emaciation and general depression increase, and there may occasionally be diarrhoea or constipation and slight fever. At this stage, or even earlier, death may occur. The flukes usually live about 9 months in the sheep and then die and pass out through the intestine, but some may live up to 5 years and in one case a survival time of 11 years has been recorded. If the animals recover, the symptoms gradually abate, but the wool later shows a 'break' in the part grown during the illness, and the lesions in the liver are never completely repaired.

In the case of cattle, the most characteristic signs are digestive distur-bances. Constipation is marked and the faeces are passed with difficulty, being hard and brittle. Diarrhoea is seen only in the extreme stages. Emaciation increases rapidly, while dullness and weakness soon lead to prostration, especially in calves.

Diagnosis is confirmed by finding the eggs in the faeces. They must be distinguished from the eggs of other flukes, especially the large eggs of paramphistomes. The *Fasciola* egg has a yellow shell with an indistinct operculum, and the embryonic cells are also rather indistinct. The paramphistome eggs as a rule have transparent shells and distinct oper-cula; their embryonic cells are clear and there is frequently a small knob at the posterior pole, while the eggs themselves are often larger than those of the liver-fluke.

Treatment

Carbon tetrachloride. This compound has been in use for approximately 40 years for the treatment of *F. hepatica* infection. It is extensively used in sheep, a routine dose of 1 ml. being satisfactory for strategic control and this may be increased to 5 ml. for the control of outbreaks of the disease. Carbon tetrachloride is not recommended for cattle which may show severe intoxication after its use. At a dose of 1 ml. per animal it is essentially effective only against the adult flukes, those aged 10 weeks or more, and has little effect on those aged 8 weeks or younger. At a dose of 10 ml. per sheep flukes as young as 5 weeks may be eliminated. The drug may be given in a gelatin capsule or mixed with some bland oil, such as liquid paraffin, in the ratio of 1 to 4, a dose of 5 ml. of the mixture being given to sheep.

Toxicity of carbon tetrachloride. In general sheep tolerate carbon tetra-chloride well, though occasional cases of carbon tetrachloride poisoning are by no means uncommon and occasionally several deaths may occur in a flock treated with the drug. Setchell (1962) in a study of the deaths which occurred in 185 flocks of sheep following administration of carbon tetrachloride concluded that no single environmental factor was consis-tently associated with the mortality. The availability of plants containing oxalate and unusually cold weather probably increased the susceptibility and in fact any form of stress might do so. Carbon tetrachloride poisoning in sheep causes kidney and liver disfunction and Gallagher (1961) reported the chemical pathology of poisoning as damage to cell structure by the lipid solvent action of carbon tetrachloride resulting in the loss of cytoplasmic constituents from the cell and later a loss of mitochondria. Cell death follows a failure of respiration due to the loss of co-enzymes from the mitochondria. Other work has shown that it is possible to prevent carbon tetrachloride poisoning by administering the precursors of the pyridine nucleotides, nicotinic acid or tryptophane. A marked fall in serum calcium may occur in lactating ewes 96 hours after administration of carbon tetrachloride (Downey, 1960) and clinical cases of toxicity may be saved by the intravenous injection of calcium borogluconate. Prior treatment with nicotinic acid may afford some protection from the toxic effects.

Intramuscular administration of carbon tetrachloride. This method of administration reduces the risk of toxicity seen with oral administration. The method has been used for many years in Central European countries and in the Soviet Union and more recently the technique has gained popularity elsewhere in the world. For sheep the equivalent of 1–2 ml. of carbon tetrachloride in a bland oil such as liquid paraffin has given efficient results, resulting in a high efficacy against mature parasites. In cattle doses of 5–15 ml. per kg. in liquid paraffin or other bland oil have been utilised. High levels of activity have been reported.

One disadvantage of intramuscular medication is the production of necrosis or abscesses at the injection site and in a few cases this may lead to temporary or even permanent lameness. In cattle extreme pain and excitement may occur following injection but these may be controlled by the incorporation of a local anaesthetic in the injection.

Hexachloroethane. Though used since 1926 in Europe this compound first received world wide recognition following Olsen's (1943) demonstration of the value of a hexachloroethane bentonite suspension for liver fluke infection in cattle. At a single dose of 220 ml. per kg. Olsen (1947a,b) reported a 92 per cent efficiency and other studies have shown that the compound has little action on immature flukes. It is generally well-tolerated by cattle, even in high doses, though occasional fatalities may occur. Liver damage appears to be a predisposing factor and the feeding of root crops may increase the sensitivity.

Hexachloroethane may also be used in sheep, dosages varying from 20 to 30 g. per animal.

Hexachlorophene. This may be used for both cattle and sheep. It is given by oral or subcutaneous route. Kendal & Parfitt (1962) reported that in sheep it had a partial effect on flukes 2 weeks of age and completely removed flukes 3–4 weeks of age at a dose of 40 mg. per kg. Consequently, the compound should be useful for the control of acute fascioliasis. For sheep a dose of 15–20 mg. per kg. is generally recommended for routine use and this is usually well tolerated. For acute fascioliasis, 40 mg. per kg. may be employed. In cattle, 15–20 mg. per kg. have been employed.

Hetol (1,4-bis-trichloromethyl-benzol). Lämmler (1960) suggested a field therapeutic dose of this drug of 150 mg. per kg. for sheep, this level giving satisfactory results. Behrens (1960) recommended a dose of 5 g. to lambs, 5–6 months of age, and 10 g. to older sheep. For cattle a dose of 125 mg. per kg. has been reported to be effective by the above authors.

The drug is more effective against adult flukes than immatures and, in general, the compound is well tolerated by both cattle and sheep at the recommended dosages.

Freon-112 (Arcton) (Difluorotetrachloroethane). Workers in the Soviet Union have investigated the action of this compound in sheep and cattle. It is essentially effective against adult flukes but it is reported to have a high efficacy. For sheep Boray & Pearson (1960) used a dosage of 330–660 ml. per kg. in field trials and eliminated the vast majority of flukes. The action against immature flukes was incomplete. In cattle, Hashizume et al. (1961) recommend a dose of 100 ml. per kg.

The drug is well tolerated by both sheep and cattle.

Bithionol (2,2'-thiobis-(4,6-dichlorophenol)). This compound has been evaluated in cattle only. Ueno et al. (1960) suggested a dose of 30–35 mg. per kg. for general use, this producing 66–88 per cent efficacy.

Prophylaxis. For discussions of the epidemiology and control of fascioliasis the reader should refer to Gordon (1955), Boray (1963) and Soulsby (1965). Possible sources of infection of the snails are: animals that have been treated but are still passing out eggs; animals with undetected light infections that are passing out eggs; eggs on the pastures that survive mild winters and infect snails the following year; eggs derived from hosts other than sheep or cattle, among which the rabbit is an important source difficult to control. Possible sources of infection of farm animals are not only cercariae escaping from the snails during any one year, but also cercariae that may have survived inside snails that may survive through the winter. Detection of light infections and effective treatment of infected animals, whether they show symptoms of fascioliasis or not, are therefore important. To control infection of farm animals with cercariae, grazing on wet pastures favourable to the snails or on the margins of pools or slow-running streams should be prevented, either by keeping the animals off these areas or by fencing off the dangerous areas. Good drainage and cutting of vegetation that gives the snails shelter will also help. Infected pastures should not be used for making hay.

Molluscicides. A detailed list of molluscicides, together with their indications is given by Faust & Russel (1964).

It has been found that a solution of 1 in 100,000 of copper sulphate kills snails in 8 hours and that a solution of one in a million kills them in 24 hours. A solution of one part in one to five million parts of water is usually sufficient to kill the snails and many of their eggs and is not injurious to stock, but may kill fish. The amount of copper sulphate required depends greatly on the amount of decayed organic matter in the water, and in some cases as much as 1 : 50,000 or more must be used, so that this method may become impracticable. The treatment has to be repeated after 2–3 months in order to kill any snails that have hatched from eggs which were not destroyed at the first treatment.

In the case of moist pastures the copper sulphate is best applied in the form of a 1-2 per cent solution or as a powder mixed with 4-8 parts of sand, using from 10-30 kg. per hectare (about 10-30 lb. per acre), according to the amount of surface water present. Stock should not be grazed on treated pastures until a rain has fallen. In the case of pools, a rough estimate of the volume of water has to be made and the required amount of copper sulphate is added after it has been dissolved in a small quantity of water. The difficulty of slowly running water, in, for instance, a fountain on a hillside, can be overcome by placing at the origin of the stream a non-metallic vessel containing a strong solution of copper sulphate dripping out through a hole at the botton at a suitable rate or by suspending small bags of the chemical in the water until the snails have been killed.

Gordon *et al.* (1959) reported successful control of *Limnaea tomentosa*, the intermediate host of *F. hepatica* in Australia, with a 30 per cent w/v paste of copper pentachlorphenate applied at 10 lb. of the active ingredient per acre in 400 gallons of water by means of a boom spray carried by two men, or a fire-fighting pump, preliminary drainage and removal or destruction of vegetation from the area treated being essential.

F. gigantica Cobbold, 1885. This is the common liver fluke of domestic stock in Africa; it occurs frequently in the Indian sub-continent, Formosa and has also been reported from Hawaii and the Philippines. In studies of the distribution of *Fasciola* species in Pakistan, Kendall (1954) found *F. gigantica* was the predominant species but it was replaced by *F. hepatica* in the Highland areas over 4000 feet. Mixed infections with both species occurred on the boundaries of the Highland areas.

F. gigantica resembles *F. hepatica* but is readily recognized by its larger size being 25-75 mm. in length and up to 12 mm. in breadth. The anterior cone is smaller than that of *F. hepatica*, the shoulders are not as prominent and the body is more transparent. The eggs measure 156-197 μ by 90-104 μ.

Life-cycle. Kendall (1965) has summarised the present information regarding the intermediate hosts of *F. gigantica*. He considers the fluke to be transmitted throughout the world by members of the super species *Lymnaea auricularia*. In the Indian sub-continent the race *rufescens* is responsible, and in Malaysia the race *rubiginosa*. With regard to the African snail host, which is commonly regarded as *Lymnaea natalensis*, Kendall suggests that this is not specifically distinguishable from *L. auricularia rufescens*. The host in East Africa, *L. caillaudi*, is regarded as synonymous with *L. natalensis*. In general there is no evidence of a common vector for *F. hepatica* and *F. gigantica*, development of one species failing to take place in the snail host of the other. However, in Hawaii, Alicata (1938) has reported the development of *F. gigantica* in *L. (fossaria) ollula* and this may also serve as an intermediate host for *F. hepatica*.

The snail hosts of *F. gigantica* are aquatic forms living in fairly large permanent bodies of water which contain abundant vegetation. Still or slightly moving clear water provides the most satisfactory habitat. They occur at sea level and at high altitudes and there is little evidence that the snail vectors of *F. gigantica* can aestivate (unlike the snail hosts of *F. hepatica*).

The development in the snail is comparable to that of *F. hepatica* in *L. truncatula* except that it takes longer. Thus at 26°C eggs of *F. gigantica* hatch in 17 days. In the warm season in East Africa, 75 days are required for development in the snail, this being extended to 175 days in the cold season. Critical studies of the development of the parthenitae of *F. gigantica* have been conducted by Dinnik & Dinnik (1964); these authors found that one to six first generation rediae may develop from a sporocyst of *F. gigantica* at 26°C, each redia producing daughter rediae and then cercariae.

Pathogenicity. This is essentially the same as that of *F. hepatica*, the acute and chronic form of infection occurring in sheep, though in cattle only the chronic form occurs.

Treatment and Control. Similar treatments are employed as for *F. hepatica*. Control is based on the similar principles to *F. hepatica* but since the molluscan vector is an aquatic form, its habitats may be more difficult to treat with molliscicides than for the control of *F. hepatica* snails. In some areas, the use of molliscicides may be contra-indicated since the large bodies of water are also important fishing areas. Infection may be avoided by grazing livestock on higher ground and avoiding lakes, swamps and dams though in many parts of the world these are used as watering places for the livestock. A detailed consideration of the control measures applicable in Africa is given by Coyle (1959) who, amongst other things, recommends the piping of water to water-troughs rather than using the dams or lakes themselves for watering places for stock. The use of bore holes and a hydraulic ram to pump water to a higher level than the large body of water is suggested. He also discusses biological control.

Genus: Fascioloides Ward, 1917

F. magna (Bassi, 1875) occurs in the liver, rarely the lungs, of cattle, horse, bison, yak, sheep and deer in North America and in cattle and deer in Europe. The worms are oval, with a rounded posterior end, and are thick and flesh-coloured. They measure 23–100 mm. long, 11–26 mm. broad and 2–4·5 mm. thick. There is no distinct anterior cone-like projection. The eggs measure 109–168 by 75–96 μ and have a protoplasmic appendage 4–21 μ in length at the pole opposite the operculum.

Life-cycle. The eggs are passed in the one-celled stage and hatch after 4 weeks or longer. About 7–8 weeks are required for development in the intermediate hosts, which are the snails *Fossaria parva*, *F. modicella*, *F. modicella rustica*, *Lymnaea bulimoides techella*, *Pseudosuccinea columella* and

Stagnicola palustris nuttalliana. The parasite wanders about in the liver of the final host until it becomes encapsulated. It reaches maturity in sheep in about 5 months.

S. palustris nuttalliana occurs in the stagnant parts of permanent or semi-permanent water which contains large amounts of dead and living vegetation. It does not survive in areas which dry up during the year. *F. parva* occurs in wet, swampy areas and it can aestivate for periods of dryness. *P. columella* is found in pools and streams as are the other species.

Pathogenicity. The behaviour and pathogenic effects of *F. magna* depend on the host it parasitizes. The normal hosts are considered to be members of the Cervidae such as moose, wapiti, white tailed deer, Northern white tailed deer, black tailed deer, elk, fallow deer, red deer, and sambar (*Cervus unicolor*). In these the parasite occurs in a fibrous cyst with fairly thin walls consisting of loose fibrous tissue. Though adjacent liver cells are destroyed by pressure atrophy the fibrous wall of the cyst abuts to normal liver cells without intermingling of fibrous tissue. The fibrous wall is vascular and both the afferent and efferent bile ducts are patent so that eggs of *F. magna* pass to the exterior. The cysts may reach up to 4 cm. in diameter and there is no marked tissue reaction or discoloration of the surrounding tissues. In long-standing cases, the cavity may become fibrosed so that the bile ducts are blocked, but usually eggs are passed for a considerable period.

In the larger Bovidae closed cysts are produced, these being seen in domestic cattle, bison, and yak in North America and the blue bull (*Boselaphus tragocamelus*) in Italy. The cyst in such animals consists of a thick, fibrous wall with both afferent and efferent ducts occluded. The outline of the cyst is not clearly differentiated from the liver tissue and there is extensive involvement of fibrosis in the surrounding parenchyma. Pigmentation may be marked giving the area a dark or black appearance. Swales (1935) suggested that the majority of trematodes fail to reach sexual maturity before being completely enclosed by the cyst. Consequently the Bovidae are unsuitable hosts for the parasite and play no major part in the dissemination of the infection.

In the sheep, which is also an abnormal host, the behaviour of *F. magna* is entirely different. Uninterrupted migration occurs and capsulation is rarely seen: rather a series of necrotic tracts with haemorrhage occurs and there is marked pigmentation in the liver parenchyma along with an adhesive peritonitis. *F. magna* may reach maturity in the sheep and lay eggs however; frequently this host is killed by a relatively few parasites and cannot be regarded as a true definitive host.

Epidemiology. *F. magna* is indigenous in North America being common in Canada and the Great Lakes Region, in the Gulf Region, and the Rocky Mountain states of the U.S.A. Sixty per cent of white tailed deer have been reported infected in Texas and in Canada, 58 per cent of elk, and 12 per cent of other deer may be infected. Domestic cattle and sheep become infected when they graze deer grazing grounds though neither play a major part in the subsequent dissemination of the infection.

Treatment and control. Little information is available regarding treatment. The newer fasciolicidal compounds which have an effect on the immature stages of trematodes may be of value in sheep and cattle. Treatment of the mature flukes may present difficulties because of the thick walled cyst.

Control consists of the elimination of snails by molluscicides. However, this presents difficulties because of the different ecological requirements of the snails which may serve as intermediate hosts. Control of Cervidae may be possible in certain areas and deer should not be moved into a clean area unless they have been demonstrated to be free of infection. Destruction of deer has been practised in a few areas.

Genus: Fasciolopsis Looss, 1899

F. buski (Lankester, 1857) occurs in the small intestine of man and pig, in the south-eastern parts of Asia, particularly in China. It is a large,

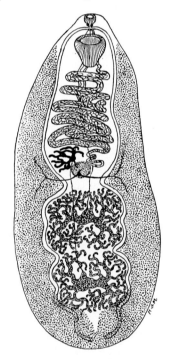

FIG. 11. *Fasciolopsis buski*, Ventral View (Original)

thick-set fluke without shoulders, rather variable in size, but usually measuring about 30–75 by 8–20 mm. The shape is elongate-oval, slightly broader posteriorly than anteriorly. The ventral sucker is situated near the anterior extremity and is much larger than the oral. The cuticle bears spines which are frequently lost. A pharynx and a short oesophagus are present, followed by the unbranched intestinal caeca, which reach almost to the posterior end of the worm. The testes are tandem, branched and posterior in position. The cirrus-sac is long and tubular, opening anterior to the ventral sucker. The ovary is branched, lying to the right of the mid-line. The vitelline glands occupy the lateral fields. The eggs have thin shells with an operculum; they are brown in colour and measure 125–140 by 70–90 μ.

Life-cycle. Similar to that of *Fasciola hepatica*, with flat, spiral-shelled snails as intermediate hosts (species of *Planorbis* and *Segmentina*). These snails feed on certain plants—the water calthrop, *Trapa natans* and *T. bicornis*, and the water chestnut, *Eliocharis tuberosa*—which are cultivated for food and are usually fertilised with human night-soil. The cercariae encyst on the tubers or nuts of these plants, which are eaten raw by the Chinese. These and possibly also other plants may carry the infection to pigs.

Pathogenicity. The parasite is chiefly of importance as a cause of disease in man. It attaches itself to the intestinal mucosa, causing a local inflammation or severer deep ulcerative lesions in heavy infections, and produces abdominal pain, diarrhoea, oedema and ascites.

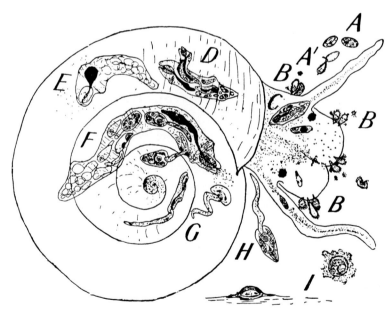

FIG. 12. *Fasciolopsis buski.* Diagram of Life-cycle (from Baylis, after Barlow)

A.	Egg	E.	Daughter redia
A'.	Miracidium escaping from egg	F.	Older daughter redia with cercariae
B,B.	Miracidia entering snail		
C.	Sporocyst	G.	Cercaria
D.	Redia with daughter redia escaping	H.	Cercaria escaping from snail
		I.	Encysted cercariae

Treatment. Carbon tetrachloride, at the usual dose rate of 0·3 ml. per kg. and administered by stomach tube, will probably produce the best results. Hexylresorcinol has been used with success in human infections. Brown *et al.* (1959) found that tetrachlorethylene was the most effective treatment of man, while ascaridol had some effect; but piperazine citrate and dithiazanine iodide had no effect.

Prophylaxis is mainly a matter of hygienic disposal of human night-soil and the faeces of pigs. The tubers and nuts of the plants mentioned should not be used as food without at least scalding them in boiling water.

Genus: Parafasciolopsis Ejsmont, 1932

P. fasciolaemorpha Ejsmont, 1932. This form occurs in the gall bladder and digestive tract of elk and wild goat in the Soviet Union and Poland. It is 3–7·5 mm. long by 1–2·5 mm. broad, the cuticle is spiny, the anterior sucker 220–285 μ, the ventral sucker 550–850μ in diameter, the egg is brownish coloured and measures 110–140 μ by 70–86 μ. The intermediate host is the snail, *Planorbis (Coretus) corneus*, which is found in deep water in areas where there is much vegetation, such as swamps. Drozdz (1963) states the parasite to be adapted to swampy habitats, deer and elk being infected when they are feeding in such areas. He records a fatal case of a massive infection with the parasite and hence it may be a parasite of importance in elk. It is unlikely however that sheep and cattle will be infected because of the association of the parasite with swampy areas.

FAMILY ECHINOSTOMATIDAE

More or less elongate flukes with a strong ventral sucker situated not far behind the smaller oral sucker. The latter is surrounded dorsally and laterally by a 'head-collar', which bears a single or double row of large spines. The cuticle is usually provided with scales or spines. The digestive tract consists of a pharynx, an oesophagus, which nearly reaches the ventral sucker, and simple intestinal caeca which extend to the posterior extremity. The genital pore opens just anterior to the ventral sucker. The testes are entire or lobed, tandem or slightly diagonal, usually situated in the posterior half of the body. A cirrus-sac is present. The ovary is anterior to the testes, median or to the right, and a receptaculum seminis is absent. The vitellaria consist of coarse follicles lying in the lateral fields and frequently extending into the central field behind the testes. Uterus anterior to the ovary, containing relatively large eggs with thin shells. Parasites in the intestine and sometimes the bile ducts of birds and mammals. The life-history is similar to that of *Fasciola hepatica*, but the cercariae frequently enter another snail, an amphibian or a fish, in which they encyst, and the final host becomes infected by ingesting the second intermediate host.

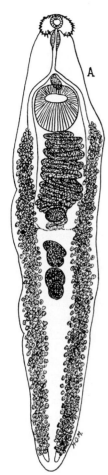

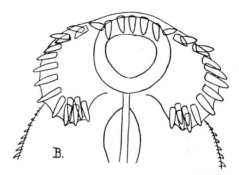

Fig. 13. *Echinostoma revolutum.* A, Ventral view; B, ventral view of anterior end, showing the head-crown (Original)

Genus: Echinostoma Rudolphi, 1809

E. revolutum (Fröhlich, 1802) occurs in the rectum and caeca of the duck, goose, and other aquatic birds, the partridge, the pigeon and the fowl, as well as in man. It is 10–22 mm. long and up to 2·25 mm. broad. The head-collar bears thirty-seven spines, of which five on either side form a group of 'corner spines', and the cuticle is spiny in the anterior region. The testes are tandem, elongate, oval or slightly lobed, situated behind the middle with the ovary anterior to them. The cirrus-sac lies between the bifurcation of the intestine and the ventral sucker and may extend slightly beyond the anterior margin of the latter. The eggs measure 90–126 by 59–71 μ.

Life-cycle. The eggs hatch after developing under favourable conditions for about 3 weeks and the miracidium penetrates into an intermediate host, *Stagnicola palustris, Helisoma trivolvis, Physa gyrina, P. occidentalis, P.*

oculans, Planorbis tenuis, Limnaea stagnalis, L. attenuate, L. (Radix) pereger or *L. swinhoei.* Cercariae are produced in 2–3 weeks and these either encyst in the snail or escape and enter another of the same or a different species, for instance *Vivipara vivipara, Sphaerium corneum, Fossaria* spp. or tadpoles. The final host becomes infected by ingesting these snails and the worms grow to adulthood in 15–19 days.

Pathogenicity. This parasite has generally been regarded as fairly harmless, but heavy infections may cause severe enteritis. Beaver (1937) reported haemorrhagic enteritis 10 days after infection of pigeons. On *post mortem* 600 flukes were found. Death in pigeons associated with several thousand echinostomes was reported by van Heelsbergen (1927a).

Diagnosis is made by finding the eggs of the worms in the faeces of the host.

Treatment. Carbon tetrachloride or tetrachlorethylene in doses of 1–2 ml., administered with about 3 ml. liquid paraffin by means of a syringe and 10 cm. of narrow rubber tubing which is pushed into the oesophagus, will probably give the best results.

Prophylaxis, should be directed towards extermination of the snails. Where possible, the birds should have access only to ponds in which the snails can be properly controlled.

Genus: Echinoparyphium Dietz, 1909

E. paraulum (Dietz, 1909) (syn. *Echinostoma columbae* Zunker, 1925; *Echinostoma paraulum* Dietz, 1909). Dawes (1946) doubts the validity of this species, which may be synonymous with *Echinostoma revolutum.* It occurs in the small intestine of the duck, the pigeon and man. It measures 6–10·5 by 0·8–1·4 mm., and the cuticle bears spines almost to the posterior extremity; but these may be lost and their absence has in some cases caused much confusion. The head-collar, which is continuous across the ventral surface, bears thirty-seven spines: twenty-seven in a double dorso-lateral row and at either end five 'corner spines'. The oral sucker measures 0·25–0·3 mm. in diameter, and the ventral 0·72–0·88 mm.; the latter lies at the end of the first quarter of the body. There is a short pre-pharynx, a pharynx and an oesophagus; the latter is 0·4–0·6 mm. long. The testes are tandem and lie in the third quarter of the body; the anterior has frequently three and the posterior four lobes. The cirrus-sac may extend back to the middle of the ventral sucker. The ovary lies just anterior to the testes. The eggs measure about 100 by 70 μ.

Life-cycle—unknown. The first intermediate host is certainly a snail and some authors suspect fish and snails as the second intermediate host.

Pathogenicity. Krause (1925) and Wetzel (1933) have observed deaths in pigeons caused by this parasite. The birds showed inappetence, thirst, diarrhoea, lassitude and progressive weakness. At *post mortem* there was a slight atrophy of the breast muscles and catarrhal enteritis with much mucus, becoming haemorrhagic behind the duodenum. The parasites were found chiefly in the middle portion of the intestine and could occur in large numbers.

Treatment. Carbon tetrachloride should be tried as for *E. revolutum.*
Prophylaxis. Extermination of the intermediate hosts is indicated.

E. recurvatum (v. Linstow, 1873) occurs in the small intestine, especially the duodenum, of the domestic duck, wild duck, fowls and pigeons. It is up to 4·5 mm. long and 0·5–0·8 mm. wide. The anterior end is curved ventrad and is armed with spines anterior to the ventral

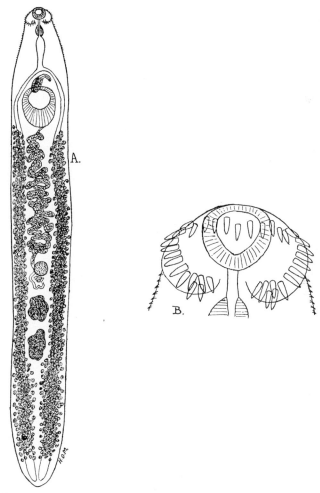

Fig. 14. *Echinoparyphium paraulum.* A, Ventral view; B, ventral view of anterior end, showing the head-crown (Original)

sucker. The head-crown has forty-five spines, of which four are corner spines on either side. The ventral sucker is 0·32–0·36 mm. wide and situated at the first quarter of the body. Testes oval, tandem, not lobed and in contact with each other. The ovary is transversely oval and the uterus is short, containing three to seven eggs, which measure 108–110 by 81–84 μ.

Life-cycle. The first intermediate hosts are *Limnaea ovata, L. auricularia, L. palustris L. stagnalis, Planorbis planorbis, P. corneus, Vivipara vivipara* etc. The frog, *Rana temporaria,* and snails, among which are *Valvata piscinalis* and *Planorbis albus,* act as second intermediate hosts. The cercariae encyst in the digestive glands of the snails and may migrate to other snails. They encyst in the kidneys of the tadpoles and even adult frogs (Harper, 1929).

Pathogenicity. Van Heelsbergen (1927b) reported emaciation, anaemia and sometimes weakness of the legs in infected fowls. At autopsy a marked enteritis with swelling of the mucosa and mucous content of the bowel was found. In the U.S.A. Annereaux (1940) reported a marked enteritis in turkeys due to *E. recurvatum* and in Great Britain Soulsby (1955) found it the cause of deaths in mute swans on the River Axe in Somerset.

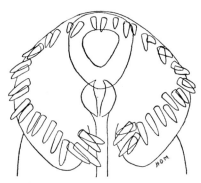

FIG. 15. *Echinoparyphium recurvatum,* Ventral View of Anterior End, showing Head-crown (Original)

Treatment. Carbon tetrachloride or tetrachlorethylene is indicated, as in the case of *Echinostoma revolutum.*

Prophylaxis should be directed towards extermination of the snail intermediate hosts, and, where possible, the birds should be prevented from ingesting infected frogs. It is obvious that it is impossible to exterminate snails everywhere without probably upsetting the water fauna, and the statement that the snails must be exterminated should be taken and applied with discretion.

Genus: Hypoderaeum Dietz, 1909

H. conoideum (Bloch, 1872) occurs in the posterior part of the small intestine of the duck, goose, swan, wild aquatic birds, fowl and pigeon. It is 5–12 mm. long and up to 2 mm. broad. The body is elongate and tapers posteriorly. The ventral sucker is relatively large and situated close to the anterior. The head-collar is weakly developed and bears forty-seven to fifty-three (usually forty-nine) spines, of which two on either side form the 'corner spines'. The anterior part of the body is well armed with spines. The oesophagus is very short. Testes elongate, slightly lobed, tandem, behind the middle. The cirrus-sac is club-shaped, reaching back almost to the posterior margin of the ventral sucker. The eggs measure 95–108 by 61–68 μ.

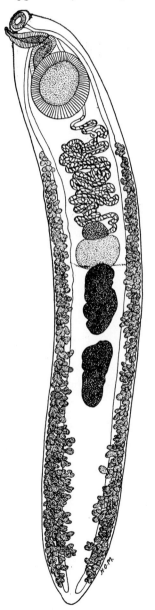

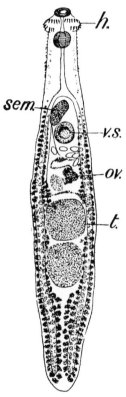

FIG. 17. *Echinochasmus perfoliatus*, Ventral View (from Baylis, after V. Rátz)

- *h.* Head-crown
- *ov.* Ovary
- *sem.* Seminal vesicle
- *t.* Testis
- *v.s.* Ventral sucker

FIG. 16. *Hypoderaeum conoideum*, Ventral View (Original)

Life-cycle. The first intermediate hosts are *Limnaea stagnalis*, *L. pereger L. ovata* and *Planorbis corneus*. Vevers (1923) has infected ducks by feeding infected *L. peregra*, showing that the cercariae in the snail are infective. That they, however, usually appear to enter a second intermediate host which carries the infection to the final host is evident from the work of Nöller & Wagner (1923), who found the cercariae encysted in the kidneys of the tadpoles and young forms of the frog *Rana esculenta*.

Pathogenicity. Localised enteritis has been noted in infected ducks (Vevers, 1923).

Genus: Echinochasmus Dietz, 1909

E. perfoliatus (v. Rátz, 1908) occurs in the intestine of the dog, cat, fox and pig in Europe and Asia. It measures 2–4 by 0·4–1 mm. The head-crown bears twenty-four spines in a single row and the anterior region of the body is spiny. The ventral sucker is nearly twice as large as

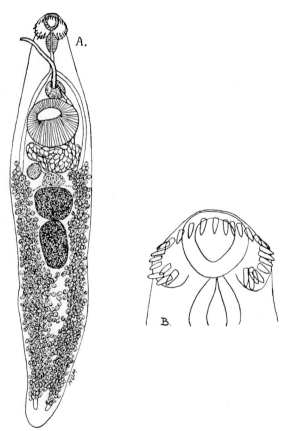

FIG. 18. *Euparyphium melis.* A, Ventral view; B, ventral view of anterior end, showing the head-crown (Original)

the oral one. The testes are large, tandem and situated behind the middle. The ovary lies to the right, anterior to the testes. The cirrus-sac lies anterior to the ventral sucker. The vitellaria extend from in front of the ventral sucker to the posterior end of the body in the lateral fields, also extending inwards behind the testes. The eggs measure 85–105 by 60–75 μ, and have a yellow colour.

Life-cycle. In Japan the primary intermediate host is the snail *Bulinus striatus japonicus* and several fresh-water fish (*Abramis brama, Esox lucius, Idus idus, Aspius aspius, Scardinius erythrophthalmus,* etc.) serve as secondary intermediate hosts.

Pathogenicity. This parasite causes severe enteritis.

Treatment. Carbon tetrachloride is indicated.

Prevention. Snails should be exterminated where this is possible and raw fish should not be fed to the animal hosts.

Genus: Euparyphium Dietz, 1909

E. melis (Schrank, 1788) occurs in the small intestine of the cat, fox, polecat, mink, pine marten, beech marten, badger, otter, weasel and hedgehog (*Erinaceus europaeus*) in Europe. The worm is elongate, measuring 3·5–12 by 1·3–3·3 mm. The head-collar bears a dorsally continuous row of twenty-seven spines, the whole ventral surface is covered with small spines, and dorsally they extend to the level of the pharynx. The oral sucker is much smaller than the ventral sucker. The latter lies in the first quarter of the body and the intestine bifurcates near its anterior border. The testes are median, tandem, entire or slightly lobed; the anterior one lies at the middle of the body. The ovary lies anterior to the testes to the right of the mid-line and the receptaculum seminis to the left. The cirrus-sac is well developed and extends dorsally to the ventral sucker. The cirrus is spiny. The vitellaria extend backwards from the level of the receptaculum seminis and almost meet behind the posterior testis. The uterus is short and the eggs measure 120–125 by 91–94 μ.

Life-cycle. According to Beaver (1941) the first intermediate host in the United States is the snail *Stagnicola emarginata angulata* and the metacercariae are found in tadpoles.

Pathogenicity. Heavy infections may be seen in the polecat without producing clinical signs. The mink, however, is very susceptible to the effects of these worms, which produce a haemorrhagic enteritis in this host.

Treatment. Carbon tetrachloride or male fern extract is indicated.

E. ilocanum (Garrison, 1908) occurs in the intestine of man in the Philippines and South East Asia. It has also been found in the dog and the Norway rat, the latter serving as a reservoir host. The first intermediate hosts are the snails *Gyraulus convexiusculus G. prashadi* and *Hippeutis* *umbilicalis.* Cercariae encyst on almost any fresh-water mollusc but *Pila luzonica*, *P. conica* and *Viviparus javanicus* are especially important since they are regarded as a delicacy and are eaten raw or at the most with a sprinkling of salt and vinegar. *The pathogenic effects* consist of inflammatory lesions of the intestinal mucosa at the site of attachment of the worms. Diarrhoea and intestinal colic may occur.

Other species of the genus include *E. jassyense* Léon & Ciurea, 1922, found in the intestine of man in Roumania, and *E. suinum* Ciurea, 1921, in the intestine of pigs in Roumania and Hungary.

FAMILY: HETEROPHYIDAE

Small trematodes, usually not over 2 mm. long and wider posteriorly than anteriorly. The body is covered with scales, decreasing in number in the posterior region. The ventral sucker is usually situated near the middle of the body and may be weak or absent. A pharynx and a long oesophagus are present and the intestinal branches reach almost to the posterior end. The genital pore opens close to the ventral sucker and is

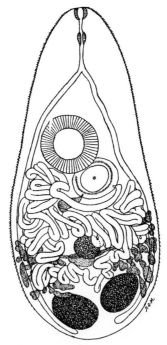

FIG. 19. *Heterophyes heterophyes*, Ventral View (Original)

frequently surrounded by a genital sucker. The testes are oval or slightly lobed, horizontal or diagonal, and situated near to the posterior end of the body. The seminal vesicle is well developed and there is no cirrus-sac. The ovary is oval or slightly lobed, anterior to the testes and median or to the right of the middle. The vitellaria are lateral and usually restricted to the posterior part. The coiled uterus is in the posterior half of the body and contains relatively few eggs. Parasites in the intestines of mammals and birds. Where known, the life-cycle includes two intermediate hosts— snails and fishes or frogs.

Genus: Heterophyes Cobbold, 1866

H. heterophyes (v. Siebold, 1852) occurs in the small intestine of the dog, cat, fox and man in Egypt and eastern Asia. It measures 1–1·7 by 0·3–0·7 mm., and is wider posteriorly than anteriorly. The ventral sucker is situated immediately anterior to the middle and is 0·23 mm. wide. The genital sucker lies directly behind it and to one side and bears an incomplete circle of seventy to eighty small rods. The testes are oval and horizontal in position. The eggs have thick shells; they are light brown in colour, provided with an operculum which fits into a slightly thickened rim of the shell, and measure 26–30 by 15–17 μ.

Life-cycle. The first intermediate hosts are the snails *Pirenella conica* in Egypt and *Cerithidia cingulata* in Japan. The second intermediate host is a fish (*Mugil cephalus, Tilapia nilotica, Aphanius fasciatus* and *Acanthogobius* spp.), in which the metacercaria is encysted. It bears a great resemblance to the adult fluke. Infection takes place through eating infected raw fish. In Egypt the fish is eaten salted as 'fessikh'. The metacercariae live up to 7 days in the salted fish. The adult starts laying eggs 9 days after infection.

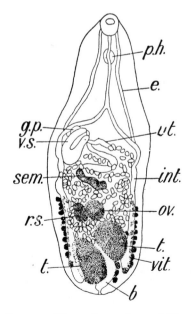

b.	Excretory bladder
e.	Excretory canal
g.p.	Genital pore
int.	Intestinal caecum
ov.	Ovary
ph.	Pharynx
r.s.	Receptaculum seminis
sem.	Seminal vesicle
t,t.	Testes
ut.	Uterus
vit.	Vitellaria
v.s.	Ventral sucker

FIG. 20. *Metagonimus yokogawai*, Ventral View (from Baylis, after Ciurea)

Pathogenicity. The flukes penetrate into the mucosa and may cause slight desquamation, but the pathogenicity of the parasites is so low that they are generally regarded as being practically harmless. In severe human cases diarrhoea may develop; this is usually intermittent and sometimes haemorrhagic.

Diagnosis is made by finding the eggs in the faeces. They have to be differentiated, especially from the eggs of *Opisthorchis*.

Treatment. Male fern extract, carbon tetrachloride, or tetrachlorethylene are recommended if treatment is necessary.

Prevention. The infection can be prevented by using no raw fish as food, while salted fish should not be used within 10 days of salting.

Genus: Metagonimus Katsurada, 1913

M. yokogawai (Katsurada, 1912) occurs in the small intestine of the dog, cat, pig, man and pelican in eastern Asia and the Balkans. Mice have been infected experimentally. The parasite measures 1–2·5 by 0·4–0·7 mm., and is wider posteriorly than anteriorly. The cuticle is armed with spines over the whole body. The ventral sucker is situated to the right of the median line and the genital pore opens in a sinus immediately anterior to it. The sinus and the sucker are surrounded by an elevated muscular ring. The testes are slightly oblique in position. The ovary is median, and the vitelline glands are composed of coarse follicles lying in the posterior parts of the lateral fields. The eggs are very similar to those of *Heterophyes* and measure 27–30 by 15–17 μ.

Life-cycle. The first intermediate host is the snail *Semisulcospira libertina* and related species. The second intermediate hosts are several species of fresh-water fish (the trout, *Plecoglossus altivelis*, also *Salmo perryi* and *Odontobutis* and *Leuciscus* spp.). The cercariae become encysted under the scales or in the tissue of the gills, fins or tail and the final host infects itself by eating these fish raw.

Pathogenicity etc., as in the case of *Heterophyes*.

Genus: Euryhelmis Poche, 1925

E. squamula (Rudolphi, 1819) occurs in the intestine of the fox, polecat, weasel and mink. The body is broad and flat, measuring about 0·6 by 1·45 mm. The oral sucker is anterior, and there are a pharynx and an oesophagus of median length. The intestinal caeca are more or less parallel to the margins of the body. The ventral sucker is situated near the middle, and is about half as large as the oral. The testes are lobed in the adult, side by side and posterior in position. The elongate cirrus-sac winds around the right side of the ventral sucker. The genital pore lies anterior to the ventral sucker. The ovary is lobed in the adult and lies anterior to the right testis, with a large receptaculum seminis in between. The uterus is coiled and lies mainly between the left testis and the ventral sucker. The vitellaria are well developed and extend along the course of the intestinal caeca (Fig. 21). The eggs measure 29–32 by 12–14 μ.

Life-cycle. Not completely known. The metacercariae are encysted in the skin of the frogs *Rana temporaria* and *Rana esculenta.*

Pathogenicity. Severe infections cause a fatal haemorrhagic enteritis in the mink.

Treatment. Male fern extract or tetrachlorethylene is effective.

Prophylaxis. The animals should be prevented from eating frogs.

Euryhelmis monorchis (Ameel, 1938) occurs in the mink in the U.S.A. It has a single testis on the same side as the ovary and the male genital organs disappear later. Its first intermediate host is the snail *Pomatiopsis lapidaria*; second intermediate hosts are the frogs *Rana clamitans, R. pipiens* and *R. palustris.*

Genus: Cryptocotyle Lühe, 1899

C. lingua (Creplin, 1825) Fischoeder, 1903, is common in the intestines of the herring gull, the greater and lesser black-backed gull, the common tern, the kittiwake, the razor bill, the Slavonic grebe and the night-heron. It also occurs in the seal, silver fox, mink, dog and cat. It is found in Europe, Canada and the U.S.A. Christensen & Roth (1949) found it in 17 per cent of dogs in Copenhagen, Cameron (1945) reported it to be the commonest trematode in fox and mink farms in Canada and McTaggert (1958) found it in mink in Scotland.

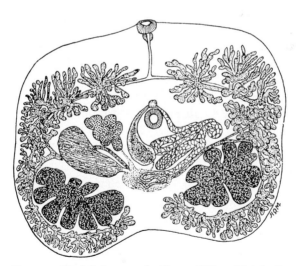

FIG. 21. *Euryhelmis squamula*, Ventral View (Original)

This species is larger than many heterophyid flukes, having a body shaped like a spatula measuring 0·5–2·0 mm. long by 0·2–0·9 mm. broad. The cuticle is spiny and the suckers are feeble, the oral one being larger than the ventral one, which is near the middle of the body and is enclosed in the genital sinus. The two branches of the intestine are long and slender. The genital atrium is near the middle of the body. The slightly lobed testes lie side by side or diagonally at the posterior end of the body, the tri-lobed ovary being in front of them and on one side of the middle line. The vitellaria fill all the space outside the intestinal caesa. The uterus has a few wide folds. The eggs measure 0·032–0·050 by 0·018–0·025 mm.

Pathogenesis. Large numbers of flukes cause a marked enteritis associated with degeneration of the epithelium, haemorrhagic erosions and the production of a large quantity of viscid mucus. Cats are less susceptible to the infection, parasites failing to attain their full size in this host.

C. concava (Creplin, 1825) Lühe, 1899, is essentially a parasite of sea birds, however, Christensen & Roth (1949) found it in fox and mink farms and also in 2 per cent of dogs in Denmark. Likewise it has been found in dogs and foxes in U.S.S.R. and Roumania.

It is a smaller species than *C. lingua* measuring 0·5–1·5 mm. by 0·35–0·88 mm. The eggs measure 30–40 μ by 16–20 μ. The molluscan intermediate host is unknown but metacercariae encyst in fish of the genera *Atherina, Gobius, Mullus* etc.

C. jejuna Nicoll, 1907, resembles **C. concava**, the eggs being 28–36 μ by 16–19 μ in size. A key for the differentiation of the three species of *Cryptocotyle* is given by Soulsby (1965). *C. jejuna* has been found in dogs experimentally infected by feeding *Gobius melanostomus*.

Both these species produce pathogenic effects similar to those seen in *C. lingua* infection.

Genus: Apophallus Lühe, 1909

A. mühlingi (Jägershiöld, 1899) Lühe, 1909, is normally a parasite of gulls and cormorants in Europe but has also been found in the intestine of cats and dogs. It is a small form, 1·2–1·6 mm. long by 0·2–0·23 mm. broad. The eggs measure 32 μ by 18 μ. The life cycle is uncompletely known but metacercariae are found in fish of the Cyprinidae family.

Genus: Rossicotrema Skrjabin, 1919

This genus is considered by some to be synonymous with the genus *Apophallus.*

R. donicum Skrjabin, 1919, occurs in the small intestine of cat, dog, fox and seal in Eastern Europe and North America. It is a small form, 0·5–1·15 mm. in length by 0·2–0·4 mm. in breadth. The cuticle is spiny and the testes are large, rounded and lie in the posterior part of the body. The eggs measure 35–40 μ by 19–24 μ.

The first intermediate hosts are unknown but metacercariae occur in fish of the Cyprinidae such as *Perca, Lucioperca* and *Scardinius* spp.

FAMILY: PLAGIORCHIDAE

These are fairly large trematodes with thick bodies. The cuticle is usually ·covered with spines. A short prepharynx, a pharynx and an oesophagus are present, and the intestinal crura are of variable length. The genital pore is anterior to the ventral sucker, usually somewhat lateral, or it may lie next to the oral sucker. Testes entire or lobed, horizontal or tandem. A cirrus-sac is present. The ovary lies in front of the testes and the ventral sucker, to the right of the middle, and may be lobed. The vitellaria lie in the lateral fields. The uterus passes backwards and forwards between the testes. Eggs numerous with thin shells.

Genus: Prosthogonimus Lühe, 1899

P. pellucidus (v. Linstow, 1873) (syn. *P. intercalandus*) occurs in the Bursa Fabricii, oviduct and posterior intestine of the fowl, duck, and various wild birds. It measures 8–9 by 4–5 mm., and is broad posteriorly. It has a pale reddish-yellow colour when fresh. The irregularly oval testes lie horizontal at the middle of the body. The genital pore is situated next to the oral sucker and the cirrus-sac is elongate, extending to near the ventral sucker. The ovary is much lobed and lies partly dorsal to the ventral sucker. The vitellaria extend from the level of the ventral sucker to the posterior ends of the testes. The operculate, dark-brown eggs bear a small spine at the pole opposite to the operculum. They measure 26–32 by 10–15 μ.

P. macrorchis Macy, 1934, is a similar species to the above occurring in the Bursa Fabricii and oviduct of domestic poultry and ducks and also wild birds in North America. It is 5–7 μ mm. in length and the testes are relatively larger than in *P. pellucidus*.

P. ovatus (Rudolphi, 1803) Lühe, 1899, is found in the Bursa Fabricii and oviduct of domestic fowl and geese and a wide variety of wild birds in Europe, Africa and Asia. It is a smaller form than the above two species measuring 3–6 mm. by 1–2 mm. The testes are slightly elongate lying side by side behind the mid part of the body. The ovary is deeply lobed and the eggs are small 22–24 μ by 13 μ.

Other species of the genus include *P. anatinus* Markow, 1902, of domestic ducks in U.S.S.R., *P. cuneatus* (Rudolphi, 1809) Braun, 1901, of the swan and *P. oviformis* Strom, 1940, of the duck in Europe.

Life-cycles. Two intermediate hosts are required, the first a water snail and the second the nymphal stage of various species of dragonflies. *Amnicola limosa porata* is the first intermediate host for *P. macrorchis*, *Bithynia teutaculata* serves *P. pellucidus* as such and *B. leachi*, *Gyraulus albus* and *G. gredleri* are the snail hosts for *P. ovatus*. Sporocysts are formed which produce cercariae without undergoing redial development, and these, being liberated from the snail, swim about in the water. They are then drawn into the anal openings of dragonfly naiads by the breathing movements of these insects. The tail of the cercaria is lost in the respiratory chamber of the naiad and the metacercaria penetrates into the muscles and encysts in the haemocoel of the nymph. Metacercariae may persist in the insect until it is mature and the final host is infected by eating either the adult dragonfly or the nymphal stage.

Several species of dragonflies may serve as hosts. In North America those of the genera *Tetragoneuria, Leucorhynia, Epicordulia* and *Mesotheronis* are concerned (Macy, 1934) and in Europe *Libellula, Platycnemis* and *Epicordulia* (Panin, 1957).

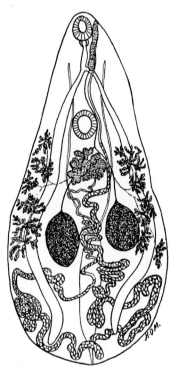

FIG. 22. *Prosthogonimus pellucidus*, Ventral View (Original)

In the final host the liberated immature trematodes migrate to the cloaca and the Bursa Fabricii where they become adult. In the mature fowl, in which the Bursa is atrophied, the parasites enter the oviduct.

Pathogenesis. P. pellucidus, as well as other species of this genus, are considered to be the most pathogenic trematode parasites of poultry in Europe and America. Fowls are mainly affected, but occasionally also ducks. In laying birds the movements of the oviduct apparently assist them to enter this organ and here they cause marked irritation, resulting in an acute inflammation of the oviduct, the production of abnormal eggs and discharges of albumen from the cloaca. The irritated oviduct readily performs retroperistaltic movements, causing broken yolks, albumen, bacteria and parasite material to enter the peritoneal cavity, where they set up peritonitis, usually with fatal results.

Clinical Signs. The disease is usually seen in spring or early summer. At first the general health is not disturbed, but several hens may begin to lay eggs with soft shells or without any shell at all. They may show a marked tendency to sit on the nest. There may be a discharge from the cloaca in the form of a milky fluid consisting chiefly of lime, which glues the feathers together around the anus. The irritated oviduct passes the eggs through so rapidly that no shell is deposited, although the lime-secreting glands act normally, and this secretion is then discharged separately. The birds become listless, the abdomen is pendulous and the legs are held widely apart in walking. Laying is suspended and the birds are obviously ill. The feathers around the cloaca are soiled with albumen, which is discharged and may contain yellowish-white strands and parasites. If peritonitis develops, the comb and wattles become cyanotic and the birds soon become prostrated and die. An 'aseptic peritonitis' may also be seen, in which case the yolk in the peritoneal cavity becomes inspissated and may obstruct the intestinal peristalsis.

Post Mortem. The oviduct shows varying degrees of inflammation according to the severity of the disease, from a catarrh to a croupous inflammation with a dirty, cheesy mass in the lumen. It may contain broken yolks and, frequently, large concrements of yolk and albumen. The parasites are not easily seen on the mucous membrane. In cases of peritonitis the abdominal cavity contains a dirty fluid and the organs are stuck together by a cheesy mass. Inspissated yolk may be present between the intestines. The serous membranes show a marked congestion and haemorrhages may be present.

Diagnosis. The eggs of the parasites can be found in large numbers in the discharges from the cloaca. In some cases the parasites may already have disappeared, but the disease continues. In such cases the worm eggs can frequently be found in the abdominal cavity at autopsy.

Treatment. No satisfactory treatment is known for removing the parasites from the oviduct. In the early stages of the disease it may be advantageous to dose the birds with carbon tetrachloride, which may remove worms still present in the intestine and prevent them from entering the oviduct.

Prophylaxis. The extermination of snails, as well as preventing the birds from eating dragonflies, as far as possible, is indicated.

Genus: Plagiorchis Lühe, 1899 (syn. Lepoderma)

Species of this genus have a more elongated body that tapers at each end. The genital opening is a little in front of the ventral sucker, usually to the left of the middle line and behind the bifurcation of the intestine. The rounded or oval testes are obliquely behind one another and the rounded ovary is near the hind end of the cirrus-sac, which is on the right side of the ventral sucker and extends behind it.

P. megalorchis Rees, 1952, was found by Rees (1952) in Wales in dead turkey poults and this author found that its first intermediate host is the snail *Limnaea pereger*, and its second intermediate hosts *Chironomus riparius*, *Culicoides stigma*, *C. nuberculosus* or *Anatopynia varius*. Rees suggests that the normal definitive host is a wild bird, possibly a gull or a heron. She concluded that *P. laricola* Skrjabin, 1924, of gulls and terns reported by Foggie (1937) from turkey poults in Northern Ireland was *P. megalorchis*.

P. lutrae Fahmy, 1954, occurs in the otter.

P. arcuatus Strom, 1924, occurs in the oviducts of fowl in Germany and U.S.S.R. It has been associated with inflammation of the oviduct.

FAMILY: NOTOCOTYLIDAE

These trematodes have no ventral sucker. The ventral surface of the body is provided with three or five rows of unicellular glands situated in groups. The cuticle is armed with fine spines anteriorly and ventrally. A pharynx is absent and the oesophagus is short, while the intestinal caeca extend to the posterior end of the body. The genital pore usually opens directly behind the oral sucker and the cirrus-sac is elongate. The testes are horizontally situated near the posterior end of the body and lateral to the intestinal caeca. The ovary lies between them. The vitelline glands occupy the lateral fields in the posterior part, anterior to the testes. The uterus forms more or less regular transverse coils extending from the ovary to the posterior end of the cirrus-sac. The eggs bear long filaments at both poles. Parasites in the intestine of aquatic birds and mammals.

Genus: Notocotylus Diesing, 1839

N. attenuatus (Rudolphi, 1809) commonly occurs in the caeca and rectum of the fowl, duck, goose and wild aquatic birds. It measures 2–5 by 0·6–1·5 mm., and is narrow anteriorly. There are three rows of ventral glands, fourteen to seventeen in the lateral rows, and fourteen to fifteen in the middle row. The vagina is half as long as the cirrus-sac. The eggs are small, 20 μ long, and bear a long filament at either pole.

Life-cycle. The intermediate hosts are the snails *Planorbis rotundatus*, *Limnaea palustris*, *L. limosa* and *Bulinus japonicus*.

Other species include *N. impricatus Szidat*, 1935, in domestic poultry in Europe and North America and *N. thienemanni* Szidat & Szidat, 1933, in domestic and wild ducks in Europe.

Genus: Catatropis Odhner, 1905

C. verrucosa (Fröhlich, 1789) occurs in the caeca of the fowl, duck, goose and wild aquatic birds. It measures 1–6 by 0·75–2 mm., and is reddish in colour. The body is rounded anteriorly and posteriorly. There are three rows of ventral glands each containing eight to twelve glands. The elliptical, reddish eggs measure 18–28 μ in length, not including the filaments, each of which is 160–200 μ long.

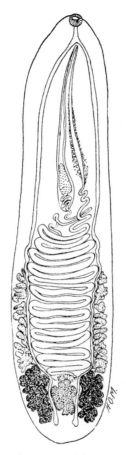

FIG. 23. *Catatropis verrucosa*, Ventral View (Original)

Life-cycle. Szidat (1930) has followed the development through the snail *Planorbis* (*Coretus*) *corneus.* The cercariae have simple tails and three eye-spots. They leave the snail and encyst on water-plants, snails etc., which may be ingested by the final host. The worms become sexually mature within a short time after infection.

Pathogenicity. The Notocotylidae are rarely associated with pathogenic effects.

Genus: Cymbiforma Yamaguti, 1933

C. indica (Bhalerao, 1942) occurs in sheep, goats and cattle in India. The parasites live in all parts of the digestive tract behind the oesophagus, but particularly the duodenum. Heavy infections are frequent. They die and disintegrate rapidly after death of the host. No pathogenic changes have been ascribed to these parasites.

They are pear-shaped and concave ventrally, measuring 0·8–2·7 by 0·31–0·96 mm. The genital opening is to the left of the midline, a short distance anterior to the middle of the body. The ovary has four distinct lobes. The eggs measure 18–37 by 11–13 μ and carry filaments at the poles.

FAMILY: BRACHYLAEMIDAE (SYN. HARMOSTOMIDAE)

More or less elongate, small or medium-sized trematodes usually with smooth bodies. A pre-pharynx and oesophagus are present and the intestinal caeca extend to the posterior end of the body. The testes are posterior in position, tandem or slightly diagonal, and the ovary lies between them. The vitellaria are follicular and occupy the lateral fields mostly behind the middle of the body. The genital pore is posterior, median or slightly lateral or even terminal or dorsal. The cirrus-sac contains a cirrus, but the seminal vesicle lies free. Parasitic in the intestine of vertebrates.

Genus: Brachylaemus Dujardin, 1843 (syn. Harmostomum)

B. commutatus (Diesing, 1858) occurs in the caeca of the fowl, pheasant, turkey, pigeon and guinea-fowl in southern Europe, North Africa and Indo-China. It measures 3·7–7·5 by 1–2 mm. The body is rounded anteriorly and tapers posteriorly. The ventral sucker lies within the anterior third of the body. The testes are irregularly rounded; the posterior one is median and the anterior one lies to the left of the mid-line, while the ovary lies to the right. The vitellaria consist of fine follicles extending in the lateral fields forwards from the level of the posterior testis. The uterus has coiled ascending and descending branches, and the genital pore is situated near the anterior border of the anterior testis in the mid-line. The eggs measure 27–32 by 13–18 μ. Dawes (1946) considers the American species *Postharmonostomum gallinum* to be identical to *B. commutatus*.

Life-cycle. The American form utilises the land snail *Eulota similaris* as an intermediate host (Alicata, 1940) though other snails such as *Subulina*, *Euhadra* and *Philomycus* spp. may serve as such. Cercariae after liberation may encyst in the same or other species of snails.

Pathogenicity. The parasites may cause an inflammation of the caeca.

B. suis (Balozet, 1936) occurs in the small intestine of the pig in Tunis and sucks blood, but is apparently not very pathogenic. The intermediate hosts are land snails, especially *Xerophila* species. The eggs are light brown and measure 30–35 by 15–17 μ.

Genus: Skrjabinotrema Orlov, Erschov & Banadin, 1934

S. ovis Orlov, Ershov and Banadin, 1934. This occurs in the posterior part of the small intestines of sheep in West China and the Steppe area of eastern U.S.S.R.

The flukes measure 0·79–1·12 by 0·32–0·7 mm. The two oval testes are large and lie diagonally, but touching each other, in the posterior part of the body, the ovary being in front of the right testis. The eggs measure 24–32 by 16–20 μ; they are slightly flattened on one side and have a large operculum at one end and a small appendage at the other.

Pathogenesis. Heavy infections may cause a catarrhal enteritis.

FAMILY: TROGLOTREMATIDAE

These medium or fairly large trematodes usually have a fleshy body, flattened or concave ventrally and convex dorsally, with a spiny cuticle. The suckers may be poorly developed and the ventral sucker is sometimes absent. A pharynx and a short oesophagus are present and the intestinal caeca do not quite reach the posterior end. The genital pore is median or slightly to the left, in front of, or behind, the ventral sucker when this is present. The testes are horizontal, at or behind the middle, elongate or deeply lobed. The cirrus-sac is usually absent. The ovary lies anterior to the right testis and is usually deeply lobed. The vitelline glands are strongly developed and almost fill the dorso-lateral aspect of the body. The uterus and eggs are variable. Parasites of carnivorous mammals and birds, usually in pairs in cysts in various parts of the body.

Genus: Paragonimus Braun, 1899

P. westermanii (Kerbert, 1878), the 'lung-fluke', occurs in the lungs and more rarely in the brain, spinal cord and other organs of the pig, dog, cat, goat, cattle, fox, pine marten, beech marten, mink, musk-rat, wild carnivores and man. The parasite is reddish-brown in colour

Fig. 24. *Paragonimus kellicotti*, Cuticular Scales (Original)

and measures 7·5–16 by 4–8 mm. The cuticle is covered with spines. The ventral sucker is situated slightly anterior to the middle. The eggs are yellowish-brown in colour and measure 75–118 by 42–67 μ; they are provided with an operculum, and the shell is thickened at the pole opposite this.

Several distinct species of *Paragonimus* are recognised by some authors: *P. westermanii* originally found in the tiger, *P. ringeri* from man in China and Japan, and *P. kellicotti* found in the cat, pig and dog in the United States, in the tiger in the Malay States and in the cat in South Africa. The main difference lies in the shape of the spines, those of *P. ringeri*

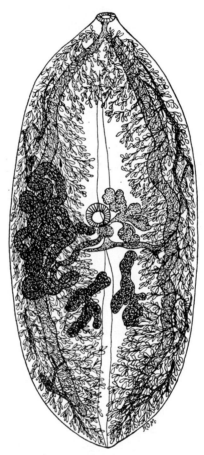

FIG. 25. *Paragonimus westermanii*, Dorsal View (Original)

being small and arranged in groups; those of *P. westermanii* are larger and have bifid points, while those of *P. kellicotti* are still larger and have a number of points each.

In the U.S.A. it is probable that the mink is the natural host, a survey by Gesinki *et al.* (1964) showing 35·48 per cent of these animals to be infected in Ohio. The muskrat (*Ondatra sibethica*) may also be a natural host.

Life-cycle. The eggs are laid in the cysts, in which the worms live and escape through connecting channels into the bronchi, or else when the cysts rupture. They pass up from the lung with the mucus and may be found in the sputum, which has a characteristic rusty colour. Animals will usually swallow the mucus, so that the eggs are found in the faeces. After development for 2–7 weeks (16 days under optimal conditions) the miracidium escapes and penetrates into a snail of the genus *Melania, Ampullaria luteostoma* or *Pomatiopsis lapidaria*, in which the usual further development takes place, including sporocysts, rediae and cercariae. The latter have an oval body and a very short tail. After escaping from the snail the cercariae swim about in the water and, on meeting a suitable crab or crayfish, penetrate into it and encyst. In Japan and China the following crustacea are known as secondary inter- mediate hosts: *Astacus dauricus, A. japonicus, A. similis, Eriocheir japonicus, E. sinensis, Potamon dehaani, P. obtusipes, P. sinensis* and *Sesarma dehaani*; and, in Venezuela, *Pseudotelphusa iturbei*. The final host becomes infected by eating the infected crustacea or by drinking water in which the meta- cercariae occur, after they have escaped from these intermediate hosts. The metacercariae escape from the crustacea when these are injured and may live in water for 3 weeks.

After being liberated in the intestine the young fluke penetrates through the wall and wanders through the peritoneal cavity and diaphragm, entering the lungs from the pleural cavity. They may also enter other organs, such as the brain, from this location. It arrives in the bronchioles, where the host forms a cyst wall around it, and grows adult. The pre- patent period is 5–6 weeks. The cysts in the lungs apparently develop from dilated small bronchioles: they are lined with stratified epithelium and are usually connected by fine channels with the bronchi, through which the eggs are discharged.

Pathogenicity and Clinical signs. The parasites in the lungs are not usually of great importance, but those lodged in the brain and other organs may cause trouble. In the lungs the parasitic cyst is surrounded by diffuse connective tissue which encroaches on the lung parenchyma. The cyst wall is infiltrated with leucocytes and giant cells. Eggs may be present in the lung tissue, where they cause small pseudotubercles to develop.

In animals the cyst usually contains two parasites, surrounded by a purulent fluid mixed with blood and the eggs. In lung infections there is a cough and the eggs may be found in the sputum in large num- bers. Parasitic cysts in other parts of the body may work their way to a surface like the intestinal mucosa, the epithelium of the bile-ducts or the skin, where the eggs are discharged and ulcers form which heal with great difficulty.

Diagnosis of lung cases is readily made by finding the eggs in the sputum or faeces. In other cases diagnosis may be extremely difficult. A complement fixation test for diagnosis has been developed by Yokogawa *et al.* (1962) and skin-sensitizing antibodies have been detected and utilised for an intradermal test (Yokogawa *et al.*, 1957).

Treatment. Workers in Japan have demonstrated the efficacy of Bithionol (2·2′-thiobis[4·6-dichlorophenol]) in human subjects. Doses of 1·5–2·5 g. (according to age) are given on alternate days for 3–4 weeks.

Emetine hydrochloride has been used but some workers believe it has limited value in treatment.

Prophylaxis. Fresh-water crustacea should not be eaten raw and the extermination of snails should be considered.

Genus: Collyriclum Ward 1917

C. faba (Bremser, 1831) occurs in subcutaneous cysts in the fowl and turkey as well as in several small wild birds like sparrows and starlings. It measures 3–5 by 4·5–5·5 mm. It is flattened ventrally convex dorsally and has a spiny cuticle. The oral sucker is small, with a diameter of 0·2–0·45 mm. The ventral sucker is absent. The ovary has three main lobes and each is divided into several smaller lobes. The vitellaria are situated in the anterior half of the body and consist each of about seven large follicles. The very small eggs measure 19–21 by 9–11 μ.

Life-cycle. The first intermediate hosts are probably snails. Metacercariae resembling the adults have been found in dragonflies. Only birds which have access to marshy places become infected.

Pathogenicity and clinical signs. The parasites are found mainly around the cloacal opening and, in heavier infections, also along the abdomen and thorax. They are lodged in subcutaneous cysts, 4–6 mm. in diameter. Each cyst has a central opening and contains a pair of the worms, lying with their ventral surfaces apposed. The cysts also contain a black fluid and the eggs, which are discharged through the pore. Heavy infections produce anaemia, emaciation and death.

Treatment. The cysts should be opened and the worms extracted, followed by suitable treatment of the wound.

Prophylaxis. The birds are to be kept from marshy places where they become infected.

Genus: Troglotrema Odhner, 1914

T. acutum (Leuckart, 1842) occurs in the frontal and ethmoidal sinuses of the fox, mink and polecat in Europe. The parasites are whitish in colour and measure about 3·27 by 2·25 mm. The body is thick and rounded anteriorly and has a narrow, tail-like, posterior extremity. The ventral sucker is located just anterior to the middle and is as large as the oral. The testes are entire or slightly lobed and lie just behind the middle. The genital pore opens immediately behind the ventral sucker. The ovary is spherical and lies to the right of the midline close to the ventral sucker. The eggs measure about 80 by 50 μ.

Life-cycle. Incompletely known, however frogs are suspected to be second intermediate hosts.

Pathogenicity. The parasites may live in pairs in cysts or, particularly in

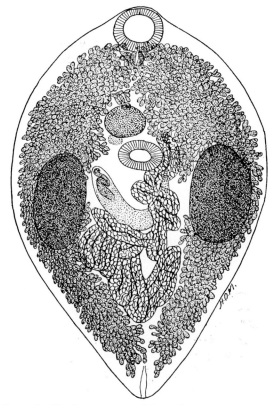

FIG. 26. *Troglotrema acutum*, Ventral View (Original)

the fox, they are found freely attached to the mucosa. In the mink and the polecat the parasites cause decalcification and atrophy of the bony walls of the sinuses and eventually perforation. Cysts may break open to the exterior or into the brain cavity.

Treatment—unknown.

Prophylaxis. The animals should be prevented from eating infected frogs.

Genus: Nanophyetus Chapin, 1927

N. salmincola (Chapin, 1926) (syn. *Troglotrema salmincola*) is a small trematode, 0·5–1·1 mm. long, which occurs in the north-west Pacific area of the United States in the small intestine of the dog, coyote (*Canis lestes*), racoon, mink and lynx (*Lynx fasciatus*), and has been experimentally transmitted to foxes and other Carnivora as well as to guinea-pigs and white rats. Witenberg (1932) considers that *N. schikhobalowi* (Skrjabin & Podjapolska, 1931), which was found in man, is identical with *N. salmincola*. The worms are white or cream in colour. The testes are large, oval and lie ventral and lateral to the posterior ends of the intestinal caeca, behind the middle of the body. There is a large cirrus-sac and the genital pore is situated a short distance behind the ventral sucker. The vitellaria are composed of large follicles and lie mainly laterally and dorsally. The ovary is spherical and situated behind and to the right of the ventral sucker. The eggs measure about 64–80 by 34–50 μ; they are yellowish-brown and have an indistinct operculum.

Life-cycle. The eggs are passed in the faeces of the host and hatch in 3 months or longer, depending on the temperature. The first intermediate hosts are snails of the genus *Goniobasis*. In the Pacific north-west of North America the species *G. plicifera plicifera* and *G. plicifera silicula* are concerned. A redia stage occurs in the life-cycle and the liberated cercariae swim in the water for a while and later penetrate into fish of the salmon family, encysting in the kidneys, muscles and other organs. The salmon *Salmo clarkii, S. irrideus Salvelinus fontinalis* and *Oncorhynchus* spp. are commonly infected. The cysts are 0·17–0·255 mm. in diameter and remain viable in fish stored at temperatures above freezing-point for $3\frac{1}{2}$ months, but are rapidly killed by freezing. Infection of the final host occurs when infected fish is eaten. The parasites grow adult in a short time; dogs pass eggs 5 days after infection.

Pathogenicity. The trematodes penetrate deeply into the mucosa of the duodenum or attach to the mucosa of other parts of the small or large intestine. In large numbers a superficial enteritis is produced and this may lead to a haemorrhagic enteritis. However, the real importance of *N. salmincola* lies in its ability to transmit the agent of 'salmon poisoning', *Neorickettsia helminthoeca*. In addition, a closely related rickettsia, that of 'Elokomin fluke fever', is also transmitted by the parasite.

'Salmon poisoning' frequently produces severe and fatal infections in dogs, foxes and other animals. Following an incubation period of 6–10 days there is a sudden onset of fever and a complete loss of appetite. Within a few days, purulent discharges from the eyes occur, vomiting is marked and there is a profuse diarrhoea, which may be haemorrhagic. Mortality varies from 50 to 90 per cent of infected animals, but recovered animals are immune to reinfection.

Elokomin fluke fever, which is immunologically distinct from salmon poisoning, causes a condition resembling infectious mononucleosis of man with generalised lymphadenopathy and an increase in circulating mononuclear cells.

Metacercariae of *N. salmincola* may remain viable in salmon for at least 5 years and also transmit the rickettsial infections for this period. At one time it was thought that the migration of salmon to the sea resulted in loss of infection, however, it is now known that this is not so and the rickettsia may be obtained from salmon taken in sea water.

Treatment. Since the main disease entity is caused by a rickettsia anthelmintic compounds will be of little avail. Tetracyclene and serum therapy is indicated. Anthelmintic treatment for the flukes alone utilises carbon tetrachloride, extract of male fern and tetrachloroethylene.

Prophylaxis. No infected fish should be fed in a raw or undercooked state. If such fish is accidentally eaten, apomorphine can be given, and it is stated to have prevented the disease when administered as long as 3 hours after infected fish had been eaten.

FAMILY: CYCLOCOELIDAE

These trematodes are medium-sized to large and flattened. The oral sucker is absent and there is usually also no ventral sucker. The mouth is anterior; there is a muscular pharynx and the intestinal caeca are simple or branched and are joined together posteriorly. The genital pore opens a short distance behind the mouth. The copulatory organs are weakly developed. Testes diagonal, entire or lobed. Ovary not lobed and situated between, or anterior to, the testes. The vitellaria occupy the lateral fields, meeting posteriorly like the intestinal caeca. The uterus has numerous transverse coils filling the central field. It contains numerous eggs which develop in the uterus, increasing in size, and the miracidium has characteristic eye-spots. Parasites of aquatic birds, usually in the body cavity, air-sacs or nasal cavity.

Genus: Typhlocoelum Stossich, 1902

T. cymbium (Diesing, 1850) (syn. *Tracheophilus sisowi*) occurs in the trachea and bronchi of domestic and wild ducks. It measures 6–11·5 by about 3 mm. The body is widest at the middle and the ends are rounded. The intestinal ring has short median branches. The testes are not lobed and lie diagonally in the posterior part of the body and the ovary lies at the same level as, or a little in front of, the anterior testis. The eggs measure 122 by 63 μ.

Life-cycle. Szidat (1933) found that the miracidium which hatches from the egg and swims about in the water contains a single redia. When a suitable snail is reached the redia alone enters it, while the miracidium dies off. *Helisoma trivolvis* and species of *Planorbis* are the chief intermediate hosts. There is no sporocyst stage. The redia, which settles down near the albuminous gland of the snail, begins to produce small numbers of cercariae after about 11 days. The cercariae have no tail and can be recognised by the complete intestinal ring; they are provided with a ventral sucker and an anterior boring apparatus. They do not leave the snail, but encyst in it after having escaped from the redia. The birds become infected by ingesting the infected snails. The larval worms probably reach the bronchi via the bloodstream, because they have been found in the lung tissue 4 days after infection. Szidat found the first eggs in the faeces 2–3 months after infection.

Pathogenicity. The parasites cause obstruction of the trachea and the birds may die of asphyxia.

Treatment. None.

Prophylaxis. The birds should be kept away from suspected water and the extermination of snails may be considered.

Two other trematodes which belong to this family and may be harmful are *Typhlocoelum cucumerinum* (Neumann, 1909) (*T. obovale*), which occurs in the trachea, air-sacs and oesophagus of ducks and related wild birds, causing dyspnoea and asphyxia, and *Hyptiasmus tumidus* (Kossack, 1911) (*H. arcuatus*), which is found in the nasal and orbital sinuses of ducks and geese, causing a catarrh.

FAMILY: PARAMPHISTOMATIDAE

These trematodes are usually thick and circular in transverse section. The ventral (posterior) sucker is situated at or close to the posterior extremity and may be very strongly developed. A large ventral pouch may be present. The anterior sucker sometimes has a pair of posterior pockets. A pharynx is absent, but the oesophagus is present and the intestinal caeca are simple. The cuticle is spineless. The genital pore opens ventrally, median, in the anterior third. The testes are frequently lobed and usually anterior to the small ovary. The vitelline glands are lateral and are, as a rule, strongly developed. The uterus runs forwards in the dorsal part of the body and is coiled. Parasites of fishes, amphibia, reptiles, birds and mammals.

A large number of species have been described from the rumen and reticulum of cattle, antelope, buffaloes, sheep and goats and from the colon of equines. The taxonomy of the paramphistomes is complex. It is discussed, with the relevant literature, by Näsmark (1937) and Dawes (1946) and check lists of the paramphistomes which occur in cattle and sheep are given by Soulsby (1965). The various genera of the family are discussed below and these are followed by an account of the life-cycles, pathogenicity etc.

Genus: Paramphistomum Fischoeder, 1901

P. cervi (Schrank, 1790). Substantial confusion exists regarding the true position of *P. cervi*. Dawes (1936) regarded this species synonymous with *P. explanatum* and later he (Dawes, 1946) synonymised several other species with *P. cervi*, these including *P. microbothrium*, *P. liorchis* and *P. ichikawai*.

However, Dawes' opinion has not been generally accepted and various authors regard the above species as valid. To avoid confusion, and without prejudice to the situation, a similar attitude will be adopted here.

The adult form occurs in the rumen and reticulum of sheep, goats and cattle in various parts of the world. It may be cosmopolitan in distribution but there is increasing evidence that a re-evaluation of earlier reports of its existence in some countries is necessary. Thus, in Australia, Durie (1951) found that the species formerly known as *P. cervi* and *Cotylophoron cotylophorum* comprise, in fact, *Calicophoron calicophorum*, *Ceylonocotyle streptocoelium* and *P. ichikawai*. In South Africa Swart (1954) reported *P. explanatum* to be *C. calicophorum*. The colour of live adult specimens is light red. It is one of the 'conical flukes' which are pear-shaped, slightly concave ventrally and convex dorsally, with a large posterior subterminal sucker. The worm measures about 5–13 by 2–5 mm. The genital pore is situated at the end of the anterior third of the body. The testes are slightly lobed and tandem, anterior to the ovary. The vitellaria are in compact groups between the pharynx and the posterior sucker. The eggs measure 114–176 by 73–100 μ.

Other species of the genus *Paramphistomum* include *P. gotoi* Fukui, 1922, of cattle in India and Japan, *P. hiberniae* Willmott, 1950, of cattle in Scotland, Ireland and Holland, *P. ichikawai* Fukui, 1922, of sheep and cattle in Japan and Australia, *P. liorchis* Fischoeder, 1901, of cattle in North America (Florida, Louisiana), *P. microbothrioides* Price & McIntosh, 1944, of cattle in U.S.A., *P. microbothrium* Fischoeder, 1901, of sheep and cattle in Africa, *P. orthocoelium* Fischoeder, 1901, of sheep, cattle and zebu in India and *P. scotiae* Willmott, 1950, of cattle in Scotland and Ireland.

Genus: Cotylophoron Stiles & Goldberger, 1910

C. cotylophorum (Fischoeder, 1901); (Näsmark, 1937) occurs in the rumen and reticulum of the sheep, goat, cattle and many other rumi-

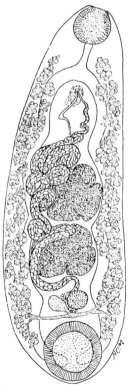

FIG. 27. *Cotylophoran cotylophorum*, Ventral View (Original)

nants. It closely resembles *P. cervi*, but there is a genital sucker surrounding the genital pore. The eggs measure 125–135 by 61–68 μ. Dawes (1936) names this species *Paramphistomum cotylophorum* (Fischoeder, 1901) and regards the whole genus *Cotylophoron* as being synonymous with the genus *Paramphistomum*.

Genus: Calicophoron Näsmark, 1937

C. calicophorum (Fischoeder, 1901; Näsmark, 1937). This species occurs in sheep and cattle in India, Australia, and South Africa. A further species in this genus is *C. ijimai* (Fukui, 1922) of sheep in India, Africa and New Zealand. Eggs of the former measure a mean of 115 μ by 69 μ.

Genus: Ceylonocotyle Näsmark, 1937

C. streptocoelium (Fischoeder, 1901; Näsmark, 1937) (= *Paramphistomum streptocoelium*, Fischoeder, 1901). This species is found in cattle, sheep and antelope in India and Australia. The eggs measure a mean size of 148 μ by 74 μ.

Genus: Gigantocotyle Näsmark, 1937

G. explanatum Näsmark, 1937, occurs in the bile ducts, gall bladder and duodenum of cattle and buffalo in India and Malaya.

Genus: Gastrothylax Poirier, 1883

G. crumenifer (Creplin, 1847) occurs in the rumen of sheep, cattle, zebu and buffalo in India, Ceylon and China. It is red when fresh, elongate, circular in transverse section and measures 9–18 by 5 mm. The worms of this genus differ from all other Digenea in having a very large ventral pouch, opening anteriorly and extending over the whole ventral surface up to the posterior sucker, which is large and terminal and has a raised border. The terminal oval sucker is small. The genital pore opens into the pouch, half-way between the pharynx and the intestinal bifurcation. The intestinal caeca end at about the level of the anterior border of the testes, which are lobed and horizontal, with the ovary behind them. The uterus crosses from right to left at about the middle of the body. The eggs measure 115–135 by 66–70 μ.

Genus: Fischoederius Stiles & Goldberger, 1910

F. elongatus (Poirier, 1883) occurs in the rumen of cattle and other *Bovidae*. It is 10–20 mm. long, and the breadth is about one-quarter of the length. It closely resembles *Gastrothylax*, but one testis lies dorsal to the other and the uterus runs forward in the midline. The intestinal caeca are not widely separated and end a short distance behind the middle of the body. The eggs measure 125–152 by 65–75 μ.

F. cobboldi (Poirier, 1883) differs from the preceding species in being only 8–10 mm. long, while the intestinal caeca end at the posterior border of the posterior testis. This worm occurs in the rumen of cattle, zebu and gayal in India. The eggs measure about 110–120 by 60–75 μ.

Genus: Carmyerius Stiles & Goldberger, 1910

C. spatiosus (Brandes, 1898) occurs in the rumen of cattle, zebu and antelopes in India and Africa and is 9–12 mm. long, It differs from *Fischoederius* in that the testes are horizontal. The posterior sucker is relatively small and spherical. The intestinal caeca reach the end of the second third of the body. The eggs measure 115–125 by 60–65 μ.

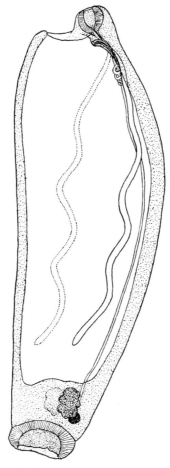

Fig. 28. *Carmyerius spatiosus*, Lateral View (Original)

C. gregarius (Looss, 1896) is found in the buffalo and cattle in India. It is 7–10 mm. long, and the intestinal caeca end a short distance behind the middle of the body.

Genus: Gastrodiscus Leuckart, 1877

G. aegyptiacus (Cobbold, 1876) occurs in the large and small intestines of equines, pig and warthog in Africa and India. It is pink in colour when fresh, and measures 9–17 by 8–11 mm. There is an anterior, more or less cylindrical, part which is up to 4 mm. long and 2·5 mm. wide, while the rest of the body is saucer-shaped, with the margins curved inwards. The ventral surface is covered by a large number of regularly arranged papillae. The posterior sucker is small and subterminal. The oral sucker has two postero-lateral pouches. The intestine branches at the anterior border of the wide portion and the caeca continue to near the hind end of the body. The testes are lobed, slightly diagonal and lie behind the middle with the ovary posterior to them. The vitellaria occupy the lateral fields. The genital pore opens at the level of the intestinal bifurcation. The eggs are oval and measure 131–139 by 78–90 μ.

G. secundus Looss, 1907. This species is found in the colon of the horse in India.

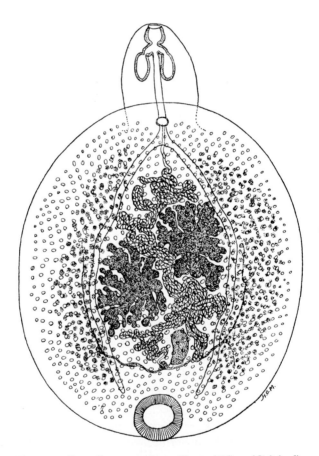

Fig. 29. *Gastrodiscus aeygptiacus*, Ventral View (Original)

Genus: Gastrodiscoides Leiper, 1913

G. hominis (Lewis & McConnell, 1876) Leiper, 1913 (= *Gastrodiscus hominis* (Lewis & McConnell, 1876) (Fischoeder, 1902)). The species occurs in the caecum of man and in the colon of the pig in India. The pig may be a reservoir host for the infection of man.

Genus: Pseudodiscus Sonsino, 1895

P. collinsi (Cobbold, 1875), Stiles and Goldberger, 1910. Varma (1957) found that this species, which occurs in the colon, was the commonest species in horses in India. Other species of the genus occur in the colon of equines.

Life-cycles of Paramphistomes. The life-cycle of the different species is generally similar. The composite eggs are clear (unlike those of *Fasciola* spp.), operculate and in the early stages of segmentation when passed in the faeces. The development time to the miracidium varies with the species (e.g. at 27°C *P. ichikawai* egg hatches in 12 days while that of *C. streptocoelium* takes 17 days to reach this stage).

Liberated miracidia swim in the surrounding water and enter a species of water snail, penetration of the snail occurring by way of the pneumostome and then through the posterior wall of the mantle cavity. However, penetration of the exposed soft parts of the snail may also occur. Young snails are more susceptible than old because the mantle cavity is completely filled with water and the pulmonary aperture permanently open.

Numerous snails have been reported as intermediate hosts, the following list indicates some of them.

Some Snail Hosts of Paramphistomes

  Paramphistomum cervi—*Bulinas liratus, B. mariei, Bulinus* spp., *Glyptanisus gilberti, Indoplanorbis exustus, Lymnaea bilimoides techella, Planorbis planorbis, Pseudosuccinea columella.*
  P. microbothrioides—*Fossaria modicella, F. parva.*
  P. microbothrium—As for *P. cervi* also *B. alluaudi.*
  P. ichikawai—*Segnetilia alphena.*
  Cotylophoron cotylophorum—*B. schakoi, B. verreauxi, F. modicella, F. parva, I. exustus.*
  Calicophoron calicophorum—*B. tropicus, Pygmanisus pelorius.*
  Ceylonocotyle streptocoelium—*Glyptanisus gilberti.*
  Gastrodiscus aegyptiacus—*Cleopatra* spp.

Further development in the snail is similar in all species and that of *Ceylonocotyle streptocoelium* given by Durie (1953) will serve as a typical life-cycle. Following penetration of the mantle cavity the miracidia lose their ciliated covering and by 12 hours an elongate sporocyst (93 μ by 53 μ) is present. Growth during the next few days is marked and by 11 days the sporocysts are mature and contain a maximum of eight rediae each. The rediae are liberated on the tenth to eleventh day of infection and undergo marked growth so that by the twenty-first day of infection they measure 0·5–1 mm. in length and contain fifteen to thirty cercariae. Daughter rediae may be formed under certain circumstances.

Cercariae are released from the rediae in an immature state and they require a period of maturation in the snail tissues before being shed. This is 13 days at 27°C (Durie, 1953). Mature cercariae are dark brown in colour and possess two distinct eye spots. They are shed during the hours of daylight being discharged within 30 minutes when a snail is stimulated by strong light. Liberated cercariae (*Cercariae pigmentata* Sonsino, 1892) are readily recognised as 'amphistome' because of the presence of anterior and posterior suckers. They have a moderately long, simple tail and the pair of eye spots. They are active for several hours but ultimately they encyst on herbage or other objects in the water. Encystment is complete in about 10 minutes and the now metacercaria gradually darkens to an almost black colour. Such stages remain viable for about 3 months.

Infection of the final host is by ingestion of the metacercariae with herbage. Excystation occurs in the intestine where the immature paramphistomes spend the first part of their vertebrate developmental cycle. Here they attach to the mucosa and after 6–8 weeks at this site they migrate forward through the reticulum to the rumen frequently becoming attached along the oesophageal groove. A further few weeks of development are required before maturity is reached. Durie (1953), by experimental infection, reported the prepatent periods of *Ceylonocotyle streptocoelium*, *Calicophoron calicophorum* and *Paramphistomum ichikawai* in sheep to be 48 days, 49–51 days and 80–95 days respectively.

Pathogenicity of paramphistomes. The adult forms in the forestomach are essentially nonpathogenic even though large numbers may be present. At the most there may be a localized loss of rumen papillae. In the case of *Gigantocotyle explanatum* in the bile ducts and gall bladder there may be a series of superficial haemorrhages indicating the sites of attachment but generally there is no severe pathogenic effect. In very heavy infections the liver may be pale and show a degree of fibrosis.

The immature stages of the paramphistomes in the duodenum and upper ileum are responsible for severe pathological changes. These are embedded in the mucosa and by drawing pieces of the mucosa into the suckers pinch them off causing necrosis and haemorrhage. In heavy infections a frank, haemorrhagic, duodenitis may be produced with immature flukes deeply embedded in the mucosa, sometimes reaching the muscular coat. Histologically there is extensive catarrhal and haemorrhagic inflammation of the duodenum and jejunum with destruction of the intestinal glands, degeneration of the associated lymph nodes and other organs. Associated with these lesions is an anaemia, a hypoproteinaemia, oedema and emaciation.

Clinical signs consist of profuse fluid diarrhoea, marked weakness and frequently death.

In some areas, e.g. India, South Africa, Australia, mortality may reach 80–90 per cent and extensive reports have recorded mortalities of 30–40 per cent in cattle and sheep (see reviews by Boray, 1959; Soulsby, 1965).

Diagnosis. This is based on clinical signs, the history of the area and the presence of immature paramphistomes in the fluid faeces. In some circumstances the presence of large number of paramphistome eggs in the faeces is also indicative of the disease since although the pathogenic effects are caused by the immature forms a large number of adult forms may also accompany the immature burden. At *post mortem* a marked enteritis is evident and large numbers of parasites are found in association. Clinical cases may reveal up to 30,000 immature paramphistomes.

Treatment. Numerous compounds have been tried for amphistomiasis of cattle and sheep with little success. Successful treatment has been reported with a hexachloroethane–bentonite suspension for cattle (Olsen, 1949) at a total dose of 180 g. (though other workers have failed to demonstrate its efficacy). Guilhon & Graber (1962) found that Bithionol at doses of 25–35 mg. per kg. completely removed amphistomes from cattle, Bosman *et al.* (1961) reported that a dose of 10 mg. and over per kg. of hexachlorophene to cattle and sheep removed *Paramphistomum* spp. and Horak (1962) found with *P. microbothrium* that a dose of 50 mg. per kg. to sheep of Yomesan (5-chloro-N(2-chloro-4-nitrophenyl)sali-cylamide) was 94–99 per cent effective against the small intestinal stages but even a dose of 75 mg. per kg. was only 15.9 per cent effective against the stages in the forestomachs. In a single dose of 200 mg. per kg. methyridine [2(β methoxyethyl) pyridine] was 45 per cent efficient but when given in multiple doses more than 99 per cent efficacy was reported.

Control. Since the vectors are water snails, sheep and cattle should be grazed on higher ground, the localised area of water fenced off or treated with molluscicides. Drainage of pools and swamps is a more permanent control measure.

FAMILY: STRIGEIDAE

These worms are characterised by a constriction which divides the body into an anterior, flattened or cup-shaped portion, which is an adhesive organ, and a posterior, cylindrical part. The latter contains the gonads. The ventral sucker may be poorly developed or absent, and behind it there is usually a special adhesive organ. The genital pore opens posteriorly in a depression or 'bursa copulatrix'. The testes lie tandem, with the ovary anterior to them. Cirrus-sac and pouch are usually absent. The uterus contains relatively few large eggs. The vitellaria are well developed, either in both parts of the body or only in its posterior part. Parasites in the alimentary canal, chiefly of birds. The cercariae are furcocercous, provided with a pharynx, and develop in snails from sporocysts. They enter a second intermediate host, which may be a fish, snail, leech etc.

Genus: Apatemon Szidat, 1929

A. gracilis (Rudolphi, 1819) occurs in the intestine of the pigeon, duck and wild duck in Europe. It is 1·5–2·5 mm. long by 0·4 mm. and is concave dorsally. The anterior cup-shaped part forms about one-third of the total length. It contains an adhesive organ. The cirrus and cirrus-sac are absent. The 'bursa' contains at its base a weak copulatory organ or genital cone. The vitellaria are restricted to the posterior part of the body. The eggs measure 100–110 by 75 μ.

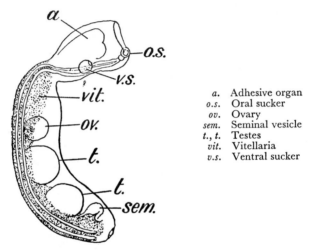

a.	Adhesive organ
o.s.	Oral sucker
ov.	Ovary
sem.	Seminal vesicle
t., t.	Testes
vit.	Vitellaria
v.s.	Ventral sucker

Fig. 30. *Apatemon gracilis*, Lateral View (from Baylis, after Brandes)

Life-cycle. The eggs are passed in the faeces of the host and the miracidium hatches under favourable conditions in about 3 weeks. After entering a suitable snail the sporocyst develops. It is very slender and about 20 mm. long. The cercariae are formed directly by the sporocysts. The secondary intermediate hosts are the leeches *Haemopis sanguisuga* and *Herpobdella atomaria*.

Genus: Parastrigea Szidat, 1928

P. robusta Szidat, 1929, occurs in the intestine of the domestic duck in Europe. It is 2–2·5 mm. long and resembles the previous species, but the anterior portion has two large, lateral expansions and a narrow opening, while the vitelline glands are mainly situated in the lateral expansions and the adhesive organ, but also partly in the posterior part of the body. The eggs measure 90–100 by 50 μ.

Life-cycle—unknown.

A number of other species are also known, especially from ducks.

Pathogenesis. The parasites attach themselves to the mucosa of the intestine by means of the anterior cup-shaped part of the body, into which they draw a number of villi, constricting them strongly at their bases. The blood vessels in the villi become markedly hyperaemic and burst, discharging the blood into the cavity, from which it is ingested by the worm. The constricted villi then degenerate and are apparently digested by the secretion of a gland in the adhesive organ. Heavy infections are associated with anaemia, a haemorrhagic enteritis and even death.

Diagnosis is made by finding the eggs in the faeces or the worms at autopsy.

Treatment. Carbon tetrachloride is indicated in doses of 1–2 ml.

Genus: Cotylurus Szidat, 1928

C. cornutus (Rud, 1809) occurs in the small intestine of the pigeon and the duck in Europe. It is only 1·2–1·5 mm. long and 0·5 mm. thick. In its morphology it resembles *Apatemon gracilis*, but the bursa contains a strong copulatory organ. The eggs measure 90–110 by 56–60 μ.

Life-cycle. The miracidia hatch in 6–8 days and penetrate into snails, *Lymnaea stagnalis* and *L. palustris*, in which cercariae develop out of the sporocysts. The cercariae are furcocercous and have a pharynx. They emerge from the first intermediate host and penetrate into other snails of the same species or other species of the genera *Lymnaea* or *Planorbis*. Pigeons become infected by ingesting infected snails. Even nestling pigeons are infected through their parents' feeding them out of their crops.

C. platycephalus (Creplin, 1825) is similar to *C. cornutus* having been found in gulls and razorbills in Europe and *C. flabelliformis* (Faust, 1925) is a North American form occuring in domestic and wild duck. The latter is a minute form, 0·56–0·85 mm. long, the two portions of the body are quite distinct and the eggs are large 100–112 μ by 68–76 μ. First intermediate hosts are snails of the genus *Lymnaea* and cercariae encyst in various *Planorbis* spp.

Pathogenesis. *Cotylurus* spp. may cause a haemorrhagic enteritis, such having been recorded in razorbills due to *C. platycephalus* (Lowe & Baylis, 1934).

FAMILY: DIPLOSTOMATIDAE

These trematodes are similar to the Strigeidae, however the anterior part of the body is more flattened and frequently ear-like processes are present on the antero-lateral parts of the forebody. The posterior part of the body is cylindrical. Parasites of birds and mammals.

Genus: Diplostomum Nordmann, 1832

D. spathaceum (Rudolphi, 1819) Olsson, 1876. This form is found in the intestine of a wide variety of gulls in Europe. The total length is

2–4 mm. The anterior region is shorter and broader than the posterior, the suckers are small and the ventral sucker is incorporated into an accessory adhesive organ which occupies about one-third of the breadth of the anterior part. The vitellaria occupy most of the posterior region and extend forward on each side of the adhesive organ. Eggs are large, 100 μ by 60 μ.

The first intermediate hosts are snails of the genus *Lymnaea* and meta-cercariae are found in a number of fresh water fish.

A heavy mortality in Black-headed gull chicks due to massive infec-tions of *D. spathaceum* has been recorded by Jennings & Soulsby (1958).

Genus: Alaria Schrank, 1788

A. alata (Goeze, 1782) Hall & Wigdor, 1918. This species is found in the intestine of dog, cat, fox and also mink in Europe, Australia and U.S.A.

It is 2–6 mm. in length and the flat expanded anterior part is much longer than the posterior cylindrical part. At the anterior lateral corners of the anterior part there are two tentacle-like processes. The suckers are very small and the adhesive organ consists of two long folds with distinct lateral margins. The vitellaria are in the anterior part of the body while the gonads are in the posterior part. The eggs measure 98–134 μ by 62–68 μ.

Life-cycle. Miracidia hatch from the eggs and swim in water, entering fresh water snails such as *Planorbis vortex* and *P. planorbis*. Sporocysts produce cercariae with bifurcated tails. Further development of *A. alata* is unknown but with other species of the genus (e.g. *A. mustelae* and *A. intermedia* in U.S.A.) cercariae encyst in the muscles of frogs. The final host may be infected by eating infected frogs but a further intermediate host (or rather paratenic host) may occur in the life cycle, in the form of a small rodent (rats, mice etc.) which may eat the infected frog and meta-cercariae are found in the rodent. Dogs, foxes etc. may then be infected by eating the rodent (Cuckler, 1940). Mature flukes are produced 10 days after infection.

Pathogenicity. A catarrhal duodenitis has been ascribed to the presence of this parasite (Erlich, 1938).

Other species of the genus include *A. canis* La Rue & Fallis, 1934 of dogs, *A. americana* Hall & Wigdor, 1918 of dog, cat and fox, *A. michiganensis* Hall & Wigdor, 1918 of dog and *A. mustelae* Bosma, 1931 of dog and cat, all of which are found in North America.

FAMILY: SCHISTOSOMATIDAE

These are elongate, unisexual and dimorphic trematodes, which in-habit the blood-vessels of their hosts. The female is slender and usually longer than the male, and the female of some species is usually carried, especially during copulation, by the latter in a ventral, gutter-like groove, the gynaecophoric canal, formed by the incurved lateral edges of the body. The suckers are weak and close together or absent. There is no pharynx and the intestinal branches usually unite posteriorly to form a single tube which extends to the hind end. The genital pore lies behind the ventral sucker. The testes form four or more lobes, situated anteriorly or posteriorly. The ovary is an elongate, compact organ, lying in front of the posterior union of the intestinal branches. The vitelline gland occupies the part of the body behind the ovary. The eggs are thin-shelled and have no operculum and those of some species have a lateral or terminal spine. They are laid by the females in the small blood vessels of the intestinal wall or the urinary bladder and pass through the tissues, leaving the host with the faeces or urine. The cercariae are furcocercous, without a pharynx, and develop from sporocysts without a redia stage. They enter the host through its skin and do not encyst.

Genus: Schistosoma Weinland, 1858

S. japonicum (Katsurada, 1904) occurs in the portal and mesenteric vessels of man as well as cattle, horse, sheep, goat, dog, cat, rabbit and pig in the Far East. The male is 9·5–20 mm. long and 0·55–0·967 mm. wide. The female is 12–26 mm. long and about 0·3 mm. thick. The suckers lie close together near the anterior end. The cuticle is spiny on the suckers and in the gynaecophoric canal. In both sexes the oesophagus is surrounded by a group of glands and the intestine bifurcates before reaching the level of the ventral sucker, again uniting in the last quarter of the body. The testes consist of six to eight lobes in a longitudinal row, lying behind the genital pore, which opens directly posterior to the ventral sucker. The ovary lies behind the middle and the vitelline gland fills the posterior quarter. The oötype is situated directly anterior to the middle, opening into the long, unfolded uterus, which extends forwards to the genital pore. The eggs are passed in the faeces of the host and measure 70–100 by 50–80 μ. They are short, oval, and may have a small lateral spine or knob.

Life-cycle. The ovigerous female penetrates deeply into the small vessels of the mucosa or sub-mucosa of the intestine, laying the eggs in the capillaries. Some eggs may be carried away by the bloodstream and are then found in the liver and other organs. They are, however, normally passed into the intestinal lumen and out in the faeces. When laid, the eggs are immature and continue their development as they pass out. The intermediate snail hosts are *Oncomelania nosophora* in Japan and the southern coast of China, *O. formosana* in Formosa, *O. hupensis* in south and southeastern China and *O. quadrasi* in the Philippines. There are two generations of sporocysts, the second forming the cercariae. The latter swarm out of the snail and swim about in the water. Infection takes place when the final host comes in contact with infected water; the cercariae penetrate through the skin, being assisted by the secretion of the cephalic salivary glands which digest the tissues. In this way they reach the blood and are transported via the lungs to the systemic circulation.

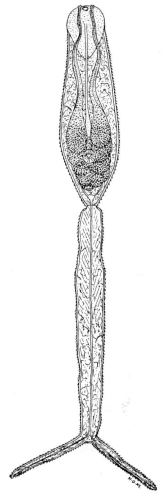

Fig. 31. Cercaria of *Schistosoma bovis* (after Mönnig)

Those that reach the abdominal vessels and pass to the portal veins develop further and become mature in about 4 weeks. The others will reach other organs in which they may produce lesions, but they eventually die and do not reach the adult stage.

Pathogenesis. The penetration of the cercariae through the skin causes a dermatitis which is most evident 24–26 hours after infection. The passage through the lungs may cause pneumonia in gross infections but usually there is a non-clinical accumulation of eosinophils and epithelioid cells. The abdominal organs, like the liver, may become congested during the early stages of the disease due to the arrival of immature worms in the intra-hepatic portal blood-vessels. The most serious damage is caused by the adult parasites in the egg-laying stage, due to the irritation caused by the eggs in the intestinal wall and in other organs which they may reach accidentally. The masses of eggs become surrounded by inflamed areas and an infiltration of leucocytes, especially eosinophils, giving rise to a rather characteristic type of abscess. The abscesses in the intestinal wall usually burst, discharging their contents into the lumen of the gut, and this is followed by healing through the formation of scar tissue. The main clinical signs resulting from these pathological changes is diarrhoea with the eggs of the parasites in the faeces, frequently accompanied by mucus and blood.

In the liver the abscesses become encapsulated and will finally calcify, a large number of such foci leading to enlargement of the organ, marked cirrhosis and ascites. The spleen and mesenteric lymph glands are usually also affected, becoming congested and showing an increase of fibrous tissue.

Post Mortem. Anaemia and emaciation are marked. Ascites is usually present. The intestinal wall is much thickened, showing the presence of scar tissue and frequently papillomatous growths of the mucosa. Cirrhosis of the liver is a conspicuous lesion and the walls of the portal veins are thickened. The mesentery, the mesenteric lymph glands and the spleen are frequently altered on account of the presence of an abnormal amount of connective tissue. Pigment is seen especially in the liver and spleen. A search should be made for the parasites while the intestine is still attached to the mesentery, as they are not easily found after exenteration of the organ.

Diagnosis. The clinical signs alone will not suffice to arrive at a definite diagnosis, but they should indicate the necessity of faeces examination, which will reveal the eggs of the parasites.

Prophylaxis. Control of the snail intermediate hosts is difficult. The methods used to prevent human infection and to control the snails with molluscicides are described in publications of the W.H.O. (see W.H.O. Chronicle, 1959). A list of molluscicides, with their indications, is given by Faust & Russel (1964). Human excreta should be properly treated before being used as fertiliser. Night-soil should be allowed to ferment, in order to kill the eggs, before it is spread on the fields. Human infection may come from snails infected with miracidia derived from eggs passed out by domesticated and wild animals, so that prophylaxis should attempt to control these sources of human infection by suitable management and treatment of these reservoir hosts, so far as this is possible. In a study of the relative importance of animals as reservoirs of infection for humans Pesigan et al. (1958) concluded that the dog and cow populations presented a serious source of infection whereas other animals such as goat, dog and buffalo played a comparatively minor role.

S. bovis (Sonsino, 1876) occurs in the portal and mesenteric vessels of cattle, sheep, goats, the sitatunga (*Limnotragus spekei*) and more rarely equines in Southern Europe (Sardinia), Southern Asia and Africa. Blackie (1933) records this parasite also from the baboon (*Papio porcarius*) in Southern Rhodesia, and he was able to infect the grey monkey (*Cercopithecus pygerythrus*). MacHattie *et al.* (1933), concluded that this parasite does not occur in man and that reported cases were infected with *S. haematobium*, a human parasite. Nelson (1959) concluded that infections of man by the schistosomes of domestic and wild herbivors of Africa are zoonoses of little clinical significance.

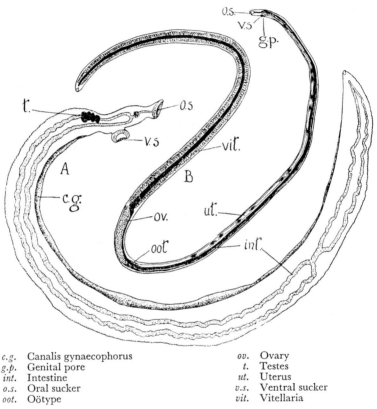

c.g.	Canalis gynaecophorus	*ov.*	Ovary
g.p.	Genital pore	*t.*	Testes
int.	Intestine	*ut.*	Uterus
o.s.	Oral sucker	*v.s.*	Ventral sucker
oot.	Oötype	*vit.*	Vitellaria

Fig. 32. *Schistosoma bovis*. A, male; B, female (Original)

The males of *S. bovis* are 9–22 mm. long and 1–2 mm. wide, depending on the degree of folding of the lateral edges. The female is 12–28 mm. long. The suckers and the body of the male behind the suckers are armed with minute spines, while the dorsal surface of the male bears small cuticular tubercles. The intestine bifurcates at the level of the ventral sucker and reunites in the female just behind the middle of the body, or sometimes farther back, being continued as a single caecum. In the male the caeca may reunite far back or not at all, or there may be several junctions between them and two posterior caeca. The male has three to six testes in a longitudinal row, situated a short distance behind the ventral sucker. The ovary is about 1 mm. long and lies at the middle of the body behind Mehlis's gland. The uterus runs forwards from this point and may contain a large number of eggs. The vitelline gland occupies as a rule the posterior half of the body behind the ovary, but in some females it may fill only the posterior quarter. The eggs are usually spindle-shaped, but small ones are frequently oval, and when passed in the faeces measure on the average 187 by 60 μ; the limits given by various authors are 132–247 μ by 38–60 μ.

Life-cycle. The known intermediate hosts are *Bulinus contortus*, *B. truncatus*, *Physopsis africana*, *P. globosa* and, in Kenya, *P. nasuta*. For a more complete account of the snail hosts and the geographical distribution of this species Malek (1961) should be consulted. Cercariae develop from daughter sporocysts which replace the redia stage. The cercaria is of the furcocercous type without a pharynx, and is armed with spines. It has four pairs of cephalic glands, two acidophil and two basophil. Infection of the host may take place through the skin, but in the case of sheep the cercariae are probably swallowed with water.

Pathogenesis. On the whole, the effects of this species resemble those of *S. japonicum*, but in the ox the worms may enter the vesical veins, and they may then cause haematuria. Haematuria has been ascribed to this parasite in the Congo (Wery, 1950). The young parasites cause some damage during migration, but most of the lesions are due to irritation produced by the eggs of the parasites in the intestine and other organs and the blood-sucking habits of the worms. According to Le Roux (1929), the eggs in the intestinal wall are surrounded by leucocytes, but neither erosions nor necrosis of the mucosa are seen nor has he found any papillomatous growths of the mucosa, as described by other authors. The affected animals become anaemic, lose condition and show alternate diarrhoea and constipation, gradually wasting away until death takes place. The faeces contain blood and mucus and the eggs can be found in them in large numbers.

Post Mortem. Anaemia and emaciation are present and there may be ascites and hydropericard. A characteristic feature is the marked grey pigmentation of the lungs and liver. The parasites in the mesenteric veins should be searched for before the intestine is exenterated. The liver may be larger or smaller than normal, depending on the stage of the disease, and is markedly cirrhotic in older cases, the surface being conspicuously uneven. On microscopical examination there is pigment in the liver and numerous eggs may be found, surrounded by cellular infiltration and fibrous tissue. The intestine shows the presence of eggs in its wall in the form of grey clusters or thickenings which are opaque and grating to the knife. The mucosa usually shows small haemorrhages and the submucosa may be thickened. The spleen may be slightly swollen and pigmented and the pancreas and lymph glands are usually pigmented.

S. mattheei (Veglia & Le Roux, 1929). This species was formerly regarded as being synonymous with *S. bovis*, but it is now known that it is a distinct species. It is differentiated from *S. bovis* on morphological and pathological grounds (see Soulsby, 1965). The eggs in the faeces are 170–280 μ by 72–84 μ and *S. mattheei* is restricted to the alimentary canal whereas *S. bovis* may occur in the urogenital system.

The intermediate host is *Physopsis globosa* which occurs in still or slowly running muddy water with abundant vegetation, snails being most abundant on the under surface of water plants.

The pathogenesis of *S. mattheei* is detailed by Le Roux (1929) who describes excessive fibrosis and pigmentation of the liver and pseudo-tubercle formation with pigmentation of the lungs.

Human infection with this parasite in South Africa and East Africa has been reported by Pitchford (1959).

S. mansoni (Sambon, 1907). This species is found in man throughout tropical Africa and was imported in African slaves to Brazil, Venezuela and the West Indies. Nelson (1961) found it in the baboon in Kenya and states that pigs are also susceptible to it, although natural infections of pigs have not yet been found.

S. rodhaini Brumpt, 1931. This species occurs chiefly in rodents, but Deramée *et al.* (1953) showed that dogs and cats are susceptible to infection with it and Nelson (1961) states that it causes serious disease in dogs in Ruanda-Urundi.

S. spindale Montgomery, 1906 (syn. *S. spindalis*), occurs in the mesenteric veins of cattle, goats, sheep, dog, and zebu (*Bos bubalis*) in India and Sumatra. It does not occur in Africa. The male is 5·6–13·5 mm. long and the female 7·18–16·2 mm. There are three to seven testes. The eggs measure 160–400 by 70–90 μ and are elongate, flattened on one side and have a terminal spine. They are usually passed in the faeces, but sometimes also in the urine. The intermediate hosts are snails of the genus *Planorbis, Indoplanorbis exustus, Lymnaea acuminata* and *L. luteola*.

S. nasalis Rao, 1932, closely resembles *S. spindale*. It causes nasal granuloma ('snoring disease') of cattle, goats and horses in India. The male is 6·3–11 mm. long, coarsely tuberculate, and has two to six testes. The female is 5–11 mm long. The eggs are boomerang-shaped, 336–581 by 50–80 μ. Intermediate hosts are *Lymnaea luteola, L. acuminata* and *Indoplanorbis exustus*. The parasites develop in the veins of the nasal mucosa, causing a marked rhinitis with a muco-purulent discharge. The mucosa is studded with small abscesses which contain the eggs of the worms, and later shows much fibrous tissue and proliferating epithelium. Clinical signs of coryza with sneezing are succeeded by dyspnoea and snoring. Good results have been obtained from injections of Antimosan and tartar emetic.

S. indicum Montgomery, 1906, occurs in the portal, pancreatic, pelvic, hepatic and mesenteric veins of sheep, goats, cattle, equines and camels in India. The male is 5–19 mm. long and the female 6–22 mm. There are five to twelve testes. The eggs are oval with a terminal spine and measure 57–140 by 18–72 μ. They are passed in the faeces of the host. The intermediate host is the snail *Indoplanorbis exustus*. The eggs cause nodules in various organs and cirrhosis of the liver with debility, especially in horses. A re-evaluation of this species is given by Srivastava & Dutt (1962).

S. suis Rao & Ayyar, 1933, occurs in the pig and the dog in India. It may be identical with *S. incognitum* of Chandler, 1926. The egg is yellowish-brown, suboval with one side flattened, with a small, stout spine inclining towards the flattened side. In the uterus it measures about 90 by 41 μ.

Treatment of Schistosomiasis. A detailed account is given by the World Health Organization (1966) of the present status of therapy of schistosomiasis, with particular reference to the important human species, *S. mansoni*, *S. haematobium* and *S. japonicum*. This publication should be consulted also for the many factors which should be taken into account during therapy.

Generally the therapy of animal schistosomiasis has followed that for the human infections. Tartar emetic has been used extensively for nasal schistosomiasis (*S. nasalis*) but the danger of toxicity is great and the dose should not exceed 2 mg. per kg. Naik (1942) recommends this treatment be given daily for 6 days. Using sodium antimony tartrate Alwar (1962) found that a dose of 1·5 mg. per kg. in 10 per cent glucose, three times daily for two consecutive days cured eleven of twelve animals with nasal schistosomiasis and in further studies a dose of 2 mg. per kg. twice daily for 2 days was similarly effective. Studies by Rao *et al.* (1962) with Trichlorphon (*O,O,*-dimethyl-2,2,2-trichloro-1-hydroxymethyl phosphonate) indicated that good clinical improvement could be obtained with a dose of 30–40 mg. per kg. given three times.

Antimosan has been used for nasal schistosomiasis in cattle, Biswal & Das (1956) reporting it to be useful in the buffalo when six daily injections of 1·7 mg. per kg. were given.

Genus: Ornithobilharzia Ohdner, 1912

In species of this genus, the intestinal caeca tend to anastomose in front of the median posterior intestinal caecum and the ovary forms a spiral in the anterior region of the body, the testes being very numerous and the uterus short, containing only one egg at a time.

Ornithobilharzia bomfordi (Montgomery, 1906) occurs in the mesenteric veins of the zebu (*Bos bubalis*) in India. The male is 6–9 mm. long and the female 3–7·3 mm. The male has about sixty testes and the female has a long posterior caecum. The eggs are oval with a posterior spine and measure 100–136 by 44–60 μ. They are found in the faeces of the host.

O. turkestanicum (Skrjabin, 1913) (syn. *O. turkestanica*) occurs in the mesenteric veins of sheep, goat, camel, horse, donkey, mule, water buffalo, cattle and the cat in Russian Turkestan, Kazakstan, Mongolia, Iraq and France. It is a small species, the male being 4·2–8 mm. long and the female 3·4–8 mm. There are seventy to eighty testes and the ovary is spirally coiled. The intestinal caecum of the female is about three times as long as the divided portion. The uterus contains one egg at a time. The eggs measure 72–77 by 18–26 μ. They have a terminal spine and a short appendage at the other end. It is of little significance in large animals, but leads to permanent debility in sheep and goats, causing marked liver cirrhosis and nodules in the intestines. The intermediate host is the snail *Lymnaea tenera euphratica*.

Genus: Bilharziella Looss, 1899

B. polonica (Kowalewski, 1896) occurs in the mesenteric and pelvic veins of wild and domestic ducks in Europe and North America. The body is flattened in both sexes and usually lancet-shaped in the posterior half, the gynaecophoric canal being rudimentary. The male is about 4 mm. long and 0·52 mm. wide, and the female is 2·1 mm. long and 0·25 mm. wide. The intestinal branches reunite near the middle of the body, forming a caecum which runs a zigzag course to the posterior extremity. The male genital pore opens to the left of the mid-line, near the middle of the body. The testes are very numerous; one lies anterior to the reunion of the intestinal branches and the rest are arranged in a row on either side of the caecum. The median female genital pore is just behind the ventral sucker. The folded, elongate ovary lies in front of the posterior union of the intestinal caeca. The short uterus contains one egg at a time. The eggs have a long, narrow, anterior elongation and are swollen posteriorly with a terminal spine; they measure 0·4 by 0·1 mm.

Life-cycle. The eggs are laid in the small vessels of the intestinal wall with the narrow part directed towards the lumen of the gut. They gradually penetrate through the wall and are passed out in the faeces. Such eggs are still in the early stages of development. The intermediate host is the snail *Planorbis (Coretus) corneus*, according to Szidat (1929). The cercariae are of the usual type and have a pair of pigmented eye-spots. There are three pairs of basophil and three pairs of acidophil cephalic glands. Infection takes place through the mouth and skin.

Pathogenicity. The eggs have been found in the wall of the intestine, where they may occasionally produce inflammatory processes with infiltration of leucocytes and connective tissue proliferation. Eggs may get into the pancreas, spleen and kidneys, but in these organs they die. The parasite is apparently not very pathogenic.

Schistosome dermatitis. The condition is variously known as 'swimmer's itch', 'clam digger's itch', 'cercarial dermatitis', 'Gulf coast itch', 'sea bather's eruption', 'lakeside disease' (Japan), 'Badedermatitis' (Germany), and 'gale des nageurs' (France). It is caused by the penetration of cercariae of non-human schistosomes into the skin of man producing, on first exposure, a mild erythema and oedema, but on repeated exposure a marked reaction with pruritis, vesicle formation and marked papule formation.

A number of species of schistosomes have been incriminated. Thus *Trichobilharzia ocellata,* which occurs in wild water fowl, was demonstrated by Cort (1928) to cause the condition and since then *T. stagnicolae* and *T. physellae* have been shown to be responsible in the Great Lakes region of North America and *Austrobilharzia variglandis* of ducks and terns causes the condition in Florida and Hawaii. Schistosomes of animals may be responsible in some cases and Malek (1961) has suggested the cercariae of *Heterobilharzia americana* (a parasite of racoon, nutria and dog in Louisiana) as a possible cause of 'water dermatitis' in that area. Buckley (1938) has indicated that the cercariae of *S. spindale* of the water buffalo may be the cause of 'rice paddy itch' in Malaysia.

The condition has been studied extensively on an experimental basis (see Batten, 1956).

REFERENCES

TREMATODA, GENERAL

BJÖRKMAN, N. & THORSELL, W. (1964). On the fine structure and resorptive function of the cuticle of the liver fluke *Fasciola hepatica* L. *Exp. Cell Res.*, **33**, 319–329
DAWES, B. (1946). *The Trematoda—with Special Reference to British and Other European Forms.* Cambridge University Press
KAGAN, I. G. (1966). Mechanisms of immunity in trematode infection. In *The Biology of Parasites* (Ed. by E. J. L. Soulsby) pp. 227–299 New York: Academic Press
READ, C. P. (1966). Nutrition of intestinal helminths. In *The Biology of Parasites* (Ed. by E. J. L. Soulsby) pp. 101–126 New York: Academic Press
SILVERMAN, P. H. (1965). *In vitro* cultivation procedures for parasitic helminths. In *Advances in Parasitology* (Ed. by B. Dawes) Vol. **3**, pp. 159–222 London: Academic Press
SMYTH, J. D. & CLEGG, J. A. (1959). Egg-shell formation in Trematodes and Cestodes. *Expl. Parasit.*, **8**, 286–323
THORSELL, W. & BJÖRKMAN, N. (1965). Morphological and biochemical studies on absorption and secretion of the alimentary tract of *Fasciola hepatica* L. *J. Parasit.*, **51**, 217–223

DICRODOELIIDAE, OPISTHORCHIIDAE

BASCH, P. F. (1966). Patterns of transmission of the trematode *Eurytrema pancreatum* in Malaysia. *Am. J. vet. Res.*, **27**, 234–240
DENTON, J. F. (1944). Studies on the life history of *Eurytrema procyonis* Denton, 1942. *J. Parasit.* **30**, 277–286
ENIGK, K. & DÜWELL, D. (1963). Die Wirksamkeit von Hetolin auf den Dicrocoelium-Befall in Schaf, Rind und Pferd. *Dt. tierärztl. Wschr.*, **70**, 377–381
ERHARDT, A. (1932). Chemotherapeutische Untersuchungen an der Opisthorchiasis der Katzen. *Arch. Schiffs u. Tropenhyg.*, **36**, 22–31
HOHORST, W. & GRAEFE, G. (1961). Ameisen-obligatorische Zwischenwirte des Lanzettegels (*Dicrocoelium dendriticum*). *Naturwissenschaften*, **48**, 229
KRULL, W. H. (1958). The migratory route of the metacercaria of *Dicocoelium dendriticum* (Rudolphi, 1819) Looss, 1899 (Dicrocoeliidae) in the definite host. *Cornell Vet.*, **48**, 17–24
KRULL, W. H. & MAPES, C. R. (1953). Studies on the biology of *Dicrocoelium dendriticum* (Rudolphi, 1819) Looss, 1899 (Trematoda; Dicrocoeliidae) including its relation to the intermediate host, *Cionella lubrica* (Müller). IX. Notes on the cyst, metacercaria, and infection in the ant *Formica fusca. Cornell Vet.*, **43**, 389–410

LÄMMLER, G. (1963). Die Experimentalchemotherapie der Dicrocoeliose mit Hetolin. *Dt.*
tierärztl. Wschr., **70**, 373–377
LEAM, G. & WALKER, I. E. (1963). The occurrence of *Platynosomum fastosum* in domestic cats in
the Bahamas. *Vet. Rec.*, **75**, 46–47
LIENERT, E. (1962). Hexachlorophene (G-11) is extremely efficient in cats and dogs naturally
infected with the liver fluke *Opisthorchis tenuicollis* (Rudolphi, 1819) Stiles and Hassal, 1896.
Wien. tierärztl. Mschr., **49**, 353–359
MALDONADO, J. F. (1945). The life history and biology of *Platynosomum fastosum* Kossak, 1910
(Trematoda; Dicrocoeliidae). *Puerto Rico J. publ. Hlth trop. Med.*, **21**, 17–60
PHILLIPSON, R. F. & McFADZEAN, J. A. (1962). Clonorchis, Opisthorchis and Paragonimus
gel diffusion studies. *Trans. R. Soc. trop. Med. Hyg.*, **56**, 13
SADUN, E. H., WALTON, B. C., BUCK, A. A. & LEE, B. K. (1959). The use of purified antigens in
the diagnosis of *Clonorchis sinensis* by means of intradermal and complement fixation test.
J. Parasit., **45**, 129–134
SAWADA, T., NAGATA, Y., TAKEI, K. & SATO, S. (1964). Studies on the substance responsible
for the skin tests on clonorchiasis. *Jap. J. exp. Med.*, **34**, 315–322
SCHUURMANS-STEKHOVEN, J. H. (1931). Der zweite Zwischenwirt von *Pseudamphistomum truncat-*
um (Rud.) nebst Beobachtung über andere Trematodenlarven. *Z. Parasitenk.*, **3**, 747–764
SHELDON, W. G. (1966). Pancreatic flukes (*Eurytrema procyonis*) in domestic cats. *J. Am. vet. med.*
Ass., **148**, 251–253
ŠIBALIĆ, S., MLADENOVIĆ, Ž. & SLAVICA, M. (1963). Delovanje Thiabendazole—A na *Dicro-*
coelium dendriticum u Ovaca. *Vet. Glasn.*, **17**, 1041–1046
SOULSBY, E. J. L. (1965). *Textbook of Veterinary Clinical Parasitology*, Vol. I. Oxford: Blackwell
Scientific Publication
STOLL, N. R. (1947). This wormy world. *J. Parasit.*, **33**, 1–18
SVADZHIAN, P. K. (1954). On the determination of the intermediate host of *Dicrocoelium lanceatum*
(Stiles and Hassall, 1895) under Armenian conditions. *Dokl. Akad. Nauk armjan. S.S.S.R.*
19, 153–156
TANG, C. C. (1950). Studies on the life history of *Eurytrema pancreaticum* Janson, 1889. *J. Parasit.*,
36, 559–573
TUBANGUI, M. A. (1925). Metazoan parasites of Philippine domesticated animals. *Philipp.*
J. Sci., **28**, 11–37
VOGEL, H. (1932). Ueber den ersten Zwischenwirt und die Zerkarie von *Opisthorchis felineus*
Riv. *Arch. Schiffs u. Tropenhyg.*, **36**, 558–561
YAMAGUCHI, T., UOHARA, K. & SHINOTO, M. (1962). Treatment of *Clonorchiasis sinensis* with
Pankiller (Dithiazanine iodine). *Jap. J. Parasit.*, **11**, 30–38

FASCIOLIDAE

ALICATA, J. E. (1938). Observations on the life history of *Fasciola gigantica*, the common liver
fluke of cattle in Hawaii, and the intermediate host *Fossaria ollula*. *Bull. Hawaii agric. exp. Stn.*,
No. 80
BEHRENS, H. (1960). Behandlung des Lebergelbefalls der Schafe mit Hetol. *Dt. tierärztl. Wschr.*
67, 467–470
BERGHEN, P. (1964). Some Lymnaeidae as intermediate hosts of *Fasciola hepatica* in Belgium.
Exp. Parasit., **15**, 118–124
BORAY, J. (1963). The ecology of *Fasciola hepatica* with particular reference to its intermediate
host in Australia. *Proc. 17th Wld vet. Congr. Hannover*, **1**, 709–715
BORAY, J. C. & PEARSON, I. G. (1960). The anthelmintic efficiency of tetrachlorodifluorethane
in sheep infested with *Fasciola hepatica*. *Aust. vet. J.*, **36**, 331–337
BROWN, H. W. *et al.* (1959). The treatment of *Fasciolopsis buski* infections with dithiazanine iodide
1-bromo-naphthol-(2), Ascaridol, Piperazine and Tetrachlorethylene. *J. Formosan med. Ass.*,
58, 992–798
COYLE, T. J. (1959). Control of Fascioliasis in Uganda. In *Symposium on Helminthiasis in Domestic*
Animals, C.C.T.A. Nairobi, No. 49, p. 67–80. I.A.C.E.D.
DAWES, B. (1960). A study of the miracidium of *Fasciola hepatica* and an account of the mode of
penetration of the sporocyst into *Limnaea truncatula*. In *Lilro Homenaje at Dr. Eduardo Caballero y*
Caballero, pp. 95–11. Mexico DF: Escuela Nacional de Ciencias Biologicas
DAWES, B. (1963). Hyperplasia of the bile duct in Fascioliasis and its relation to the problem
of nutrition in the liver fluke, *Fasciola hepatica* L. *Parasitology*, **53**, 123–133
DINNIK, J. A. & DINNIK, N. N. (1964). The influence of temperature on the succession of redial
and cercarial generations of *Fasciola gigantica* in a snail host. *Parasitology*, **54**, 59–65
DOWNEY, N. E. (1960). Serum calcium and magnesium levels in ewes following the admission
of carbon tetrachloride. *Vet. Rec.*, **72**, 598–600
DROZDZ, J. (1963). Naturalne ognisko parafasciolopsozy w Wojewodztwie Bialostockun.
Wiad. parazyt., **9**, 129–132
FAUST, E. C. & RUSSEL, P. F. (1964). *Craig and Faust's Clinical Parasitology*, 7th edn. Philadelphia:
Lea & Febiger
GALLAGHER, C. H. (1961). The pathology and prophylaxis of poisoning by carbon tetrachloride.
Aust. vet. J., **37**, 131–134
GORDON, H. McL. (1955). Some aspects of Fascioliasis. *Aust. vet. J.*, **31**, 182–189

GORDON, H. McL., PEARSON, I. G., THOMPSON, B. J. & BORAY, J. C. (1959). Copper penta-chlorphenate as a molluscicide for the control of Fascioliasis. *Aust. vet. J.*, **35**, 465–473

HASHIZUME, K., NODA, R., NODA, S. & OTSUGI, T. (1961). The fasciolicidal action of tetra-chlorodifluorethane. (In Japanese) *J. Jap. vet. med. Ass.*, **14**, 472–478

HUBENDICK, B. (1951). Recent Lymnaeidae. *K. svenska VetenskAkad. Avh. Naturskydd.*, **3**, 1

HUGHES, D. L. (1963). Some studies on the host–parasite relations of *Fasciola hepatica*. Ph.D. Thesis University of London

JENNINGS, F. W., MULLIGAN, W. & URQUHART, G. M. (1956). Radioisotope studies on the anemia produced by infection with *Fasciola hepatica*. *Exp. Parasit.*, **5**, 458–468

KENDALL, S. B. (1949a). Species of *Lymnaea* as intermediate hosts of *F. hepatica*. *Vet. Rec.*, **61**, 462

KENDALL, S. B. (1946b). Nutritional factors affecting the rate of development of *Fasciola hepatica* in *Limnaea truncatula*. *J. Helminth.*, **23**, 179–190

KENDALL, S. B. (1954). Fascioliasis in Pakistan. *Ann. trop. Med. Parasit.*, **48**, 307–313

KENDALL, S. B. (1965). Relationships between the species of *Fasciola* and their molluscan hosts. In *Advances in Parasitology*, Vol. 3, pp. 59–98 (Ed. by B. Dawes). London: Academic Press

KENDALL, S. B. & OLLERENSHAW, C. B. (1963). The effect of nutrition on the growth of *Fasciola hepatica* in its snail host. *Proc. Nutr. Soc.*, **22**, 41–46

KENDALL, S. B. & PARFITT, J. W. (1962). The chemotherapy of Fascioliasis. *Brit. vet. J.*, **118**, 1–10

LÄMMLER, G. (1960). Chemotherapeutische Untersuchungen mit Hetol, einem neuen, hoch-wirksamen Leberegelmittel. *Dt. tierärztl. Wschr.*, **67**, 408–413

OLLERENSHAW, C. B. (1959). The ecology of the liver fluke (*Fasciola hepatica*). *Vet Rec.*, **71**, 957–965

OLSEN, O. W. (1943). Preliminary observations on hexachlorethane for controlling the common liver fluke, *Fasciola hepatica*, in cattle. *J. Am. vet. med. Ass.*, **102**, 433–436

OLSEN, O. W. (1947a). Hexachloroethane-bentonite suspension for controlling the common liver fluke, *Fasciola hepatica*, in cattle in the Gulf Coast Region of Texas. *Am. J. vet. Res.*, **8**, 353–366

OLSEN, O. W. (1947b). Longevity of metacercariae of *Fasciola hepatica* on pastures in the upper coastal region of Texas and its relationship to liver fluke control. *J. Parasit.*, **31**, 36–42.

ROWCLIFFE, S. A. & OLLERENSHAW, C. B. (1960). Observations on the bionomics of the egg of *Fasciola hepatica*. *Ann. trop. Med. Parasit.*, **54**, 172–181

SETCHELL, B. P. (1962). Poisoning of sheep with anthelmintic doses of carbon tetrachloride. I. A summary of the histories of 185 mortalities. *Aust. vet. J.*, **38**, 487–490, 491–494

SINCLAIR, K. B. (1964). Studies on the anaemia of ovine Fascioliasis. *Br. vet. J.*, **120**, 212–222

SINCLAIR, K. B. (1965). Iron metabolism in ovine Fascioliasis. *Br. vet. J.*, **121**, 451–461

SOULSBY, E. J. L. (1965). *Textbook of Veterinary Clinical Parasitology*, Vol. I, *Helminths*. Oxford: Blackwell Scientific Publications

SWALES, W. E. (1935). The life cycle of *Fascioloides magna* (Bassi, 1875), the large liver fluke of ruminants, in Canada, with observations on the bionomics of the larval stages and the inter-mediate hosts, pathology of *Fascioloidiasis magna*, and control measures. *Can. J. Res.*, **12**, 177–215

TAYLOR, E. L. (1949). The epidemiology of Fascioliasis in Britain. *Proc. 14th Int. vet. Congr. London*, **2**, 81–87

TAYLOR, E. L. (1951). Parasitic bronchitis in cattle. *Vet. Rec.* **63**, 859–873

UENO, H., WATANABE, S. & FUJITA, J. (1960). Studies on anthelmintics of common liver fluke. II. Anthelmintic effect of bithionol on bovine liver fluke. (In Japanese) *J. Jap. vet. med. Ass.* **13**, 151–155

WIKERHAUSER, T. (1960). A rapid method for determining the viability of *Fasciola hepatica* metacercariae. *Am. J. vet. Res.*, **21**, 895–897

ECHINOSTOMATIDAE

ANNEREAUX, R. F. (1940). A note on *Echinoparyphium recurvatum* (von Linstow) parasitic in California turkeys. *J. Am. vet. med. Ass.*, **96**, 62–64

BEAVER, P. C. (1937). Experimental studies on *E. revolutum* (Froel.), a fluke from birds and mammals. *Illinois biol. Monogr.*, **15**, 1–96

BEAVER, P. C. (1941). Studies on the life history of *Euparyphium melis* (Trematoda: Echinostom-idae). *J. Parasit.*, **27**, 35–44

DAWES, B. (1946). *The Trematoda*. Cambridge University Press

HARPER, W. F. (1929). On the structure and life history of British fresh-water larval trematodes. *Parasitology*, **21**, 189–219

VAN HEELSBERGEN, T. (1927a). Echinostomiasis bij de duif door Echinostoma. *Tijdschr. Diergeneesk.*, **54**, 414–416

VAN HEELSBERGEN, T. (1927b). Echinostomiasis bij kippen door Echinoparyphium. *Tijdschr. Diergeneesk.*, **54**, 413–414

KRAUSE, C. (1925). Gehäuftes Sterben bei Tauben durch Echinostomiden. *Berl. tierärztl. Wschr.*, **41**, 262–263

NÖLLER, W. & WAGNER, O. (1923). Der Wasserfrosch als zweiter Zwischenwirt eines Trema-toden von Ente und Huhn. *Berl. tierärztl. Wschr.*, **39**, 463

SOULSBY, E. J. L. (1955). Deaths in swans associated with trematode infection. *Br. Vet. J.*, **111**, 498–500
VEVERS, G. M. (1923). Observations on the life-histories of *Hypodaerium conoideum* (Bloch) and *Echinostomum revolutiom* (Froel): Trematode parasites of the domestic duck. *Ann. appl. Biol.*, **10**, 134–136
WETZEL, R. (1933). Zum Wirt-Parasitverhältnis des Saugwurmes *Echinoparyphium paraulum* in der Taube. *Dt. tierärztl. Wschr.*, **41**, 772–775

HETEROPHYIDAE, PLAGIORCHIDAE, NOTOCOTYLIDAE, CYCLOCOELIDAE, TROGLOTREMATIDAE

ALICATA, J. E. (1940). The life cycle of *Postharmostomum gallinum*, the cecal fluke of poultry. *J. Parasit.*, **26**, 135–143
CAMERON, T. W. M. (1945). Fish-carried parasites in Canada. I. Parasites carried by freshwater fish. *Can. J. comp. Med.*, **9**, 245–254, 283–286, 302–311
CHRISTENSEN, N. O. & ROTH, H. (1949). Investigation on internal parasites of dogs. *Yearbook: Royal Veterinary and Agricultural College, Copenhagen, Denmark*
DAWES, B. (1946). *The Trematoda*. Cambridge University Press
FOGGIE, A. (1937). An outbreak of parasitic necrosis in turkeys caused by *Plagiorchis laricola* (Skrjabin). *J. Helminth.*, **15**, 35–36
GESINSKI, R., THOMAS, R. E. & GALLICCHIO, V. (1964). Survey of *Paragonimus* in Ohio mink. *J. Parasit.*, **50**, 151
MACY, R. W. (1934). Studies on the taxonomy, morphology and biology of *Prosthogonimus macrorchis* Macy, a common oviduct fluke of domestic fowls in North America. *Univ. Minn. agric. Exp. Stn. Tech. Bull.*, No. 98
McTAGGERT, H. S. (1958). *Cryptocotyle lingua* in British mink. *Nature, Lond.*, **181**, 651
PANIN, W. J. (1957). Variability of the morphological characters and its importance in the systematisation of suckers of the genus *Prosthogoniums* (Lühe, 1909). *Trudy Inst. Zool., Alma-Ata.*, **7**, 170–215
REES, F. G. (1952). The structure of the adult and larval stages of *Plagiorchis* (*Multiglandularis*) *megalorchis* n. nom. from the turkey and an experimental demonstration of the life history. *Parasitology*, **42**, 92–113
SOULSBY, E. J. L. (1965). *Textbook of Veterinary Clinical Parasitology*, Vol. I, Helminths. Oxford: Blackwell Scientific Publications
SZIDAT, L. (1930). Die Parasiten des Hausgeflügels. 4. *Notocotylus* Diesing und *Catatropis* Odhner, Zwei, die Blinddärme des Geflügels bewohnende Monostome Trematodengattung, ihre Entwicklung und Übertragung. *Arch. Geflügelk.*, **5**, 105–111
SZIDAT, L. (1933). Über die Entwicklung und den Infektionmodus von *Tracheophilus sisowi* Skrj. eines Luftröhrenschmarotzers der Enten aus der Trematodenfamilie der Zyklozöliden. *Tierärztl. Rdsch.*, **39**, 95–99
WITENBERG, G. G. (1932). On the anatomy and systematic position of the causative agent of so-called salmon poisoning. *J. Parasit.*, **18**, 258–263.
YOKOGAWA, M., TSUJI, M. & OKURA, T. (1962). Studies on the complement fixation test with paragonimiasis on the method of criterion of care. *Jap. J. Parasit.*, **11**, 117–122
YOKOGAWA, M., YOSHIMURA, H., OSHIMA, T. & KIHATA, M. (1957). Immunological study on paragonimiasis. III. Passive transfer (P–K) experiments on human skins. *J. agric. Met. Tokyo*, **6**, 449–457

PARAMPHISTOMATIDAE

BORAY, J. C. (1959). Studies on intestinal amphistomosis in cattle. *Aust. vet. J.*, **35**, 282–287
BOSMAN, C. J., THOROLD, P. W. & PURCHASE, H. S. (1961). Investigation into and the development of hexachlorophene as an anthelmintic. *Jl. S. Afr. vet. med. Ass.*, **32**, 227–233
DAWES, B. (1936). On a collection of Paramphistomidae from Malaya, with revision of the genera *Paramphistomum* Fischoeder, 1901 and *Gastrothylax* Poirier, 1883. *Parasitology*, **28**, 330–354
DAWES, B. (1946). *The Trematoda*. Cambridge University Press
DURIE, P. H. (1951). The paramphistomes (Trematoda) of Australian ruminants. I. Systematics. *Proc. Linn. Soc. N.S.W.*, **76**, 41–48
DURIE, P. H. (1953). The paramphistomes (Trematoda) of Australian ruminants. II. The life history of *Ceylonocotyle streptocoelium* (Fischoeder) Näsmark and of *Paramphistomum ichikawai* Fukui. *Aust. J. Zool.*, **1**, 193–222
GUILHON, J. & GRABER, M. (1962). Action du Bithionol sur les amphistomes et sur *Fasciola gigantica*. *Bull. Acad. vet. Fr.*, **35**, 275–278
HORAK, I. G. (1962). Studies on Paramphistomiasis. IV. Modified critical and controlled anthelmintic tests on the conical fluke *Paramphistomum microbothrium*. *Jl. S. Afri. vet. med. Ass.*, **33**, 203–208
NÄSMARK, K. E. (1937). Revision of the Trematode Family Paramphistomidae. *Zool. Bidr. Upps.*, **16**, 301–565
OLSEN, O. W. (1949). Action of hexachlorethane-bentonite suspension on the rumen fluke, *Paramphistomum*. *Vet. Med.*, **44**, 108–109
SOULSBY, E. J. L. (1965). *Textbook of Veterinary Clinical Parasitology*. Oxford: Blackwell Scientific Publications

SWART, P. J. (1954). The identity of so-called *Paramphistomum cervi* and *P. explanatum*, two common species of ruminant trematodes in South Africa. *Onderstepoort J. vet. Res.*, **26**, 463–473

VARMA, A. K. (1957). On a collection of paramphistomes from domesticated animals in Bihar. *Indian J. vet. Sci.*, **27**, 67–76

STREGEIDAE, DIPLOSTOMATIDAE AND SCHISTOSOMATIDAE

ALWAR, V. S. (1962). Further studies on intensive treatment of nasal schistosomiasis in cattle. *Indian vet. J.*, **39**, 33–39

BATTEN, P. J. (1956). The histopathology of swimmers itch. I. The skin lesions of *Schistosomatium douthitti* and *Gigantobilharzia huronensis* in the unsensitized mouse. *Am. J. Pathol.*, **32**, 363–377

BISWAL, G. & DAS, L. N. (1956). Observations on the treatment of nasal schistosomiasis in cattle and buffaloes in Orissa. *Indian Vet. J.*, **33**, 204–216

BLACKIE, W. K. (1933). A helminthological survey of Southern Rhodesia. Memoir Series No. 5. London School of Hygiene and Tropical Medicine

BUCKLEY, J. J. C. (1938). On a dermatitis in Malays caused by the cercariae of *Schistosoma spindale* Montgomery, 1906. *J. Helminth.*, **14**, 117–120

CORT, W. W. (1928). Schistosome dermatitis in the U.S. (Michigan). *J. Am. med. Ass.*, **90**, 1027–1029

CUCKLER, A. C. (1940). Studies on the migration and development of *Alaria* spp. (Trematoda: Strigeata) in the definitive host. *J. Parasit.*, **26**, (Suppl.), 36

DERAMÉE, O., THIENPONT, D., FAIN, A. & JADIN, J. (1953). Sur un foyer de bilharziose canine a *Schistosoma rodhaini* Brumpt au Ruanda-Urundi; note preliminaire. *Anns Soc. belge méd. trop.*, **33**, 207–209

ERLICH, I. (1938). Paraziticka fauna posa s podrucja grada Zagreba. (Die parasitäre Fauna der Hunde vom Gebiete der Stadt Zagreb. German summary). *Vet. Arh.*, **8**, 531–571

FAUST, E. C. & RUSSEL, P. F. (1964). *Craig and Faust's Clinical Parasitology*. 7th edn. Philadelphia: Lea & Febiger

JENNINGS, A. R. & SOULSBY, E. J. L. (1958). Disease in a colony of blackheaded gulls *Larus ridibundus*. *Ibis*, **100**, 305–312

LE ROUX, P. L. (1929). Notes on the life-cycle of *Schistosoma mattheei* and observations on the control and eradication of schistosomiasis in Man and animals. *15th Rep. Dir. vet. Serv., Dept Agric. Un. S. Afr.*, **1**, 407–438

LOWE, P. R. & BAYLIS, H. A. (1934). On a flock of razorbills in Middlesex found to be infested with intestinal flukes with a parasitological report. *Br. Birds.*, **28**, 188–190

MACHATTIE, C., MILLS, E. A. & CHADWICK, C. R. (1933). Can sheep and cattle act as reservoirs of human schistosomiasis? *Trans. Rev. Soc. trop. Med. Hyg.*, **27**, 173–184

MALEK, E. A. (1961). The biology of mammalian and bird schistosomes. *Bull. Tulane med. Fac.*, **20**, 181–207

NAIK, R. N. (1942). Experiment on the control of nasal granuloma. *Indian J. vet. Sci.*, **12**, 150–159

NELSON, G. S. (1959). *I.A.C.E.D. Symposium on Helminthiasis in Domestic Animals, Nairobi.*, pp. 61–66. C.C.T.A.

NELSON, G. S. (1961). Personal communication

PESIGAN, T. P., FAROOG, M., HAIRSTON, N. G., JAUREGUE, J. J., GARCIA, E. G., SANTOS, A. T., SANTOS, B. C. & BESA, A. A. (1958). Studies on *Schistosoma japonicum* infection in the Philippines. I. General considerations and epidemiology. *Bull Wld Hlth Org.*, **18**, 345–455

PITCHFORD, R. J. (1959). Cattle schistosomiasis in Man in the Eastern Transvaal. *Trans. R. Soc. trop. Med. Hyg.*, **53**, 285–290

RAO, N. S. K., SINGH, B. K. & MURTHY, K. S. (1962). Nasal schistosomiasis in cattle—treatment with oral administration of Neguvon. *Indian vet. J.*, **39**, 484–487

SOULSBY, E. J. L. (1965). *Textbook of Veterinary Clinical Parasitology*. Oxford: Blackwell Scientific Publications

SRIVASTAVA, H. D. & DUTT, S. C. (1962). Studies on *Schistosoma indicum*. Research Series No. 34. Indian Council of Agricultural Research. New Delhi

SZIDAT, L. (1929). Die Parasiten des Hausgeflügels. 3. *Bilharziella polonika* Kow., ein im Blut schmarotzender Trematode unserer Enten, seine Entwicklung und Uebertragung. *Arch. Geflügelk.*, **3**, 78–87

WERY, J. E. (1950). La Schistosomiase Bovine au Runanda-Urundi. *Annls. Soc. belge méd. trop.*, **30**, 1613–1614

WORLD HEALTH ORGANIZATION (1959). Molluscicides in the control of bilharziasis. *Wd Hlth Org. Chron.*, **13**, 33–38

WORLD HEALTH ORGANIZATION (1966). Chemotherapy of bilharziasis. *Technical Report Series* No. 317. Geneva

Cestodes

CLASS: CESTODA

The class Cestoda is divided by Wardle & McLeod (1952) into eleven orders. Of these, nine are parasitic in annelids, fishes, amphibia or reptiles and need not be considered in this book. The remaining two orders include species parasitic in domesticated animals and man. They are:

ORDER: PSEUDOPHYLLIDEA

Most of the species of this order are parasitic in fish, but one species of them, belonging to the family Diphyllobothriidae, namely *Diphyllobothrium latum* (*Dibothriocephalus latus*), is parasitic in the dog, fox, cat and most fish-eating mammals, including man. It is described below.

ORDER: CYCLOPHYLLIDEA

To this order belong all the other species of tapeworms described in this book. The description of Cestoda that follows also applies chiefly to species of this order.

Tapeworms are hermaphrodite, endoparasitic worms with an elongate, flat body and without a body-cavity or an alimentary canal. The body consists of a head or *scolex*, usually provided with suckers and hooks, and a *strobila*, which consists of a number of segments or *proglottides*. Between the scolex and the strobila there may be a short unsegmented portion that is often called the neck. Each proglottis usually contains one or two sets of male and female reproductive organs. The life-cycle is indirect, requiring one or more intermediate hosts.

Morphology. Cestodes vary in size from a few millimetres to several metres in length. The scolex is usually more or less globular and bears two or four suckers with muscular walls which may be armed with hooks. Anteriorly the scolex may be armed with a protrusible part, the *rostellum*, which may bear one or more rows of hooks. These hooks vary much in shape, but generally they may consist of a handle, a guard and a blade. The hooks are sometimes lost, especially when they are small.

The strobila may consist of a few or numerous proglottides, and these vary considerably in shape and size in different species. They are formed behind the head, so that the anterior ones are the youngest, and they increase in size and the development of their internal parts progresses as they are pushed farther and farther away from the scolex by the younger segments.

The structure of the body is somewhat similar to that of the trematodes. The body is covered by a 'cuticle', but this is more properly termed a tegument since it is not comparable with a cuticular structure seen in other animal groups (Read, 1966). There is much evidence that the tegument is the major absorptive structure in cestodes and evidence of a physiological activity is given by the presence of mitochondria, phosphatases, indophenol oxidase and several other hydrolytic and oxidative enzymes (Read, 1966). Electronmicroscopy has shown the integument to possess surface villi which are bounded on the outer surface by a tri-laminate membrane and possess an inner core of supporting microtubular

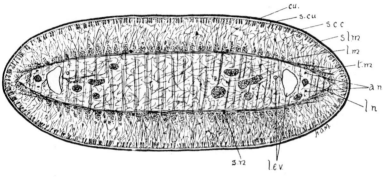

a.n.	Accessory nerves	*s.c.c.*	Subcuticular cells
cu.	Cuticula	*s.cu.*	Subcuticula
l.e.v.	Longitudinal excretory vessels	*s.l.m.*	Subcuticular longitudinal muscles
l.m.	Longitudinal muscles	*s.n.*	Submedian nerve
l.n.	Lateral nerve	*t.m.*	Transverse muscles

Fig. 33. Transverse Section of a Cestode: Diagrammatic (Original)

structures which Lumsden (1965) has compared to microvilli of other absorptive cells, e.g. those of the vertebrate intestine. A review of the absorptive functions of cestodes is given by Read *et al.* (1963) and Read (1966). Beneath the tegument the body is filled with a parenchyma similar to that of the trematodes. In this lie more centrally, strong bundles of longitudinal muscle fibres. Internal to these there is a thinner layer of transverse muscles which divide the body into outer cortical and inner medullary portions. Dorso-ventral muscles are also present, but are weakly developed. The medulla contains the excretory, nervous and reproductive organs.

The excretory system consists of flame-cells and efferent canals as in the trematodes. There are usually, on either side, two longitudinal canals, a larger central and a smaller dorsal, each pair being connected by a transverse vessel in the posterior part of the proglottis, and all are joined together by transverse loops in the scolex. Frequently a small bladder occurs in the terminal segment, but it is lost when this segment is detached and then the canals open separately.

The central part of the nervous system is situated in the scolex and consists of several ganglia and commissures, from which two large and several smaller nerve trunks run through the strobila. The main trunks are lateral to the large excretory canals.

The male genital organs are the first to develop in the young proglottides. Segments in which the reproductive organs have become mature and functional are called *mature* segments. When the eggs have been fertilised, either by cross- or self-fertilisation of individual segments, the reproductive organs degenerate, leaving only the uterus, full of

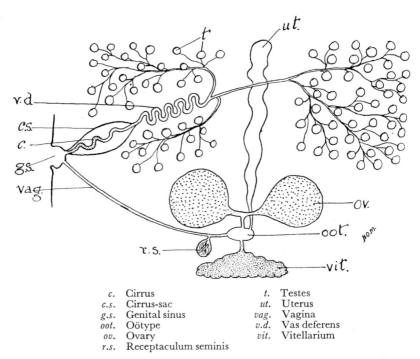

c.	Cirrus	*t.*	Testes
c.s.	Cirrus-sac	*ut.*	Uterus
g.s.	Genital sinus	*vag.*	Vagina
oot.	Oötype	*v.d.*	Vas deferens
ov.	Ovary	*vit.*	Vitellarium
r.s.	Receptaculum seminis		

FIG. 34. Reproductive Organs of a Cestode: Diagrammatic (Original)

fertilised eggs, and segments that have reached this stage are called *gravid* segments. Gravid segments are passed out of the host, either singly or in chains, and the eggs are set free by disintegration of the gravid segments or by expression of the eggs through a pore in the uterus.

The male organs consist of one, or a few or more usually a large number, of testes, discharging into vasa efferentia, which join to form a vas deferens. This may form a seminal vesicle and ends in a cirrus which is surrounded by a cirrus-sac. The male and female genital pores frequently lie close together in a shallow sinus on the lateral margin of the proglottis (most

Cyclophyllidea), or on the ventral surface (many *Diphyllobothriidae*), and self-fertilisation of individual segments may occur.

The female pore leads into a vagina, a narrow duct which frequently bears a seminal receptacle and ends where it is joined by the oviduct and the vitelline duct, in the oötype, which is surrounded by Mehlis's glands. The ovary is single and usually lobed. The vitelline gland is usually compact in the *Cyclophyllidea*, but in some cases it is divided into follicles, especially in the *Diphyllobothriidae*. From the oötype the uterus arises. It may open distally and discharge the eggs, but more usually it ends blindly and assumes various shapes as it becomes filled. The uterus may persist as a protective envelope for the eggs, or the eggs may pass from it into protective envelopes which may be: (a) *egg-capsules*, which are formed by the uterus itself; (b) *paruterine organs*, which appear in species of the families Anoplocephalidae and Davaneidae. Paruterine organs may be formed by denser parenchyma near the uterus into which the eggs pass; or they may arise as dilatations of the uterus in which the eggs may remain after the uterus has disappeared, or the eggs may pass from these dilatations into fibrous envelopes formed by the parenchyma called *egg-pouches*. Whatever their method of formation, egg-capsules, egg-pouches and paruterine organs all perform the function of protecting the fertilised eggs. For a discussion of the formation of the egg shell in cestodes and trematodes, see Smyth & Clegg (1959).

In most cases the embryonic development takes place in the uterus and the eggs, when they are laid, contain a spherical or ovoid embryo called the *oncosphere*. With the *Pseudophyllidea* the egg is operculate and resembles that of a trematode. A period of embryonation is required before the stage (*coracidium*) comparable to the oncosphere is produced. The oncosphere has three, rarely five, pairs of hooks and is known as the *hexacanth embryo*. Wardle & McLeod (1952) discuss the development of the egg. The egg of the cyclophyllidean forms initially is bounded by a capsule which is easily lost when the egg is passed from the uterus. Beneath the capsule is a vitelline layer which contains the yolk cells in the early stage of development but these disintegrate leaving a thin membraned structure. Beneath this is the *embryophore* which has variously been referred to as the 'egg-shell' or 'oncosphere coat'. These terms are strictly invalid but are, nevertheless, in common usage. Beneath the embryophore is the oncospheral membrane which finally encloses the oncosphere. Various modifications can occur with the latter two membranes. In the Anoplocephalidae the outermost forms the pyriform apparatus described below (p. 95); in the Taeniidae these two envelopes are connected by septa, so that the covering of the eggs of Taeniidae has a characteristic radially-striated appearance, although strictly speaking they have no shell. The eggs of *Diphyllobothrium latum* escape continuously into the intestine of the host through the open uterine pore of this species; those of the Cyclophyllidea, which have no uterine pore, pass out inside the gravid proglottides and are liberated by injuries done to these proglottides, or by their disintegration, or, in *Taenia saginata* and some other species, through openings made into the uterus when the gravid proglottis is detached, the eggs being then exuded in a milky fluid as the active proglottis moves about outside the host.

Development. The *Diphyllobothriidae* rather resemble the trematodes in their development and will be treated later. In the *Cyclophyllidea* the egg hatches after having been swallowed by the intermediate host, and the hexacanth embryo penetrates into the intestinal wall in order to reach a suitable part of the body for its further development. Here it grows into a cyst composed of an outer cuticle and an inner germinal layer, containing a cavity filled with fluid. It develops one or more heads on its wall or in special brood-capsules. The wall forms an invagination, at the bottom of which the rostellum with the hooks and the suckers develop in such a way that the head is at first turned outside inwards, but it soon rises up in the lumen of the invaginated part, where it usually remains. It is thus surrounded by two walls, with the cavity of the cyst, filled with fluid, between them. This bladderworm, as it is called, is ready for further development in the final host as soon as the hooks and suckers are sufficiently developed to enable the parasite to attach itself in the intestine.

The common form of cyclophyllidean bladderworms can be classified as follows:

Cysticercus: a bladderworm with a large vesicle and one head; usually found in vertebrates.

Cysticercoid: a small vesicle, practically without a cavity, and one head; usually found in invertebrates.

Cercocystis: a cysticercoid with a tail-like appendage to the vesicle.

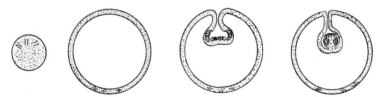

FIG. 35. Stages in the Development of a Cysticercus (Original)

Cryptocystis: a cysticercoid that has lost its tail-like appendage.

Tetrathyridium (Dithyridium): an elongate larva with a solid body into which the head is invaginated (see Mesocestoididae below).

Coenurus: usually a large cyst containing fluid, with a number of heads developing on the wall.

Echinococcus: a large cyst containing fluid, which does not usually develop heads directly on its walls, but forms here instead other cysts, called *brood-capsules*, in which the heads normally develop.

The bladderworm is passively transferred to the final host when the latter ingests the infected intermediate host. After its arrival in the intestine the bladderworm evaginates its head and attaches it to the mucosa. The bladder is discarded and the proglottides develop. In *Hymenolepis nana*, a parasite of man, mice and the rat, these hosts act as both final and intermediate hosts, because the cysticercoid develops in the mucosa of the intestine and proceeds with its development to the adult stage in the same host. Cysticercoids will also develop in various species of fleas and beetles, which can act as intermediate hosts.

A review of the biology of cestode life-cycles, including an account of embryonation, hatching and development is given by Smyth (1963).

ORDER: CYCLOPHYLLIDAE

Fourteen families of the order have been recognised. The species found in domesticated animals and man belong to the following six families:

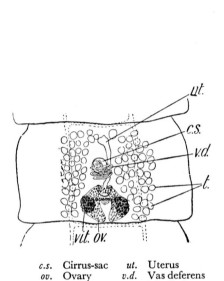

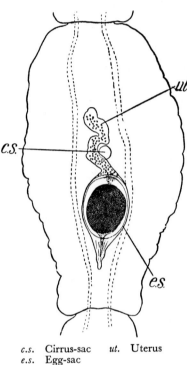

c.s.	Cirrus-sac	ut.	Uterus
ov.	Ovary	v.d.	Vas deferens
t.	Testes	vit.	Vitellarium

FIG. 36. *Mesocestoides lineatus*, Mature Segment, Dorsal View (after Baylis)

c.s.	Cirrus-sac	ut.	Uterus
e.s.	Egg-sac		

FIG. 37. *Mesocestoides lineatus*, Gravid Segment, Dorsal View (after Baylis)

FAMILY: MESOCESTOIDIDAE

This family is characterised by the presence of four suckers, the absence of a rostellum and hooks, the median ventral position of the genital pore and the presence of two yolk glands. The eggs become enclosed in a thick-walled par-uterine organ formed from the parenchyma.

Genus: Mesocestoides Vaillant, 1863

M. lineatus (Goeze, 1782) occurs in the small intestine of the dog, cat, fox, beech marten, mink and wild carnivores in Europe, Asia and Africa. The scolex is large and the suckers are elongate oval. The worm is 30–250 cm. long and has a maximum width of 3 mm. The mature segments each contain a single set of reproductive organs. The cirrus-sac and the vagina open close together near the midline on the ventral surface. There are about fifty testes, lying on either side of the longitudinal excretory canals. The ovary and the vitelline gland are bilobed and posterior in position. The eggs are oval and measure 40–60 by 35–43 μ.

Life-cycle. Two intermediate hosts are required. The first is a coprophagous insect, oribatid mites of the genus *Trichoribates* serving as such in the U.S.S.R. A cysticercoid is produced in these and when the infected mite is eaten by a second intermediate host (dog, cat, birds, reptiles, amphibians) a tetrathyridium (*Dithyridium*) is formed. This is a slender worm like structure 1–2 cm. in length, which when eaten by the final host becomes adult in 16–20 days. The tetrathyridium may persist, in an encapsulated form, in the second intermediate host for some time. Wardle & McLeod (1952) consider its second larva is *Tetrathyridium bailleti* (*T. elongatum*).

Treatment. See *Taenia* spp. of dogs.

Dithyridium variabile (Diesing, 1850) is a larval form which occurs in small cysts under the skin of the fowl, turkey and wild birds.

FAMILY: ANOPLOCEPHALIDAE

The worms of this family have neither rostellum nor hooks. The proglottides are usually wider than long and each has one or two sets of genital organs. The genital pores are marginal. The testes are usually numerous. The uterus may persist or be replaced by egg pouches, or the eggs may pass into one or more par-uterine organs. Each egg has three coverings, an outermost vitelline membrane, a middle albuminous coat, and an innermost chitinous membrane, which is frequently pear shaped, bearing on one side a pair of hooked projections which may cross one another, this structure being called the *pyriform apparatus*. The known intermediate hosts are mites of the Family *Oribatidae*.

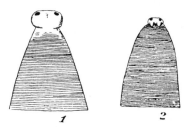

FIG. 38. 1, *Anoplocephala magna*, Anterior End; 2, *A. perfoliata*, Anterior End (after Mönnig)

Genus: Anoplocephala E. Blanchard, 1848

A. magna (Abildgaard, 1789) occurs in the small intestine and rarely in the stomach of equines. It measures up to 80 cm. in length and 2 cm wide. The scolex is large, 4–6 mm. wide, with suckers opening anteriorly.

There is usually a short neck and the segments are very short. The genital organs are single and the pores are unilateral. The main stem of the uterus is transverse, with anterior and posterior branches. The eggs have a pyriform apparatus and measure 50–60 μ.

A. perfoliata (Goeze, 1782) occurs in the small and large intestine of equines. It measures up to 8 by 1·2 cm. It differs from the preceding species in having a smaller head, 2–3 mm. in diameter, provided with a small lappet behind each sucker, while the segments are exceedingly short. The eggs measure 65–80 μ.

Genus: Paranoplocephala Lühe, 1910

P. mamillana (Mehlis, 1831) occurs in the small intestine and occasionally the stomach of the horse. It measures only 6–50 by 4–6 mm. The openings of the suckers are slit-like and situated dorsally and ventrally. The eggs measure about 51 by 37 μ.

Life-cycles of Anoplocephala *spp.* Oribatid mites serve as intermediate hosts. For *A. perfoliata, Scheloribates laevigatus, S. latipes, Galumna obvious, G. nervosus, Achiperia* spp. and *Ceratozetes* spp. have been experimentally infected, for *A. magna, S. laevigatus* and *S. latipes* are concerned and for *P. mamillana, G. obvious* and *Allogalumna longipluma* are concerned. Cysticercoids are produced in these mites. Adult tapeworms are found 4–6 weeks after ingestion of infected mites with herbage.

Pathogenesis. Light infections in horses produce no clinical signs, but large numbers may cause ill health, unthriftiness and even death. *A. perfoliata* frequently localises near the ileo-caecal valve which may show ulceration, oedema and occasionally a marked excess of granulation tissue. This may lead to partial occlusion of the ileocaecal valve. In rare, acute, massive infections of young horses, an acute catarrhal or ulcerative enteritis may occur. *A. magna* is probably the most pathogenic of the three species, heavy infections producing catarrhal or haemorrhagic enteritis. *P. mamillana* is seldom responsible for ill health.

Treatment. Male fern, Kamala and Oil of Chenopodium have been used. Fukui *et al.* (1960) found Bithionol effective at a dose of 7 mg. per kg.

Genus: Moniezia R. Blanchard, 1891

M. expansa (Rudolphi, 1810) occurs in the small intestine of sheep, goat, cattle and several other ruminants in most parts of the world. It may reach a length of 600 cm. and a width of 1·6 cm. The scolex is 0·36–0·8 mm. wide, with prominent suckers. The segments are broader than long and each contains two sets of genital organs. The ovaries and the vitelline glands form a ring on either side, median to the longitudinal excretory canals, while the testes are distributed throughout the central field or they may be concentrated towards the sides. At its posterior border each proglottis contains a row of interproglottidal glands, arranged around small pits. The eggs are somewhat triangular in shape, containing a well-developed pyriform apparatus, and measure 56–67 μ in diameter.

M. benedeni (Moniez, 1879) occurs in ruminants, chiefly cattle, and differs from *M. expansa* in being broader (up to 2·6 cm.), and in having the interproglottidal glands arranged in a short, continuous row close to the mid-line of the segment.

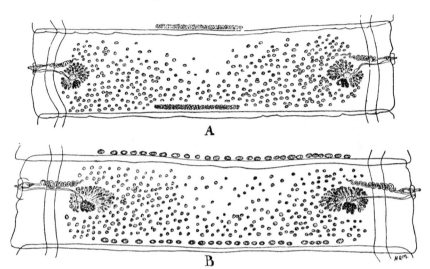

FIG. 39. A, *Moniezia benedeni*, Mature Segment: B, *M. expansa*, Mature Segment (Original)

Life-cycle. Cysticercoids develop in oribatid mites of the genera *Galumna, Oribatula, Peloribates Protoscheloribates, Scheloribates Scutovertex* and *Zygoribatula*. The life-cycle in such mites was originally discovered by Stunkard (1937) and since then more than two dozen mites have been shown to serve as natural or experimental hosts. The ability to infect experimentally does not necessarily indicate that the species of oribatid mite is concerned with natural transmission. Thus Rayski (1949) found only *Scutovertex minutus* naturally infected (in Scotland) though other species found could be infected experimentally. Lambs become infected very early in life and may pass ripe segments when they are 6 weeks old. The worms apparently do not live longer than about 3 months in the host.

Pathogenicity. As a rule only lambs, kids and calves under 6 months of age are substantially infected. A wide divergence of opinion exists regarding the pathogenic effects of the *Moniezia* spp. in sheep and cattle. There is little doubt that light infections are of little importance. Some authors, especially from the U.S.S.R., ascribe severe pathogenic effects to the tapeworms but workers in the U.S.A. (e.g. Hawkins, 1946; Kates & Goldberg, 1951) have failed to detect any serious effect from even apparently substantial burdens. There are, in fact, very little critical data available but it can be imagined that heavy infections, in which the small intestine is virtually a solid mass of tapeworms, are causing at least some degree of ill health. Because of the large size of the cestodes their presence is obvious and frequently the true underlying cause of the parasitism, small trichostrongyles, is overlooked.

Diagnosis. The presence in the faeces of ripe segments, which resemble cooked rice grains and from which *Moniezia* eggs can be identified, indicates the presence of tapeworms.

Treatment. Copper sulphate has been used for many years. A dose of 10–100 ml. of a 1 per cent solution is recommended. Copper sulphate and nicotine sulphate mixtures have also been widely used (1·8 g. per animal). Lead arsenate (0·5–1·0 g. in gelatine capsule), arsenic trisulphide (0·5g.) and tin arsenate (200 mg. per sheep) have all been used, generally with success. Of the newer compounds for tapeworms, dichlorophen (300–600 mg. per kg.), Yomesan (75 mg. per kg.) and cupric acetoarsenite (5·5 mg. per kg.) have been used with good results.

Genus: Cittotaenia Riehm, 1881

C. ctenoides (Railliet, 1890) occurs in the small intestine of the rabbit in Europe. It may grow up to 80 cm. long and 1 cm. wide. The scolex is about 0·5 mm. broad. A short neck is present. The proglottides are all much broader than long and each contains two sets of genital organs. The genital pores are situated in the posterior quarters of the proglottides. On either side there is a group of sixty to eighty testes behind the ovary. The cirrus pouch is 0·2 mm. long. The eggs have a pyriform apparatus and measure about 64 μ in diameter.

C. denticulata (Rudolphi, 1804) occurs in the rabbit in Europe. It has no neck and the scolex measures 0·8 mm. in diameter.

C. pectinata (Goeze, 1782) occurs in hares and rabbits in Europe, Asia and America. Its scolex is about 0·25 mm. in diameter and a neck is present.

Life-cycle. The intermediate hosts are oribatid mites.

Pathogenicity. Heavy infections of these tapeworms, especially *C. ctenoides*, frequently cause digestive disturbances, emaciation and even death amongst rabbits.

Treatment. Male fern extract at the rate of 0·3 g. per kg. bodyweight is effective. No information is available on the value of dichlorophen for the *Cittotaenia* spp., but it is worthy of trial.

Genus: Avitellina Gough, 1911

Several species of this genus have been described and the question of their identity is not definitely settled. They are discussed by Wardle & McLeod (1952). They occur in the small intestine of sheep, goats, cattle and other ruminants in Africa, Italy and India. They are 3 m. long or longer and about 3 mm. wide. The scolex measures up to 2 mm. in diameter. The proglottides are very short and not well marked, so that the worm appears macroscopically to be unsegmented. Posteriorly there is a median opaque line formed by the uterus and eggs, while the wide excretory canals on either side show as transparent lines. The ripe portion of the body is narrow and almost cylindrical. The genital organs are single and the pores irregularly alternating. There are groups of testes on either side of the excretory canals. Vitelline glands are absent. The eggs in the ripe segments pass into large thick-walled par-uterine organs, one to each segment. They have no pyriform apparatus. The diameter of the eggs, including their outer envelope, is about 220 μ. Development possibly occurs in psocids (bark lice, dust lice, book lice).

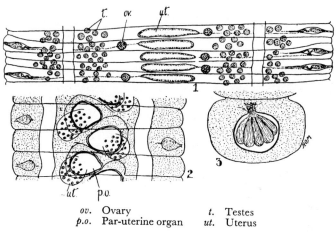

ov. Ovary	*t.* Testes
p.o. Par-uterine organ	*ut.* Uterus

FIG. 40. *Avitellina centripunctate:* 1, Mature Proglottides: 2, Gravid Proglottides, Eggs passing into Par-uterine Organs; 3, 'Ripe' Proglottis, Par-uterine Organ with Eggs in Bunches (Original)

Pathogenicity. These tapeworms are not as pathogenic as the Moniezias, but when they occur in large numbers clinical effects may be produced. They occur more frequently in adult animals than the Moniezias.

Genus: Stilesia Railliet, 1893

S. hepatica Wolffhügel, 1903, occurs in the bile ducts of sheep, goat, cattle and wild ruminants in Africa and is very common in certain parts. Complete specimens are rarely obtained, as the parasites creep into the fine bile ducts and the strobila breaks easily. They are about 20–50 cm. long and up to 2 mm. wide. The scolex is large, with prominent suckers, and is often followed by a broad neck about 2 mm. long. The segments are short but usually well visible. The genital organs are single. There are about eleven testes on either side, mainly median to the excretory canals. Vitelline glands are absent. The uterus consists of two portions united by a transverse duct. Each segment forms two par-uterine organs. The ovoid eggs have no pyriform apparatus. They measure, including the outer envelope, 260 by 160–190 μ.

Pathogenicity. *Stilesia hepatica* occurs in animals of all ages. It is practically non-pathogenic. Cases of extremely heavy infections are often seen in perfectly healthy sheep. Although the bile ducts may be practically occluded, or even form sac-like dilatations filled with the worms, no icterus or other symptoms are seen. In affected livers there may be slight cirrhosis and the walls of the bile ducts are usually thickened.

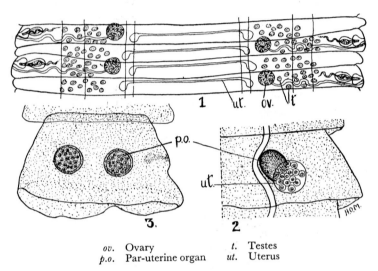

| *ov.* | Ovary | *t.* | Testes |
| *p.o.* | Par-uterine organ | *ut.* | Uterus |

FIG. 41. *Stilesia hepatica:* 1, Mature Proglottides; 2, Half of Gravid Proglottis, Eggs passing into Par-uterine Organ; 3, 'Ripe' Proglottis, Eggs in Par-uterine Organs (Original)

Such livers have to be condemned at meat inspection, and this is the only practical significance of the parasite.

S. globipunctata (Rivolta, 1874) occurs in the small intestine of the sheep and goat in Europe and India. It is 45–60 cm. long and up to 2·5 mm. wide. It has four to seven testes on either side, lateral to the excretory canals.

Genus: Thysanosoma Diesing, 1835

T. actinioides Diesing, 1835, the 'fringed tapeworm', occurs in the bile ducts, pancreatic ducts and small intestine of sheep, cattle and deer in America, especially the western parts of the United States and also in South America, but it does not occur outside the western hemisphere. It measures 15–30 cm. by 8 mm. The scolex is up to 1·5 mm. wide. The segments are short and conspicuously fringed posteriorly. Each segment contains two sets of genital organs and the testes lie in the median field. Several paruterine organs are formed in each segment and the eggs have no pyriform apparatus.

Life-cycle. Work by Allen (1959) demonstrated that cysticercoids could be recovered from laboratory reared psocids which had been fed egg capsules containing oncospheres. As yet it has not been possible to induce infections in cattle or sheep with infected psocids.

Pathogenicity. The pathogenicity of this parasite has apparently been over-estimated. The symptoms of selenium (loco) poisoning and other diseases have been ascribed to it in the past (Christenson, 1931). It may partly obstruct the flow of bile and pancreatic juice and cause digestive disorders and unthriftiness.

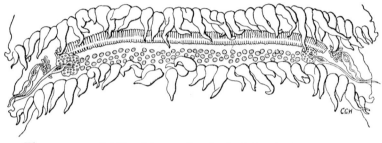

FIG. 42. *Thysanosoma actinioides,* Mature Proglottis (after Fuhrmann in Kükenthal)

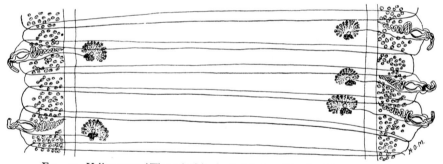

FIG. 43. *Helictometra (Thysaniezia) giardi,* Mature Proglottides (Original)

Diagnosis is made by finding the ripe segments and eggs in the faeces.

Treatment. Ryff *et al.* (1950) found that 550 mg. per kg. bodyweight of dichlorophen (diphenthane-70) was effective for the removal of this species from sheep on full feed and that 110 mg. per kg. bodyweight was enough after starvation of the sheep for 24 hours. Allen *et al.* (1962) reported that bithionol at a dose of 220 mg. per kg. cleared the majority of sheep of infection while 175 mg. per kg. substantially reduced infection.

Genus: Thysaniezia Skrjabin, 1926

T. giardi (Moniez, 1879) occurs in the small intestine of sheep, goat and cattle in Europe, Africa and America. It grows to about 200 cm. long and

12 mm. wide, the width varying greatly in different specimens. The scolex is often small, but may measure over 1 mm. in diameter. The segments are short and each contains a single set of genital organs, very rarely two, the pores alternating irregularly. The testes are lateral to the excretory canals. The side of the segment which contains the cirrus-sac bulges out, thus giving the margin of the worm an irregular appearance. The eggs, which are devoid of a pyriform apparatus, pass from the uterus into a large number of small paruterine organs. The ripe segments found in the faeces are therefore readily distinguishable from those of *Moniezia*.

Life-cycle. Potemkina (1944) has reported that the Oribatid mites *Galumna obvious* and *Scheloribates laevigatus* serve as intermediate hosts. However other workers in the U.S.S.R. (see Svadzhian, 1963) failed to confirm this previous work, rather finding that cysticercoids could be recovered from psocids when they were fed egg capsules of *T. giardi*.

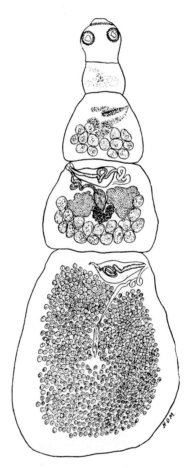

FIG. 44. *Davainea proglattina*, Complete Specimen (Original)

Pathogenicity. This worm occurs in young and adult animals, but is rarely seen in numbers sufficiently large to produce clinical signs. It is the most frequent tapeworm of adult cattle in South Africa.

Treatment and Prevention. Probably as in the case of *Moniezia.*

FAMILY: DAVAINEIDAE

These cestodes are characterised by the presence on the rostellum of numerous small, hammer-shaped hooks. The suckers are usually also provided with hooks. Genital organs usually single. The eggs may pass into egg-capsules (*Raillietina*) formed by the uterus or into a par-uterine organ formed from denser parenchyma near the uterus, or the uterus may persist. Parasites of birds chiefly.

Genus: Davainea Blanchard, 1891

D. proglottina (Davaine, 1860) occurs in the duodenal loop of the small intestine of the fowl, pigeon and other gallinaceous birds in most parts of the world. It has only four to nine proglottides and is 0·5–3 mm. long. The rostellum bears eighty to ninety-four hooks, 7–8 μ long, and the suckers have a few rows of small hooks which are easily lost. The genital pores are regularly alternating. The eggs lie singly in the parenchyma of the ripe segments and measure 28–40 μ in diameter.

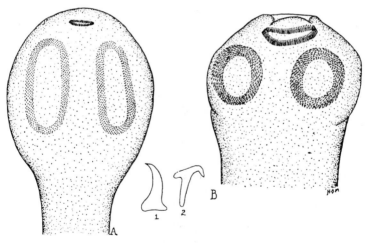

FIG. 45. A, *Raillietina tetragona*, Scolex; B, *R. echinobothrida*, Scolex; 1, Hook from Sucker; 2, Hook from Rostellum of B (Original)

Life-cycle. The ripe segments are passed in the faeces and the eggs hatch after having been swallowed by slugs of the genera *Limax, Arion, Cepoea* and *Agriolimax*, in which the embryo develops into a cysticercoid in about 3 weeks during the summer. Fowls become infected by ingesting the infected slugs. The adult stage is reached in the fowl in about 14 days.

The onchospheres remain viable for about 5 days in moist surroundings, but are rapidly killed by frost and drying. The ripe proglottides are positively phototropic and climb up moist grass blades, where they are eaten by the slugs.

Pathogenicity and Treatment. See pp. 108–109.

Genus: Raillietina Fuhrmann, 1920

More than 200 species have been described in this genus which has been divided into several sub-genera to accommodate them (see Wardle & McLeod, 1952). In the sub-genus *Raillietina* the genital pores are unilateral and there are the egg-pouches formed from the parenchyma, each of which contains several eggs.

R. (R.) tetragona (Molin, 1858) occurs in the small intestine of the fowl, guinea-fowl, pigeon and pea-fowl, and is cosmopolitan in distribution. It is one of the largest of the fowl tape-worms, measuring up to 25 cm. in length. It has a long, thin neck and a small scolex with 100 minute hooks, 6–8 μ long, in one row on the rostellum. The suckers are oval in shape and armed with eight to ten rows of small hooks, which may be lost. The egg pouches each contain six to twelve eggs, the diameter of which is 25–50 μ, and the pouches extend laterally to the excretory vessels. This species is difficult to distinguish from *R. echinobothrida*. The oval shape of the suckers and the weaker armature of the scolex are conspicuous when the two worms are compared to each other.

Life-cycle. The intermediate hosts are *Musca domestica* and ants of the genera *Tetramorium* and *Pheidole*.

Pathogenicity and Treatment. See pp. 108–109.

R. (R.) echinobothrida (Megnin, 1880) occurs in the small intestine of the fowl in most parts of the world. In shape and size it resembles *R. tetragona*. The rostellum bears 200 hooks, 10–13 μ long, in two rows, and the suckers are armed with eight to ten rows of hooks, all of which are about twice as large as those of the latter species, and the scolex has the appearance of being more heavily armed, while the suckers are circular in outline. The genital pores are as a rule unilateral, but in occasional specimens they are alternating. The gravid segments frequently separate at the middle, forming small windows in the posterior part of the worm.

Life-cycle. The ants *Tetramorium caespitum* and *Pheidole vinelandica* serve as hosts for the cysticercoids in North America. In Europe the ants *T. caespitum*, *T. semilaeve* and *P. pallidula* have been incriminated as vectors. Artificially infected birds passed the first ripe segments after 19–20 days.

Pathogenicity and Treatment. See pp. 108–109.

In the sub-genus *Skrjabinia* the genital pores alternate irregularly and the egg-capsules usually contain one egg each.

R. (S.) cesticillus (Molin, 1858) occurs in the small intestine of the fowl, guinea-fowl and turkey, and is cosmopolitan in distribution. It is the most commonly found member of the genus. It may grow up to 13 cm., but is usually not much over 4 cm. long. The worm is easily recognised by the absence of a neck and the large scolex which bears a wide rostellum, armed with 400–500 small hooks. The suckers are inconspicuous and unarmed. The egg-capsule contains one egg only and each egg has a diameter of 75–88 μ.

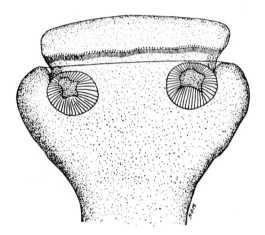

FIG. 46. *Raillietina cesticillus*, Scolex (Original)

Life-cycle. The intermediate hosts are *Musca domestica* and beetles of the genera *Calathus, Amara, Pterostichus, Bradycellus, Harpalus, Poecilus, Zabrus* (in Europe) and *Anisotarsus, Choeridium Cratacanthus, Calathus, Stenolaphus, Stenocellus, Amara* and *Selenophorus* (in North America). Development in the fowl takes 19–20 days.

Pathogenicity and Treatment. See pp. 108–109.

Quite a number of other species of this genus are known from domestic birds, but are not very common.

Genus: Cotugnia Diamare, 1893

C. digonopora (Pasquale, 1890) occurs in the small intestine of the fowl in Europe, Africa and Asia. It is up to 107 mm. long. Like the other species of this genus, it has two sets of genital organs in each segment. The rostellum bears two rows of small hooks and the suckers are unarmed.

Life-cycle—unknown.

Pathogenicity and Treatment. See pp. 108–109.

C. fastigata (Meggit, 1920), occurs in the duck in Burma and **C. cuneata** (Meggit, 1924), in the pigeon in Burma and India.

Genus: Houttuynia Fuhrmann, 1920

H. struthionis (Houttuyn, 1773) occurs in the small intestine of the ostrich. Several species of this genus have been described from the ostrich, but probably they are identical. A similar parasite occurs in the South American rhea. The worms grow up to 60 cm. long and 9 mm. wide. The scolex is 1–2 mm. wide and bears a double row of about 160 large and small hooks. The large hooks are 0·077 mm. long and the small ones 0·063 mm. The genital pores are unilateral. In the gravid segments the eggs are contained in parenchymatous capsules, about fifteen to twenty-five in each.

Life-cycle—unknown.

Pathogenicity. The parasite is seen especially in ostrich chicks, causing unthriftiness, emaciation and sometimes diarrhoea. The affected chicks are inactive, lose their appetite and often die. Numerous chicks may be lost where the infection is severe. The adult birds are frequently carriers of the infection, but rarely show any symptoms.

Treatment. No very satisfactory remedy is known, but the newer compounds such as tin dilaurate or dichlorophen (see p. 109) are indicated.

Prophylaxis. It has been found expedient in practice to raise the chicks in runs planted with lucerne as far away as possible from the adult birds. When the chicks have to run with the hen, the paddock should be cleaned of droppings daily and all insects should be exterminated.

FAMILY: DILEPIDIDAE

In this family the rostellum is usually provided with hooks, but the suckers may or may not be unarmed. Genital organs single or double. The testes are numerous. The uterus may be sac-like or branched and persist or the eggs pass into parenchymatous capsules or paruterine organs.

Genus: Amoebotaenia Cohn, 1899

A. sphenoides (Railliet, 1892) occurs in the small intestine of the fowl in most parts of the world. It is a small worm with an elongate, triangular shape, rarely over 4 mm. long and 1 mm. wide. The rostellum bears twelve to fourteen hooks with a characteristic shape and there are about twenty proglottides. The testes are twelve or more in number and lie near the posterior border of the segment. The uterus is sac-like and slightly-lobed.

Life-cycle. The intermediate hosts are earthworms of the genera *Eisenia, Pheretina Ocnerodrilus* and *Allolobophora*, in which the cysticercoid develops in about 14 days. Fowls acquire the infection frequently after rains when the earthworms come to the surface. The worms grow adult in the fowl in 4 weeks.

Pathogenicity and Treatment. See pp. 108–109.

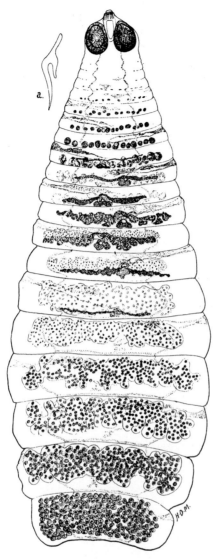

FIG. 47. *Amoebotaenia sphenoides*, Complete Specimen;
a, Rostellar hook, much enlarged (after Mönnig)

Genus: Choanotaenia Railliett, 1896

C. infundibulum (Bloch, 1779) occurs in the small intestine of the fowl and turkey. It is up to 20 cm. long and the segments are markedly wider posteriorly than anteriorly, giving the worm a characteristic shape. The scolex bears sixteen to twenty slender hooks. The genital pores alternate irregularly and open near to the anterior border of the segment. There are twenty-five to sixty testes, situated posteriorly. The uterus is persistent and strongly lobed.

Life-cycle. The intermediate hosts are the house fly, *Musca domestica,* and beetles of the genera *Geotrupes, Aphodius, Calathus* and *Tribolium.*

Tapeworm Infections of Poultry

Pathogenicity. The tapeworms most often found in poultry and related birds belong to the genera *Davainea, Raillietina, Amoebotaenia* and *Choanotaenia* and the pathogenicity of the different species varies greatly. *Davainea proglottina,* although it is the smallest, is the most harmful. It penetrates deeply into the mucosa and produces a marked enteritis, which is frequently haemorrhagic in heavy infections. *Raillietina tetragona* and *R. echinobothrida* follow next in order of pathogenicity. The young worms of the latter species penetrate with their anterior ends deeply into the

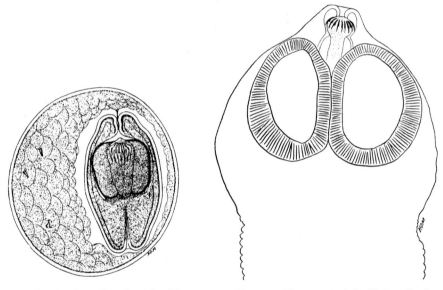

FIG. 48. *Amoebotaenia sphenoides*, Mature   FIG. 49. *Choanotaenia infundibulum*, Scolex
Cysticercoid (after Mönnig)   (Original)

mucosa and submucosa of the duodenum, causing the formation of nodules, which must be differentiated from tubercular nodules. They are visible from the peritoneal surface and contain necrotic tissue and leucocytes. During the early stages the young worms can be found hanging out into the lumen of the gut. Later the adult parasites are found in the posterior part of the small intestine. The other species are not very harmful unless the infection is severe, when marked clinical signs may be produced. *Amoebotaenia sphenoides* is practically harmless under normal conditions.

Clinical signs. Young birds are most frequently affected. They show loss of appetite, droopiness, usually thirst, emaciation and anaemia. Heavy infections may cause the death of young birds. In the case of laying birds egg-production is decreased or suspended. *Davainea proglottina* causes diarrhoea, the faeces being discoloured by blood pigments. This species and sometimes also others have been associated with nervous disorders or partial or complete paralysis but there is no strong evidence that the tapeworms are associated with such entities.

Diagnosis. The clinical signs and the presence of large numbers of tapeworm segments or eggs in the faeces will indicate the cause of the disease. A daily rhythm in the production of ripe segments has been noted in the case of *Davainea proglottina* and *Raillietina cesticillus*, the majority of segments being passed in the early part of the afternoon. It is, however, much more satisfactory to conduct an autopsy on a few representative members of the flock. Then an enteritis is evident. Nodules may be present (*R. echinobothrida*). Since *D. proglottina* is very small it is advisable to examine a sample of mucosal scraping microscopically.

Treatment. Several tin compounds have been found effective, however, di-*N*-butyl tin dilaurate is the one most commonly employed. It is highly effective against the *Raillietina* spp. when given in the food at the

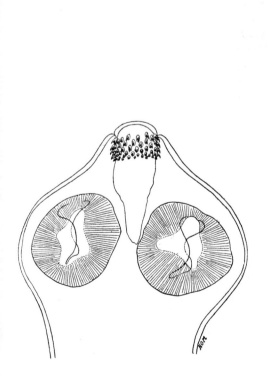
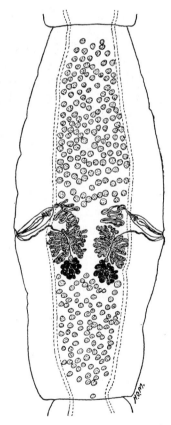

FIG. 50. *Dipylidium caninum*, Scolex (Original)

FIG. 51. *Dipylidium caninum*, Mature Proglottis (Original)

rate of 250 mg. per kg. for 48 hours, and when given at the level of 500 mg. per kg. it is also highly effective against *Davainea* and *Amoebotaenia* spp. (Edgar, 1956). Di-*N*-butyl tin oxide has been shown effective at 65 mg. per kg.

Hexachlorophene has high activity against *R. cesticillus*, a single dose of 50–100 mg. per bird being 90 per cent or more efficient. Dichlorophen has been used for the *Raillietina* spp. by Guilhon & Graber (1963) with success: 300 mg. per kg. being satisfactory for *R. tetragona* and *R. echinobothrida*, but 700–800 mg. are required for *R. cesticillus*.

Prophylaxis. As the life-cycles of the parasites indicate, birds on free range are more liable to become infected than those that are kept in pens. However, badly constructed poultry houses may allow beetles and ants to accumulate in them. As far as possible, the intermediate hosts should be exterminated. The soil may be treated with molluscicides to destroy snails or with insecticides such as benzene hexachloride, chlordone or parathion to kill the arthropod intermediate hosts.

Genus: Dipylidium Leuckart, 1863

D. caninum (Linnaeus, 1758) occurs in the small intestine of the dog, cat, fox, and occasionally in man. It has a world-wide distribution, and is the commonest tapeworm of dogs in most parts of the world. The parasite may be up to 50 cm. long, and usually has a light reddish-yellow colour. The mature, and even more the gravid, proglottides have a characteristic elongate, oval shape, resembling cucumber seeds. The rostellum bears three to four rows of small, rose-thorn-shaped hooks. Each segment contains two sets of genital organs. The numerous testes are distributed throughout the medullary parenchyma. The ovaries and vitelline gland form a mass on either side, resembling a bunch of grapes in shape. In the gravid segments the eggs lie in egg-capsules, each containing up to twenty eggs.

Several other species of the genus exist, e.g. *D. sexcoronatum* von Ratz, 1900, occurs principally in the cat and appears to be a distinct species while others *D. gracile* Millzner, 1926, *D. compactum* Millzner, 1926, *D. diffusum* Millzner, 1926, and *D. buencaminoi* Tubangui, 1925, may be synonyms of *D. caninum*.

Life-cycle. The ripe segments are voided with the faeces or they may leave the host spontaneously, as do those of some other cestodes. In the latter case the segment may crawl about actively, disseminating its eggs as it moves along. The intermediate hosts are the dog flea, *Ctenocephalides canis*, the cat flea, *C. felis*, and the human flea, *Pulex irritans*. The dog louse, *Trichodectes canis*, has also been incriminated but this is more readily a host for *D. sexcoronatum*. The larval stages of the fleas become infected by swallowing the eggs, and the cysticercoids develop in them after the fleas have reached the adult stage. The final host acquires the parasite by swallowing the infected flea, while the human cases, which occur mainly in young children, are probably due to the accidental ingestion of such fleas when the children play with dogs or cats.

Treatment. See p. 133.

Related to *Dipylidium* are the genera *Joyeuxiella* and *Diplopylidium*. Species of both these genera occur in cats. In *Joyeuxiella* the rostellum bears a large number of rows of hooks resembling those of *Dipylidium*, while *Diplopylidium* has a few rows of hooks with the guard and handle well developed. In both genera the egg-capsules contain only one egg each. They develop apparently through dung beetles, and use lizards and other reptiles as secondary intermediate hosts.

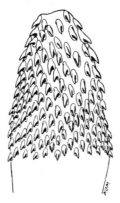

Fig. 52. *Joyeuxiella fuhrmanni*, Rostellum (Original)

Genus: Metroliasthes Ransom, 1900

M. lucida Ransom, 1900, is a rather rare parasite occurring in the small intestine of the fowl and turkey in North America, India and Africa. It is about 20 mm. long and 1·5 mm. wide. The scolex is devoid of a rostellum and hooks. The genital pores are single, irregularly alternating and often prominent. There are thirty to forty testes in each proglottis. In the gravid segments the eggs pass into a large paruterine organ. The intermediate hosts are grasshoppers of the genera *Chorthippus*, *Paroxya* and *Melanoplus*.

FAMILY: HYMENOLEPIDIDAE

These cestodes are usually provided with a rostellum which bears a single row of hooks, but the suckers are usually unarmed. The genital pores are unilateral, rarely double. The genital organs are as a rule single and the testes are few in number, mostly three per segment. The uterus is generally persistent and sac-like. The eggs are enclosed in three envelopes.

Genus: Hymenolepis Weinland, 1858

This genus contains a large number of species which occur chiefly in domestic and wild birds. They are rather difficult to distinguish, but a generic diagnosis is sufficient for most practical purposes. Further details may be found in Wardle & McLeod (1952). The worms are usually narrow and thread-like in appearance, and there are three testes in each mature segment. The ovary shows as a fourth globular body, and the cirrus-sac and receptaculum seminis may also be large.

H. lanceolata is a large species, measuring up to 130 mm. long and 18 mm. in width. The proglottides are much broader than they are long. It occurs in ducks and geese, and is one of the most harmful parasites of this group.

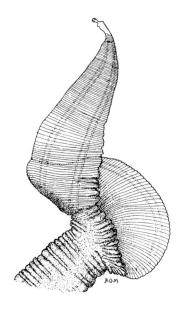

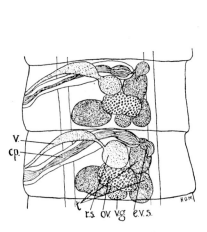

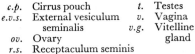

c.p.	Cirrus pouch	*t.*	Testes
e.v.s.	External vesiculum	*v.*	Vagina
	seminalis	*v.g.*	Vitelline
ov.	Ovary		gland
r.s.	Receptaculum seminis		

Fig. 53. *Hymenolepis carioca*, Mature Proglottides (Original)

Fig. 54. *Fimbriaria fasciolaris*, Scolex and Pseudoscolex (Original)

Life-cycle. The intermediate hosts are fresh-water crustacea, usually Copepoda, among which *Cyclops strenuus* has been experimentally infected.

H. carioca is one of the commonest species found in the fowl. It has an unarmed scolex and is transmitted, according to American workers, by the beetles *Aphodius granarius*, *Choeridium histeroides*, *Hister-14-striatus* and probably *Anisotarsus agilis*.

Hymenolepis diminuta. This species occurs in rats and mice and has been recorded in man. It is 2–6 cm. long or longer and the scolex has no hooks. Its intermediate hosts are the larvae, nymphs and adults of various species of moths, earwigs, cockroaches, fleas, beetles and millipedes.

Hymenolepis nana (von Siebold, 1852) (= *H. fraterna*) is the dwarf tapeworm of man, rats and mice; the entire worm is only 25–40 mm. long. A variety of it occurs in rats and mice, but human infection is usually derived from other human beings. It may be numerous and common in children. In man the oncospheres hatch out of the ingested eggs in the small intestine, penetrate into the intestinal villi and develop there, later leaving these to become attached to other villi lower down the intestine, where they develop into mature worms. Continuous heavy infection in man is explained on the basis of internal auto-infection. There is therefore no intermediate host, but it has been shown that the variety in mice can use fleas and beetles (*Tenebrio*) as intermediate hosts.

Treatment. For *H. nana* in man dithiazanine has given good results and quinacrine hydrochloride (mepacrine, Atabrine) is also effective. Filix-mas has some effect. For infections of laboratory rats or mice lead arsenates and dichlorophen may be tried and are said to be not toxic to mice. Also effective, but liable to be toxic to mice, are mepacrine, dibutyl tin dilaurate and kamala (Crowley, 1961).

Pathogenicity. Heavy infections of these parasites may cause enteritis, anorexia, headaches, anal pruritus and abdominal distress.

Genus: Fimbriaria Fröhlich, 1802

F. fascialaris (Pallas, 1781) occurs in the small intestine of the fowl, duck, goose and many wild birds. It varies in length from 25 to 425 mm. The scolex is small and provided with ten hooks, but it is usually lost and the anterior portion of the body forms a folded expansion or 'pseudo-scolex', by means of which the parasite attaches itself. Externally the body is finely segmented, but this does not correspond to the internal arrangement of the organs. The genital pores are unilateral, and there are three testes to each set of genital organs. The uterus is continuous throughout the strobila and posteriorly breaks up into tubules, which each contain several eggs. The latter measure 35–45 μ in diameter.

Life-cycle. The cysticercoid has been found in the copepods, *Diaptomus vulgaris* and *Cyclops* spp.

FAMILY: TAENIIDAE

The *Taeniidae* are usually large tapeworms. The gravid segments are longer than they are wide. The rostellum is usually armed with a double row of large and small hooks which have a characteristic shape. The genital pores are single and irregularly alternating. There are, as a rule, a large number of testes, and the ovary is situated in the posterior part of the proglottis. The uterus has a median longitudinal stem and lateral branches. The egg is usually seen in the faeces without its shell, but is surrounded by two envelopes separated by septa, so that the egg-envelope looks thick and radially striated. The larval stage is a cysticercus, a coenurus or an echinococcus (hydatid) cyst.

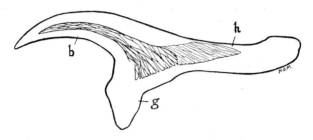

b Blade   *g* Guard   *h* Handle

FIG. 55. Rostellar Hook of a *Taenia* (Original)

Genus: Taenia Linnaeus, 1758

T. solium Linnaeus, 1758, occurs in the small intestine of man. The parasite is of veterinary importance because the larval stage is found in the pig and dog. The worm is usually 3–5 mm. long, rarely up to 8 mm. The scolex is 0·6–1 mm. wide, and the rostellum bears twenty-two to thirty-two hooks in two rows, one row of large hooks measuring 0·14–0·18 mm., and one of small hooks measuring 0·11–0·14 mm. The gravid segments are 10–12 mm. long by 5–6 mm. wide. The ovary is in the

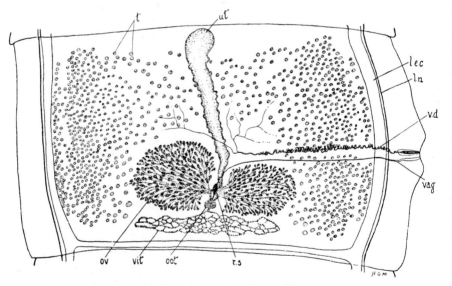

l.e.c.	Longitudinal excretory canal	*t.* Testes
l.n.	Lateral nerve	*ut.* Uterus
oot.	Oötype and Mehlis' gland	*vag.* Vagina
ov.	Ovary	*vit.* Vitellarium
r.s.	Receptaculum seminis	*v.d.* Vas deferens

FIG. 56. *Taenia solium*, Mature Proglottis (Original)

posterior third of the proglottid and has two lobes and an accessory third lobe. The uterus has seven to twelve side-branches on either side. The egg is roughly spherical, measuring 42 μ in diameter. The gravid segments, which each contain about 40,000 eggs, are frequently detached in short chains and are passed in the faeces of the host. The worm may live in man for up to 25 years, and more than one may be present in an individual.

Life-cycle. When the eggs are ingested by a pig the hexacanth embryo hatches in the intestine. The physiology of the hatching process of taeniid eggs has been reviewed by Smyth (1963). The initial mechanism consists of the release of the oncosphere which is effected by digestion of the cement substance which holds together the prismatic blocks that make up the embryophore. The conditions required to digest vary with the species of tapeworm; with *T. pisiformis*, *H. taeniaeformis* and *E. granulosus* it readily occurs in pancreatin but not pepsin though with *T. saginata* pancreatin is ineffective but hatching occurs by successive treatment of eggs with acid-pepsin and 'intestinal juice' (Silverman, 1954). Following release of the oncosphere, activation then takes place, this being dependent on the presence of bile, various bile salts being concerned in the process. The now activated embryo tears its way out of the oncospheral membrane, possibly aided by secretions from the penetration gland and then penetrates into the intestinal wall. The oncosphere finally enters the submucosal blood vessels and is carried to the liver and subsequently is disseminated throughout the body. In the case of *T. solium* the principal location of the cysticerci is the striated muscles, however, cysticerci may also develop in other organs such as lungs, liver, kidney or brain. Such cysticerci are called *Cysticercus cellulosae*. Man becomes infected with the adult worm by eating raw pork which contains viable cysticerci.

Besides the pig, a number of other animals have been mentioned as intermediate hosts, including sheep, goat, cattle, various other ruminants, horse, dog, bear and monkeys, but the identification of the cysticerci was probably erroneous in many cases. The pig is the major intermediate host of this parasite though occasionally the dog or sheep may harbour the cysticercus. The cysticercus can, however, also develop in man. Human infection with cysticerci may occur by the ingestion of eggs in contaminated food, by unclean habits such as dirty fingers being placed in the mouth or by reversed peristalsis whereby eggs in the bowel are carried forward to the duodenum or stomach and here are stimulated to hatch.

Cysticerci may be found in every organ of the body of man but are most common in the subcutaneous tissue, then the eye and then the brain. Larvae which reach the brain develop in the ventricles or superficially and frequently they become racemose in character, then being referred to as *Cysticercus racemosus*. Frequently little reaction occurs to the cysticercus while it is alive but on its death, and associated with the marked tissue reaction which occurs, a variety of CNS disorders may be evident, some of which may be rapidly fatal.

Man can therefore be both the intermediate and the definitive host of this tapeworm.

The cysticercus requires about 10 weeks for its complete development in the pig. After about 2 months the bladderworm is already infective, as the suckers and hooks are sufficiently well-developed to allow the scolex to attach itself. The fully developed cysticercus measures up to 20 by 10 mm., and contains an invaginated scolex which resembles that of the adult worm. It is situated in the intermuscular connective tissue and is surrounded by a relatively thin connective tissue capsule formed by the host. Immature cysts may be detected as early as 2 weeks after infection, however development of the scolex is required before the cysticercus is detected with ease. In meat inspection, cysts over 6 weeks of age are usually readily detected.

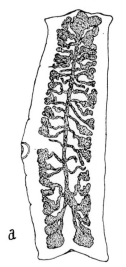
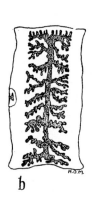

FIG. 57. Gravid Segments of a. *Taenia saginata*; b, *Taenia solium*. × 1¾ (after Mönnig)

The cysticerci are found chiefly in the muscles of the heart, tongue, forearm, thigh and neck, but may also occur in many other parts of the body. The longevity of *C. cellulosae* is not known with certainty but it probably remains viable for one or more years. In meat inspection the incidence of degenerated or calcified cysts is low, this possibly being a function of the age at which pigs are usually slaughtered.

Clinical signs. Infected pigs show no signs as a rule. Increased sensitivity of the snout, paralysis of the tongue or convulsions have been described. Dogs with cysts in the brain may show symptoms resembling those of rabies.

Diagnosis. The cysticerci can sometimes be felt under the tongue of the animal, but a negative finding is not conclusive. Most usually the infection in pigs is detected at meat inspection. Serological tests have been attempted with the swine infection but, due to non-specific reactions, are at present of very little value. In the human field serological tests have been used for the diagnosis of cerebral cysticercosis these including interfacial precipitin tests and haemagglutination tests (Biagi *et al.*, 1961).

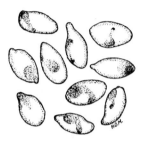

FIG. 58. *Cysticercus cellulosae*, as seen in Transmitted Light. × 1½ (Original)

This work suggested that antigens from *C. cellulosae* and *C. racemosus* were specific for their respective types of cysticercosis. Radiographic diagnosis is also employed in the human field.

Treatment and Prophylaxis. The most satisfactory compound for the human infection is *Yomesan* (5-chloro-N-(2 chloro-4-nitrophenyl) salicyclamide). It is highly effective and has low toxicity. Dichlorophen is also effective. There are no compounds which are effective against the cysticercus.

Because man acquires his infection only by consuming raw, undercooked or insufficiently cured pork or ham, and the pig is infected through the eggs passed in the faeces of infected persons, prophylaxis is a matter of education, hygiene and proper meat inspection. The parasite is consequently rare in those countries in which such measures are practised and frequent in others where the population is ignorant of the facts, facilities for meat inspection are insufficient and pigs run about freely.

Cysticercus cellulosae may be killed by freezing pork at 14–18°F continuously for 4 days, but chilling the meat at 32°F is not sufficient, and the cysts may remain viable in chilled meat for 70 days. Heating the pork at 113–122°F kills the cysts, but roasting may fail to kill cysts at the centre of a large joint. Pickling of pork may also fail to kill the cysts, especially if the pieces pickled are large. The cysts can survive for 6 weeks after the death of the host and decomposition of the pork does not necessarily kill them. Pigs may acquire massive infections, because the gravid segments of *T. solium*, unlike those of *T. saginata*, are not active and may remain in and about the faeces, so that the eggs may be concentrated in these. Stoll (1947) estimated that, at that time, about 2½ million people in the world were infected, most of them being inhabitants of Africa, Asia and the U.S.S.R. In most countries this worm is therefore of greater importance as an economic problem of the pig-breeder than as a human parasite.

Pigs should not run on free range where human excreta may be found, and all persons concerned in pig-raising should be regularly examined and treated for tapeworms if necessary.

T. saginata Goeze, 1782, occurs in the small intestine of man, while the intermedate stage is found in cattle. This worm is usually 4–8 rarely up to 15 m. long. The scolex is 1·5–2 mm. wide, and has neither rostellum nor hooks. This species is frequently placed in the sub-genus *Taeniarhynchus* because of these features. There may be one to two thousand proglottides in the chain. The gravid segments are 16–20 mm. long and 4–7 mm. wide, and contain each about 100,000 eggs. They are usually shed singly and may leave the host spontaneously, and may crawl about the body, clothes and beds of human beings. The gravid uterus has fifteen to thirty-five or more lateral branches on either side, and these branches may subdivide. The egg is roughly spherical, and measures 30–50 by 20–30 μ. Stoll (1947) estimated that about 38·9 million people in the world were infected with this species at the time when he made his estimations, most of them being inhabitants of Africa, Asia, and the U.S.S.R.

Life-cycle. This is similar to that of *T. solium*, but cattle act as intermediate hosts. Several other ruminants, including sheep, goat, llama etc., have been recorded as carriers of the bladderworm, *Cysticercus bovis*, but the correctness of at least some of the identifications is doubtful. The cysticercus has been reported in man but it is likely that the majority of such identifications are inaccuracies. It requires about 18 weeks for its complete development in the bovine, but is infective already somewhat earlier. The fully-grown bladderworm is milky-white and round or oval and measures 7·5–9 by 5·5 mm. and is usually situated in the intermuscular connective tissue, surrounded by a connective tissue capsule, however cysticerci may also occur, especially in heavy infections in other organs such as liver, lungs, kidney and abdominal fat. Cases of infection in calves suspected to have occurred before birth have been reported McManus (1960).

It has been stated in the past that the muscles of predilection are the masseters, heart, diaphragm and tongue. Apart from the heart, which usually shows some cysticerci, even in light infections the cysts may occur in any muscle of the body and there appears to be no specific predilection.

Cysticerci commence to degenerate 4–6 months after infection and by 9 months a substantial number may be dead. This depends on the mass of the original infection and also on the age of the animal when it was infected. Heavy artificial infections are usually dead and calcified by 9 months (Penfold, 1937) but with lighter infections cysticerci may remain viable for 2 years or more (see Soulsby, 1965). In East Africa viable cysticerci may remain viable in animals for up to 5 years.

Soulsby (1961) reported that a degree of immunological unresponsiveness to the infection could be induced in calves if they were infected within a few days of birth. This was indicated by a lack of the normal antibody response and a lack of immunity to re-infection when the calves were challenged with eggs 9 months after the initial infection. Calves infected at 4–6 months of age showed a good antibody response and a high order of immunity to challenge 9 months after infection.

Diagnosis is made after the animal has been slaughtered by finding the cysticerci with unarmed heads. *Ante-mortem* diagnosis is not possible except by serological methods, which are, however, not sufficiently specific to be of much value.

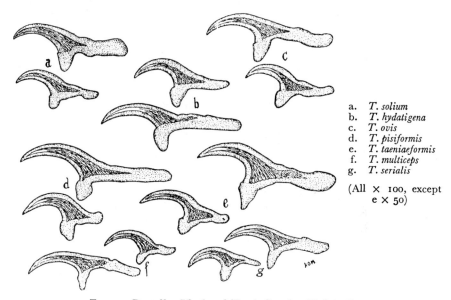

a. *T. solium*
b. *T. hydatigena*
c. *T. ovis*
d. *T. pisiformis*
e. *T. taeniaeformis*
f. *T. multiceps*
g. *T. serialis*

(All × 100, except e × 50)

Fig. 59. Rostellar Hooks of *Taenia* Species (Original)

Treatment and Prophylaxis. As in the case of *C. cellulosae*. Eggs may remain viable for 71 days in liquid manure, 16 days in city sewage, 33 days in river water and 159 days on pastures (Jepson & Roth, 1949). Australian workers quoted by Seddon (1950) found that the eggs may remain alive on pastures for at least 8 weeks and on dry, sunny pastures for 14½ weeks. Other studies have shown that eggs will live in liquid manure for more than 10 weeks and on pastures not subjected to drying for more than 20 weeks. Human manure or sewage should, therefore, not be used to manure pasture on which cattle may graze and the direct contamination of pasture by human defaecation should, if possible, be prevented. Silverman & Griffiths (1955) reviewed methods of sewage disposal in Britain in relation to the dissemination of the eggs of *T.*

saginata. They concluded that many sewage disposal plants may fail to kill the eggs and that seagulls may disseminate viable eggs of *T. saginata.* The adult tapeworm is commoner all over the world than is *T. solium,* possibly because the diagnosis of measles in cattle is more difficult than the diagnosis of *C. cellulosae* in pigs, and consequently lightly-infected carcasses are passed for human consumption. The discovery of dead or degenerate cysts by meat inspection does not guarantee that all the cysts in the carcass are dead. The cysticercus is killed by cooking *all parts* of the meat to 135°F or more, i.e. till the meat is uniformly grey, and by low temperatures which freeze the liquid in the bladder, for which up to 10 days at −8° to −10°C are necessary.

T. hydatigena Pallas, 1766 (syn. *T. marginata*) occurs in the small intestine of the dog, pine marten, stoat, weasel, polecat, related wild carnivora like the jackal, and perhaps in the cat. This is a large worm, measuring 75–500 cm. long. The rostellum bears twenty-six to forty-four hooks in two rows, the large hooks being 0·17–0·22 mm. long and the small ones 0·11–0·16 mm. The gravid segments measure 10–14 by 4–7 mm., and the uterus has five to ten branches on either side. The elliptical eggs measure 38–39 by 34–35 μ.

It must be pointed out that the identification of the *Taenia* species of Carnivora is not an easy matter and should be left to a specialist.

Life-cycle. The intermediate stage is known as *Cysticercus tenuicollis* and occurs normally in the peritoneal cavity of sheep, goat, cattle, pig, squirrel, hamster and wild ruminants. It has also been recorded from the dog, cat, rodents, monkeys and man, but the correctness of these latter records is uncertain. The hexacanth embryos, after hatching in the intestine, reach the liver via the blood and break out of the portal vessels. Occasionally they may pass into the posterior vena cava and be transported to other parts of the body, but usually they burrow small channels in the liver parenchyma, eventually reaching the surface of that organ, and enter the peritoneal cavity after about 3–4 weeks. The stages in the liver may measure up to 8·5 by 5 mm. and resemble unripe cucumber seeds. There is an invagination at one end, but the scolex is not yet developed. The adult bladderworm may be found anywhere in the abdominal cavity, lying in a delicate cyst formed by the peritoneum. The vesicle may be 5 cm. or more in diameter and contains a watery fluid and a scolex invaginated into a long neck. The final host becomes infected by ingesting the cysticercus.

Pathogenicity and Symptoms. The effects of the adult parasite resemble those of other adult Taenias (see page 133), but the cysticerci may cause a serious disease. They break down the liver parenchyma during their migration, causing haemorrhages and leaving behind them a track of detritus. A few larvae cause no appreciable damage nor clinical signs, but in heavy infections the liver lesions may be so extensive or the haemorrhages so severe that the animal dies. Peritonitis is frequently present. The condition is usually seen only in young animals. The course of the disease may be so acute that hardly any clinical signs are seen. In less rapidly fatal cases the animal is markedly depressed, weak, and the appetite is lost. If peritonitis develops, the temperature is elevated and ascites may be present. The adult cysticercus usually causes no harm to the host. Sweatman & Plummer (1957) studied the biology and pathological effects of this species in lambs and swine.

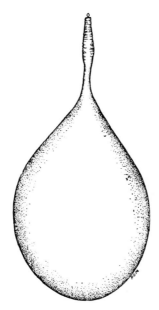

FIG. 60. *Cysticercus tenuicollis* with the Head Everted; Natural Size (Original)

Post Mortem. The main lesions are seen in the liver, which shows on section, and frequently also on the uneven surface, a number of dark-red foci and streaks which have a diameter of about 2 mm. The organ may be fragile in consistence and the young worms are found in the burrows. Lesions associated with peritonitis may be present. Foci of bronchopneumonia and pleuritis have been described, being due to young cysticerci which entered the lungs.

Prophylaxis. Hepatitis cysticercosa cannot be treated except by nursing the animal. The condition should be prevented by regular treatment of dogs for tapeworms (see p. 133) and by destroying cysticerci found in slaughtered animals.

T. pisiformis (Bloch, 1780) (syn. *T. serrata*) occurs in the small intestine of the dog, fox, several wild Carnivora and rarely the cat. It may grow up to 200 cm. long. The rostellum bears thirty-four to forty-eight hooks in two rows, the large hooks being 0·225- 0·294 mm. long and the small ones 0·132–0·177 mm. The gravid segments measure 8–10 by

4–5 mm., and the uterus has eight to fourteen lateral branches on either side. The elliptical eggs measure 37 by 32 μ.

Life-cycle. Similar to that of *T. hydatigena*, but the intermediate hosts in this case are rodents, chiefly rabbits and hares. The young stages, after having developed in the liver for about 15–30 days, penetrate through the parenchyma of this organ and the adult bladderworm is found in the peritoneal cavity attached to the viscera. It is a small cyst, about the size of a pea.

Pathogenicity and Symptoms. The effects of the adult parasites resemble those of other adult Taenias, but heavy infections with the cysticerci may cause hepatitis, as in the case of *C. tenuicollis*. The affected animal may die suddenly, or in more chronic cases it is inactive and emaciation develops as the result of digestive disturbances.

Prophylaxis. Where rabbits are bred, dogs should not have access to uncooked meat or offal derived from them. Similarly dogs should not be allowed to contaminate rabbit food.

T. ovis (Cobbold, 1869) occurs in the small intestine of the dog and fox in many parts of the world. It grows to about 1 m. in length. The rostellum bears twenty-four to thirty-six hooks, of which the large ones are 0·156–0·188 mm. long and the small ones 0·096–0·128 mm. The uterus in the gravid proglottides has twenty to twenty-five lateral branches on either side. The oval eggs measure 34 by 24–28 μ.

Life-cycle. Similar to that of *C. cellulosae*. The cysticercus, *C. ovis*, found in sheep and goats, mainly under the epicardium and the pleura of the diaphragm, but also in other muscles and organs. It grows mature in about 3 months and is about the same size as *C. cellulosae*. The tapeworm grows adult in the dog in 7 weeks.

Pathogenicity. The parasite is not very frequent and its main significance is that the cysticercus may be mistaken for *C. cellulosae*. This probably accounts for some of the records of the pork measle in sheep.

Hydatigera taeniaeformis (Batsch, 1786) (syn. *T. crassicollis*) occurs in the small intestine of the cat and other related carnivores, including the stoat, the fox and the lynx (*Lynx unita*), and is of cosmopolitan distribution. It is 50–60 cm. long and has a characteristic appearance on account of the absence of a neck and the bell-shaped posterior proglottides. The scolex is 1·7 mm. wide and bears a large rostellum with twenty-six to fifty-two, usually thirty-four, hooks. The large hooks are 0·38–0·42 mm. long and the small ones 0·25–0·27 mm. The suckers are prominent, facing outwards and forwards. The spherical eggs measure 31–37 μ in diameter.

Life-cycle. The bladderworm stage, *Cysticercus fasciolaris*, develops in the livers of the intermediate hosts, which are rodents, chiefly rats and mice, and also the rabbit, the squirrel and the muskrat. The vesicle is small and the scolex is not invaginated, but is connected to the vesicle by a segmented strobila, so that the whole larva looks like a small tapeworm (strobilocercus). When the cysticercus is ingested by the final host the vesicle and a fraction of the strobila are digested off and the remaining part of the strobila with its attached scolex develop in 42 days or so into the adult tapeworm.

Pathogenicity. The tapeworm penetrates with its head deeply into the mucosa, even causing perforation in rare cases. It has been described as causing severe digestive disturbance. The cysticercus appears to be fairly harmless, at least in rats, even when it occurs in large numbers. It has been associated with malignant growths in the liver of rats.

T. krabbei Moniez, 1789, is a tapeworm of the dog occurring in northern countries. The intermediate stage, *Cysticercus tarandi*, is found in the muscles of reindeer. The worm is about 26 cm. long or longer. There are twenty-six to thirty-four hooks, the large ones being 0·148–0·17 mm. long and the small ones 0·085–0·12 mm. The mature segments are much broader than long, and the organs are compressed and transversely elongated. The uterus has nine to ten lateral branches on either side.

Genus: Multiceps Goeze, 1782

The only constant difference between this genus and the genus *Taenia* is the fact that the larval stage of species of the genus *Multiceps* produces numerous, single tapeworm heads on the inner wall of the bladderworm (Fig. 61), which is called a *Coenurus*.

M. multiceps (Leske, 1780) occurs in the small intestine of the dog, coyote, fox and jackal, and is found in most parts of the world. It is 40–100 cm. long and has a small head, 0·8 mm. in diameter. There are twenty-two to thirty-two hooks: the large ones are 0·15–0·17 mm. long and the small ones 0·09–0·13 mm. The gravid segments measure 8–12 by 3–4 mm., and the uterus has nine to twenty-six lateral branches on either side. The eggs have a diameter of 29–37 μ.

Life-cycle. The intermediate stage, *Coenurus cerebralis*, develops in the brain and spinal cord of the sheep, goat, cattle, horse and other ungulates and has also been found in man. The embryos, after hatching in the intestine, pass via the bloodstream to various parts of the body. Only those that reach the central nervous system will develop; the others soon die off. The young cysts wander about in the brain before settling down and are fully developed in 7–8 months. The fully grown cyst measures 5 cm. or more in diameter. It has a delicate, translucent wall, and bears on its inner surface a number of heads which may amount to several hundred, and each resembles the scolex of the adult worm. The final host acquires the infection by ingesting the bladderworm, and all or most of the fully formed heads develop into tapeworms.

Pathogenesis and Clinical signs. The effects of the adults resemble those of adult Taenias, but the coenurus stage causes the disease called 'gid', 'sturdy', 'staggers' etc. in sheep and calves. From about 1 to 3 weeks after infection, when the young worms wander about in the brain, the sheep may show an elevated temperature and other signs associated with a cortical encephalitis or meningitis. This will, however, happen only when several parasites invade the brain simultaneously, and in many cases these preliminary signs do not appear. Quite exceptionally an animal may die at this stage owing to a very severe infection.

The characteristic clinical signs of the disease are seen from about 2 to 7 months after infection. The animal performs forced movements, vary-

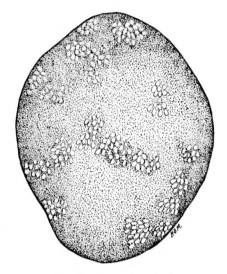

FIG. 61. *Caenurus cerebralis*

ing in nature with the position of the parasite in the central nervous system. Most frequently the cyst is situated in the parietal region on the surface of one of the cerebral hemispheres. The animal then holds its head to one side and turns in a circle towards the affected side. Many such sheep are blind in the eye on the opposite side. If the parasite is lodged in the anterior part of the brain, the head is held against the chest and the animal steps high ('trotters'), or it may walk in a straight line until it meets an obstacle and then remain motionless for a time. The cyst may also occur in a ventricle, in which case the movements are to some extent the reverse of those described. If the cyst presses on the cerebellum, the animal is in a hyperaesthetic condition, easily frightened, and it has a jerky or staggering gait in the hind legs which gradually grows worse and finally leads to prostration. The sight of the animal and the expression of its eyes are frequently affected, and grinding of the teeth, salivation, complete loss of balance and convulsions may be seen. All these may be intermittent. Sometimes the cyst is localised in the lumbar region of the spinal cord, causing progressive paresis of one or

PLATE I

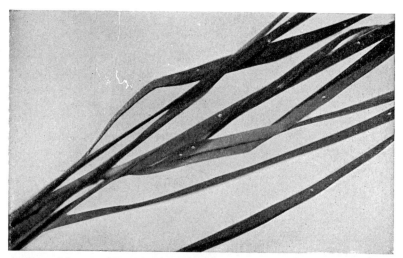

A. Cercarial cysts of *Fasciola hepatica* (about 0·2 mm in diameter) attached to blades of grass. A mucoid substance secreted by the cystogenous cells forms a cyst wall round the cercaria and attaches it firmly to vegetation. (H. Thornton)

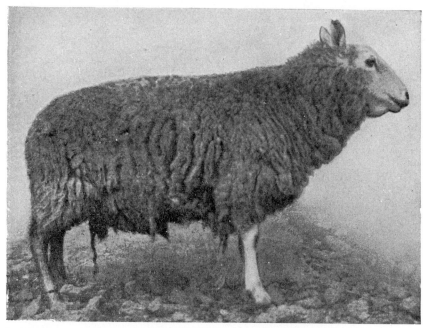

B. Half-bred ewe showing oedema of throat ('bottle neck') and dry, loose wool. the result of liver fluke infestation. Similar symptoms may be seen in severe roundworm infestation of the stomach and intestines. (W. Lyle Stewart)

PLATE II

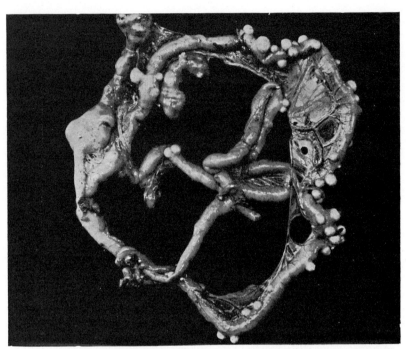

Nodular tapeworm disease of small intestine of fowl caused by *Raillietina echinobothrida*. (K. D. Downham)

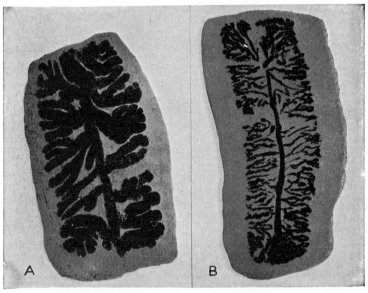

A. Segment of *Taenia solium*; and B, segment of *Taenia saginata*, showing gravid uteri and their lateral branches. × 6. (Dr. A. Jepsen)

PLATE III

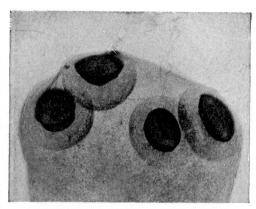

A. Microphotograph of the head of *Taenia saginata* showing elliptical suckers and absence of rostellum and hooklets. × 80. (Dr. J. F. Brailsford)

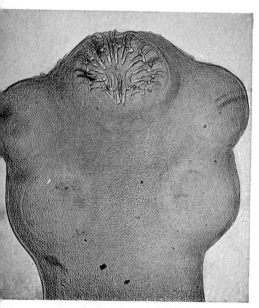

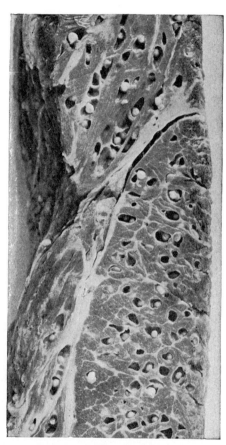

Microphotograph of scolex of *Cysticercus cellulosae* wing four suckers and rostellum of hooklets. × 100. (Dr. J. F. Brailsford)

C. Pork showing extensive invasion of muscle by *Cysticercus cellulosae*. Fibrous capsules have formed round the cysts and remain patent when the cyst is removed. The rounded white cysts contain the invaginated scolices. Natural size. (Dr. J. F. Brailsford)

PLATE IV

A. Degenerated cysts of *Cysticercus bovis* in wall of left ventricle of ox heart. One cyst, indicated by arrow, is visible beneath the epicardium. (E. F. McCleery)

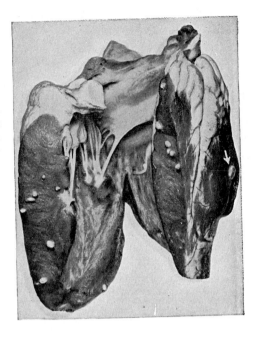

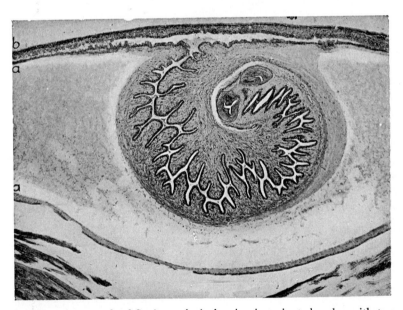

B. Microphotograph of *Cysticercus bovis* showing invaginated scolex with two suckers apparent; (a,a) tail bladder; (b) connective tissue capsule. × 28. (H. Thornton)

PLATE V

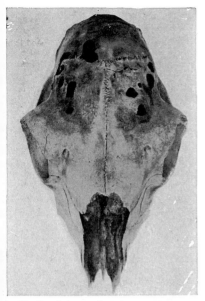

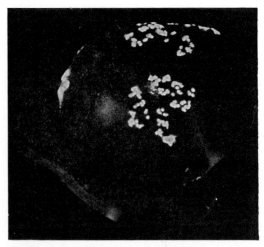

B. *Multiceps multiceps* cyst removed from sheep brain illustrated in C. Numerous scolices are seen as white clusters on the inner wall of the cyst. × 2. (W. P. Blount)

A. Skull of sheep showing perforation caused by *Multiceps multiceps*. (Original)

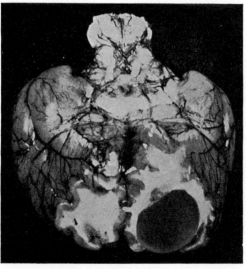

C. Brain of sheep affected with sturdy. The base of the brain is uppermost, and one large *Multiceps multiceps* cyst can be seen in the region of the olfactory bulb of the left cerebral hemisphere. Cysts in this position are usually manifested by symptoms of forward movements with strongly flexed head. (W. P. Blount)

PLATE VI

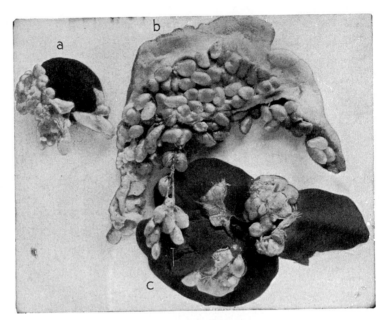

A. Abdominal viscera of rabbit showing subserous distribution of cysts
of *Cysticercus pisiformis* in (a) kidney; (b) omentum; (c) liver. (Dr. J. F.
Brailsford)

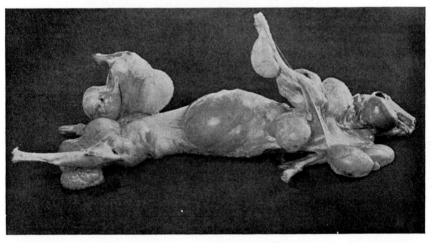

B. Rabbit extensively affected with *Multiceps serialis* cysts. (Crown copyright)

PLATE VII

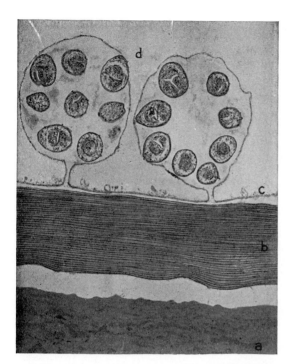

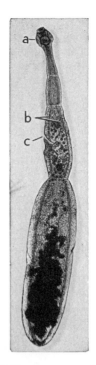

A. Microphotograph of wall of a fertile hydatid cyst from sheep liver. (a) Connective tissue capsule formed by reaction of host; (b) external cuticular membrane; (c) internal germinal layer attached to which are (d) two brood capsules each containing eight scolices. × 50. (H. Thornton)

B. *Echinococcus granulosus:* (a) Head with four suckers and double crown of hooklets; (b) excretory canal of second segment; (c) genital pore. The black mass in the terminal segment is the uterus filled with ripe ova. × 11. (H. Thornton)

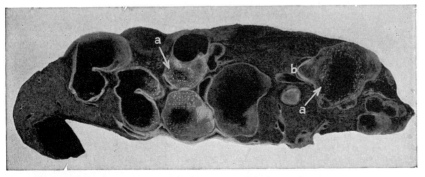

C. Section of sheep liver showing fertile hydatid cysts. The white spots on the germinal layer at (a,a) are brood capsules and at (b) a growing cyst is assuming an irregular shape as it orientates round a bile duct. (H. Thornton)

PLATE VIII

Extensive infestation of small intestine of pig with *Ascaris lumbricoides* (var. *suis*). A, Unopened intestine; B, same intestine opened. The presence of the parasites in the intestine is frequently associated with a reddish slime and a distinctive odour on the wall of the intestine. (Dr. A. Jepsen)

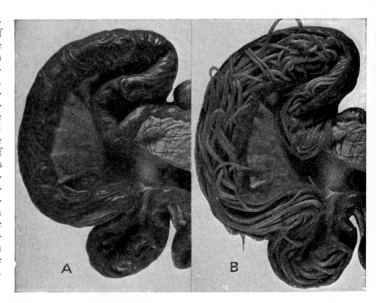

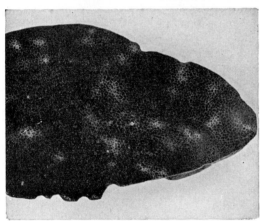

C. Lobe of pig liver, anterior surface, showing numerous milk spots caused by larvae of *Ascaris lumbricoides* (var. *suis*).
(H. Thornton)

D. Two pigs from same litter and aged $5\frac{1}{4}$ months; the pig on the left is stunted by severe *Ascaris* infection. (R. Daubney)

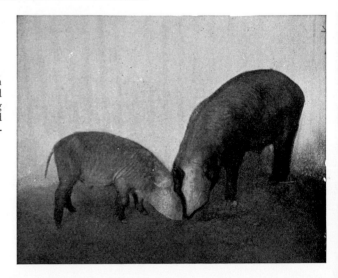

both hind limbs and of the pelvic organs. The animal soon becomes indifferent to food and water, wanders from the flock, and eventually dies of emaciation or through direct affection of a vital nerve centre.

If the parasite is situated on the surface of the brain, the skull undergoes pressure atrophy, even to the extent of perforation, so that on examination the affected part can be localised, as it yields to pressure. Such manipulation causes pain and may incite a spell of clinical signs.

Diagnosis. The clinical signs must be differentiated from those caused by blindness and other conditions affecting the brain, like a depressed fracture of the skull, meningitis, tumours, abscesses, poisoning by certain plants (e.g. *Matricaria nigellaefolia*, which causes 'pushing disease' in cattle), louping ill and heartwater, for which the history of the case, locality etc., are of great importance. It is frequently, however, not possible to arrive at a definite diagnosis except by conducting a *post mortem* examination.

Post mortem. Animals which die in the early stages show an inflammation of the meninges and a number of sinuous tracks on the surface of the brain, at the ends of which the young bladderworms can be found.

Animals which die in the later stages of the disease are emaciated and may be anaemic. One or more coenuri may be found on or in the brain, often lying in a cavity produced by pressure and surrounded by necrotic material. Or they may be found in the vertebral canal, especially in the lumbar, cervical or medullary regions. There may be local pressure atrophy or perforation of the skull. In old cases the cyst has sometimes degenerated and can be identified only by finding the hooks.

Treatment. If the cyst is situated on the surface of the brain and can be located, especially by palpation, it can be removed after trephining or by means of a special trocar and cannula. In other cases treatment is useless and the animal should be slaughtered before it becomes too emaciated.

Prophylaxis. The bladderworms found in carcasses of affected animals should be destroyed, to prevent the final hosts from eating them. It is advisable to kill infected sheep, as they are easy prey for wild Carnivora and serve to spread the infection. Dogs should be treated regularly for tapeworms and wild Carnivora, which may act as intermediate hosts, should be destroyed. It is probable that in some countries the infection is kept going between antelopes and carnivores, since occasionally epizootics of gid are seen in sheep even where no dogs are present.

Multiceps gaigeri Hall, 1916, occurs in the small intestine of the dog in various parts of the world. It measures up to 182 cm. in length, and the rostellum bears twenty-eight to thirty-two hooks. The large ones are 0·16—0·18 mm. long and the small ones 0·115–0·15 mm. The gravid uterus has twelve to fifteen lateral branches on either side.

Life-cycle. The intermediate stage, which is a coenurus, resembles *Coenurus cerebralis*, and is of about the same size and appearance; it

6

develops in the intermuscular connective tissue, nervous system and other organs of the goat.

Pathogenicity. The parasite is not very common and has little significance. When it occurs in the central nervous system it may cause gid.

Multiceps serialis Gervais, 1847, is a tapeworm of the dog and fox and has a cosmopolitan distribution. It grows to a length of 72 cm. and the scolex bears two rows of twenty-six to thirty-two hooks. The large hooks are 0·135–0·175 mm. long and the small ones 0·078–0·12 mm. The gravid uterus has twenty to twenty-five lateral branches on either side. The elliptical eggs measure 31–34 by 29–30 μ.

It is not easy to differentiate the various species of the genus *Multiceps* and Clapham (1942) has suggested that they be classified together as *Taenia (Multicep) multiceps*. In addition she envisages that the coenurus stage can occur in the CNS, connective tissue, abdominal cavity and elsewhere, the form adopted in any host being an individual characteristic.

Life-cycle. The intermediate stage, *Coenurus serialis*, develops in the intermuscular connective tissue of the hare, rabbit, coypu and squirrel and has also been found in man. The full-grown cyst is usually ovoid in shape and about 4 cm. long, but may be larger. It develops a number of scolices, which are arranged in lines radiating from a centre and are invaginated into their necks. Internal as well as external daughter bladders may be formed, and these are also able to produce scolices. The dog acquires the infection by eating the raw flesh of infected rodents.

Pathogenesis. This multiceps is not very pathogenic, but severe infections in fur-bearing animals may be important.

Treatment and Prophylaxis. Dogs and foxes can be treated for the tapeworm (see p. 133) and dogs should not have access to places where fur-bearing rodents are bred. Infected rodents must not be fed to the final hosts.

Genus: Echinococcus Rudolphi, 1801

Echinococcus granulosus (Batsch, 1786). This species is found in the small intestine of the dog, dingo (*Canis dingo*), jackal (*C. aureus*) and wolf (*C. lupus*). The coyote (*C. latrans*) may become infected but it is a poor host. In the past it was considered that the fox was also a host for *E. granulosus*, however such reports almost certainly refer to *Echinococcus multitocularis* (see below). Gemmel (1959) attempted to infect foxes (*Vulpes vulpes*) with dog material and although some became infected with very light burdens (maximum forty-five compared with 14,493 in dog controls) ova were never produced in the infected foxes. Odd infections have been reported in other fox species such as *V. fulva* in Canada and *V. corsac* in the Soviet Union. The host range of *E. granulosus* and the biochemical basis for the specificity is discussed by Smyth (1964).

Studies of *E. granulosus* by Sweatman & Williams (1963), Williams & Sweatman (1963) and Dailey & Sweatman (1965) have resulted in these authors dividing the species into a number of sub-species. The criteria for this are morphological and biological. The sub-species described are *E. granulosus granulosus* (cosmopolitan distribution; cysts in sheep, bovine, pig and white mice), *E. granulosus canadensis* (dog and reindeer in North Western Canada; poor or no development of cysts in sheep, pigs or mice)

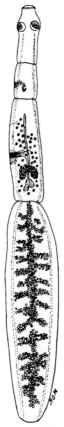

FIG. 62. *Echinococcus granulosus*, Entire Specimen (Original)

E. granulosus borealis (timber wolves and moose, also deer in boreal North America; poor development of cysts in sheep and mice) and *E. granulosus equinus* (probably cosmopolitan; in dogs and horses; cysts rarely develop in sheep but do in mice). The detailed morphology of the sub-species is given by the above authors.

The typical description of *E. granulosus* is as follows. It is $2 \cdot 1$–$5 \cdot 02$ μ long and usually has only three proglottids, the terminal one being usually more than half the length of the whole worm. The sexually mature segment is the penultimate one, the gravid one being the last segment. The scolex has two rows of hooklets, varying from thirty to sixty in number, the large ones being $33 \cdot 2$–$39 \cdot 8$ μ and the smaller ones $22 \cdot 1$–34 μ long. The genital pores alternate irregularly and are usually behind the middle of the proglottid, seldom at its middle. There are thirty-eight to fifty-two testes in each segment. The ovary is not acinous and is kidney-shaped. The uterus of the gravid segment has lateral diverticula. The eggs are the typical *Taenia* eggs and they measure 32–36 by 25–30 μ. The embryonic egg shell is slightly ovoid.

Life-cycle. After the eggs have been ingested by the intermediate host they hatch in the intestine and the embryos migrate to the blood stream, which carries them to various organs. The intermediate hosts include man, domestic mammals as well as numerous wild mammals. An extensive intermediate host list is given by Smyth (1964). The dog is only very rarely an intermediate host, this possibly being associated with the composition of dog bile (see Smyth, 1963). The embryo grows into a large vesicle, 5–10 cm. or more in diameter, known as an echinococcus or 'hydatid' cyst. Although this is the more usual size, much larger cysts

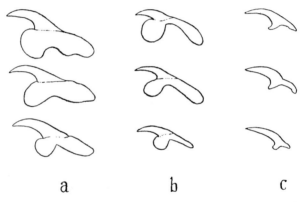

a   b   c

FIG. 63. Rostellar Hooks of *Echinococcus granulosus*: *a*, Large hooks; *b*, small hooks; *c*, hooks from bladderworm (Original)

have been found in man. One of the largest of these was 50 cm. (20 in.) in diameter and contained 3½ gallons of fluid. Typical hydatid cysts have a fairly thick cuticle, concentrically laminated, and an internal germinal layer. The latter produces numerous small vesicles or brood capsules about 5–6 months after infection, and scolices are formed in these and perhaps also on the germinal layer directly. Each brood capsule may contain up to forty scolices invaginated into their neck portions and attached to the wall by stalks. The scolices and their stalks are covered by a cuticular layer. The brood capsules may become detached from the wall of the vesicle and float freely in the vesicular fluid, giving rise to the term 'hydatid sand'. They may rupture and turn inside out. The final host acquires the infection by ingesting fertile hydatids. Factors, such as the biochemistry of the bile, which determine host specificity of *E. granulosus* are extensively discussed by Smyth & Haslewood (1963). The worm grows adult in the dog in 6–7 weeks.

All hydatid cysts do not form scolices; a large percentage are frequently sterile. In cattle 90 per cent may be sterile, in pigs about 20 per cent, and in sheep 8 per cent.

The hydatid cyst is filled with a clear to pale yellow fluid containing from 17 mg. to over 200 mg. of protein per 100 ml. There is a striking similarity of proteins of hydatid fluid to those of the serum of the host (Goodchild & Kagan, 1961). Cysts in liver may contain bile pigments while those in the kidney may contain traces of urine. A more detailed consideration of the chemical composition and metabolism of the cyst and the scolices is given by Smyth (1964). Cysts have been found in practically all organs, but in domestic animals they occur chiefly in the lungs and liver.

The cyst is normally spherical in shape, but its shape depends on the organ in which it grows, because it is moulded by resistant tissues; for instance, in the liver by the bile ducts. An echinococcus cyst growing in bone is a reticular structure which fills the Haversian and marrow canals. It causes erosion of the bone and may predispose to fracture. Such cysts usually do not form scolices except where they reach the surface and are able to grow normally.

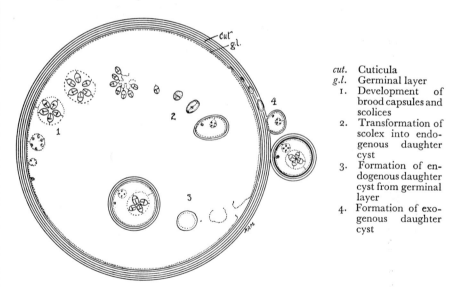

cut. Cuticula
g.l. Germinal layer
1.   Development of brood capsules and scolices
2.   Transformation of scolex into endogenous daughter cyst
3.   Formation of endogenous daughter cyst from germinal layer
4.   Formation of exogenous daughter cyst

FIG. 64. *Echinococcus granulosus*, Diagrammatic Representation of a Hydatid Cyst (Original)

Multiplication of the echinococcus can take place in various ways. Endogenous daughter cysts may be formed from detached fragments of the germinal layer or from brood capsules or scolices, the latter being able to undergo regressive changes and develop into cysts. The daughter cyst is covered with cuticle and lined with a germinal layer and it can produce brood capsules, scolices and granddaughter cysts, like the

original bladder. Exogenous daughter cysts are formed by budding out-
ward. This usually happens when a piece of the germinal layer becomes
enclosed in the cuticle due to uneven growth. As the cuticle is shed on
the outside and formed inside, the enclosed tissue will gradually move
outwards and there give rise to a new bladder.

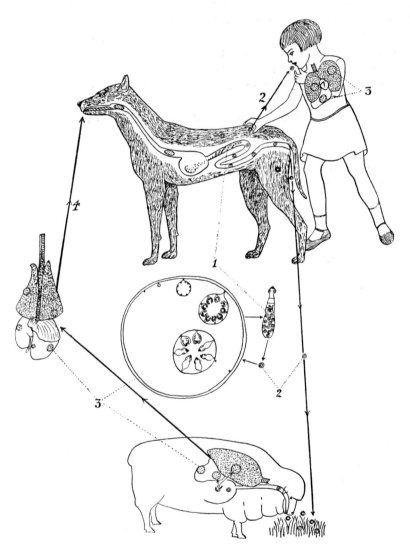

FIG. 65. *Echinococcus granulosus*, Life-cycle (Original)

The cyst may burst into a cavity—for instance, the peritoneum—and
the liberated scolices, brood capsules and germinal layer can all form
new bladders.

Pathogenicity. The adult tapeworm is comparatively harmless to the dog, except when it occurs in large numbers, in which case a marked enteritis may be produced.

The harmfulness of the hydatid cyst naturally depends on the organ in which it is situated and the severity of the infection. As the cysts gradually increase in size they may impair the health of the host and cause dyspnoea when they occur in the lungs, or digestive disturbances and possibly ascites when the liver is infected. In domestic animals disease due to hydatid cysts is rare, but in the human being it is more dangerous on account of the frequent development of exogenous daughter cysts which escape into the peritoneal cavity from the liver, or leakage from primary cysts, both giving rise to multiple omental cysts. The significance of domestic animals as hosts of this parasite is therefore mainly that they act as reservoirs of the infection for man.

Diagnosis of hydatid infection in animals is rarely made in the living subject. When the liver is infected it may be enlarged and a fluctuating cyst may be determined by percussion. In the lungs percussion may also lead to the detection of a cyst. Immunodiagnostic tests are widely used in human medicine. The more recent ones are the haemagglutination and flocculation techniques, but complement fixation and skin tests are still widely used. The haemagglutination test is very sensitive, cyst fluid from swine being the antigen of choice. In a low percentage of patients positive reactions may occur in the absence of hydatid infection, this being due to auto-antibodies induced by hepatic disease which cross react with host antigens in the cyst fluid.

Immunology. Extensive analyses of the hydatid cyst have been carried out using gel precipitation and immuno-electrophoretic techniques. Twenty-three different hydatid antigens have been detected so far, but it is unlikely that these represent the whole array. Kagan & Norman (1963), in an analysis of these reported four of parasite origin, six of host origin and thirteen of undetermined origin.

Early studies of vaccination were carried out by Turner *et al.* (1935, 1936) who reported successful immunisation of dogs against the adult tapeworm with hydatid cyst material. More recent work by Gemmel (1962) has indicated that good immunity can be induced by the injection of hatched oncospheres into dogs.

Treatment and Prophylaxis. Compounds of value for *E. granulosus* are discussed on p. 133.

For the treatment of infections with hydatid cysts the only method known is surgical removal of them, when this is possible.

Preventive measures include regular treatment of dogs for tapeworms and the destruction of hydatids found in slaughtered animals. It should be borne in mind that wild Carnivora in zoological gardens and menageries may be a great danger when infected with *Echinococcus* tapeworms, and all meat fed to them should be carefully inspected. Dogs should get no raw offal to eat. Particular attention should be given to sheepdogs, and persons handling sheep must remember that the *Echinococcus* eggs tend to stick to the fleece, from which they may be transferred to human beings.

E. multilocularis (Leuckart, 1863) Vogel, 1955. According to Vogel (1957) this species includes *E. sibiricensis* which is considered to be a sub-species or geographical race of *E. multilocularis*. *E. multilocularis* differs from *E. granulosus* as follows:

(a) It is rather smaller, its length varying from 1·2 to 3·7 mm.; (b) it has three to five proglottids, the terminal one measuring less than half the length of the whole worm; (c) the sexually mature segment is the third; (d) the hooks are smaller and differ in shape; (e) the genital pore is in front of the middle of each segment; (f) there are fewer (fourteen to thirty-one) testes; (g) the ovary is acinous and has two lobes united by a small isthmus; (h) the uterus of the gravid segment has no lateral diverticula; (i) the range of definitive hosts is wider, the adult worm being found in the small intestine of the dog, fox and house cat.

In Alaska the Arctic fox (*Alopex lagopus*) and the dog are definitive hosts.

The intermediate host in Southern Europe is the field mouse *Microtus arvalis* while in the Alaskan region the tundra vole (*Microtus oeconomus*), the ground squirrel (*Clitellus undulatus*), the shrew (*Sorex jacksoni*) and the field mouse (*Clethrionomys tutilis*) serve as such. Monkeys and pigs have been infected experimentally.

Man is infected with the hydatid stage of *E. multilocularis* by the ingestion of eggs in the faeces of the definitive host which have contaminated such things as fruit and vegetables. Thus foxes hunt mice and rodents in woods, fruit gardens and orchards and wind-fall fruit and berries provide vehicles for infection. In the Alaskan area the close association of man with his sledge dogs and hunting dogs permits contamination of food and drink and trappers may become infected when the pelt of a fox is being removed.

Pathogenesis, Prophylaxis and Treatment. The hydatid cyst is usually found in the liver of man, but it may attack the lungs or other organs. Its slow infiltration of the organs attacked may cause symptoms resembling those of a slow-growing carcinoma. Because the cyst is not encapsulated, its surgical removal is difficult or impossible and the prognosis is usually grave. No effective drug treatment is known. In areas in which the infection is endemic measures should be taken to avoid the ingestion, especially by children, of soil contaminated by the faeces of dogs, foxes and wolves.

Other species of Echinococcus. Several other species have been described and these include *E. oligarthus* (Diesing, 1863) found in the jaguar and puma in South America, *E. lycaontes* Ortlepp, 1934, from the cape hunting dog (*Lycaon pictus*) in South Africa, *E. felidis* Ortlepp, 1934, from the lion in South Africa and *E. cameroni* Ortlepp, 1934, also from the lion in South Africa. A detailed consideration of these and other species is given by Sweatman & Williams (1963) and Smyth & Smyth (1964).

TAPEWORM INFECTIONS OF DOGS AND CATS

Pathogenesis. In general, adult cestodes are not very harmful to dogs and cats. The clinical signs are vague consisting of mild gastro-intestinal upsets but in heavy infections of young animals there may be persistent diarrhoea, possibly alternating with constipation. Gravid segments may migrate through the anal sphincter and then migrate in the perianal region. The gravid segments of *D. caninum* may undulate around on the dog's coat or on carpets for some time after passing from the dog. Irritation of the anal sphincter may occur inducing the dog to drag its anus over the ground.

D. caninum infection of children has been reported; usually only one worm is present and may be associated with mild gastro-intestinal upsets.

Diagnosis. Gravid segments are usually seen in the faeces. These should be examined to determine the genus of the parasite. In the absence of gravid segments the faeces should be examined by flotation techniques after thorough mixing of the sample to disperse any eggs present. Though the eggs of *D. caninum* can be readily recognised by the 'egg nests' the eggs of the *Taenia* spp. cannot be easily differentiated and for practical purposes a diagnosis of *Taenia* spp. is all that can be made. This is based on general size and the possession of a striated 'shell'.

A positive diagnosis of *E. granulosus* is made following purgation with arecoline at a dose of 0·5–1·0 grains per dog. The evacuated faeces are examined under low power for the minute tapeworms.

Treatment. A wide range of compounds is now available for treatment.

Arecoline hydrobromide. Given orally at the rate of 1–2 mg. per kg. Prior fasting is advised and treatment may be followed with an enema. It is unsafe for cats. Efficacy 90–100 per cent for common *Taenia* spp. and *D. caninum*, similarly against *E. granulosus*.

Arecoline acetarsol (Nemural: 3-acetylamino-4-hydroxyphenylarsonic acid N-methyl-tetrahydro-1-methylnicotinate). Given orally at the rate of 1 mg. per kg. Unsafe for cats under 6 months and puppies under 3 months. Generally effective against the common tapeworms and good action against *E. granulosus*. The drug produces purgation and when this does not occur the anthelmintic action is poor.

Dichlorophen (5:5'-dichloro-2:2' dihydroxydiphenylmethane). Given orally at the rate of 200 mg. per kg. No dietary restrictions are necessary with its use. Highly effective against the common tapeworms. Activity against *E. granulosus* poor.

Anthelin (N-methyl-tetrahydromethylnicotinate-*p*-carboxyphenylstibonic acid). Given orally at a dose of 10 mg. per kg. Good effect against the common tapeworms. Action variable against *E. granulosus* but generally equal to Arecoline hydrobromide. Vomiting may occur following treatment.

Yomesan (5-chloro-N-(2 chloro-4-nitrophenyl) salicylamide). Given orally at the rate of 50 mg. per kg. Higher doses may be used with safety. The compound is highly effective against the common tapeworms. Higher doses (300 mg. per kg.) are necessary for a satisfactory effect against *E. granulosus*.

Bunamidine hydrochloride (Scoloban) is a recently developed compound for the treatment of tapeworms in dogs and cats. It has high efficiency against the common *Taenia* spp., *Dipylidium*, and *Echinococcus*, causing destruction and disintegration of the tapeworm, including the scolex. No preparative treatment is necessary and the compound has a wide margin of safety. The dosage rate is 25–30 mg. per kg.

Prophylaxis. The regular treatment of dogs and cats for tapeworms is a major part of any control programme. Dogs should not be fed raw offal of slaughtered animals nor the entrails of rabbits when they are dressed after being hunted. In the case of *D. caninum* an essential part of prophylaxis is the elimination of fleas from kennels. These should be thoroughly cleaned and treated with insecticides.

ORDER: PSEUDOPHYLLIDEA

Species of this order may vary from a few millimetres to 30 m. or more in length. The scolex has, instead of suckers, narrow, deep grooves, weaker than suckers, called *bothria*. Typically there is one dorsal and one ventral bothrium, but bothria may be absent or poorly developed. There are no hooks on the scolex. The 'neck' is inconspicuous or absent. Usually there is only one set of hermaphrodite reproductive organs in

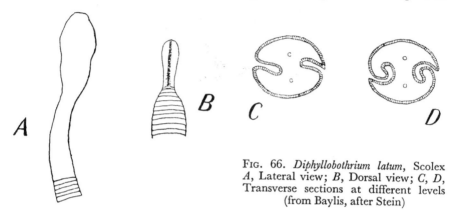

FIG. 66. *Diphyllobothrium latum,* Scolex *A,* Lateral view; *B,* Dorsal view; *C, D,* Transverse sections at different levels (from Baylis, after Stein)

each segment, though some species have two sets. The numerous testes and the vitellaria are scattered and the ovary is bilobed. The gravid uterus is usually a sinuous tube. There is a permanent uterine pore opening on the ventral side of the proglottis. The eggs are usually operculated and they may be mistaken for those of trematodes.

FAMILY: DIPHYLLOBOTHRIIDAE

Genus: Diphyllobothrium Cobbold, 1858

D. latum (Linnaeus, 1758) occurs in the small intestine of man, dog, pig, cat, fox, polar bear and other fish-eating animals in many parts of the world. Its length varies from 2 to 10 m. (6 tu 33 ft.) and it may develop 3000 segments or more. Specimens as long as 18–20 m. have been recorded. Its colour, when it is fresh, is yellowish-grey, with dark, central markings caused by the uterus and eggs. The scolex is almond-shaped, 2–3 mm. long, provided with dorsal and ventral, elongate bothridia. The neck varies in length with the state of contraction. The anterior proglottides are broader than long and the posterior ones square. There are a large number of testes lying dorsally in the lateral parts of the proglottides, and the vas deferens winds forwards to the cirrus, opening in the mid-line on the ventral surface. The vagina opens immediately behind the cirrus and runs straight back to join the oviduct. The ovary

is bilobed, lying in the posterior region. The vitellaria are follicular and
are situated in the lateral regions of the cortex. The rosette-shaped uterus
winds forwards from the oötype to the uterine pore, opening behind the

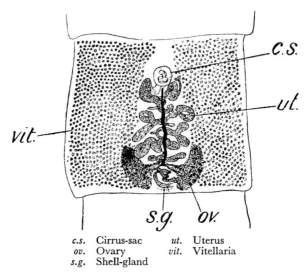

c.s.	Cirrus-sac	*ut.*	Uterus
ov.	Ovary	*vit.*	Vitellaria
s.g.	Shell-gland		

Fig. 67. *Diphyllobothrium latum,* Mature Segment (from Baylis, after Stephens)

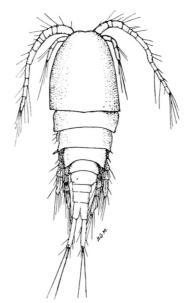

Fig. 68. *Cyclops strenuus,* Dorsal View (Original)

genital pore. The eggs are light brown, operculate and measure 67–71
by 44–45 μ. They are found in the faeces of the host.

    Life-cycle. The eggs develop for several weeks after leaving the body of
the host, before the first larval stage, the *coracidium* is ready to hatch in

water. The coracidium consists of an oncosphere (with six hooks) covered with a ciliated embryophore. It swims about in the water and dies fairly soon unless it is ingested by a suitable crustacean. *Cyclops strenuus, Diaptomus gracilis* and several other species of these two genera are known to act as the first intermediate hosts. In their body-cavity a larval stage, a procercoid, develops in 2–3 weeks. If the copepod is then swallowed

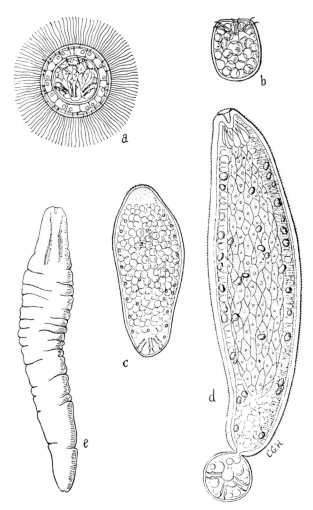

Fig. 69. *Diphyllobothrium latum*, Developmental Stages *a*, Coracidium; *b*, onchosphere from body cavity of *Cyclops*, 5 days after passage through intestinal wall; *c*, young procercoid from body cavity of *Cyclops*; *d*, mature procercoid; *e*, young plerocercoid from body-cavity of pike

by a suitable fresh-water fish, the larval worm penetrates through the intestine to the muscles or other organs, where it develops into a plerocercoid. This is an elongate, solid larval stage with a head resembling that of the adult. It is 1–2 cm. long. A large number of fishes are known to act as secondary intermediate hosts, including pike, trout, salmon and perch. The final host becomes infected through eating raw or insufficiently cooked fish or raw caviare. The worm grows adult in dogs in about 4 weeks.

Pathogenicity. The pathogenicity of this parasite for dogs and cats is not well known and it is chiefly important as a parasite of man, who is apparently its normal host. It has been shown that only a small percentage of the eggs passed by dogs will hatch, while a much larger percentage of those of human origin develop and the worms reared in dogs are generally smaller than those from human cases.

In man the worm produces severe anaemia. Von Bonsdorff (1956) has demonstrated that *D. latum* assimilates large quantities of vitamin B_{12}, competing with the host for this. This occurs especially when the worm is situated more anterior than usual in the digestive tract (e.g. in duodenum). When the available supply of B_{12} is severely depleted pernicious anaemia results.

By no means all infected persons develop anaemia and there are several aspects of the pathogenesis which still require investigation.

Treatment and Prophylaxis. For human infections it is claimed that quinacrine hydrochloride (mepacrine) gives excellent results. Yomesan has been reported to be highly effective against *D. latum* (Knorr, 1960). This drug may also be used for dogs; in addition arecoline hydrobromide has been used. The infection can be avoided by preventing the animals from eating raw or insufficiently cooked fish, and this is of course an important measure in the control of the parasite as far as man is concerned.

Genus: Spirometra Mueller, 1937

Members of this genus are closely related to the genus *Diphyllobothrium*. The major points of difference, which are summarised by Bearup (1953), are the eggs have more pointed ends than in *Diphyllobothrium*, the uterine coils form a spiral of two to seven coils rather than a rosette, the orifices of the cirrus and the vagina open separately rather than in a common sinus, the first intermediate hosts are species of *Cyclopidae* and the second intermediate hosts are frogs, snakes and mammals rather than fish.

The larval stage in vertebrates is referred to as a *sparganum*. This is a white, ribbon-like wrinkled plerocercoid which may have bothridia-like grooves at the anterior end. They may increase in number by transverse division but with one exception they do not branch. The exception is *Sparganum proliferum* which is found in man in Japan and Formosa, in the muscles and connective tissue. It may be a whitish ribbon 12 by 2·5 mm. or it may bud off irregular branches and the buds may detach and establish themselves in numerous cysts all over the body. The adult stage of *Sparganum proliferum* is possibly *Spirometra ranarum* but with several spargana the adult stage is not known. In the past, there has been a tendency to give such forms a specific name (e.g. *S. proliferum*) but their true entity must await the identification of adult forms raised in the defir.ive host(s). Wardle & McLeod (1952) discuss the confusion of the forms.

Spirometra mansoni (Cobbold, 1882) Joyeux, 1928. This is found in dogs and cats in the Far East. Procercoids occur in *Cyclops* spp. and the sparganum (*Sparganum mansoni*), which is 6–35 cm. in length, occurs in the connective tissue of frogs and snakes. Human infection, especially of the eye may occur. In south-east Asia, the flesh of frogs is considered to be a remedy for eye disease and if the frog is infected with spargana these invade the human flesh causing a marked local reaction. Human infection may also be acquired by the ingestion of infected *Cyclops* spp. or by the ingestion of raw flesh of frogs, snakes etc., in this case the sparganum migrates through the bowel wall to the inner organs.

Spirometra mansonoides Mueller, 1935. This is found in the cat, bobcat and occasionally the dog in North America. Procercoids occur in *Cyclops* species such as *C. leukarti*, *C. viridis* and *C. bicuspidatus* and spargana in rats, snakes and also wild mice. In studies on themselves, Mueller & Coulston (1941) demonstrated that the spargana migrated extensively causing local induration, urticaria and oedema. The larval stages in these persons grew from 2 to 15 mm. in 50–60 days. When the spargana were fed to a cat, adult · orms were recovered.

Spirometra erinacei (Rudolphi, 1819). Occurs in cats and foxes in the Far East and in Australia. Many wild pigs from western New South Wales are affected with spargana, probably acquiring the infection either from infected crustacea or from infected frogs etc., since such pigs live near water. *S. erinacei* is present in wild foxes in this area (Gordon et al., 1954).

Kotlan (1923) described *Dibothriocephalus raillieti* from the pig in Hungary, however this identification was based upon the larval stage only and the exact identity is unknown. Sparganosis of pigs has also been recorded in south-east Asia and Madagascar.

REFERENCES

CESTODES—GENERAL

LUMSDEN, R. D. (1965). Quoted by Read, C. P. (1966)
READ, C. P. (1966). Nutrition of intestinal helminths. *Biology of Parasites* (Ed. E. J. L. Soulsby) New York: Academic Press.
READ, C. P. and SIMMONS, J. E., Jr. (1963). Biochemistry and physiology of tapeworms. *Physiol. Rev.*, **43**, 263–305
SMYTH, J. D. (1963). *The Biology of Cestode Life Cycles.* Tech. Comm. No. 34, Commonwealth Bureau of Helminthology. Farnham Royal, England: Commonwealth Agricultural Bureaux
SMYTH, J. D. and CLEGG, J. A. (1959). Egg-shell formation in trematodes and cestodes. *Exp. Parasit.*, **8**, 286–323
WARDLE, R. A. and MCLEOD, J. A. (1952). *The Zoology of Tapeworms.* Minneapolis: University of Minnesota Press.

MESOCESTOIDIDAE, ANOPLOCEPHALIDAE, DAVAINEIDAE, DILEPIDIDAE, HYMENOLEPIDIDAE

ALLEN, R. W. (1959). Preliminary notes on the larval development of the fringed tapeworm of sheep *Thysanosoma actinioides* Diesing, 1834, in Psocids (Psocoptera: Corodentia). *J. Parasit.*, **45**, 537–538

ALLEN, R. W., ENZIE, F. D. and SAMSON, K. S. (1962). The effects of bithionol and other compounds on the fringed tapeworm, *Thysanosoma actinioides*, of sheep. *Am. J. vet. Res.*, **23**, 236–240

CHRISTENSON, R. O. (1931). An analysis of reputed pathogenicity of *Thysanosoma actinioides* in adult sheep. *J. agric. Res.*, **42**, 245–249

CROWLEY, J. (1961). An *in vivo* screening method for anthelmintic activity using *Hymenolepis nava* var. *fraterna* in mice. *Parasitology*, **51**, 339–345

EDGAR, S. A. (1956), The removal of chicken tapeworms by di-n-butyl tin dilaurate. *Poult. Sci.*, **35**, 64–73

FUKUI, M., KANEKO, C. & OGAWA, A. (1960). Studies on equine tapeworms and their intermediate hosts. II. Studies on removal effects of bithionol, bithionol acetate, and dichlorophen for equine tapeworm, *Anoplocephala perfoliata*. *Kiseichugaku Zasshi (Jap. J. Parasit.)*, **9**, 217–223

GUILHON, J. and GRABER, M. (1963). Action du dichlorophene sur les cestodes du poulet. *Bull. Acad. vet. Fr.*, **36**, 249–251

HAWKINS, P. A. (1946). Studies of sheep parasites. VII. *Moniezia expansa* infections. *J. Parasit.*, **32** (sect. 2), 14

KATES, K. C. and GOLDBERG, A. (1951). The pathogenicity of the common sheep tapeworm, *Moniezia expansa*. *Proc. helminth. Soc. Wash.*, **18**, 87–101

POTEMKINA, V. A. (1944). Contribution to the study of the development of *Thysaniezia ovilla* (Rivolto, 1878) a tapeworm parasite in ruminants. *Dokl. Akad. Nauk SSSR*, **43**, 43–44

RAYSKI, C. (1949). Observations on the life-history of *Moniezia* with special reference to the bionomics of the oribatid mites. *Proc. XIVth Int. vet. Congr. Lond.*, **2**, 51–55 (1952)

RYFF, J. F., BROWNE, J., STODDARD, H. L. & HONESS, R. F. (1950). Removal of the Fringed tapeworm from sheep. *J. Am. vet. med. Ass.*, **177**, 471–473

STUNKARD, H. W. (1937). The life cycle of *Moniezia expansa*. *Science, N.Y.*, **86**, 312

SVADZHIAN, P. K. (1963). Development of *Thysaneizia giardi* (Moniez, 1879) in the bodies of insects of the order of Psocids (Psocoptera). *Dokl. Akad. Nauk armyan. SSSR*, **36**, 303–306

WARDLE, R. A. and McLEOD, J. A. (1952). *The Zoology of Tapeworms*. Minneapolis: University of Minnesota Press

TAENIIDAE

BIAGI, F., NAVARRETE, F., PINA, A., SANTIAGO, A. M. & TAPIA, L. (1961). Estudio de tres reacciones serologicas en el diagnostico de la cisticercosis. *Rev. med. Hosp. gen.*, **25**, 501–508

CLAPHAM, P. A. (1942). On identifying *Multiceps* spp. by measurement of the large hook. *J. Helminth.*, **20**, 31–40

DAILEY, M. D. & SWEATMAN, G. K. (1965). The taxonomy of *Echinococcus granulosus* in the donkey and dromedary in Lebanon and Syria. *Ann. Trop. Med. Parasit.* **59**, 463–477

GEMMEL, M. A. (1959). Hydatid disease in Australia. IV. Observations on the incidence of *Echinococcus granulosus* on stations and farms in endemic regions of New South Wales. *Aust. vet. J.*, **35**, 396–402

GEMMEL, M. A. (1962). Natural and acquired immunity factors interfering with development during the rapid growth phase of *Echinococcus granulosus* in dog. *Immunology*, **5**, 496–503

GOODCHILD, C. G. & KAGAN, I. G. (1961). Comparison of proteins in hydatid fluid and serum by means of electrophoresis. *J. Parasit.*, **47**, 178–180

JEPSEN, A. & ROTH, H. (1949). Epizootiology of *Cysticercus bovis*—resistance of the eggs of *Taenia saginata*. *Proc. 14th Int. vet. Congr. Lond.*, **2**, 43–50

KAGAN, I. G. & NORMAN, L. (1963). Analysis of helminth antigens (*Echinococcus granulosus* and *Schistosoma mansoni*) by agar gell methods. *Ann. N.Y. Acad. Sci.*, **113**, 130–153

McMANUS, D. (1960). Prenatal infection of calves with *Cysticercus bovis*. *Vet. Rec.*, **72**, 847–848

PENFOLD, H. B. (1937). The life history of *Cysticercus bovis* in the tissues of the ox. *Med. J. Aust.*, **1**, 579–583

SEDDON, H. R. (1950). *Diseases of Animals in Australia*, Part 1. Helminth Infestations. Publication No. 5. Commonwealth of Australia, Department of Health, Service Publications (Division of Veterinary Hygiene) No. 6

SILVERMAN, P. H. (1954). Studies on the biology of some tapeworms of the genus *Taenia*. I. Factors affecting hatching and activation of taeniid ova, and some criteria of their viability. *Ann. trop. Med. Parasit.*, **48**, 207–215

SILVERMAN, P. H. & GRIFFITHS, R. B. (1955). A review of methods of sewage disposal in Great Britain, with special reference to the epizootiology of *Cysticerus bovis*. *Ann. trop. Med. Parasit.*, **49**, 436–450

SMYTH, J. D. (1963). The biology of cestode life-cycles. Tech. Comm. No. 34, Commonwealth Bureau of Helminthology. Farnham Royal, England: Commonwealth Agricultural Bureaux

SMYTH, J. D. (1964). The biology of the hydatid organism. *Advances in Parasitology*, Vol. 2. (Ed. by B. Dawes). New York and London: Academic Press.

SMYTH, J. D. & HASLEWOOD, G. A. D. (1963). The biochemistry of bile as a factor in determining host specificity in intestinal parasites, with particular reference to *Echinococcus granulosus*. *Ann. N.Y. Acad. Sci.*, **113**, 234–260

REFERENCES 141

SMYTH, J. D. & SMYTH, M. M. (1964). Natural and experimental hosts of *Echinococcus granulosus* and *E. multilocularis*, with comments on the genetics of speciation in the genus *Echinococcus Parasitology*, **54**, 493–514
SOULSBY, E. J. L. (1961). *Zjawiska Immunologiczine w Przebiegninwazji Robakow Parazytnichzych* Warszawa: Polska Akademia Nauk
SOULSBY, E. J. L. (1965), *Textbook of Veterinary Clinical Parasitology*. Vol. I. *Helminths*. Oxford: Blackwell Scientific Publications
STOLL, N. R. (1947). This wormy world. *J. Parasit.*, **33**, 1–18.
SWEATMAN, G. K. & PLUMMER, P. J. G. (1957). The biology and pathology of the tapeworm *Taenia hydatigena* in domestic and wild hosts. *Can. J. Zool.*, **35**, 93–109
SWEATMAN, G. K. & WILLIAMS, R. J. (1963). Comparative studies on the biology and morphology of *Echinococcus granulosus* from domestic livestock, moose and reindeer. *Parasitology*, **53**, 339–390
TURNER, E. L., BERBERIAN, D. A. & DENNIS, E. W. (1935). Successful artificial immunization of dogs against *Taenia echinococcus*, *Proc. Soc. expt. Biol. Med.*, **30**, 618–619
TURNER, E. L., BERBERIAN, D. A. & DENNIS, E. W. (1936). The production of artificial immunity in dogs against *Echinococcus granulosus*. *J. Parasit.*, **22**, 14–28
VOGEL, H, (1957). Ueber die Spizifische Natur und die Entwicklung des Alveolar-Echinococcus in Europa. *Arch. Int. Hidatid.*, **16**, 517–522
WILLIAMS, R. J. & SWEATMAN, G. K. (1963). On the transmission, biology and morphology of *Echinococcus granulosus equinus*, a new subspecies of hydatid tapeworms in horses in Great Britain. *Parasitology*, **53**, 391–407

PSEUDOPHYLLIDEA

BEARUP, A. J. (1953). Life history of a spirometrid tapeworm, causing sparganosis in feral pigs, *Aust. vet. J.*, **29**, 217–224
VON BONSDORFF, B. (1956). *Diphyllobothrium latum* as a casue of pernicious anemia. *Exp. Parasit.*, **5**, 207–230
GORDON, H. McL., FORSYTH, B. A. & ROBINSON, M. (1954). Sparganosis in feral pigs in New South Wales, *Aust. vet. J.*, **30**, 135–138
KNORR, R. (1960). Bandwurmbehandlung mit Yomesan bei 36 Patienten. *Med. Klin.* **55**, 1937–1938
KOTLAN, A. (1923), Ueber *Sparganum raillieti* Ratz und den zugehörigen geschlechtsreifen Bandwurm, *Dibothriocephalus raillieti* Ratz. *Centralbl. Bakt. Abt. I.* (orig.), **90**, 272–285
MUELLER, J. F. & COULSTON, F. (1941). Experimental human infection with the sparganum larva of *Spirometra mansonoides* (Mueller, 1935). *Am. J. trop. Med. Hyg.*, **21**, 399–425
WARDLE, R. A. & McLEOD, J. A. (1952). *The Zoology of Tapeworms*. Minneapolis: University of Minnesota Press

Nematodes

THE Nematodes are free-living or parasitic, unsegmented worms, usually cylindrical and elongate in shape. An alimentary canal is present. With a few exceptions the sexes are separate and the life-cycle may be direct or include an intermediate host.

Morphology. The shape of the body is elongate, cylindrical and tapering at the extremities. A few exceptions occur; for instance, the females of *Tetrameres*, which swell up after copulation, becoming almost spherical, and those of *Simondsia*, in which the posterior part of the body also assumes a globular shape.

The body is unsegmented, but the cuticula which forms the covering is usually provided with circular annulations not readily visible to the naked eye, or it may be smooth or have longitudinal striations. The cuticula is relatively thick in nematodes and is continuous with the cuticular lining of the buccal cavity, the oesophagus, the rectum and the distal portions of the genital ducts. It may form special adhesive structures; for instance, hooks (*Rictularia*, *Tetrameres* males), simple or more complicated thickenings (*Gongylonema*, *Acuaria*) or a cephalic collar (*Physaloptera*). Many species have lateral cuticular flattened expansions, called *alae*, especially in the cervical region (*Toxascaris*, *Physocephalus*, *Oesophagostomum*), and in most species the males bear cuticular expansions at the posterior extremity. Electron microscopy studies of the cuticula of various nematodes show, in general, a number of layers consisting of an outer membrane, a cortical layer, a matrix and fibre layers. These layers are divisible into about nine separate layers. There are a number of differences between species (see Bird, 1957; Hinz, 1963; Lee, 1965).

The cuticula is formed by an underlying subcuticular layer, called the *hypodermis*. This usually consists of cells in the free-living forms and of a matrix containing a number of nuclei in the parasitic forms. This layer forms four longitudinal thickenings on the inner aspect, situated dorsally, ventrally and laterally and known as the 'longitudinal lines'. The lateral lines contain the longitudinal canals of the excretory system. The cuticle is not significantly permeable to small molecules of nutritional significance (e.g. glucose or amino acids) though the basis of this determination is based mainly on *Ascaris*. In *Ascaridia galli* it has been demonstrated that glucose and alanine do enter through the cuticle and much needs to be done regarding the nutritional significance of the cuticle in other groups. The cuticle, is, however, penetrated by certain anthelmintics.

The muscular layer, which follows next and lines the body cavity, consists of a number of cells having a basal contractile portion which is tranversely striated, and a cytoplasmic portion which contains the nucleus and is connected to the nerve trunks running in the dorsal or ventral line. The muscular layer is divided into four quadrants by the longitudinal lines.

The mouth is anterior, sometimes sub-dorsal or sub-ventral, and is usually surrounded by lips. The original forms apparently had three lips, one dorsal and two ventral, each bearing two sensory papillae. This arrangement still persists in most free-living and some parasitic forms (*Ascaroidea*). In other forms there are two lips, each bearing three papillae,

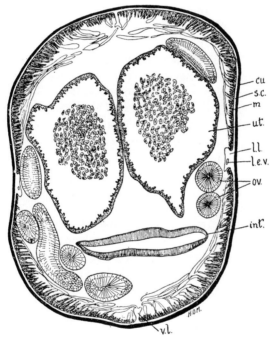

cu.	Cuticula	*ov.*	Ovary
int.	Intestine	*s.c.*	Subcuticula
l.e.v.	Longitudinal excretory vessel	*ut.*	Uterus
l.l.	Lateral line	*v.l.*	Ventral line
m.	Muscular layer		

FIG. 70. *Ascaris equorum*, Transverse Section of Female (Original)

and these lips may be sub-divided into three parts each (*Spiruroidea*), or the lips may disappear completely (*Strongyloidea, Filarioidea*), and the papillae stand around the mouth opening. Though difficult to see in some parasitic forms, a pair of depressions occur on each side of the head end, lying lateral or posterior lateral to other specialised head structures.

These are the *amphids* and are probably chemoreceptors. They are well supplied with nerve fibres and may be associated with a glandular structure. Comparable organs, the *phasmids*, are placed in the posterior extremity in many forms. These occur posterior to the anus and glands are usually associated with the organelles. The possession, or otherwise, of *phasmids* is the basis of the classification of Nematodes into the *Phasmidia* (with) or *Aphasmidia* (without).

In the forms without lips secondary structures may develop in their place. The *Strongylidae*, for instance, develop *leaf-crowns* which consist of a large number of fine, pointed processes which arise from the rim of the mouth opening (external leaf-crown) or the rim of the buccal capsule (internal leaf-crown). The mouth may lead into a *buccal capsule*, which has thick cuticular walls and may contain special tooth-like structures, or into a *pharynx*, which is usually cylindrical and surrounded by muscular tissue, or directly into the *oesophagus*. The oesophagus of nematodes shows variations of structure that are used for the classification of species. It is a strongly muscular organ with a triradiate lumen which is thickly lined with cuticula, and divides the wall into one dorsal and two subventral sectors, corresponding to the primitive arrangement of the lips. The wall of the oesophagus contains three *oesophageal glands*, one in each sector, which secrete digestive enzymes. The dorsal gland opens into the mouth and the others into the lumen of the oesophagus. Posteriorly the oesophagus may have a bulbar swelling called the *oesophageal bulb*, which contains a valvular apparatus (e.g. *Heterakis*). The muscles of the oesophagus dilate its lumen, so that it sucks in liquid food which is passed into the intestine. In the blood-sucking Ancylostomidae its pumping pulsations may achieve a rate of 120 or more a minute. In order to prevent regurgitation the oesophagus may be separated from the intestine by three valves. In other species the posterior part of the oesophagus may be non-muscular and has a structure that is possibly glandular; it is called the *ventriculus* (e.g. Anisakinae). In the non-parasitic first larvae of many species of nematodes and the individuals of the non-parasitic generations of the Rhabditata described below the oesophagus has a club-shaped anterior portion connected by a narrow neck with a pear-shaped posterior bulb. An oesophagus of this type is called a *rhabditiform* oesophagus to distinguish it from the type of oesophagus which is club-shaped without a posterior bulb, the latter being called a *filariform* oesophagus. A filariform oesophagus is found in the second and later larvae of nematodes and in the individuals of parasitic generations of the Rhabditata. The intestine is a simple tube with a non-muscular wall, composed of a single layer of columnar cells standing on a basal membrane. It leads into the rectum, which is lined with cuticula and into which the genital duct opens in the male; the latter, therefore, has a cloaca.

The gut plays an important role in absorption of nutrients. Electronmicroscopy has shown the gut cells as possessing microvilli which are identical with the 'bacillary layer' seen under the light microscope. In *Ascaris* the microvilli contain adenosine triphosphate (Tanaka, 1961). It is probable that the gut has both a secretory and absorptive function. Active transport of glucose by the gut of *Ascaris* has been demonstrated (see Read, 1966) this being rapidly converted to trehalose but apparently not in the gut cells. An accumulation of amino acids into the gut tissue has been demonstrated (histidine, methionine, glycine, valine) but there

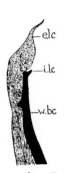

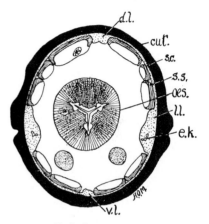

e.l.c.	External leaf-crown	*cut.*	Cuticula
i.l.c.	Internal leaf-crown	*d.l.*	Dorsal line
w.b.c.	Wall of buccal capsule.	*e.c.*	Excretory canal
		l.l.	Lateral line
		m.c.	Muscle cell
		aes.	Oesophagus
		s.c.	Subcuticula
		v.l.	Ventralline.

Fig. 71. *Strongylus equinus*, Section through Rim of Buccal Capsule (Original)

Fig. 72. *Strongylus equinus*, Section through Oesophageal Region (Original)

is as yet no firm evidence that active transport is involved. Read (1966) concludes that the uptake is mediated by a process having some specificity since some amino acids competitively inhibited the uptake of others.

The part of the body behind the anal or cloacal opening is called the tail.

The region between the layer of muscle-cells and the alimentary canal is called the *perienteric* space. It is filled by tissue, composed of very few cells, in which there are large intracellular spaces containing the *perienteric fluid*, which contains proteins, fats, glucose, enzymes and, in some species, haemoglobin. In *Ascaris* four large cells with numerous processes ending in terminal knobs, called the stellate cells or *phagocytic organs*, ingest, in an amoeboid manner, bacteria and other material experimentally introduced into the perienteric space. There are similar cells in other species (e.g. *Strongylus equinus*) and also free phagocytic cells in the perienteric fluid.

The excretory system opens by a ventral pore situated a short distance behind the anterior extremity and consists of a pair of unbranched lateral longitudinal vessels embedded in the hypodermis which do not end in flame-cells as the excretory tubes of flatworms do. The function of the lateral canals is not fully known and they may not be completely excretory. In *Ascaris* these canals are joined by a transverse canal behind the perioesophageal nerve ring to form an H-shaped system. Variations of this type occur. The right-hand canal may, for instance, be absent in Anisakinae and there are no lateral canals in the Trichurata and Dioctophymata.

The nervous system consists of a number of ganglia connected by fibres, forming the *nerve ring* which surrounds the oesophagus. From this central organ six nerve trunks arise anteriorly and posteriorly, the principal ones running in the dorsal and ventral lines. Solitary ganglia occur in other parts of the body; for instance, an anal ganglion. The sense organs are (1) around the mouth, the amphids, as already described; (2) a pair called the *cervical papillae* or *deirids*, which project through the cuticle at the sides of the oesophagus and are probably tactile (e.g. in *Oesophagostomum*; (3) frequently a lateral or sub-dorsal pair near the middle of the body; (4) on the posterior extremity of the male, the genital papillae, which are mostly paired and may have long stalks supporting the caudal alae or the copulatory bursae of the strongyles. In the latter case the stalks contain muscle fibres and the papillae are arranged according to the definite system described below. The female may also bear a pair of papillae on the tail or in the region of the vulva; (5) the phasmids, as already described.

The sexes are usually separate. In the parasitic nematodes the function of reproduction is markedly developed and there is much variation in the genital organs. Sexual dimorphism is sometimes very marked. Apart from other differences, the males are frequently smaller than the females.

The male organs are composed of a single testis in the parasitic and most free-living forms, a vas deferens, sometimes a seminal vesicle and a muscular ejaculatory duct which opens into the cloaca. In most species there are one or two spicules lying in sheaths which also open into the cloaca. These organs are cuticular, often pigmented, and they vary in shape and size and are of great value in determination of the species. They serve during copulation for attachment and probably also to expand the vagina and direct the flow of sperms. The spicules are moved by special muscles and in many cases the wall of the cloaca is provided with cuticular thickenings which guide the spicules. Such a thickening on the dorsal wall is called a gubernaculum. Less frequently there is one on the ventral wall, known as a telamon.

In the female the vulva was originally posterior and there were two uteri and two ovaries running forward (prodelph). Some free-living and also some parasitic forms have only one uterus and ovary. On the other hand, the uteri may be subdivided, so that forms with up to sixteen uteri are known. The vulva may be found in various positions, even quite close to the anterior extremity (*Oxyuridae, Filariidae*) and the uteri may run in opposite directions (amphidelph) or both run backwards (opistho-delph). The ovary is proximally a solid, cylindrical organ containing a number of cells, which divide to form the ova and further on arrange themselves around a central rhachis, from which they later become detached. They pass through an oviduct to the seminal receptacle, a small dilated part of the organ in which spermatozoa are stored and fertilisation takes place. This is followed by the uterus, in which the egg-shells are formed and the embryo may develop. The uteri are usually connected to the vagina by muscular ovijectors, or one for both uteri, lined with cuticula like the vagina. The vulva is usually situated on the ventral surface. Some nematodes are oviparous, others are ovoviviparous or viviparous. The eggs vary greatly in shape and size, a fact which is of great importance in making a specific diagnosis by faeces examination. The parasitic nematodes are very prolific and a female may lay several thousand eggs per day.

Development. The original egg cell divides into two, then four and so on, and the embryo passes through a morula stage and later through a 'tadpole' stage, in which the anterior end is broad and the embryo is bent double. Eventually the larva is fully formed and ready to hatch. Normally four moults or ecdyses, in which the whole cuticle is shed and replaced by a new one, take place before the adult stage is reached, but in some cases a moult may be omitted. Each period between two moults consists of two phases: one in which the worm feeds and grows, and the second during which it becomes inactive, or lethargic, while structural changes take place in the body in preparation for the next moult (the lethargus). The larval worm becomes infective for the final host as a rule after the second moult, and in those species which are free-living up to this stage the cuticle of the second moult is usually retained as a protective sheath until the worm has entered its host. The infective stage may, in certain species, be reached in the egg-shell. In species which use an intermediate host, the infective larva develops inside this host.

Infection of the host in which the adult nematodes occur may therefore be effected by (a) an active, non-parasitic third larva which enters the host through its mouth (e.g. *Strongylus*); (b) a passive infective egg containing a second or third infective larva (e.g. *Ascaris*); (c) an intermediate host in which the infective larva develops. In these instances the intermediate host is either eaten by the definitive host (e.g. *Metastrongylus*) or it conveys the infective larva to the definitive host and the infective larva then penetrates through the skin of the definitive host (e.g. *Filarioidea*).

The third and fourth ecdyses take place in the final host, after which the worms are in the adult stage and grow to maturity.

Various types of life-cycles are found among the nematodes, depending to some extent on the degree of adaptation to a parasitic existence that has been reached. The most specialised species (e.g. *Trichinella*) have no period of free existence at all. The life-cycles may therefore be classified as follows:

I. *Without an intermediate host*

(i) Eggs hatch in the open and larvae are free-living for a time; infective larvae are active, e.g. most *Strongylidae* and *Trichostrongylidae*. Entry into the host is through the mouth with food and water, but the infective larvae of some species can penetrate the host's skin as well as entering through its mouth (*Ancylostoma, Bunostomum*).

(ii) Eggs develop in the open but do not hatch there; infective larvae are passive inside the egg. Entry into the host is made only through its mouth, e.g. *Ascaridae*.

II. *With an intermediate host*

(i) Eggs hatch or the worms are viviparous and the larva enters the intermediate host after a short free existence, e.g. *Metastrongylidae, Habronema* spp. Intermediate host is eaten by the definitive host.

(ii) Eggs do not hatch and are ingested by the intermediate host, e.g. *Spiruroidea*. Intermediate host is eaten by the definitive host.

(iii) The worms are viviparous and the larvae enter the blood of the host, from which they are taken up by a blood-sucking intermediate host, inside which the infective larva develops. When the intermediate host sucks the blood of the definitive host, the infective larvae break out of the proboscis of the intermediate host and penetrate into the definitive host through its skin, e.g. *Filarioidea*.

After having entered the final host many nematodes migrate through the body before settling down in their normal habitat, and some of them do much harm in a mechanical way during this process.

CLASSIFICATION OF THE NEMATODES

Within recent years there has been a consolidation of the classification of the nematodes into the system originally proposed by Chitwood & Chitwood (1933, 1937). This system which divides the nematodes into two major groups *Phasmidia* and *Aphasmidia*, has been accepted to a major degree by the helminthologists of the Soviet Union and it is probable that more work has been done on systematic parasitology in that country than in any other. Consequently, it has been decided to adopt the Russian system for the revision of this book. This, of course, means discarding the Baylis & Daubney (1927) system which has been a feature of the several editions of the book; there does, however, seem little justification for retaining it, especially in the light of modern knowledge of systematics.

With the exception of the classification of the Spiruroidea for which the system of Dolfus & Chabaud (1957) has been used the rest of the classification has been drawn from the several volumes on *Essentials of Nematology* (1949–1963) edited by Academician K. I. Skrjabin. Only the groups of immediate interest are included in the classification.

PHYLUM: NEMATHELMINTHES SCHNEIDER, 1873

Class	NEMATODA Rudolphi, 1808
Subclass	PHASMIDIA Chitwood & Chitwood, 1933
Order	RHABDITIDA Chitwood, 1933
Suborder	RHABDITATA Chitwood, 1933
Superfamily	Rhabditoidea Travassos, 1920
Family	*Rhabditidae* Oerley, 1880
Family	*Strongyloididae* Chitwood & McIntosh, 1934
Suborder	STRONGYLATA Railliet and Henry, 1913
Superfamily	Strongyloidea Weinland, 1858
Family	*Strongylidae* Baird, 1853
Family	*Trichonematidae* Witenberg, 1925
Family	*Amidostomidae* Baylis & Daubney, 1926
Family	*Ancylostomatidae* Looss, 1905
Family	*Stephanuridae* Travassos & Vogelsang, 1933
Family	*Syngamidae* Leiper, 1912
Superfamily	Trichostrongyloidea Cram, 1927
Family	*Trichostrongylidae* Leiper, 1912
Family	*Ollulanidae* Skrjabin & Schikhobalova, 1952
Family	*Dictyocaulidae* Skrjabin, 1941
Superfamily	Metastrongyloidea Lane, 1917
Family	*Metastrongylidae* Leiper, 1908
Family	*Protostrongylidae* Leiper, 1926
Family	*Crenosomatidae* Schulz, 1951
Family	*Filaroididae* Schulz, 1951
Order	ASCARIDIDA Skrjabin & Schulz, 1940
Suborder	ASCARIDATA Skrjabin, 1915
Superfamily	Ascaroidea Railliet & Henry, 1915
Family	*Ascaridae* Baird, 1853
Family	*Ascardiidae* Skrjabin & Mosgovoy, 1953
Superfamily	Anisakoidea Mosgovoy, 1950
Family	*Anisakidae* Skrjabin & Karokhin, 1945
Suborder	OXYURATA Skrjabin, 1923
Superfamily	Oxyuroidea Railliet, 1916
Family	*Oxyuridae* Cobbold, 1864
Family	*Kathlaniidae* Travassos, 1918
Superfamily	Subuluroidea Travassos, 1930
Family	*Heterakidae* Railliet & Henry, 1914
Family	*Subuluridae* York & Maplestone, 1926

Order	SPIRURIDA Chitwood, 1933
Suborder	SPIRURATA Railliet, 1913
Superfamily	Spiruroidea Railliet & Henry, 1915
Family	*Spiruridae* Oerley, 1885
Family	*Thelaziidae* Railliet, 1916
Family	*Tetrameridae* Travassos, 1924
Family	*Acuaridae* Seurat, 1913
Superfamily	Physalopteroidea Sobolev, 1949
Family	*Physalopteridae* Leiper, 1909
Family	*Gnathostomatidae* Railliet, 1895
Suborder	FILARIATA Skrjabin, 1915
Superfamily	Filaroidea Weinland, 1858
Family	*Filariidae* Cobbold, 1864
Family	*Setariidae* Skrjabin & Schikhobalova, 1945
Suborder	CAMALLANATA Chitwood, 1936; Skrjabin & Schulz, 1940
Superfamily	Dracunculoidea Cameron, 1934
Family	*Dracunculidae* Leiper, 1912
Subclass	APHASMIDIA Chitwood & Chitwood, 1933
Order	TRICHOCEPHALIDA Skrjabin & Schulz, 1928; Spassky, 1954
Suborder	TRICHURATA Neveu-Lemaire, 1936 (syn. *Trichocephalata*, Skrjabin & Schulz, 1928)
Family	*Trichuridae* Railliet, 1915 (syn. *Trichocephalidae*, Baird, 1853)
Family	*Capillariidae* Neveu-Lemair, 1936
Family	*Trichinellidae* Ward, 1907
Suborder	DIOCTOPHYMATA Skrjabin, 1927
Family	*Dioctophymidae* Railliet, 1915
Family	*Soboliphymidae* Petrov, 1930

THE PHASMID NEMATODES

SUBCLASS: PHASMIDIA Chitwood & Chitwood, 1933

Nematodes with phasmids present. Amphids pore-like and labial in position. Males commonly possess caudal alae.

ORDER: ASCARIDIDA Skrjabin & Schulz, 1940

Probably have arisen from Rhabditoidea; possess three large lips; caudal alae when present are laterally placed.

SUBORDER: ASCARIDATA Skrjabin, 1915

Superfamily: Ascaroidea Railliet & Henry, 1915

Mostly large nematodes. Mouth surrounded by three large lips; no buccal capsule, oesophagus usually lacks posterior bulb; intestine may have caeca; tail of female blunt, of male frequently coiled; two spicules in the male; life cycle may be direct or indirect.

Family: Ascaridae Baird, 1853

Genera of importance: Ascaris, Parascaris, Toxascaris

These are usually relatively large worms with three well-developed lips, one dorsal and two subventral, each of which usually bears two papillae. Between the bases of these lips there may be smaller lips, called interlabia. The inner surface of each lip may bear a dentigerous ridge of small teeth. There is no buccal capsule or pharynx. The oesophagus is usually club-shaped, muscular, and without a posterior bulb. The tail of the male is usually without well-developed caudal alae, but it usually bears numerous caudal papillae. The male has paired spicules and the vulva of the female is in front of the middle of the body. The females are oviparous and produce a large number of eggs, which are usually unsegmented when they are laid. The eggs are oval or sub-globular and the shell is in most cases thick.

Hatching mechanisms in Ascarids. The processes involved in the hatching of eggs consist of a stimulus from the host which acts on a 'receptor' in the infective egg, this causes a resumption of development from the previous stage of resting and the secretion of 'hatching fluid'. Hatching fluid contains various enzymes which attack the layers of the egg shell and subsequently the infective larval stage emerges.

Studies with *Ascaris lumbricoides*, *Toxocara cati* and *Ascaridia galli* have indicated that dissolved CO_2 and undissociated carbonic acid comprise

151

the host stimulus, though strongly reducing conditions and a satisfactory pH are also necessary. Under *in vitro* conditions the reducing conditions can be produced by cysteine, glutathionine, sodium dithionite or sulphur dioxide (Fairbairn, 1961). The optimal concentration of undissociated carbonic acid plus dissolved CO_2 is of the order of 0.25–0.5×10^{-3} M at pH 7.3 (Rogers, 1960).

Hatching fluid of *Ascaris suum* contains an esterase and a chitinase which attack the lipid and chitin in the egg shell. One of the first effects after stimulation is an increased permeability of the vitelline membrane which allows the enzymes to reach the shell.

Genus: Ascaris Linnaeus, 1758

A. suum Goeze, 1782. This species is cosmopolitan in distribution, occurring in the pig. Immature specimens, sometimes described as *A. ovis*, are occasionally found in sheep and cattle and the parasite has also been reported from certain squirrels and the dog.

For many years this species was considered synonymous with the human parasite *A. lumbricoides* Linnaeus, 1758, however there is now some evidence that they are distinct species. Serological differences have been reported in the carbohydrate fractions of the two (Campbell, 1937); Sprent (1952) has described morphological differences in the denticulation of the lips of the two forms and epidemiological studies in areas where human and swine ascariasis is common failed to indicate any evidence of cross-infection. However, there is also some evidence against this view, thus the chromosomes are identical, gametogenesis is similar and patent infections with the human form can be induced in pigs under appropriate circumstances. In a summary of much of the evidence, Taffs (1961) concluded that the two forms should be considered as distinct. It would seem appropriate at the present time to consider them distinct but further study may necessitate a revision of this opinion.

The males measure 15–25 cm. by about 3 mm. and the females up to 41 cm. by 5 cm. The cuticle is relatively thick and the worms are fairly rigid. The dorsal lip bears two double papillae and each ventro-lateral lip one double subventral and a small lateral papilla. Each lip bears on its inner surface a row of minute denticles. The oesophagus is about 6.5 mm. long and simple in shape. The spicules of the male are about 2 mm. long and stout. There are a large number of pre-cloacal papillae, some of them standing in pairs on either side; of the postcloacal papillae, two pairs are double and three single. The vulva opens near the end of the first third of the body. The vagina is short and leads into two posteriorly-directed uteri. The eggs are oval, measuring 50–75 by 40–50 μ. They have thick shells and the albuminous layer bears prominent projections.

Life-cycle. It has been estimated that a female may lay as many as 200,000 eggs per day. The eggs are passed in the faeces of the host and develop to the infective stage in 10 days or longer, depending on the temperature. The eggs are very resistant to adverse conditions, like drying or freezing, and to chemicals, and they may remain viable for as long as 5 years, or perhaps longer, but hot, dry conditions, such as those prevailing in sandy soil with direct sunlight, kill them in a few weeks. During its development the larva moults once in the egg-shell to become the second larva and this is the infective larva which infects another host. The larvae rarely hatch and infection usually takes place through ingestion of the eggs with food or water or from the soiled skin of the mother in the case of sucking pigs.

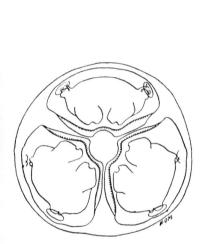
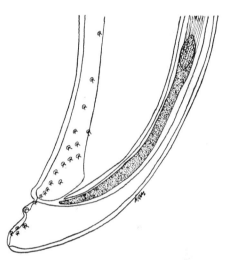

FIG. 73. *Ascaris suum*, Anterior View of Head (Original)

FIG. 74. *Ascaris suum*, Hind End of Male, Lateral View, showing One Spicule (Original)

The ingested eggs hatch in the intestine and the larvae burrow into the wall of the gut. They may pass through into the peritoneal cavity and thence to the liver; but the majority reach this organ by way of the hepato-portal blood stream. They may arrive in the liver 24 hours after the eggs have been ingested, or even earlier. From the liver they are carried by the blood through the heart to the lungs, where they are arrested in the capillaries, although some may pass through into the arterial circulation and reach other organs like the spleen and kidneys. The majority of larvae moult to the third larval stage between the fourth and fifth day after infection. At this time many larvae are still in the liver though a good proportion are migrating to the lungs and may be in the lungs. The act of moulting initiates a period of marked growth and development and this is also associated with the migration of larvae to the lungs.

Larvae break out of the alveolar capillary into the alveolus and pass through the alveolar duct to the small bronchioles and then gradually ascend the bronchial tree. As the infection continues, larger numbers of larvae are found more and more towards the anterior end of the large bronchi and trachea. Larvae then migrate from the trachea to the pharynx when they are swallowed and third stage larvae arrive in the intestine seven to eight days after infection. Douvres (1967) states that the moult to the fourth larval stage occurs about the 10th day, in the intestine, this being contrary to the views of Roberts (1934) who stated that this moult occurred in the respiratory system and that only fourth stage larvae were able to survive the acid environment of the stomach. At this time larvae measure 1·2–1·4 mm. Large numbers of fourth stage larvae are present in the small intestine between the 14th and 21st day after infection and by 21 days they measure 4·5–6·5 mm. The moult to the fifth stage, or young adult, occurs 21–29 days after infection. Maturity occurs after 50–55 days and eggs appear in the faeces at 60–62 days.

A detailed account of the morphology and sizes of different developmental stages is given by Soulsby (1965).

The eggs of *A. suum* will hatch and the larvae migrate in many animal species, including man. Much work has been done with *A. suum* infections in guinea-pigs, rabbits, rats and mice and in these the migratory cycle is much the same as in the pig. There are slight differences in size of larvae from various animals, thus larvae from mice are smaller than those from swine. Normally *A. suum* does not mature in such animals though Berger *et al.* (1961) have reported this in the rabbit.

Migration of *A. suum* in the human occurs also but patent infections do not appear to take place commonly, although accidental human infection in laboratory workers using *A. suum* has been noticed. The development of *A. lumbricoides* in swine has received more attention and patent infections of the human form have been produced. deBoer (1935) produced it in young piglets, this work being confirmed by Soulsby (1961) using baby pigs deprived of colostrum.

The mode of migration of *A. suum* in laboratory animals, especially the white mouse, has received attention by Sprent (1956, 1959). Essentially this parasite follows the 'tracheal' route of migration. Other forms, such as *Toxocara canis* behave differently, undergoing 'somatic' migration in which they fail to break out of the alveolar capillaries into the alveoli, but rather are carried to the systemic circulation and distributed throughout the body (see p. 160).

There is no evidence of prenatal infection in *A. suum*.

Pathogenesis. During the migratory period the larvae are able to do much damage if the infection is heavy. Destruction of tissue and haemorrhage may occur in the liver, especially around the intralobular veins, but the most important lesions are produced in the lungs, where the larvae cause numerous small haemorrhages into the alveoli and bronchioles, followed by desquamation of the alveolar epithelium, oedema and infiltration of the surrounding pulmonary parenchyma with eosinophiles and other cells. In heavy infections death from severe lung damage may occur 6–15 days after infection. Under field conditions, however, it is unlikely that a single large lethal dose would be acquired. Nevertheless marked pathological changes are seen in the lungs and these are due to repeated infections, the lesions of oedema, emphysema and haemorrhage being due to a hypersensitive state resembling asthma.

The adult parasites in the intestine cause a catarrhal enteritis, however there is a lack of critical information on the pathogenic effects of the adult parasites. The worms may be so numerous that they may become twisted into bundles in such a way that intestinal obstruction occurs. Ascarids have the habit of wandering about and they may enter the stomach and be vomited, or wander up the bile duct into the liver, causing biliary stasis, or block up the bile ducts, or they may even perforate the intestine and produce peritonitis.

Clinical signs. The clinical signs of ascariasis in pigs depend on the severity of the infection. Young pigs are chiefly affected. New-born pigs which become heavily infected may show signs of pneumonia, especially a cough and exudate into the lungs. In less severe cases the animals cough and their growth is stunted. Heavy infections with adult worms produce diarrhoea, this having a marked effect on growth rate.

The migration of *A. suum* larvae in the pig may enhance latent infections of enzootic (virus) pneumonia.

Post Mortem. The liver shows varying degrees of fibrosis, which may be localised in the form of 'milk spots'. These are usually whitish in colour but may be haemorrhagic indicating a more recent nature. In chronic infections the liver may be markedly fibrotic. Varying degrees of pneumonia or bronchitis may be found or only a number of petechial haemorrhages in the lungs. The larvae can be found by pressing small bits of lung tissue between two slides and examining these under a low magnification, or by teasing up portions of the organ in warm saline. Small haemorrhagic or necrotic foci may also be seen in other organs. In the intestine worms of various ages may be found and some may have become lodged in the bile ducts.

Diagnosis. During the early stages of the disease the pulmonary signs will indicate the possible aetiological factor and larvae may be found in the sputum. *Ascaris* eggs will be found in the faeces of the older pigs or in the soil on which the animals are kept. Unfertilised eggs are frequently seen, and they are significant when only female worms are present in large numbers. Apparently fertilisation has to be repeated at intervals and unfertilised eggs may be laid even when males are present. Such eggs are variable in shape, elongate or triangular, and contain numerous vacuoles and large granules.

Treatment. Sodium fluoride will remove 90 per cent of mature and immature ascarids and it has been widely used. It must not be given with a wet feed, because it may then be toxic; nor should it be given with whole grain. It mixes well only with ground grain, wheat meal or oat-meal. It is not very palatable and is best given in the morning after starvation for 24 hours. It should not be given to pigs in poor condition. It can be used for group treatment, provided that the weights of the pigs in each group are not markedly different and that precautions are taken to allow the pigs to have equal opportunities to get to the feed. It can be given to pregnant sows. Satisfactory results are obtained when sodium fluoride is mixed with dry feed at the rate of 0·1–0·15 g. per lb. bodyweight. Another method of administration is to mix sodium fluoride as 1 per cent of the whole day's feed and to give this day's feed in three parts, in the morning, at mid-day and in the evening. This dose may be repeated, if necessary, after 4 weeks to remove parasites which have matured since the first treatment.

Piperazine compounds. These are widely used for the removal of ascarids in swine. A number of salts are available (e.g. piperazine citrate, adipate, dihydro-chloride etc.) and all have a wide margin of safety. They are usually administered in the food, 100–300 or 400 mg. per kg. giving excellent results.

Cadmium compounds. Cadmium oxide and cadmium anthranilate are effective in the removal of *A. suum* at a concentration of 0·01–0·02 per cent in the food for 3 days. Levels above 0·03 per cent are unpalatable.

Thiabendazole. A mixture of 0·1–0·4 per cent in the feed has been reported to eliminate adult worms and also to have an effect on migrating larvae (Egerton, 1961).

Hygromycin. Within recent years this has been extensively used as a feed additive for the control of ascariasis in pigs. Critical tests showed that 6000 units per lb. of feed was 98 per cent effective when fed over a period of 3 weeks. For general feeding a rate of 12 million units of hygromycin per 1 ton of feed is recommended, this being fed for 60 days but may be continued for 100 days or even for the life of the pig.

Prophylaxis. Owing to the longevity of the eggs and their resistance to disinfectants it is not feasible to disinfect a plot on which infected pigs have been kept. The eggs survive best in damp, dirty and overcrowded quarters, so that cleanliness and good management are important. The animals should be removed to a temporary enclosure for treatment and transferred to fresh ground within 10 days, before any eggs passed by them can have become infective. Sties with concrete floors can be kept relatively clean by scrubbing out with boiling water and soda every 10 days or longer, depending on the temperature.

Young pigs are more susceptible to infection and require special attention. After the age of 4–5 months pigs are less seriously affected by ascariasis, however these animals and sows may remain sources of infection for the younger pigs.

The most important preventive measures are therefore those concerned with the protection of the young pigs immediately after birth or later.

A very satisfactory system, which was devised by Ransom in America, is known as the MacLean County System. The sow is treated for ascarids a little time before farrowing and then within a few days of farrowing is thoroughly washed and scrubbed in order to remove any eggs adhering to the body, and is then placed in the farrowing pen. The latter has a concrete floor and has been prepared by thoroughly scrubbing the floor and walls with boiling water, soda and a hard broom. Within 10 days of farrowing the sow and her litter are carted to a clean field planted with rape or other suitable crop. After weaning the sow is removed and the young pigs grow up in safety.

Genus: Parascaris Yorke & Maplestone, 1926

Parascaris equorum (Goeze, 1782) Yorke & Maplestone, 1926 (syn. *Ascaris megalocephala, Ascaris equorum*), occurs in the small intestine of equines, including the zebra, and perhaps also cattle. The males are 15–28 cm. long and the females up to 50 cm. by 8 mm. This is a rigid, stout worm with a large head. The three main lips are separated by three small intermediate lips and are divided into anterior and posterior portions by horizontal grooves on their medial surfaces. The male tail has small lateral alae. There are two double and three single pairs of postcloacal papillae, a large number of precloacal paired papillae and a

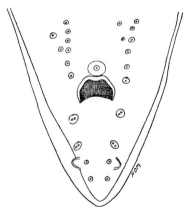

FIG. 75. *Parascaris equorum*, Hind End of Male, Ventral View (Original)

single median papilla on the anterior border of the cloaca. The spicules are about 2–2·5 mm. long. The vulva is situated at the end of the first quarter of the body. The eggs are sub-globular with a thick, pitted albuminous layer and measure 90–100 μ in diameter.

Life-cycle. Similar to that of *A. suum*. The worms reach maturity in about 12 weeks after infection.

Pathogenicity and Clinical signs. Foals especially suffer from this parasite, sometimes massive burdens being present (more than 1000 worms). The

7

worms cause a catarrhal enteritis which produces diarrhoea which may be foetid in odour and pale in colour. Flatulence is common. There is general malaise, debility and the coat is harsh. Complications may occur due to the migration of adult worms to aberrant sites such as the bile duct, they may penetrate the bowel wall and cause local or generalised peritonitis or may 'ball up' and cause an obstruction.

Diagnosis can be made by finding the eggs in the faeces. They can be readily distinguished from the eggs of other equine worms.

Treatment. Carbon bisulphide is administered, after fasting for 18 hours, by stomach tube or in capsules at the rate of 5 ml. per 100 kg. A purgative should not be given; it may cause excessive purgation; nor should oily substances or phenothiazine be given with this drug. The worms are passed for several days after treatment.

Piperazine. The several salts of piperazine (e.g. adipate, citrate, carbo-dithioic acid etc.) are highly effective and relatively non-toxic. At a dose rate of 100 mg. of piperazine base per kg. 100 per cent efficacy can be expected. Immature ascarids are also removed at this dose level.

Thiabendazole. A dose of 44 mg. per kg. has been shown to be highly effective.

Prophylaxis. Attention should be paid to the young foals at the time of birth, and the foal should run with its mother in a clean paddock. Boxes in which mares foal should be thoroughly cleaned before the event. Brood mares should be treated for ascarids before foaling. It should be remembered that foals have a habit of licking the faeces of their dams and may ingest eggs in this manner. These eggs will, however, be harmless if the eggs have not lain on the ground for the 6 weeks or so required for the development of infective second larvae in them. Frequent removal of the droppings from paddocks and other places, where this is possible, will therefore remove this source of infection. Stables should be cleaned frequently, and clean water and food supplied in such a way that contamination is not likely to occur. Manure disposal plays an important part, since practically all worm eggs and larvae will be killed by the heat generated during fermentation of the manure.

A. columnaris Leidy, 1856 occurs in the small intestine of the skunk, stoat, weasel and the Siberian polecat (*Putorius eversmanni*). The males are up to 9 cm. and the females up to 22·5 cm. long. The spicules are about 0·4 mm. long. The vulva is situated at the end of the first quarter of the body. The eggs have finely pitted shells and are subglobular, measuring 88–90 by 66–68 μ.

Life-cycle. Mice act as intermediate hosts. Sprent (1955) has shown that the larvae of *A. columnaris* and also of *A. devosi* cause an encephalitis in mice.

Genus: Toxascaris Leiper, 1907

T. leonina (v. Linstow, 1902) Leiper, 1907 (syn. *T. limbata*) occurs in the small intestine of the dog, cat, fox and wild Canidae and Felidae in most parts of the world. The anterior part of the body is provided with large cervical alae and is bent dorsad. The cervical alae of species of this genus, and also those of the genus *Toxocara* described below, give the anterior ends of species of these two genera an arrow-like appearance. For this reason they are sometimes called arrow-worms or arrow-headed worms. The males are up to 7 cm. long and the females up to 10 cm. The female genital organs lie behind the level of the vulva. The tail of the male is simple and the spicules are 0·7–1·5 mm. long. The eggs are slightly oval, with smooth shells, and measure 75–85 by 60–75 μ.

Life-cycle. The infective stage is the egg containing a second stage larva. This, under optimal conditions outside the host, is reached in 3–6 days. Following ingestion and hatching, second stage larvae enter the wall of the intestine and remain in this site and this stage for about 2 weeks. Moulting to the third stage larvae commences about 11 days after infection and is followed fairly quickly by a moult to the fourth larval stage. Fourth stage larvae are present in numbers 3–5 weeks after infection and may measure up to 8 mm. in length. At this stage they are in the mucosa and the lumen of the intestine. Fifth stage larvae are produced about 6 weeks after infection and eggs are produced from 74 days onwards.

No migration of larvae occurs, as compared with *Toxocara canis* (see below).

Larvae of *T. leonina* may occur in mice. In this animal, third stage larvae are distributed in many tissues and if an infected mouse is eaten by a dog or cat, the larvae are digested from the mouse tissues and develop to maturity in the wall and lumen of the intestine of the final host.

Whereas larvae in the dog and cat are restricted to the intestine, in the mouse they migrate out of this site being distributed all over the body. Sprent (1959) considers this indicative that intermediate hosts are fully utilised in the life history of the parasite.

FAMILY: ANISAKIDAE SKRJABIN & KAROKHIN, 1945

Genera of importance: Toxocara, Neoascaris, Porrocaecum, Contracaecum

Members of this family possess one or more of the following structures at the base of the oesophagus: a posterior granular ventriculus—*Toxocara, Neoascaris*; a posterior ventriculus and an anterior caecum projecting forward alongside the oesophagus—*Porrocaecum*; a posterior ventriculus, an anterior caecum and a posterior appendix projecting backwards from the ventriculus—*Contracaecum*.

Parasites of carnivors, felines, ruminants and, in case of the latter two genera, of birds, fishes and reptiles.

Genus: Toxocara Stiles, 1905

T. canis (Werner, 1782) occurs in the small intestine of the dog and fox. It is larger than the previous species, the males being up to 10 cm. long and the females up to 18 cm. Large cervical alae are present and the body is anteriorly bend ventrad. The female genital organs extend anteriorly and posteriorly to the vulvar region. The male tail has a terminal narrow appendage and caudal alae. The spicules are 0·75–0·95 mm. long. The eggs are subglobular, with thick, finely pitted shells, and measure about 90 by 75 μ.

Life-cycle. The life-cycle of *T. canis* is a classical example of the somatic route of migration of ascarids. Eggs reach the infective stage in 10–15 days, under optimal conditions, and following ingestion they hatch (see p. 151) in the small intestine. Eight days after infection, second stage larvae are to be found in various tissues of the body (e.g. liver, lungs, kidneys) and at this stage they have undergone no development (Sprent, 1958). Such larvae can become resident in the somatic tissues of the adult dog and remain there for some time. The subsequent history of such larvae is not completely clear but during pregnancy they are mobilised and they migrate to the foetus giving rise to prenatal infection. Douglas & Baker (1959) noted that this mobilisation did not occur before the forty-second day of pregnancy and also that larvae had to be acquired by the pregnant bitch at least 14 days prior to this if prenatal infection were to occur. Not all larvae are mobilised at each pregnancy and some may remain to undergo the process at subsequent pregnancies. The duration of larvae in bitches may be long and animals infected for up to 385 days may still be capable of transmitting infection to puppies. The factor(s) which induce mobilisation and migration are as yet unknown, however, it seems reasonable to suppose that the mechanism may have a hormonal basis. When larvae reach the liver of the foetus it is likely that they moult to become third stage larvae. At birth of the puppy, third stage larvae are present in the lungs and they continue to appear here during the first week of life. The moult to the fourth stage also takes place in the first week of life when larvae are in the lungs or, subsequently, the stomach. By the end of the second week after birth, larvae moult to the fifth stage, being 5–7 mm. in length at this time. Subsequently, growth is rapid and the adult form may be present by the end of the third week, though an increasing number mature in the next week or two. Patency of prenatal infections varies from 23 to 40 days after birth. From this life-cycle it is seen that development in the bitch is 'somatic' in character, while in the late foetal stage and in the neonate it is 'tracheal' in character. It would seem that the ability to undergo 'tracheal' migration ceases with larvae that have infected puppies older than about 3 weeks. Sprent (1958) was able to create patent infection in puppies 1–3 weeks of age by feeding infective eggs, but when puppies 5 weeks of age were fed eggs, larvae were distributed in the somatic tissues and failed to reach the intestine. Thus there is a short period in the life of the puppy when it can be infected directly but otherwise infection is via the prenatal route. An exception to this occurs when rodents infected with the larvae of *T. canis* are ingested by dogs. This latter mode of infection is probably not an important source of infection for *T. canis*.

Several workers have reported the occurrence of eggs in the faeces of bitches shortly after parturition. Baker & Douglas (1959) ascribe this to a 'weakening of the immunity' at parturition which permits larvae to pass through the lungs and complete their development in the intestine. However, Sprent (1961) states it may be due to the habit of the bitch of licking the faeces of the puppies and, by so doing, ingesting immature worms which are shed in the faeces of the puppy. These undergo no migration in the bitch and mature in her intestine. Such post-parturient infections are eliminated a few weeks after they are acquired.

T. cati (Schrank, 1788) Brumpt, 1927 (syn. *T. mystax*) (Zeder, 1800) occurs in the small intestine of the cat and wild Felidae. The cervical alae are very broad and are striated. The males are 3–6 cm. and the females 4–10 cm. long. The spicules are 1·63–2·08 mm. long. The diameter of the eggs is 65–75 μ.

Life-cycle. Infection occurs by the ingestion of eggs containing an infective second stage larva. For the first 2 days, larvae are found in the stomach wall where they measure 360–460 μ. By the third day some are found in the liver and lungs and by the fifth day they are to be found in the lungs and tracheal washings. Larvae which have passed through the tracheal route are found in the stomach wall by the tenth day, though, many are still to be found in the lungs, and by the twenty-first day the number in the stomach wall has greatly increased and larvae are also found in the stomach contents and intestinal contents. Subsequently, the number of larvae in the intestinal contents increases while the number in the lungs and stomach decreases.

The migration is accomplished by larvae in the second stage and third stage larvae do not occur until larvae have returned to the digestive tract. The majority of third stage larvae occur in the stomach wall while fourth stage larvae occur in the stomach contents, the bowel wall and bowel contents.

Mouse infections also play an important part in the life cycle. In these, larvae remain as second stage forms but when an infected mouse is eaten by a cat the larvae liberated by digestion enter the stomach wall of the cat and develop to third stage larvae. From 21 days onwards they are found in the intestinal wall and contents as fourth stage larvae.

As well as mice acting as 'intermediate hosts', second stage larvae may be found in the tissues of earthworms, cockroaches, chickens, sheep and other animals fed infective eggs. Sprent (1956) considers the parasite to be well adapted to the Felidae in that the larger members of the family may acquire the infection by predation on ruminants etc., while the smaller members may acquire the parasite by ingestion of small rodents or invertebrates.

ASCARIASIS IN DOGS, CATS AND FUR-BEARING ANIMALS

Pathogenesis. Heavy infections are most commonly seen in kennels and catteries and, under conditions of poor hygiene, heavy infection of young animals may occur.

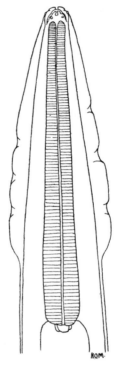

FIG. 76. *Toxocara canis*, Anterior End, Dorsal View (Original)

Heavy prenatal infection with *T. canis* may lead to the death of whole litters of puppies. Though the migration of larvae through the lungs of the new born puppy may cause pneumonia, this is uncommon and the more usual effect is a progressive malaise associated with vomiting and diarrhoea. The maturing worms in the stomach and intestine irritate these organs so that finally each meal is rejected. The puppy often becomes covered with stale vomit, it may suffer from inhalation pneumonia and, in all, presents an abject picture of despair. Death frequently occurs 2–3 weeks after birth.

In less severe infection of *T. canis* and in infections of *T. leonina* and *T. cati* there is general unthriftiness, a pot-bellied appearance, intermittent diarrhoea and possibly anaemia.

Adult worms, on occasion, migrate to aberrant sites, such as the bile duct or through the bowel wall, and in these cases the pathogenesis depends on the site of the worm.

Nervous disorders are frequently associated with roundworm infection of dogs. The mechanisms responsible for these effects have yet to be clarified, however, they may result from irritation of the bowel by the worms or may be due to local sensitisation of the central nervous system on the death of aberrant larvae, clinical signs of nervous disorders arising when materials from the adult worms are absorbed into the general circulation.

Clinical signs. The animals are unthrifty and either pot-bellied or the abdomen is tucked up, the coat is dull and harsh, there is usually emaciation, often anaemia, restlessness and diarrhoea or constipation. Death due to acute intestinal obstruction may occur. In the case of foxes the most dangerous period is during the first few weeks of life, especially from the second to the fourth. Extreme pot-belliedness of fox pups, which is not infrequent, indicates the presence of ascarids in the peritoneal cavity, the worms having reached this situation during migration.

Diagnosis is made on the basis of the clinical signs and is confirmed by finding the eggs in the faeces.

Treatment. Chenopodium oil at the rate of o·1 ml. per kg., given in, or followed by, a large dose of castor oil, produces excellent results.

Piperazine. Salts of piperazine, which are well tolerated by dogs and cats, are highly effective against the dog and cat ascarids. Piperazine adipate at a dose of 100 mg. per kg. is highly effective against adult forms and at the dose of 200 mg. per kg. will remove immature worms from puppies 1–2 weeks of age. This allows for the control of prenatally acquired infections.

There is no effect by the piperazine salts against larvae in the body of the bitch.

Diethylcarbamazine. Though one of the older compounds this, at a dose of 50 mg. per kg., is highly effective in a single dose against the dog and cat ascarids.

Thenium [(N:N-dimethyl-N-2-phenoxyethyl-N-2′ thenylammonium) *p* chlorobenzene sulphonate] when combined with piperazine and given on the morning and evening of one day is 98 per cent or more effective against *T. canis.*

Prophylaxis. Good hygiene is essential in kennels and catteries. With *T. leonina* and *T. cati* where infection leads directly to a patent infection the parasites can be eliminated by regular treatment of dogs or cats and by frequent thorough cleansing of the premises. Earth exercise areas should be either fenced off or made impervious.

With *T. canis*, in which prenatal infection plays an important part in the life cycle, the situation is different and more difficult. The bitch may harbour 'dormant' larvae in her tissues for several months or years, transmitting the infection to several litters of puppies. Immediate tactical control consists of recognising and anticipating prenatal infection and treating puppies with piperazine within 2 weeks of birth. More long-term control consists of regular treatments to lower or eliminate contamination of the environment and also measures to eliminate an established environmental contamination. This is best achieved by providing impervious surfaces to the kennels so that they may be thoroughly and regularly cleaned. The eggs of the dog and cat ascarids may remain viable for several months, consequently a cursory or token disinfection is of little value.

Since rodents may play an important part in the life cycles of the parasites, these should be exterminated from the kennels.

Visceral Larva Migrans

This condition is mainly caused by the larvae of *T. canis* though the larval stages of *T. leonina*, *T. cati*, *Capillaria hepatica* (of rodents) and *Lagochilascaris minor* (of wild felines) etc. have also been incriminated. Petter (1960) has compiled a list of hosts of ascarids which may be responsible for causing the visceral larva migrans syndrome. The entity is characterised by chronic granulomatous (usually eosinophilic) lesions, associated with larvae of the above parasites, in the inner organs of children, especially the liver, lungs, brain, sometimes the eye and also elsewhere. In the child, larvae migrate in the 'somatic' manner, as they would for example in a rodent, and on repeated infection large numbers may occur in the body of the child. Recently Beaver (1966) has reported on one case which had 300 larvae per gram of liver!

The pathological entity consists of an enlarged liver with eosinophilic granulomatous lesions, pulmonary infiltration, intermittent fever, loss of weight, loss of appetite and a persistent cough. However, the clinical picture varies greatly though a relatively constant feature is a high (50 per cent) and persistent circulating eosinophilia. The eye lesions caused by these larvae have received considerable attention in recent years, especially since they often resemble a retinoblastoma. A mistaken diagnosis may result, and on several occasions has resulted, in unnecessary enucleation of the eyeball.

The condition is most usually seen in children under 4 years of age. Children of this age frequently adopt the habit of dirt eating and where soil is heavily contaminated with *Toxocara* eggs (e.g. soil around doorsteps etc.) the ingestion of even moderate amounts of soil may result in the intake of large numbers of infective eggs. Since it is common to give young puppies to children as playmates, a special hazard may arise since it is the young puppy which is preferentially infected with *T. canis*. However, doorstep and garden soil contaminated by domestic pets is not the sole danger. There is a much wider public health problem which has yet to be recognised by the general public at large. It is the extensive fouling of public parks, playgrounds and sidewalks with the faeces of domestic pets, especially in large cities. Though modern-day man has largely solved the problems of mass hygiene, he has yet to provide a solution to the disposal of the excreta of his pets.

The specific diagnosis of visceral larva migrans is based on the demonstration of the lesions and the larvae in biopsy material. Immuno-diagnostic tests are not, as yet, specific enough to be used as a sole means of diagnosis, however, they are a useful adjunct to diagnosis. A detailed account of visceral larva migrans is given by Beaver (1956, 1966) and is discussed in relation to the veterinary aspect by Soulsby (1965).

Visceral larva migrans also occurs in other animals. Sprent (1955) has extensively studied the migration of dog and cat ascarids in experimental animals. Done et al. (1960) reported brain and spinal cord lesions in pigs infected with T. canis: clinical signs of illness occurring about 22 days after infection were associated with encapsulation and death of larvae. Roneus (1963) has reported on the migration of T. cati larvae in pigs.

Genus: Porrocaecum Railliet & Henry, 1912

P. crassum (Deslongchamps, 1824) occurs in the intestine of domestic and wild ducks. The male is 12–30 mm. in length and the female 40–55 mm. Worms reddish white in colour. A short anterior caecum arises from the gut; the tail of the male is conical and there are no caudal alae. Eggs ellipsoidal, reticulated and measure 85 by 110 μ. Life-cycle includes an earthworm in which third stage larvae occur in the ventral blood vessels.

P. ensicaudatum (Zeder, 1800) is a similar form occurring in passerine birds.

Genus: Contracaecum Railliet & Henry, 1912

C. spiculigerum (Rudolphi, 1809) occurs in ducks, geese, swans and a wide variety of water fowl. Male 32–45 mm. in length, female 24–64 mm. An oesophageal appendix and an anterior caecum are present. Eggs spherical, 50–52 μ. Related forms use crustacea as intermediate hosts.

Larval forms of *Porrocaecum* and *Contracaecum* spp. of fish may be encountered in meat inspection.

Genus: Neoascaris Travassos, 1927

Neoascaris vitulorum (Goeze, 1782) Travassos, 1927 (syn. *Ascaris vitulorum*) occurs in the small intestine of cattle, zebu and the Indian buffalo, and is found in many parts of the world. The males measure up to 25 cm. by 5 mm. and the females 30 cm. by 6 mm. The cuticle is not as thick as that of other large ascarids, and these worms therefore have a soft, translucent appearance. The body does not taper much towards the extremities. There are three lips, broad at the base and narrow anteriorly. The oesophagus is 3–4·5 mm. long and has a posterior, granular ventriculus. The tail of the male usually forms a small spike-like appendage. There are about five pairs of post-cloacal papillae; the anterior pair is large and double. The pre-cloacal papillae are variable in number. The spicules are 0·99–1·25 mm. long. The vulva is situated about one-eighth of the body length from the anterior end. The eggs are subglobular, provided with a finely pitted albuminous layer and measure 75–95 by 60–75 μ.

Life-cycle. There are many indications that *N. vitulorum* behaves similarly to *Toxocara canis* in that larvae undergo somatic migration in the tissues (as opposed to the tracheal migration) and create prenatal infection. Under natural conditions mature parasites may be found in calves aged 10–42 days and Lee (1959) reported that mature worms were restricted to the first 4 or 5 months of calfhood. Attempts to induce patent infections by post-natal infections have generally been unsuccessful with the exception of animals infected a few hours after birth. On the other hand, patent infections in calves have been produced by feeding infective eggs to pregnant cows (see Soulsby, 1965). In animals infected after birth, extensive migration of larvae occurs in organs such as liver, lungs and kidneys, indicating that the life cycle is not comparable to that of *A. suum.*

Pathogenicity. Severe clinical effects have been ascribed to *N. vitulorum,* however, much of the work is unsupported by critical experimental data. It has been reported as a serious pathogen of calves in Africa, Philippines, Ceylon and India, clinical signs being diarrhoea and emaciation. Frequently the breath of the animal has a butyric odour. In contrast to the above, Lee (1959) was unable to observe any clinical difference between infected or non-infected calves.

Diagnosis can be made by finding the eggs in the faeces.

Treatment. Lee (1956), treating cattle in Africa, obtained good results with piperazine at a dose of 220 mg. per kg.

Prophylaxis. Regular treatment of infected animals should be combined with hygienic conditions for cattle.

FAMILY: ASCARIDIIDAE SKRJABIN & MOSGOVOY, 1953

Parasites of this family have a mouth surrounded by three lips, there is no posterior bulb to the oesophagus. Males possess a preanal sucker. Parasites of birds.

Genus: Ascaridia Dujardin, 1845

A. galli (Schrank, 1788) (syn. *A. lineata, A. perspicillum*) occurs in the small intestine of the fowl, guinea-fowl, turkey, goose, and various wild birds in most parts of the world. Male 50–76 mm., female 72–116 mm. long. There are three large lips and the oesophagus has no posterior bulb. The tail of the male has small alae and bears ten pairs of papillae, most of which are short and thick. There is a circular pre-cloacal sucker with a thick cuticular rim. The spicules are sub-equal, 1–2·4 mm. long. The vulva is situated a short distance anterior to the middle of the body. The eggs are oval, with smooth shells, and are unsegmented when laid. They measure 73–92 by 45–57 μ.

Life-cycle. The eggs are passed in the faeces of the host and develop in the open, reaching the infective stage in about 10 days, or longer. The egg then contains a fully developed second stage larva and is fairly resistant to adverse conditions. The eggs can remain viable for over 3 months in shaded places, but are rapidly killed by dry, hot weather, even when they are 6 in. deep under the soil exposed to sunlight. Infection takes place by ingestion of the eggs with food or water. Earthworms may ingest the eggs and may, when they are swallowed by the birds, transmit the infection mechanically.

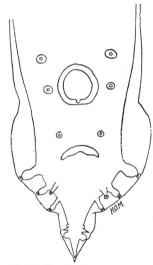

FIG. 77. *Ascaridia galli*, Hind end of Male, Ventral View (Original)

The eggs hatch in the intestine of the host and the larvae live for the first 8 days or so in the lumen of the intestine. The majority are then found in the intestinal mucosa from the eighth to the seventeenth day. Subsequently the larvae re-enter the lumen and reach maturity in 6–8 weeks, this depending on the age of the chicken. The moult to the third larval stage occurs about 8 days after infection, that to the fourth stage at 14–15 days. These moults may be delayed if larvae spend too long in the tissues (Tugwell & Ackert, 1952).

Pathogenicity. Young birds are more susceptible to infection than adult birds or others that have had a previous infection. Dietary deficiencies, such as those of vitamins A, B and B_{12}, various minerals and proteins, predispose to heavier infections. Chickens over 3 months of age are more resistant to infection and this may be associated with a marked increase in goblet cells in the gut mucosa about this time. Ackert *et al.* (1939) demonstrated a factor in duodenal mucin which inhibited the growth of larvae.

Pathogenesis and Clinical signs. Marked lesions may be produced when large numbers of the young parasites penetrate into the duodenal mucosa. They cause haemorrhage and enteritis and the birds become anaemic and suffer from diarrhoea. The birds become unthrifty, markedly emaciated, generally weak and egg production is decreased. In heavy infections intestinal obstruction may occur.

Post Mortem. A haemorrhagic enteritis may be seen and larval worms, which are about 7 mm. long are found in the mucosa. In other cases the carcass is emaciated and anaemic and the worms are found in the intestine. Occasionally viable or calcified parasites may be found in the albumin portion of eggs.

Diagnosis can be made by finding the eggs in the faeces or the worms in the intestine at autopsy.

Treatment. The piperazine compounds are highly effective against *A. galli* infections. Several salts may be used: they are given in the feed or drinking water. Thus piperazine adipate at a dose rate of 300–440 mg. per kg. in the feed is 94–100 per cent efficient; 440 mg. of piperazine citrate per liter of water for 24 hours has a similar efficiency and piperazine carbodithioic acid is effective at similar dose rates. The drug has no effect on growth or egg production at therapeutic levels.

Phenothiazine is variable in its effect and up to 2200 mg. per kg. must be given for even moderate efficiency.

Other, older, compounds are nicotine sulphate, pyrethrum, oil of chenopodium etc., but these are seldom used now.

Hygromycin B at the rate of 8 g. per ton of feed administered for 8 weeks has been reported as highly effective in controlling *A. galli* infection.

Prophylaxis. Special attention should be paid to the young birds. When birds are kept out of doors, young birds should be separated from the old and the poultry runs should be well drained. Rotation of poultry runs is highly desirable.

Heavy burdens of *A. galli* may occur in birds kept in deep-litter houses, especially when excess moisture occurs. Attention should be paid to ventilation, feeding troughs and drinking water appliances. Periodically, the litter around the feeding and water area should be mixed with dry litter in other parts of the house.

Prior to each new batch of chickens being placed in the litter house, the litter should be stacked for several days to allow heating and sterilisation.

A. columbae (Gmelin, 1790) (syn. *A. maculosa*) occurs in domestic and wild pigeons. It is, like the previous species, a large worm, the male being 16–70 mm. and the female 20–95 mm. long, but apparently not very pathogenic. The eggs measure 80–90 by 40–50 μ. Enormous numbers of worms may be present in pigeons that show no clinical signs.

SUBORDER: OXYURATA SKRJABIN, 1923

SUPERFAMILY: OXYUROIDEA RAILLIET, 1916

Nematodes with the ventrolateral papillae rudimentary or absent. Males with two, one or no spicules. Oesophagus possessing a posterior bulb.

FAMILY: OXYURIDAE COBBOLD, 1864

These are medium-sized or small worms with three inconspicuous lips. The oesophagus has a well-developed posterior bulb. The male bears a number of large papillae around the cloacal opening. The females are usually much larger than the males and have long, tapering tails. The vulva is situated near the anterior end of the body. The eggs are usually flattened on one side and development takes place without an intermediate host.

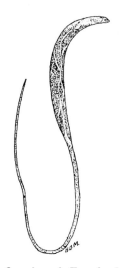

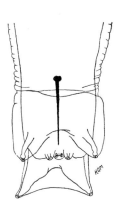

FIG. 78. *Oxyuris equi*, Female, Natural Size (Original)

FIG. 79. *Oxyuris equi*, Hind End of Male, Ventral View (Original)

Genus: Oxyuris Rudolphi, 1803

O. equi (Schrank, 1788) (syn. *O. curvula, O. mastigodes*) occurs in the large intestine of equines in all parts of the world. The male is 9–12 mm. long and the female up to 150 mm. The oesophagus is narrow at the middle and the bulb is not distinctly marked off. The male has one pin-shaped spicule which is 0·12–0·165 mm. long and the tail bears two pairs of large and a few small papillae. The young females are almost white in colour, slightly curved and have relatively short, pointed tails.

The mature females have a slatey-grey or brownish colour and narrow tails which may be more than three times as long as the rest of the body. The eggs are elongate, slightly flattened on one side, provided with a plug at one pole, and measure about 90 by 42 μ.

Life-cycle. The males and young females inhabit the caecum and large colon. After fertilisation the mature females wander down to the rectum and crawl out through the anal opening with the anterior parts of their bodies. The eggs are laid in clusters on the skin in the perineal region. Development of the egg is rapid, reaching the infective stage in 3-5 days. The infective stage may be reached on the perineal region or, more usually, the egg falls off to the ground. Eggs probably survive for several weeks in moist surroundings but desiccation is rapidly lethal.

Infection is by ingestion of the infective eggs on fodder and bedding. Infective larvae are liberated in the small intestine and third stage larvae are found in the mucosal crypts of the ventral colon and caecum. Fourth stage larvae are produced about 8-10 days after infection: these possess a large buccal capsule and browse on the mucosa. The sexually mature adult stage is reached about 4-5 months after infection.

Pathogenesis. The fourth stage larva feeds on the intestinal mucosa of the host. The adult worms are, however, not found attached and probably feed on the intestinal contents. The chief feature of oxyuriasis in equines is the anal pruritus produced by the egg-laying females.

Clinical signs. The irritation caused by the anal pruritus produces restlessness and improper feeding, which results in loss of condition and a dull coat. The animal rubs the base of its tail against any suitable object, causing the hairs to break off and the tail to acquire an ungroomed appearance.

Diagnosis. The clinical signs should lead to an examination of the perineal region, where cream-coloured masses of eggs will be found. These should be removed and identified under the microscope. The condition should be differentiated from mange and anal pruritus due to other causes.

Treatment. Piperazine compounds are highly effective against adult *O. equi.* At a dose of 400 mg. per kg. it is 100 per cent effective.

Thiabendazole is the drug of choice: 25, 50 and 100 mg. per kg. removes all mature *O. equi* and the higher doses will eliminate up to 62 per cent of immature forms.

Control of *O. equi* depends on good hygiene in stables. Bedding should be removed frequently and feeding appliances constructed so that they are not contaminated by bedding. A clean supply of water should be available.

Genus: Enterobius Leach, 1853

E. vermicularis (Linnaeus, 1785). This is the human pinworm or seat worm. As well as the human, it may occur in higher primates such as the chimpanzee. It never occurs in the dog or cat.

The worms are cream-coloured and slender, the male measuring 2–5 mm. and the female 8–13 mm. The female has a long pointed tail: otherwise the parasites resemble *Oxyuris equi*.

Adult worms occur in the caecum, appendix and ascending colon. Gravid females migrate posteriorly and deposit eggs on the perianal and perineal regions. The eggs become infective within a day or so and further infection is by ingestion of infective embryonated eggs, mature worms being produced about 2 months after infection.

The gravid females produce an intense pruritus. This causes restlessness, insomnia and various effects on behaviour including inattention, lack of cooperation and possibly a feeling of shame and inferiority.

Genus: Passalurus Dujardin, 1845

P. ambiguus (Rudolphi, 1819) occurs in the caecum and the colon of rabbits, hares and other rodents. Male 4·3–5 mm., female 9–11 mm. long. The lips are inconspicuous and the cervical alae are small. The oesophagus has a prebulbar swelling and a strong bulb. The male tail has a whip-like appendix and small caudal alae supported by papillae. The spicule is simple and 0·09–0·12 mm. long. The female has a tapering tail 3·4–4·5 mm. long and the cuticle of its distal extremity is marked with about forty circular striations. The vulva opens 1·54–1·89 mm. from the anterior extremity. The eggs are flattened on one side and measure 95–103 by 43 μ.

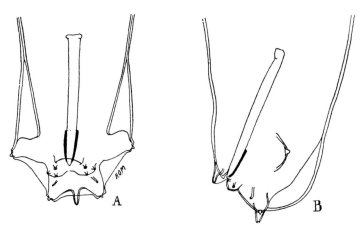

FIG. 80. *Skrjabinema ovis*, Hind End of Male (Original) A, ventral view; B, lateral view

Life-cycle. Development is direct and infection occurs through the ingestion of infective eggs. The young stages are found in the mucosa of the small intestine and the caecum.

Pathogenicity, etc. These worms sometimes occur in enormous numbers in young rabbits, but appear to be relatively harmless.

Genus: Skrjabinema Vereschagin, 1926

This genus contains several species of small worms measuring about 3–8 mm. in length, which occur in the caeca of ruminants. They have three large, complicated lips and three small intermediate lips. The oesophagus is cylindrical and terminates in a large spherical bulb. The tail of the male is bluntly rounded and has a cuticular caudal expansion supported by two pairs of processes. There is a single spicule in the male. The life-cycle is direct. Eggs are fully embryonated when deposited by the female on the perianal skin. The prepatent period is about 25 days.

S. ovis (Skrjabin, 1915) has been found in the sheep, goat and antelopes in several countries, and *S. alata* (Mönnig, 1932) in the sheep in South Africa. These worms are apparently not pathogenic, but they may be mistaken for young forms of other nematodes, such as *Oesophagostomum columbianum.*

FAMILY: KATHILANIIDAE TRAVASSOS, 1918

Oxyuroidea with the isthmus of the oesophagus sub-spherical: oesophagus terminated by a bulb. Parasites of the large intestine of equines, apes and tortoises.

Genus: Probstmayria Ransom, 1907

P. vivipara (Probstmayr, 1865). This is a minute nematode living in the colon of horses. It measures 2–2·9 mm. in length. The females are viviparous and give birth to larvae almost as large as the adults. As a result of this almost unique method of reproduction, infections may be enormous, but the worms are not known to be pathogenic.

SUPERFAMILY: SUBULUROIDEA TRAVASSOS, 1930

FAMILY: HETERAKIDAE RAILLIET & HENRY, 1914

Medium sized to small worms with three lips round the mouth, a small buccal or pharynx. Lateral alae extending down the body. Oesophagus in three parts—a short pharynx, a cylindrical, middle part and a bulbous posterior part with a valvular apparatus. A pre-anal sucker at the tail end of the male which has a chitinous rim. Many anal papillae.

Genus: Heterakis Dujardin, 1845

H. gallinarum (Schrank, 1788) Madsen, 1949 (syn. *H. papillosa, H. vesicularis, H. gallinae*) occurs in the caeca of the fowl, guinea-fowl, pea-fowl, turkey, duck, goose and numerous other birds. The male is

7–13 mm. long and the female 10–15 mm. There are large lateral alae extending some distance down the sides of the body. The oesophagus has a strong posterior bulb. The tail of the male is provided with large alae, a prominent, circular, pre-cloacal sucker and twelve pairs of papillae. The spicules are unequal, the right being slender and 2 mm. long, while the left has broad alae and measures 0·65–0·7 mm. The vulva opens directly behind the middle of the body. The eggs have thick, smooth shells; they measure 65–80 × 35–46 μ and are unsegmented when laid.

Life-cycle. The eggs develop in the open and reach the infective second larval stage in 14 days or longer. They are very resistant. When the

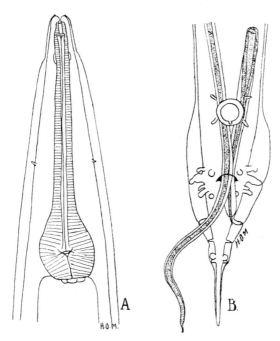

FIG. 81. *Heterakis gallinarum*: A, anterior end, dorsal view; B, hind end of male, ventral view (Original)

host swallows an infective egg the larva hatches in the intestine after 1–2 hours. Baker (1933) states that up to about the fourth day the young worms are rather closely associated with the caecal mucosa and some injury to the glandular epithelium may occur. Osipov (1957) considers that second stage larvae spend 2–5 days in the glandular epithelium before continuing their development in the lumen. They moult to the third stage on the sixth day after infection, the fourth stage on the tenth day and the fifth stage on the fifteenth day. The first eggs are passed in the faeces of the bird after 24–30 days. Baker found that the presence of blackhead in the host causes considerable retardation of development and fewer worms develop than in healthy birds.

Other species of this genus which occurs in the fowl are:

H. brevispiculum Gendre, 1911. Spicules equal, 0·4 mm. long, each with a barb near the tip.

H. putaustralis Lane, 1914 (syn. *H. beramporia*). Spicules sub-equal, the right 0·32–0·55, the left 0·26–0·36 mm. long, both alate, the left angulated near the tip. In fowls in Asia.

H. dispar (Schrank, 1790) occurs in the goose and duck. The males are 11–18 mm. long and the females 16–23 mm. The sub-equal spicules are 0·04–0·05 mm. long.

Pathogenicity and Clinical signs. The direct effects of *H. gallinarum* are slight and only in heavy infections may there be a thickening of the caecal mucosa with a number of petechial haemorrhages on the surface. Even so, no marked ill effects are ascribable to such infections. With *H. isolonche* on the other hand, marked lesions are produced in the caecum of the pheasant. These consist of a nodular typhlitis which leads to diarrhoea, wasting, emaciation and death. Frequently the nodules coalesce to form large necrotic centres. All stages of *H. isolonche* may be found in the lesions.

The principal economic importance of *H. gallinarum* lies in its role as a carrier of *Histomonas meleagridis*, the causal agent of 'blackhead', or enterohepatitis, of turkeys. The protozoan may remain viable in the egg of *H. gallinarum* for a long time, possibly as long as the egg remains viable. It is also thought that the shelter of the helminth egg allows passage of the protozoan through the anterior part of the digestive tract, which normally is lethal to the blackhead organism.

Diagnosis is made by finding the eggs in the faeces. Caecal faeces have to be examined and the eggs must be differentiated from those of *Ascaridia galli* and other related worms.

Treatment and Prophylaxis. Phenothiazine is 80–100 per cent effective when given at the rate of up to 1 g. per bird.

FAMILY: SUBULURIDAE YORK AND MAPLESTONE, 1926

Oxyuroidea with mouth with no lips or lips poorly visible. Buccal capsule present and frequently teeth are present in it. Oesophagus with a posterior bulb. Pre-anal sucker present, slit like, without a chitinous rim.

Genus: Subulura Molin, 1860

S. brumpti (Lopez Neyra, 1922) occurs in the caeca of the fowl, turkey, guinea-fowl and wild related birds in Africa, South America and Spain. The males are 6·9–10 mm. long and the females 9–17·5 mm. Lateral alae are present. The small buccal capsule has three teeth at its base. The oesophagus has a small swelling posteriorly, followed by a deep constriction and then a spherical bulb. The tail of the male is provided with large lateral alae and is curved ventrad. The pre-cloacal sucker is an elongate slit, surrounded by radiating muscle fibres. There are ten pairs of small caudal papillae. The spicules are equal, alate and 1·3–1·5 mm. long. The vulva is situated just anterior to the middle of the body. The eggs are subglobular with smooth shells, and contain a fully developed embryo when laid. They measure 52–64 by 41–49 μ.

Life-cycle. The intermediate hosts are various beetles of the genera *Blaps, Gonocephalum* and *Dermestes* and the cockroach *Blatella germanica.*

Pathogenicity. Apparently not marked.

S. differens (Sonsino, 1890) is a similar form occurring in the fowl and guinea-fowl in Southern Europe, Africa and Brazil.

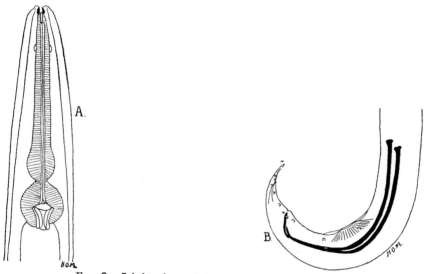

FIG. 82. *Subulura brumpti*, A, anterior end, dorsal view, B, hind end of male, lateral view.

ORDER: RHABDITIDA CHITWOOD, 1933

SUBORDER: RHABDITATA CHITWOOD, 1933

SUPERFAMILY: RHADITOIDEA TRAVASSOS, 1920

Forms with an oesophagus with a long anterior cylindrical portion (sometimes a median bulbar swelling) and a posterior bulb with a valvular apparatus. Cephalic papillae consisting of an inner circle of six and an outer circle of ten. Oral stylet absent. Excretory system symmetrical and 'H' shaped: mainly free-living forms, or forms parasitic in invertebrates, amphibians, reptiles etc.

FAMILY: RHABDITIDAE OERLEY, 1880

Mainly free-living forms, some parasitic in arthropods, earthworms, molluscs etc. Small buccal cavity, three or six tips. Oesophagus rhabditiform, i.e. an anterior wide portion, then a narrow shorter portion and terminated by a spherical posterior bulb with valves. Females oviparous or viviparous.

Genus: Rhabditis Dujardin, 1845

R. strongyloides (Leuckart, 1883) is a free-living nematode which may in rare cases invade the skin, but probably only when the latter is already damaged. Chitwood (1932) describes the affection in a dog. The skin of the affected areas is red, denuded, partly covered with crusts, and there are pustules surrounded by red zones, as well as nodules. The pustules contain typical *Rhabditis* larvae, 596–600 μ long.

FAMILY: STRONGYLOIDIDAE CHITWOOD & McINTOSH, 1934

Free-living generation saprophytic, parasitic generation in gut of vertebrates. Free-living generation with oesophagus with a valvulated bulb. Parasitic generation with markedly elongated cylindrical oesophagus. Heterogenetic.

Genus: Strongyloides Grassi, 1879

This genus contains several species which live partly as parasites in domestic animals. The parasitic forms are parthenogenetic and their eggs may give rise, outside the host, directly to infective larvae of another parasitic generation or to a free-living generation of minute males and females. The oesophagus in the free-living generation is rhabditiform. The vulva is near the middle of the body, the eggs are few, but large, and have thin shells. This non-parasitic generation produces a parasitic generation. The oesophagus of the parasitic generation is not rhabditiform but is cylindrical, without a posterior bulb (filariform). The infective larvae of the parasitic generation are able to penetrate through the skin of the host and pass with the blood to the lungs, thence up the trachea to the pharynx and on to the intestine. The adult parasitic worms are characterised by their female genital organs and by the relatively long oesophagus.

S. papillosus (Wedl, 1856) occurs in the small intestine of the sheep, goat, cattle, rabbit and wild ruminants. Similar worms have been found in various fur-bearing animals, including the mink. It is 3·5–6 mm. long and 0·05–0·06 mm. thick. The oesophagus is 0·6–0·8 mm. long. The eggs have rather blunt ends and thin shells. They measure 40–60 by 20–25 μ and contain fully developed embryos when passed in the faeces of the host.

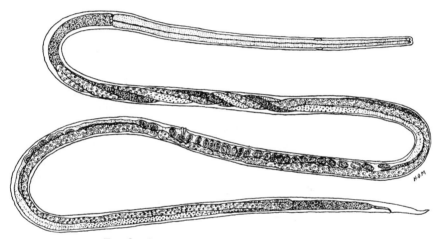

FIG. 83. *Strongyloides westeri*, Female (Original)

S. westeri Ihle, 1917 occurs in the small intestine of the horse, pig and zebra. It is up to 9 mm. long and 0·08–0·095 mm. thick. The oesophagus is 1·2–1·5 mm. long and the eggs measure 40–52 by 32–40 μ.

S. stercoralis (Bavay, 1876) occurs in the small intestine of man, dog, fox and cat. The parasitic female is about 2·2 mm. long and 0·034 mm. thick. The parasitic male is 0·7 mm. long. The oesophagus is 0·6 mm. long. The eggs measure 50–58 by 30–34 μ, but most usually rhabditiform larvae are found in fresh faeces.

S. cati Rogers, 1939 (syn. *S. planiceps*) occurs in the small intestine of the cat. It is 2·37–3·33 mm. long. The eggs measure 57·6–64 by 23–40 μ and are poorly developed when passed in the faeces.

S. ransomi Schwartz & Alicata, 1930 occurs in the small intestine of the pig. It is 3·33–4·49 mm. long. The eggs measure 45–55 by 26–35 μ.

S. avium Cram, 1929 occurs in the small intestine and the caeca of the fowl, turkey and some wild birds. It is 2·2 mm. long. The oesophagus is 0·7 mm. long and the eggs measure 52–56 by 36–40 μ.

Life-cycles. The parthenogenetic female is found buried in the mucosa of the small intestine. This form is triploid in character and produces thin-shelled transparent eggs which are passed in the faeces, except in the case of *S. stercoralis* where the eggs hatch in the intestine and first stage larvae are found in the faeces. The first stage larvae may either develop directly to become third stage infective larvae (homogonic cycle) or they may develop to free-living males and females which subsequently produce infective larvae (heterogonic cycle). When environmental conditions are satisfactory (e.g. warmth, humidity etc.) the heterogonic cycle occurs but when environmental conditions are unfavourable the homogonic cycle predominates.

In the heterogonic cycle the first stage larvae are rapidly transformed so that within 48 hours sexually mature free-living males and females occur. Following copulation, the free-living female produces eggs which hatch in a few hours and these larvae metamorphose to become infective larvae. There is much evidence to indicate that only one generation of larvae is produced by the free-living females; though copulation may occur several times, up to thirty-five eggs being produced after each mating, a total of about 180 eggs being produced per worm (Premvati, 1958).

In the homogonic cycle, first stage larvae metamorphose rapidly to become infective larvae, as little as 24 hours being required for this at 27°C.

Studies on the genetics of *Strongyloides* by Chang & Graham (1957) and Little (1962) have indicated that the parasitic female has a triploid number of chromosomes, the free-living female a diploid number, the free-living male being haploid and the infective larva, triploid. Chang & Graham (1957) described three types of eggs from the parthenogenetic female, some triploid, some diploid and some haploid. Little (1962) showed that haploid eggs developed to free-living males and he suggested that the diploid eggs produced either infective larvae (directly) or free-living females. It would seem, however, that a triploid egg would be necessary in the life-cycle if adult parasitic females were to arise from the direct life-cycle.

In the past there has been much debate concerning the factors which determine whether the direct or the indirect cycle are undergone. At one time it was considered that the environmental conditions played a major part in inducing the first stage larvae to go one way or the other. Of course, such an idea would necessitate both a recognition and a reaction system in the first stage larvae. It is more likely that all stages are produced initially, this being determined genetically in the egg, and the success or otherwise of each developmental stage is determined by the environmental conditions. Thus, when conditions are adverse, only the first stage larvae which are triploid survive to produce infective larvae, but when conditions are favourable, larvae of all three genetic types survive.

Infection of the vertebrate host is mainly by skin penetration, though oral infection may occur. Larvae reach a skin capillary or venule and are carried by the blood to the lungs. Here they break out into the alveoli, migrate up the smaller bronchioles to the bronchi and trachea and then descend the oesophagus to the intestine where they mature. The prepatent period is 5–7 days.

Recently Monocol & Batte (1966) have demonstrated with *S. ransomi* of the pig that transcolostral infection may occur (see below).

In human infection hyper-infection and auto-infection may occur. In the former, first stage larvae in the bowel metamorphose to infective larvae, these penetrate the bowel wall and undergo a lung migration as before. In auto-infection the transformed larvae are voided in the faeces and these penetrate the skin of the perianal and perineal regions and continue the lung migration as before. There is little evidence for these modes of infection with the *Strongyloides* spp. of animals.

The infective larva of *Strongyloides* has no protective sheath (compare Strongyle infective larvae) and does not resist desiccation. The oesphagus is extended for more than a third of the body length from the anterior end and the tail is distinctly bifid.

Pathogenicity and clinical signs. Experimental studies of the pathogenicity of *S. papillosus* by Turner (1959) showed that exposure of lambs to 100,000 or more larvae caused death in 13–41 days. Pathological changes included erosion of the intestinal mucosa, fluid gut contents and the clinical signs consisted of anorexia, loss of weight, diarrhoea and a moderate anaemia. Field outbreaks of disease were associated with a catarrhal enteritis of the upper small intestine but fatalities were few. The larvae of *S. papillosus* are associated with the introduction of the organisms of 'foot rot' into the skin around the feet of sheep (Beveridge, 1934).

Severe infections of *S. stercoralis* may occur in dogs, especially in puppies. The condition is most commonly seen in summer when the weather is hot and humid and is frequently a kennel problem. Lesions consist of a catarrhal inflammation of the small intestine while in severe infections there may be necrosis and sloughing of the mucosa. Dogs show moderate to severe diarrhoea which may be blood stained. Dehydration, followed by death, may occur.

Pathological manifestations of *S. ransomi* are usually seen in young suckling pigs, infection being acquired either orally, free infective larvae adhering to the udder and teats or by skin penetration from larvae in the litter and soil. Nevertheless, heavy infections of piglets also occur under circumstances in which neither of these modes of infection are likely to operate and recently Monocoe & Batte (1966) have demonstrated passage of larvae with the colostrum into the newborn pig. Piglets removed from sows prior to suckling and subsequently fed cows milk developed no infection; those fed colostrum without treatment developed infection but those fed filtered colostrum failed to develop infection. Larvae of *Strongyloides* were recovered from the residue after filtration. Following transcolostral infection patent infections were evident in 4 days. Mortality in young piglets may reach 50 per cent: the chief clinical signs are initially anorexia then diarrhoea, which soon becomes continuous and frequently haemorrhagic.

Skin lesions may be seen (Ippen, 1953) but pulmonary disorders are not frequent in natural outbreaks of the disease. Nevertheless, they can be produced experimentally (Supperer & Pfeiffer, 1960).

S. westeri in foals produces diarrhoea which may be acute. The parasite may be responsible for a high incidence of scouring in nursing foals. Foals usually develop a satisfactory immunity to the infection at 15-23 weeks after birth but in the donkey, heavy infections have been recorded at the age of 9-12 months (Pande & Rao, 1960).

Immunology of Strongyloides infections. Much experimental work has been carried out on the immune response to *Strongyloides* (see Soulsby, 1965). Essentially a few infections lead to a marked immunity and in domestic animals this is exemplified by the fact that only young animals are severely affected by the parasite.

Diagnosis. This is made by demonstrating the eggs or larvae (dogs) in the faeces.

Treatment

Sheep. A dose of 180 mg. per kg. methyridine given subcutaneously is more than 90 per cent effective.

Thiabendazole—75 mg. per kg. orally is highly effective. Other compounds which may be used are Dowco 105 [O-methyl-O-(4 tert.-butyl-2-chlorophenyl)ethylphosphoramidothioate] (200 mg. per kg.), Bayer 21/199 (coumaphos, Co-Ral) [O-O-diethyl-O-(3-chloro-4-methyl-7-coumarinyl) phosphorothioate] (25 mg. per kg.) and haloxon [O,O,-di-(2-chlorethyl)-O-(3-chloro-4-methyl-coumarin-7yl)phosphate] (30–55 mg. per kg.).

Pigs. Gentian violet has been used in the past; a dose of 50–70 mg. per kg. being given twice daily for 3 days. *Thiabendazole* is highly effective at the rate of 50 mg. per kg. mixed in the food.

Dogs. Various compounds have been used over years, including diethylcarbamazine (100 mg. per kg.), gentian violet (65 mg. three times daily for 10 days), dithiazanine (ten daily doses of 5 mg. per kg.) and pyrvinium pamoate (20 mg. per kg. per day for 5 days, 5 days rest and then another 5 days treatment). Unpublished reports indicate that thiabendazole at a dose of 50–75 mg. per kg. is highly effective.

Horses. Though no critical trials have been conducted with thiabendazole, it is likely it will be highly effective.

Prophylaxis. Since the infective larvae are not resistant to desiccation, the infection can best be prevented by providing clean, dry quarters and pastures for the animals. Mink are best protected by keeping them on raised wire-netting floors.

ORDER: RHABDITIDA CHITWOOD, 1933

SUBORDER: STRONGYLATA RAILLIET & HENRY, 1913

Nematodes with six, three or no lips, usually small if present. Corona radiata (leaf-crowns) may be present. Female reproductive system well developed, uterus with well-developed muscular ovejectors. Males with bursa and rays usually well developed. Oesophagus club-shaped in adult parasites.

Superfamilies of importance in this suborder include Strongyloidea, Trichostrongyloidea and Metastrongyloidea.

SUPERFAMILY: STRONGYLOIDEA WEINLAND, 1858

Worms with mouth well developed, often the oral opening is surrounded by corona radiata. Teeth or cutting plates may occur in the buccal cavity. Copulatory bursa on the posterior end of the male worms well developed. This structure consists of cuticular alae which usually form two lateral lobes and a dorsal lobe, enclosing the posterior extremity, and are supported by modified caudal papillae, known as the 'bursal rays'. These rays contain muscle fibres and are arranged in a definite order. There are two ventral rays; a ventro-ventral and a latero-ventral; three lateral rays; an antero-lateral (externo-lateral), a medio-lateral and a postero-lateral; and a set of dorsal rays usually comprising an externo-dorsal on either side of the single or divided dorsal ray (see Fig. 84). The hind end of the male enclosed in the bursa is called the 'genital cone'. There are usually two equal spicules, and a gubernaculum, as well as a telamon, may be present. The families of importance in this superfamily include Strongylidae, Trichonematidae, Syngamidae, Stephanuridae, Ancylostomatidae and Amidostomatidae.

FAMILY: STRONGYLIDAE BAIRD, 1853

There is a well-developed globoid buccal capsule on the dorsal wall of which there may be a median thickening, called the *dorsal gutter*, which carries the duct of the dorsal oesophageal gland. The anterior margin of the buccal capsule usually bears leaf-like cuticular structures called the *leaf-crowns* or *corona radiata*. There may be an external leaf-crown round the mouth opening and an internal leaf-crown on the inner wall of the buccal capsule a little further back. The supposed resemblance of these fringes to a palisade gave origin to the term 'palisade worms' formerly given to these species. The anterior margin of the buccal capsule does not bear teeth or cutting plates, but teeth may be present in the depth of the buccal capsule. The male bursa is strongly developed and has typical

181

rays. The life-cycle is direct in all known cases. Genera of importance include *Strongylus, Triodontophorus, Craterostomum   Oesophegodontus, Codiostomum, Chabertia*.

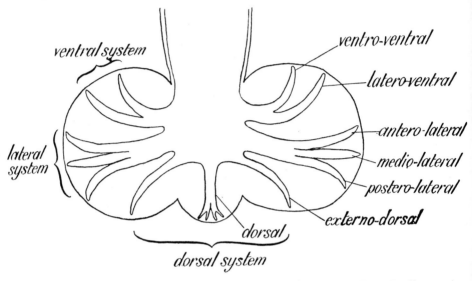

FIG. 84. Diagram of the Copulatory Bursa of the Strongylidae (from Baylis, 1929)

Genus: Strongylus Müller, 1780

S. equinus Müller, 1780 occurs in the caecum and colon of equines, including the zebra. The worms are fairly rigid and dark grey in colour; sometimes the red colour of the blood in the intestine can be seen. The male is 26–35 mm. long and the female 38–47 mm. by about 2 mm. thick. The head end is not marked off from the rest of the body. The buccal capsule is oval in outline and there are external and internal leaf-crowns. At the base of the buccal capsule there is a large dorsal tooth with a bifid tip and two smaller sub-ventral teeth. The dorsal oesophageal gland opens into the buccal capsule through a number of pores situated in a thickened ridge, the dorsal gutter, formed by the wall of the buccal capsule. The male has two simple, slender spicules. The vulva lies 12–14 mm. from the posterior extremity and the uteri are of the amphidelph type. The eggs are oval, thin-shelled, segmenting when laid, and measure 70–85 by 40–47 μ.

S. edentatus (Looss, 1900) also occurs in the large intestine of equines. The male is 23–28 mm. long and the female 33–44 mm. by about 2 mm. broad. This worm resembles *S. equinus* macroscopically, but the head is somewhat wider than the following portion of the body. The buccal capsule is wider anteriorly than at the middle and contains no teeth.

S. vulgaris (Looss, 1900) occurs in the large intestine of equines. The male is 14–16 mm. long and the female 20–24 mm. by about 1·4 mm. thick. This worm is distinctly smaller than the two preceding species.

The buccal capsule is roughly oval and contains two ear-shaped dorsal teeth at its base. The elements of the external leaf-crown are fringed at their distal extremities.

Life-cycles of Strongylus spp.

Bionomics of Strongyle larvae. The eggs of the parasites are passed in the faeces in the early stages of segmentation. The egg is thin shelled, composed of an outer chitinous shell and an inner delicate vitelline membrane. Usually there is a wide fluid cavity between the inner membrane and the cell mass. The shape of the egg is that of a regular ellipse. Embryonation

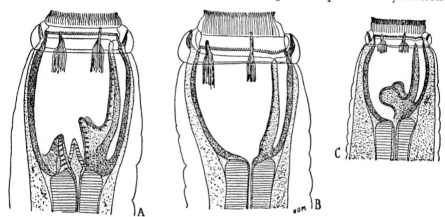

FIG. 85. Anterior End, Dorso-Lateral View, of A, *Strongylus equinus*; B, *S. edentatus*; C, *S. vulgaris* (Original)

commences immediately but is dependent on suitable environmental conditions such as moisture, oxygen and a favourable temperature. At about 26°C a first stage larva is produced in 20–24 hours; this hatches from the egg to become a free-living stage. Development to the first larval stage may be inhibited by several factors, temperature and lack of moisture being the two major ones. At temperatures below 7·2°C (45°F) development is extremely slow and the majority of eggs fail to develop to the pre-hatch stage. However, these which do so may hatch if the temperature is raised to above 9°C (48·2°F). Eggs which have not undergone embryonation do not readily survive temperatures below 0°C but if they have reached the pre-hatch stage they may survive for several weeks at low temperatures. Desiccation is generally lethal to eggs which have not undergone development to the pre-hatch stage, however those which do so may remain viable for several weeks in a state of resistant dormancy. Upon the return of moist conditions, hatching can occur within a few minutes.

After hatching from the egg, the larva is in the first stage and is characterised by having a rhabditiform oesophagus. It feeds apparently mainly on bacteria and grows, but soon enters a lethargic state in preparation for the first moult, from which the second-stage larva emerges. This has a less rhabditiform oesophagus than the first-stage larva. The process of feeding and growth is repeated, followed by lethargy. The old cuticle is separated off, but is not shed; it remains as a sheath round the third larva. This sheathed, third larva is the only larval stage that can infect a new host and is therefore called the infective larva. It has a club-shaped oesophagus.

The habits of the infective larva are different from those of the earlier stages. It does not feed, and exists on the reserve food granules stored in its intestinal cells. As soon as these are exhausted the larva dies. The larva does not actively enter the host, but is swallowed with food, or sometimes water, and its habits are of such a nature that they increase the possibility of finding a host. These habits can be described as the normal responses to a number of external stimuli, and the following are the most important: (i) The larva is said to be negatively geotropic because it crawls up blades of grass or other herbage. (ii) It is positively phototropic to a mild light, but is repelled by strong sunlight. The larva will therefore crawl up blades of grass only in the early morning, towards the evening and at other times of the day in dull weather. At night some of the larvae may descend to the soil. Moisture is necessary for these migrations, as the larvae are unable to crawl on a dry surface, but a very thin film of water suffices. (iii) There is a certain amount of response to heat; migration is more active in warm than in cold weather.

The sheath affords some protection against adverse conditions. One of the most lethal factors is desiccation, larvae failing to survive more than a few days when this is marked. However, on pasture the local microclimate at the soil surface may not be dry as the general environment and larvae may survive for much longer under these conditions. Some larvae may penetrate the soil, where they survive more readily than on the surface. In loose, sandy soil they are able to move more easily and to penetrate deeper than in fine clay soil, so that from this point of view sandy soil is favourable. In water the larvae sink to the bottom and may live for a month or more, depending on the temperature and the presence of other organisms which appear to affect them.

Taking all these factors together, the length of life of a larva in a pasture is favourably affected by moisture, shade and a relatively low temperature. Since the larvae do not feed and have only a limited amount of food reserves, conditions favourable for migration, like warmth, marked daily fluctuations in the intensity of light and loose soil, lead to rapid exhaustion and death. In general, under such conditions, as well as during dry seasons, the larvae will not live longer than about 3 months, but some may live for a year or longer in a cool climate where sufficient moisture is available in the soil. More detailed considerations of the ecology of the pre-infective and infective stages of strongyles may be found in Soulsby (1965) and Levine (1963).

Infection is by the ingestion of infective larvae. Liberation of the infective larva from the retained sheath of the second stage larva (exsheathment) occurs in the small intestine. It is probable that the mechanism of this is comparable to the exsheathment of the trichostrongyle larvae (see p. 223). Poynter (1956) has shown that the infective larvae of several species of horse strongyles could be induced by exposing them to fresh equine duodenal contents at 38°C. Various species of *Escherichia* bacteria appeared to be concerned with the process.

Life-cycle of S. equinus. Exsheathed infective larvae penetrate the mucosa of the caecum and colon and enter the subserosa where they cause the formation of nodules. Eleven days after infection, fourth stage larvae occur in the nodules and these migrate to the peritoneal cavity and then to the liver in which they wander for about 4 months. During this time they moult to the fifth larval stage and acquire a permanent buccal capsule, being up to 40 mm. in length. Following this they leave the liver and return to the large intestine but the route employed is unknown except that larvae may be found in the pancreas during this process. After entry into the lumen of the colon, they reach maturity, eggs being produced about 260 days after infection (Wetzel, 1941; Wetzel & Vogelsang, 1954).

Life-cycle of S. edentatus. Infective larvae enter the wall of the intestine and pass to the liver via the portal system. In the liver, fourth stage larvae are produced about 11–18 days after infection. Such fourth stage forms may migrate in the liver for up to 9 weeks and then they pass between the peritoneal layers of the hepatic ligaments to reach the parietal peritoneal region in the right abdominal flank. Late fourth and early fifth stage larvae are found in this site in association with haemorrhagic nodules which vary in size from one to several centimetres in diameter. Larvae are found here up to about 3 months after infection, but they then migrate between the layers of the mesocolon to the walls of the caecum and colon, here again causing haemorrhagic nodules. Such nodules are seen 3–5 months after infection. Eventually the young adult forms pass to the lumen and become mature. Eggs are produced about 300–320 days after infection (Wetzel, 1952; Wetzel & Dersten, 1956).

Life-cycle of S. vulgaris. Over the years there has been considerable controversy about the migratory route of the larvae of *S. vulgaris.* This has arisen because of the frequent widespread arterial lesions caused by the larvae, which in some cases, occurred as far anterior in the arterial system as the origin of the aorta. Essentially the various theories of the life-cycle can be condensed to four migratory pathways proposed by Olt (1932), Wetzel & Enigk (1938) (which was later added to by Enigk (1952)), Ershov (1949) and Farrelly (1954) (the latter being added to by Poynter (1960)).

A detailed consideration of the various propositions put forward by these various authors is given by Soulsby (1965). However, all the opinions, except that of Enigk (1952), are based on naturally infected animals. Enigk's experimental work has now been added to and confirmed by Drudge et al. (1966). The chronology of infection proposed by the German workers is as follows. Infective larvae penetrate the intestinal wall where, about 8 days after infection, fourth stage larvae are produced. Such fourth stage forms penetrate the intima of the submucosal arterioles and migrate in these vessels towards the cranial mesenteric artery. They are to be found here from the 14th day after infection onwards associated with thrombi and later aneurysms. Starting about the 45th day after infection fourth stage larvae pass back via the arterial system to the submucosa of the caecum and colon, and here become fifth stage larvae about 3 months after infection. They then enter the lumen and reach maturity, egg production occurring about 200 days after infection. Some larvae may linger as fourth or fifth stage forms in the aneurysms in the cranial mesenteric artery for several weeks after the main population has returned to the large bowel.

Drudge et al. (1966) confirmed the migratory pathway proposed by Enigk stating that shortly after penetration of the gut the larvae migrate in the intima of the mesenteric arteries, against the flow of blood, to the anterior mesenteric artery. The behaviour of the larvae accounts for the characteristic localisation of the primary lesions in the walls of the small intestine, the caecum, ventral colon and the associated arteries.

Lesions elsewhere in the arterial system may be accounted for by the proposal that a few larvae may migrate more rapidly than others and enter more distant arteries than the cranial mesenteric.

Pathogenesis of the Strongylus spp. The specific pathogenesis of the three species will be dealt with here, however since *Strongylus* spp. infections are almost always combined with *Trichonema* spp. infection, a general account of Strongyle infection of horses, together with treatment and control measures is discussed on page 192.

In their adult forms all three *Strongylus* spp. attach themselves to the mucosa of the large intestine and suck blood. In heavy infections this results in an anaemia of the normochromic, normocytic type. Lesions produced by the adult worms consist of small haemorrhagic ulcers indicating the site of attachment. Some may become confluent to produce an ulcerous patch. They are however superficial, unlike the deep ulcers produced by the *Triodontophorus* spp. The latter may occasionally break down with a fatal haemorrhage.

The larval stages of the *Strongylus* spp. may be responsible for severe pathogenic effects. The fourth and fifth larval stages of *S. vulgaris* are responsible for severe lesions in the arterial system from the aortic valves to the iliac arteries, though the majority of the lesions occur in the region of the cranial mesenteric artery and the arteries which derive from it. Extensive irregular inflammatory lesions occur in the media of the affected arteries producing an endarteritis and the formation of thrombi. Larval stages may be found embedded in the thrombus. At times thrombus formation may be marked, being large, soft friable structures extending for several centimetres in the arterial system. Detachment of such thrombi may lead to a rapidly fatal event especially if they are situated at the anterior end of the arterial system.

With the formation of the thrombus, especially in the cranial mesenteric artery, a thickening of the arterial wall occurs and progressive dilatation begins due to degeneration of elastic fibres. Ultimately a large dilated mass occurs.

The consequences of such lesions are varied. Detachment of large anterior thrombi may lead to catastrophic events such as occlusion of a coronary artery or the brachiocephalic trunk (Farrelly, 1954). Infarction of the iliac artery may lead to temporary lameness while thrombosis of a testicular artery may lead to passive congestion of one or both testicles. Infarction of the kidney has been described.

An association between cranial mesenteric artery aneurysms and colic has long been suggested. Indeed Enigk (1952) produced death in five animals due to haemorrhagic or anaemic infarction of the small and large intestine by giving 800–8000 infective larvae. Similar results were obtained by Drudge et al. (1966). However, in natural cases, it is unlikely that the massive embolism necessary to produce fatal infarction would commonly occur and since the aneurysm of the cranial mesenteric artery is produced slowly, it is likely that collateral circulations will be well established. Olt (1932) has suggested that colic may be due to the pressure of the cranial mesenteric aneurysm on associated nerve plexuses and Ottaway & Bingham (1946) confirmed this view, demonstrating degeneration of the coeliac and anterior mesenteric plexuses.

The pathogenicity of S. equinus larvae has been described by Wetzel (1941). Fatal infections caused by 4000 larvae were associated with haemorrhagic tracts in the liver and pancreas. Clinical signs consisted of colic, anorexia and general malaise. Five hundred infective larvae produced no marked clinical signs.

The larval stages of S. edentatus may be responsible for serious ill health. In acute experimental infections (3000–75,000 larvae) there is a marked peritonitis, acute toxaemia, jaundice and fever. The peritoneal cavity contains a large amount of haemorrhagic fluid and numerous haemorrhages and fibrinous deposits occur on the peritoneum. Larvae which have migrated to the sub-peritoneal region of the right flank produce haemorrhagic nodules. These reach their fullest development about 3–5 months after infection and in severe infections the abdominal cavity is dotted with such nodules. Some may break down, leading to a serious and, at times, fatal intra-peritoneal haemorrhage. At other times, an acute peritonitis occurs which may later turn septic.

Genus: Triodontophorus Looss, 1902

The four species of this genus vary from 9–25 mm. in length. The buccal capsule is sub-globular and rather thick-walled. It has three pairs of teeth and its base and a well-developed dorsal gutter. The spicules of the male end in small hooks and the vulva of the female is near the

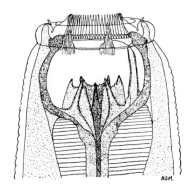

FIG. 86.   *Triodontophorus serratus*, Anterior End, Dorso-Lateral View (Original)

posterior end of the body. The developmental cycle of the *Triodontophorus* spp. is unknown but it is likely that development is restricted to the bowel mucosa.

T. tenuicollis causes the formation of ulcers, which at times may be deep and haemorrhagic, in the right dorsal colon to which bunches of the worms ιnay be found attached.

Genus: Craterostomum Boulenger, 1920

Species of this genus resemble *Triodontophorus*, but they have no teeth in the buccal capsule and the vulva of the female is further forward. Two species may be found in the large intestines of equines. The developmental cycle is unknown.

Genus: Oesophagodontus Railliet & Henry, 1902

One species of this genus, *O. robustus*, is rather rare in the large intestines of equines. The male is 15–16 mm. and the female 19–22 mm. long. There is a slight constriction between the anterior end and the rest of the body. The goblet-shaped buccal capsule has a posterior circular ridge and at its base are three tooth-like folds which do not project into the buccal capsule. There is no dorsal gutter. The developmental cycle probably resembles that of the *Trichonema* spp.

Genus: Codiostomum Railliet & Henry, 1911

C. struthionis Horst, 1885 occurs in the large intestine of the ostrich. The male is about 13 mm. long and the female 17 mm. The buccal capsule is sub-globular, strongly chitinised and provided with external and internal leaf-crowns, but there are no teeth. The dorsal gutter is well developed and reaches the anterior margin of the buccal capsule. The male bursa has a large projecting dorsal lobe and the vulva of the female is situated close to the anus.

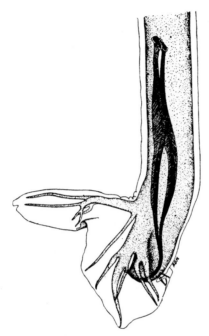

FIG. 87. *Codiostomum struthionis*, Hind End of Male, Lateral View (Original)

Life-cycle. Unknown; probably direct.

Pathogenicity. Little is known, but the parasite must be considered a dangerous one, especially when infections are heavy.

Genus: Chabertia Railliet & Henry, 1909

C. ovina (Gmelin, 1790) occurs in the colon of sheep, goats, cattle and a number of other ruminants. Male 13–14 mm. long, female 17–20 mm. long. The anterior end is curved slightly ventral and the large buccal capsule opens antero-ventrally. The oral aperture is surrounded by a double row of small cuticular elements representing the leaf-crowns. There is a shallow ventral cervical groove, and anterior to it a slightly inflated cephalic vesicle. The male bursa is well developed and the spicules are 1·3–1·7 mm. long, with a gubernaculum. The vulva of the female opens about 0·4 mm. from the posterior extremity. The eggs measure 90–105 by 50–55 μ.

Life-cycle. This is direct, and, as far as the free stages are concerned, resembles that of *Strongylus equinus*. The sheath of the infective larva has a

8

relatively long tail. Infection of the host occurs per os. No migration in the body is known. Threlkeld (1948) found that, 90 hours after infection of parasite-free lambs, the infective larvae had performed the third ecdysis and were attached to the mucosa of the upper colon or had entered its wall. There were profuse petechial haemorrhages here. The larvae were then 650 μ long, but 6 days later they were 1040 μ long and had developed a provisional buccal capsule. By the eighteenth day the larvae were sexually differentiated, the permanent buccal capsule was being formed and both sexes were 2 mm. or more long; these larvae were late fourth stage larvae and, by the twenty-fifth day, they had performed the last ecdysis to become adults. By the thirty-fourth day males and females, 7 mm. long, had well-developed sexual organs and copulation occurred on the thirty-eighth day. Eggs appeared in the faeces of the lambs 48–54 days after their infection.

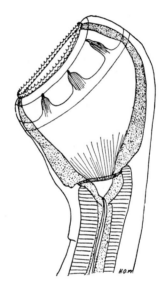

Fig. 88. *Chabertia ovina*, Anterior End, Lateral View (Original)

Pathogenesis. The worms attach themselves firmly to the mucosa of the colon by means of their buccal capsules and draw in a plug of the mucosa, chiefly the glandular layer, which is digested by the secretions of the oesophageal glands of the worm. The worms suck blood by accident only, when a blood vessel is ruptured. The adjoining parts of the mucosa show an increased activity of goblet cells and infiltration with lymphocytes and eosinophils. At autopsy the worms are found attached to the mucosa of the colon, which is congested, swollen and covered with a transparent mucus in severe cases, while punctiform haemorrhages may be present. In severe infections the sheep lose condition and may become anaemic and die. *Chabertia* infections may be responsible for a specific reduction of wool growth in sheep.

Diagnosis is made by finding the eggs in the faeces and by identification of the larvae in faecal cultures.

Treatment. Pheniothiazine (20–30 g. per animal) is usually highly effective: Thiabendazole (50 mg. per kg.) is also highly effective.

FAMILY: TRICHONEMATIDAE WITENBERG, 1925

Strongyles with a short cylindrical or annular buccal capsule, dorsal gutter short and not reaching the anterior border of the buccal capsule. Leaf-crowns present. Genera of importance include *Trichonema, Poteriostomum, Gyalocephalus, Bourgelatia* and *Oesophagostomum*.

Genus: Trichonema Cobbold, 1874
(syn. Cyathostomum; Cylicostomum)

The buccal capsule of the species of this genus is relatively short and without teeth and the dorsal gutter is short. The spicules of the males have barbed tips. The vulva of the female is near to the anus. There are about thirty-five species, the males of which vary from 4 to 17 mm. and the females from 4 to 26 mm. in length.

Life-cycle. The larvae of *Trichonema* develop in nodules in the wall of the large intestine. The duration of the stay in the mucosa varies greatly. Some larvae appear to persist in an encapsulated stage for several months, but with others the prepatent period is about 3 months (Wetzel & Vogelsang, 1954). A detailed account of the different larvae stage which occur in the mucosa is given by Soulsby (1965).

Genus: Poteriostomum Quiel, 1919

Species of this genus resemble *Trichonema*, but the externo-dorsal ray and the dorsal ray of the male bursa arise from a common trunk and the dorsal ray gives off, almost at right angles, two lateral branches near the origin of the externo-dorsal rays; the dorsal ray is cleft only to about half its length and not to its base, as it is in *Trichonema*. Two species occur in equines. The males are 9–14 mm. and the females 13–21 mm. long.

Genus: Gyalocephalus Looss, 1900

Species of this genus have a short, thick-walled buccal capsule at the base of which are thin, triangular, chitinoid plates which line the very large oesophageal funnel, from which three teeth project into the buccal capsule. There is no dorsal gutter. One species, *G. capitatus*, is rather rare in the large intestine of equines. The male is 7–8·5 mm. and the female 8·5–11 mm. long.

Pathogenesis of Trichonema spp. These parasites are often found in very large numbers in the caecum and colon of horses. The larval stages occur in nodules, chiefly in the caecum. In heavy infections the nodules may be so numerous that it is difficult to find an area of normal mucosa. The larval stages are reputed to suck blood and large numbers cause a catarrhal enteritis with a diffuse inflammation of the caecum and colon. The intestinal contents may be dark brown or black. The associated clinical signs are enteritis alternating with constipation. In the terminal stages of heavy infections, anaemia and oedema are common features.

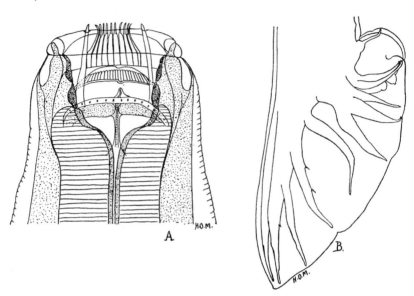

FIG. 89. *Trichonema tetracanthum.* (Original) A, Anterior end, dorsal view; B, hind end of male, lateral view.

The adult parasites live on the surface of the mucosa, feeding on the superficial layers, they do not suck blood. Large numbers produce a general catarrhal enteritis.

STRONGYLE INFECTION OF EQUINES

Though some of the equine strongyles are blood suckers and some are not, the infections are usually mixed and consequently the general clinical signs can be considered to be caused by all the worm collectively. Specific clinical signs may arise due to the larval stages of the *Strongylus* spp. (see p. 187). Enormous numbers of strongyles may be present in foals. Eggs of the worms found in the faeces of foals may come from at least two sources. They may come from worms parasitic in the foals, though these do not appear until the foals are 7–8 weeks old. Eggs may be found in the faeces of foals younger than this, or even in the meconium, but these are usually derived from the faeces of the dam licked or eaten by the foals. Foals can infect themselves from the faeces of the dam only by means of infective larvae derived from eggs in the dam's faeces, not by the eggs themselves. It is possible that foals may be infected before birth by larvae, especially those of *S. vulgaris*, present in the blood, but the occurrence of prenatal infection has not been demonstrated experimentally. Older equines develop a high resistance and may carry heavy infections without serious effects, so that they may be dangerous sources of infection. It has been estimated that a horse passing out 1000 eggs per g. of its faeces may pass out 30 million eggs a day.

In general the clinical signs develop slowly. The faeces become soft and have a bad odour. Later diarrhoea develops, the appetite diminishes, the animals become emaciated, easily exhausted and the coat is rough. Anaemia develops and may become marked and associated with oedematous swellings on the abdomen and the legs. Various degrees of the disease are seen, depending on the number of the parasites present and the condition and food of the animal. Death may occur in severe cases.

Post-Mortem. There may be anaemia and emaciation, even ascites, oedema and cachexia. Erratic forms of the parasites may be found in various organs.

In the intestine the worms are found free or attached to the mucosa, which shows numerous small red bite-marks or ulcers caused by *Triodontophorus tenuicollis*. The wall of the organ may contain nodules of various sizes, the large, haemorrhagic ones being those caused by the larvae of the large strongyles returning after migration, while the small ones are produced by the larvae of some other species which develop in the intestinal wall.

Diagnosis. The eggs of the various strongyle species of the large intestine of horses cannot be readily distinguished from one another and if accurate identification is required faecal cultures should be made to obtain third stage larvae. These may then be identified using appropriate keys (see Soulsby, 1965). As a rule the presence of oval, thin-shelled, strongyle-type eggs is sufficient for diagnosis of infection and the presence of 1000 eggs per g. of faeces, or more, is evidence that removal of the worms is necessary. The presence of an aneurysm in the cranial mesenteric artery can be determined in small horses by rectal palpation.

Treatment of Strongyle infections of horses. Phenothiazine has been used for many years with excellent results. For a detailed bibliography see Gibson (1965). A safe dose is 30–35 g. per animal. Highly effective against *Trichonema* spp. but low effect against *Strongylus* spp. at this level. Higher doses may be toxic to horses, causing anaemia and haemoglobinurea.

Low-level dosage of phenothiazine has been introduced because of toxicity of single large doses to horses. One to 2 g. of phenothiazine are given daily in food. Such doses do not reduce adult worm burden but reduce the egg output to low levels or zero and also interfere with embryonation of eggs which are passed. Low level dosage has been used extensively in Great Britain and the U.S.A. as part of control schemes, to reduce contamination of pastures and hence the intake of infective larvae by young animals. Resistant strains of helminths have been demonstrated (Gibson,

1960) but there is no evidence that this is a serious drawback to this method of usage.

Piperazine compounds are highly effective against *Trichonema* spp.; lower effect against *S. vulgaris* and *S. edentatus* and with very little effect against *S. equinus*. The four salts of piperazine, adipate, citrate, phosphate and carbodithioic acid, are more or less equally effective and are given at the rate of 200 mg. of piperazine base per kg.

Phenothiazine–Piperazine mixtures are superior to either compound alone. A mixture of 66 mg. phenothiazine and 220 mg. piperazine per kg. is highly effective against the majority of the large intestinal strongyles of horses.

Thiabendazole is highly effective. At doses of 50 mg. per kg. the three *Strongylus* spp. are more or less all removed, and all *Trichonema* spp. are removed (see Egerton *et al.*, 1962; Enigk & Stoye, 1963). The drug may be given in the feed: it is well tolerated.

Prophylaxis. The general principles of pasture management for the control of parasitic nematodes enumerated for the control of ruminant parasites·are applicable to horse parasites.

Pastures should not be overstocked or overgrazed. Special attention should be given to young horses which are more susceptible than the older ones. If possible clean pasture should be available for them. Proper disposal of manure, by allowing it to ferment in heaps, will kill the eggs and larvae by the heat of fermentation.

Regular treatment with thiabendazole will reduce the general burden of all horses. Low level dosing with phenothiazine or thiabendazole greatly assists in control measures. Usually 1–2 g. are given daily in the feed for the first 3 weeks of every month, followed by a rest period to the end of the month. In some areas of the U.S.A. low-level dosing has been carried on continuously for several years without apparent ill effect.

Genus: Bourgelatia Railliet Henry & Bauche, 1919

B. diducta Railliet Henry & Bauche, 1919 occurs in the caecum and colon of the pig in India, Indo-China and Java. The male is 9–12 mm. long and the female about 11–13·5 mm. The mouth is directed straight forwards. The buccal capsule is cylindrical and shallow, and its thick wall is divided into an anterior and a posterior portion, the latter being continuous with the lining of the wide oesophageal funnel. The external leaf-crown has twenty-one long elements projecting from the oral aperture and the internal leaf-crown has about twice as many elements. The spicules are equal, alate and about 1·3 mm. long. The vulva opens near the anus. The posterior end of the female is straight and ends in a sharp point. The eggs measure 58–77 by 36–42 μ.

Life-cycle. Probably direct.

Pathogenicity. Very little is known about the effects of this parasite on its host.

Genus: Oesophagostomum Molin, 1861

Members of this genus have a cylindrical buccal capsule, usually narrow. Leaf-crowns are present. There is a ventral cervical groove near the anterior end, anterior to which the cuticle is dilated to form a cephalic vesicle. Species parasitic in the posterior small intestine and the large intestine of cattle, sheep and pigs etc.

O. columbianum (Curtice, 1890), the 'nodular worm', occurs in the colon of the sheep, goat and a number of wild antelopes. It has been recorded once from cattle, but in this instance the identification of the worms may have been at fault. The male is 12–16·5 mm. long and the female 15–21·5 mm. by about 0·45 mm. wide. There are large cervical alae which produce a marked dorsal curvature of the anterior part of the body. The cuticle forms a mouth-collar which is fairly high, shaped like a truncate cone and separated from the rest of the body by a constriction. About 0·25 mm. from the anterior end there is a cervical groove which extends around the ventral surface to the lateral aspects of the body. The cuticle anterior to this groove is slightly inflated to form a cephalic vesicle. Immediately behind the cervical groove the cervical alae arise and their anterior extremities are pierced by the cervical papillae. The buccal

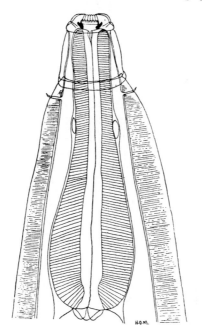

FIG. 90. *Oesophagostomum columbianum*, Anterior End, Dorsal View (Original)

capsule is shallow and wider anteriorly than posteriorly. The external leaf-crown consists of twenty to twenty-four elements and the internal has two small elements to each of the external. The male bursa is well developed and there are two equal, alate spicules, 0·77–0·86 mm. long.

The tail of the female tapers to a fine point. The vulva is situated about 0·8 mm. anterior to the anus. The vagina is very short, transverse, leading into the kidney-shaped 'pars ejectrix' of the ovijectors. The eggs have thin shells and are laid in the eight to sixteen cell stage. They measure 73–89 by 34–45 μ.

Life-cycle. The eggs are passed in the faeces of the host and the development and bionomics of the free stages are similar to those of the *Strongylus* spp. The infective stage is reached under optimum conditions in 6–7 days. None of the pre-infective stages are resistant to desiccation. After having been ingested by the host the larvae cast their sheaths and penetrate into the wall of the intestine, anywhere from the pylorus to the rectum. Here the third ecdysis takes place and the larvae grow to a length of about 1·5–2·5 mm. They now have a sub-globular buccal capsule with a dorsal tooth at the base, and the cervical groove is conspicuous. Normally they return to the lumen of the gut after 5–7 days and pass to the colon, where they grow adult after the fourth ecdysis. The first eggs are passed in the faeces of the host 41 days after infection.

Pathogenesis. In lambs, or in older sheep that have no resistance against the parasite, the larvae incite practically no reaction by their migration into the mucosa, so that eventually a large number of adult worms can be found in the colon while there are no nodules in the wall of the intestine. In other cases, probably due to previous sensitisation, the larvae pass into the submucosa and a marked reaction takes place in the form of a localised inflammation around each larva. Leucocytes, especially eosinophiles, and foreign body giant cells collect around the parasite and the focus becomes encapsulated by fibroblasts. The larvae may stay in these nodules for about 3 months, and when the contents caseate and calcify the parasite either dies or leaves the nodule, and then frequently wanders about between the muscle fibres, leaving behind it a narrow canal filled with material similar to that found in the nodules. Although the nodules usually have a small opening through which pus is discharged into the intestine, the large majority of these larvae do not find their way back into the lumen. In such cases the intestinal wall may therefore show numerous nodules and tracks, while the colon contains few adult worms.

O. columbianum is a serious pathogen of sheep, 200–300 adult worms constituting a severe infection for young sheep. Extensive nodular formation of both the small and large intestine seriously interfere with absorption, bowel movement and digestion. The nodules are frequently suppurative and may rupture to the peritoneal surface causing peritonitis and multiple adhesions. Though the adult worms do not suck blood they cause a marked thickening of the bowel wall, congestion and a large production of mucus. Infections have a profound effect on appetite and growth and also wool growth (Gordon, 1950).

On *post mortem* there is marked emaciation and an almost complete absence of fat. In heavy initial infections a large number of adult worms is seen, the mucous membrane is thickened, reddish and covered with mucus in which the worms are embedded. After repeated infections the ileum and colon may be thickly studded with nodules of various sizes, some having been converted to abscesses and containing a green to yellowish pus or caseous material.

Clinical signs. In lambs the first sign is a marked and persistent diarrhoea, which results in exhaustion and death unless the animals are removed from the infected pasture. The faeces usually have a dark green colour and contain much mucus and sometimes blood. This diarrhoea begins on the sixth day after a severe infection and coincides with the

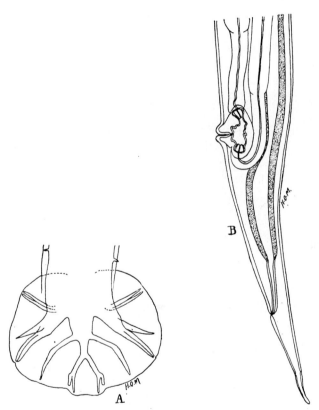

Fig. 91. *Oesophagostomum columbianum*: A, bursa of male; B, hind end of female, lateral view (Original)

time when the larvae leave the nodules. The debilitated animal shows a humped back, the action of the hind legs is stiff and the tail is often held at an angle from the body. In more chronic cases there may be an initial diarrhoea, later followed by constipation and occasional spells of diarrhoea. The animal shows progressive emaciation and general weakness. The skin becomes dry and the wool is unthrifty. The characteristic picture of chronic oesophagostomiasis in sheep is that of extreme emaciation and cachexia with atrophy of the muscles, ending in complete prostration for 1–3 days and death.

Diagnosis. Examination of the faeces may show the fourth-stage larvae in acute cases with diarrhoea or the presence of eggs in other cases. Chronic cases without adult parasites can be diagnosed only tentatively by consideration of the clinical signs together with the history. Because the eggs of *O. columbianum* cannot easily be differentiated from those of many other gastro-intestinal nematodes of sheep, faecal cultures have to be made and examined when the larvae have reached the infective stage. The infective larvae of *O. columbianum* and other species of this genus have a sheath provided with a long, whip-like tail, while the tail of the larva itself is much shorter and ends in a simple point. The sheath is rather loose and shows characteristic transverse wrinkles, which are not so marked in the case of other larvae. Approximate measurements in millimetres of some of the most important infective larvae found in sheep faeces cultures are given at the end of the book.

Treatment. *Phenothiazine* is highly effective. Dose 600–700 mg. per kg. (20–30 g. per animal).

Piperazine is highly effective at a dose of 125 mg. per kg. (4 g. per animal).

Thiabendazole is highly effective at a dose of 50 mg. per kg.

Some *organophosphorus compounds* are effective, others have little effect (see Gibson, 1965, for review).

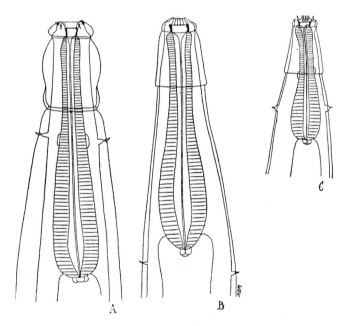

Fig. 92. Anterior End, Dorsal View, of A, *Oesophagostomum radiatum*; B, *O. venulosum*; C, *O. dentatum* (Original)

O. venulosum (Rudolphi, 1809) occurs in the colon of sheep, goat, deer and camel. The male is 11–16 mm. and the female 13–24 mm. long. There are no lateral cervical alae and the worms are therefore not curved anteriorly. The cervical papillae are situated behind the level of the oesophagus. The external leaf-crown consists of eighteen and the internal leaf-crown of thirty-six elements. The vagina of the female is 0·5–0·6 mm. long and the spicules of the male 1·1–1·5 mm.

Pathogenesis. Though *O. venulosum* is very similar to *O. columbianum* and occurs in the same site in the host, the pathogenic effects are quite different. *Oesophagostomum venulosum* is relatively harmless: infection seldom produces nodule formation. Even in heavy experimental infections the clinical effects are of a low order (Goldberg, 1952).

Treatment. As for *O. columbianum.*

O. radiatum (Rudolphi, 1803) occurs in the colon of cattle. The male is 14–17 mm. and the female 16–22 mm. long. This species is characterised by a rounded mouth-collar, a large cephalic vesicle which is constricted behind its middle, and the absence of an external leaf-crown. The internal leaf-crown consists of thirty-eight to forty minute elements. The vagina is short as it is in *O. columbianum*. The spicules of the male are 0·7–0·8 mm. long. Anantaraman (1942) described and illustrated the eggs, larvae, adults and nodules caused by this species.

Pathogenesis. The life-cycle is similar to that of *O. columbianum*. *O. radiatum* is one of the more pathogenic species of helminths of cattle when it is present in large numbers. In the acute form of the disease there is inflammation of the small and large intestine and black foetid diarrhoeic faeces are passed. The chronic disease may occur in young stock (in which it may be fatal) and in old (in which animals usually recover). Extensive nodular formation occurs, affecting the whole of the intestinal tract. This is associated firstly with intermittent diarrhoea and later with continuous purging resulting in emaciation, prostration and often death in young animals.

O. dentatum (Rudolphi, 1803). In this species the males are 8–10 mm. long and the females are 11–14 mm. The cephalic vesicle is prominent, but cervical alae are practically absent. The cervical papillae are towards the posterior end of the oesophagus. The submedian head papillae project forward conspicuously, as well as the nine elements of the external leaf-crown. The internal leaf-crown has eighteen elements. The spicules of the male are 1·15–1·3 mm. long. Other species of the genus which occur in the pig are *O. longicaudum, O. brevicaudum* and *O. georgianum* which have been recorded from North America. A key for their differentiation is given by Soulsby (1965).

The life-cycle of these species is similar to that of *O. columbianum.*

Pathogenesis. Nodule formation occurs on infection and in repeated infections a multitude of nodules may occur in the large intestine, along with large numbers of adult worms. There is a thickening of the bowel wall, a catarrhal enteritis and associated scarring and lack of growth. The infection is most commonly seen in pigs at pasture.

Treatment. Phenothiazine is highly effective at a dose of 220 mg. per kg. *Piperazine* compounds are highly effective, given at the rate of 110 mg. of piperazine base per kg. in drinking water. Hygromycin B, at the rate of 12 million units per ton of feed for 5 weeks has been shown to remove *Oesophagostomum* spp.

1 : 8 Dihydroxyanthraquinone is effective at a dose of 55 mg. per kg.

Organo-phosphorus compounds—Trichlorophon (44 mg. per kg.) and Ronnel [*O,O*-dimethyl-*O*-(2,4,5-trichlorophenyl)phosphorothioate] (100 mg. per kg.) are both highly effective.

FAMILY STEPHANURIDAE TRAVASSOS & VOGELSANG, 1933

Nematodes with a cup-shaped buccal capsule, containing teeth. Vulva near anus. Parasites of kidney and perirenal tissues. Genus of importance *Stephanurus*.

Genus: Stephanurus Diesing, 1839

S. dentatus Diesing, 1839, the 'kidney-worm' of swine, occurs in the perirenal fat, the pelvis of the kidney and the walls of the ureters, and as an erratic parasite in the liver or other abdominal organs and sometimes the thoracic organs, as well as the spinal canal of the pig; it is rarely seen in the liver of cattle and has also been reported from a donkey. The parasite is widely distributed in tropical and sub-tropical

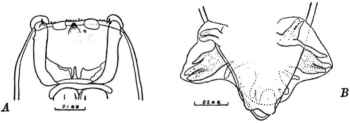

FIG. 93. *Stephanurus dentatus: A*, anterior end; *B*, posterior end of male, ventral view (from Baylis, after Daubney)

countries. Male 20–30 mm., female 30–45 mm. long. The worms are stout, the female being about 2 mm. broad, and the internal organs are partly visible through the cuticula. The buccal capsule is cup-shaped and thick-walled with six variable cusped teeth at its base. Its rim bears a leaf-crown of small elements and six external cuticular thickenings or 'epaulettes', of which the dorsal and ventral are the most prominent. The male bursa is small and its rays are short. The two spicules are equal or unequal and measure 0·66–1 mm. in length. The vulva is situated close to the anus. The eggs measure about 100 by 60 μ.

Life-Cycle. In their normal habitat the adult worms are lodged in cysts which communicate with the ureters, so that the eggs are passed out in the urine of the host. At this stage the embryo consists of about thirty-two to sixty-four cells. The development of the pre-infective stages is similar to that of *Strongylus* spp. At an optimum temperature of 26°C, and if sufficient oxygen is available, the eggs hatch after 24–36 hours and the larvae reach the infective stage about 4 days later after two ecdyses, retaining the second skin as a sheath. The eggs and all larval stages are rapidly killed by freezing and dryness. The infective larvae can live in moist surroundings up to 5 months, but the majority die off after 2–3 months. Under wet conditions they live a shorter period and they are also adversely affected by sunlight. They show little negative geotropism.

Infection of the host occurs per os or through the skin. Earthworms (e.g. *Eisenia foetida*) may serve as transport hosts. Infective larvae accumulate in masses of amoebocytes in the earthworm and probably can survive here for several weeks or months (Batte *et al.*, 1960). The sheath of the infective larva is cast soon after infection has occurred and the third ecdysis takes place about 70 hours later, either in the wall of the stomach, after oral infection, or in the skin and the abdominal muscles after pre-cutaneous infection. The fourth-stage larva possesses a buccal capsule. From both ports of entry the larvae reach the liver: after oral infection via the portal vessels in 3 days or longer, and after skin penetration via the lungs and the systemic circulation in 8–40 days. Normally the larvae escape from the hepatic vessels and wander through the liver parenchyma until they reach the surface. They wander about underneath the liver capsule and eventually, 3 months or more after infection, penetrate through the latter into the peritoneal cavity. After having reached the perirenal tissues they perforate the walls of the ureters, in order to establish connection with the external world, and then live in the renal region in cysts which communicate with the ureters through fine canals.

The migrating larvae have a marked tendency to penetrate soft tissues and many of them go astray. After percutaneous infection some remain in the pulmonary capillaries and become encapsulated in the lungs, or they may wander further and reach the pleural cavity and other thoracic organs. Frequently larvae pierce the walls of the portal vessels, the vena cava caudalis or the gastrohepatic artery, causing the formation of thrombi, and the worms may accumulate around these vessels. In the peritoneal cavity they do not all reach the perirenal tissues, but penetrate into other organs such as the spleen, psoas muscles etc.

Pathogenesis. Percutaneous infection causes the formation of nodules in the skin, with oedema and enlargement of the superficial lymph glands. These lesions disappear after 3 or 4 weeks or longer. The migrating larvae produce lesions of an acute inflammatory nature, especially in the liver. The inflammatory processes may take the form of abscesses or give rise to extensive liver cirrhosis and multiple adhesions of organs; much damage is done in this indirect way. The adult parasite itself is not markedly pathogenic and is found in cysts varying from 0·5 to 4 cm. in diameter, each cyst usually containing a pair of worms embedded in green pus. Cysts may occur in the kidney tissue. The ureter is thickened and in chronic cases may be almost occluded.

Clinical signs. The temporary subcutaneous nodules seen in the early stages of the infection may affect the host; precural nodules, for instance, may cause stiffness of the leg. Posterior paralysis has been ascribed to the parasite. The general effects are a depressed growth rate, loss of appetite and later emaciation. Where cirrhosis of the liver is marked ascites may be present. The infection is a herd problem and the general picture is one of lack of growth and wasting in the herd.

Post-mortem. Decomposition takes place rapidly in animals that have died from the results of this infection. According to the severity and the stage of the disease, there may be cutaneous nodules, pneumonic lesions, peritonitis of varying degrees with adhesions of the abdominal organs, cirrhosis and abscesses in the liver and elsewhere. Young and even adult worms may be found in cysts or abscesses in the lungs and other thoracic organs or free in the pleural cavity. A venous hyperaemia is seen in the liver, kidneys and portal and mesenteric lymph glands. The liver is enlarged and its surface is uneven on account of the presence of irregular tracks and scars, which are also found deeper in the parenchyma. Cirrhosis may be marked and ascites is then usually present. Thrombi in the hepatic blood vessels are common and they may contain young stages of the worms or these may have accumulated in the tissues surrounding the vessel. Thrombi may also occur elsewhere; they may, for instance, be associated with infarcts in the kidneys. The perirenal tissues usually show a certain degree of hypertrophy and the surface of the kidneys may bear small scars of healed abscesses. The worms are found in and around the kidneys and ureters, as described above. The portal and mesenteric lymph vessels are enlarged, while in older cases they are indurated and have uneven surfaces.

Diagnosis can be made by finding the eggs of the parasite in the urine of the pig if mature worms are present and in communication with the ureters. In other cases a definite diagnosis can be made at autopsy only. Thromba & Baisden (1960) have described a gel precipitin test for the diagnosis of non-patent *S. dentatus* infection.

Treatment. Egerton (1961) has reported that thiabendazole, when incorporated in the food at the rate of 0·1–0·4 per cent is effective in inhibiting the migration of *S. dentatus* larvae. However, Alicata (1961) could not demonstrate a beneficial effect of this drug on *S. dentatus* infections in rabbits.

Prophylaxis is largely a matter of hygiene. Pigs must be protected from larvae of the worm derived from their urine. It has been found in America that the swine sanitation system used for the control of *Ascaris suum* brought about a considerable decrease in the incidence of *S. dentatus*, and that it is expedient to provide a hard, bare strip, 1·5–2 m. wide, along the edge of the pasture and to place the shelters and troughs on a bare patch 10 m. wide at the end of the field, since the pigs mostly urinate in these places. Adequate drainage of pig pens and yards is essential. Thus muddy areas and pig wallows should be drained and filled in. Pigs should be fed on a concrete apron which should be cleaned regularly.

Alicata (1953) has reported that the treatment of soil with 'polyborate' (a mixture of sodium pentaborate tetrahydrate and sodium tetraborate pentahydrate) is successful under laboratory and field conditions in destroying the eggs and larvae of *S. dentatus*. It is applied at the rate of 5 lb. per 100 sq. ft. Each treatment lasts for about 30 days. The toxicity of polyborate for pigs is low and they may be allowed access to treated soil without ill effect. Segregation of clean, especially young, animals from infected ones and periodic unstocking of pens, which are then allowed to dry thoroughly in sunlight, are important measures.

FAMILY SYNGAMIDAE LEIPER, 1912

Nematodes with a cup-shaped buccal capsule, without leaf-crowns. Teeth may be present. Vulva in anterior part of the body. Parasites of respiratory tract.

Genera of importance include *Syngamus* and *Cyathostoma*.

Genus: Syngamus v. Siebold, 1836

S. trachea (Montagu, 1811), the 'gapeworm', occurs in the trachea of the turkey, fowl, pheasant, guinea-fowl, goose and various wild birds. The parasites are bright red in colour when fresh and the sexes are found permanently in copulation. Male 2–6 mm., female 5–20 mm. long. The mouth opening is wide, without leaf-crowns, and the buccal capsule is cup-shaped, bearing six to ten small teeth at its base. The male bursa has short, stout rays. The spicules are 0·053–0·082 mm. long, equal and simple in shape. In the female the vulva opens in the anterior third of the body, while the coils of the uterus and ovaries lie behind this level. The eggs, which measure 70–100 by 43–46 μ, are provided with a thickened operculum at either pole and are ejected from underneath the male bursa in the sixteen-celled stage.

Life-cycle. The eggs of the worms are usually coughed up and swallowed by the host, and they pass out in the faeces. The infective larva develops inside the egg, requiring, under optimal conditions of moisture and temperature, about 3 days. The larva moults twice in the egg and will hatch, if conditions are suitable, on the ninth day. The larva retains the cuticle of the previous stage as a sheath and is infective also if it has not hatched from the egg. The infective larva has a short, pointed tail and a relatively long oesophagus. It soon becomes rather inactive and shows no negative geotropism, nor is it able to resist desiccation. Infection of the host occurs per os. The infective larvae may be swallowed by earthworms, snails, slugs, flies and other arthropods, in which they become encysted and here they may live for several months or even years. Such invertebrates may become heavily infected and act as important transport hosts. According to Clapham (1935) and Morgan & Clapham (1934), passage through earthworms renders the larvae more highly infective, enabling strains from wild birds to pass to chicks more readily than is otherwise the case.

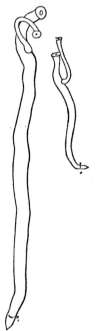

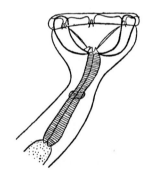

FIG. 94. *Syngamus trachea*, Outlines of two pairs of worms: on the right, female immature; on the left, female gravid (from Baylis, after Chapin)

FIG. 95. *Syngamus trachea*, Anterior End (from Baylis, after Yorke & Maplestone)

The larvae are carried by the blood to the lungs, which they may reach 6 hours after they have entered the bird-host. In the lungs they are found in the alveoli. A further ecdysis occurs on the third day after infection, after which the sexes can be differentiated. The final ecdysis occurs on the fourth or fifth day and the young worms migrate to the larger bronchi, where copulation takes place. The trachea is reached as early as the seventh day and the first eggs are found in the faeces of the host from 17–20 days after infection.

Pathogenesis. In heavy infections migration through the lungs may cause ecchymoses, oedema and even lobar pneumonia. In the trachea the worms attach themselves to the mucosa and suck blood, with consequent catarrhal tracheitis and the secretion of much mucus. The males become deeply embedded with their anterior ends in the wall of the trachea of turkeys, causing the development of nodules.

Clinical signs. Gapeworm disease chiefly affects young birds. Adult hens are not usually infected and guinea-fowl are little affected at any age. Turkeys are susceptible to infection at any age, and some authors consider them to be the natural hosts of *S. trachea*. They may be, however, dangerous carriers of the disease, from which other birds may acquire infection. Hen-chicks, goslings and pheasants suffer most from the parasites. The characteristic signs of 'gapes' are those of dyspnoea and asphyxia, occurring in spasms on account of the accumulation of mucus in the trachea. The bird shakes and tosses its head about and it may cough, or it extends the neck, opens the beak and performs gaping movements. Death results from asphyxia during such an attack or from progressive emaciation, anaemia and weakness caused by the parasite.

Post-mortem. The carcass is emaciated and anaemic and the worms are found in the posterior part of the trachea, attached to the mucosa and surrounded by mucus which may be streaked with blood.

Diagnosis can be made from the clinical signs and by finding in the faeces the characteristic eggs, which must be differentiated from those of *Capillaria*. The diagnosis will be further confirmed by finding the worms at the autopsy of a selected case.

Treatment. A good remedy is barium antimonyl tartrate. The chicks are placed in a suitable container and the powdered drug is blown into the air of the closed container several times. One ounce of the compound is sufficient for 8 cu. ft. *Cyanacethydrazide*, at a dose rate of 5 g. per 5 litres of drinking water has shown to be effective for *S. trachea* infection in pheasants. Horton-Smith *et al.* (1963) reported that a single dose of 0·3–1·5 g. per kg. of thiabendazole was significantly effective, especially against the fourth and subsequent larval stages. When given in the feed at a rate of 0·1 per cent it was also effective especially when treatment was started before the birds were infected.

Prophylaxis. Infected birds that cannot be treated should be killed and the heads, the respiratory and the digestive organs destroyed by burning. The clean birds are best removed to fresh ground. Severe outbreaks of gapeworm disease are less likely to occur if the birds are not kept for long periods on the same ground. Moist localities where earthworms, slugs and snails occur should be avoided if possible. It is difficult to control these transport hosts, but it is advantageous not to let chicks out before the dew is off the grass. Turkeys should not be kept on the same ground as chickens or even near to them. When new chicks are introduced they should be purchased out of clean flocks or otherwise quarantined and examined for the presence of the parasite. Wild birds, especially pheasants, rooks and starlings, which may harbour the parasite, should be prevented from introducing the infection into the fowl-run.

Other species of *Syngamus* in birds include *S. skrjabinomorpha* (in chickens and geese in U.S.S.R.), *S. merulae* (in blackbirds) and *S. microspiculum* in shags (*Phalacrocorax carbo*).

S. laryngeus Railliet, 1899 occurs in the larynx of cattle and buffaloes in India, Malaya and South America, and has also been reported from man. The affected animals cough and lose condition and calves especially may develop bronchitis.

S. nasicola v. Linstow, 1899 has been found in the nasal cavities of sheep, cattle, goats and deer in Brazil, Africa, Turkestan and the West Indies.

Genus: Cyathostoma E. Blanchard, 1849

C. bronchialis (Muehlig, 1884) occurs in the trachea and bronchi of the goose, duck and swan. These worms are not permanently in copula. Male 4–5·8 mm., female 16–31 mm. long. The buccal capsule is cup-shaped with six to seven teeth at its base. The male bursa is well developed and the spicules are 0·51–0·62 mm. long. The eggs measure 74–83 by 49–62 μ.

Life-cycle—unknown.

Pathogenicity. The parasite is very harmful, especially to young geese and ducks. Even two or three worms may be responsible for death by asphyxiation.

Treatment and Prophylaxis. As for *Syngamus trachea*.

FAMILY: ANCYLOSTOMATIDAE LOOSS, 1905

Strongyloidea with a well-developed buccal capsule, which is devoid of leaf-crowns, but is armed on its *ventral* margin either with teeth or with chitinous cutting plates. The anterior extremity is usually bent in a dorsal direction. The male bursa is normally developed. Most species are voracious blood-suckers and are parasitic in the small intestine.

The name Ancylostoma is derived from the Greek words *ankylos*, a hook, and *stoma*, a mouth. It was originally given by Fröhlich to a species of the genus *Uncinaria* found in a fox, because the rays of the copulatory bursa seemed to Fröhlich to be hook-like. Some authors, however, derive the name *Ancylostoma* from the fact that the anterior ends of many species are bent up dorsally to give the worm a hook-like appearance.

The species of the family Ancylostomatidae described below may be classified as follows:

SUBFAMILY: ANCYLOSTOMINAE

The buccal capsule bears on its ventral margin one to four pairs of teeth. Inside the buccal capsule there are two dorsal teeth. The dorsal gutter does not project into the cavity of the buccal cavity to form a dorsal cone. *Ancylostoma. Agriostomum.*

SUBFAMILY: NECATORINAE

The ventral margin of the buccal capsule bears, instead of teeth, cutting plates (semi-lunes), but these are usually absent from *Globocephalus.* There are also sub-ventral teeth inside the buccal capsule. Dorsal teeth are absent, but small sub-dorsal (lateral) teeth may be present. The end of the dorsal gutter carrying the duct of the dorsal oesophageal gland projects into the buccal capsule as a prominence called the *dorsal cone. Necator. Bunostomum. Gaigeria. Globocephalus. Uncinaria.*

SUBFAMILY: ANCYLOSTOMINAE STEPHENS, 1916
Genus: Ancylostoma Dubini, 1843

A. caninum (Ercolani, 1859) occurs in the small intestine of the dog, fox and very rarely also in man. It is cosmopolitan in distribution. Male 10–12 mm., female 14–16 mm. long. The worms are fairly rigid and grey or reddish in colour, depending on the presence of blood in the alimentary canal. The anterior end is bent dorsad and the oral aperture is directed antero-dorsally. The buccal capsule is deep. There is no dorsal cone. The dorsal gutter ends in a deep notch on the dorsal (posterior) margin of the buccal capsule, the ventral margin of which bears three teeth on either side. In the depth of the capsule there is a pair of triangular dorsal teeth and a pair of ventro-lateral teeth. The male bursa is well developed and the spicules are 0·8–0·95 mm. long. The vulva is situated near the junction of the second and last thirds of the body. The uteri and ovaries form numerous transverse coils in the body. The eggs measure 56–75 by 34–47 μ and contain an embryo of about eight cells when laid.

A. tubaeforme (Zeder, 1800). The normal hookworm of the cat. For many years it has been accepted the *A. caninum* occurs in the cat but studies by Biocca (1954) in Italy, by Burrows (1962) in the U.S.A., and others, demonstrated *A. tubaeforme* to be a valid species. The two species are not interchangeable between the two hosts. Apparently cosmopolitan in distribution. Male 9·5–11·0 mm., female 12·0–15 mm. Mouth capsule similar to *A. caninum*, but teeth on the ventral margin slightly larger. Spicules of the male larger than 1 mm. (1·23–1·4 mm.) (compare *A. caninum*). Eggs 55–75 μ by 34·4–44·7 μ.

A. braziliense Gomez de Faria, 1910 (syn. *A. ceylanicum,* Looss, 1911), occurs in the small intestine of the dog, cat, fox and sometimes man, and is found in most tropical and sub-tropical countries. It is slightly smaller than *A. caninum*, the males measuring 6–7·75 mm. and the females

7–10 mm. It can be differentiated from the previous species by the fact that its ventral teeth consist of a large and a small one on either side. The eggs measure 75–95 by 41–45 μ.

A. duodenale Dubini, 1843, one of the hookworms of man in Europe, north Africa, western Asia, China and Japan, has also been recorded from certain wild Carnivora and the pig. Experimental infection of young dogs and cats has been successful, but the parasite does not normally occur in these hosts. The ventral teeth of this worm consist of two large and one small one on either side.

Life-cycles. The pre-infective stages develop and react like those of *Strongylus* spp., but none of them, not even the infective larvae, are resistant to desiccation, so that they are therefore found only in moist surroundings. The infective stage is reached within a week if the temperature is suitable, and it enters the host either through the skin or through the mouth. In the former case the larvae reach the blood, which carries them via the heart to the lungs. Here the majority will become arrested in the capillaries, from which they pass, as *Ascaris* larvae do, to the alveoli and then up the respiratory passages to the pharynx and down again to the intestine, increasing in size during their migration. Some larvae may pass through the pulmonary capillaries and reach the systemic

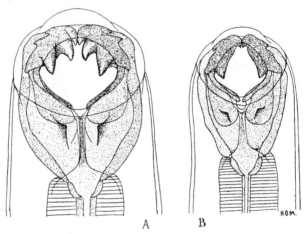

A   B

FIG. 96. Anterior End, Dorsal View, of A, *Ancylostoma caninum*; B, *A. braziliense* (Original)

circulation. They are then carried to various organs, in which they cause small haemorrhages and later die, or, in a pregnant animal, they may reach the foetus and establish a prenatal infection. In puppies, the larvae lie dormant until the puppies are born and then they grow up into adult worms. After oral infection the larvae may also migrate through the lungs, but those of *A. caninum* frequently penetrate into the wall of the stomach or intestine and remain there for a few days before they return to the lumen. The worms reach the adult stage in the host in about 5 weeks in the case of *A. duodenale* and 14–20 days in the case of *A. cani-*

num. Following prenatal infection the prepatent period is about 13 days. Transcolostral infection with *A. caninum* has been suggested by Stone and Girardeau (1966).

Pathogenesis and Treatment. See pp. 216–218.

Genus: Agriostomum Railliet, 1902

A. vryburgi Railliet, 1902 occurs in the small intestine of the zebu (*Bos indicus*) and perhaps the ox in India and Sumatra. Male 9·2–11 mm., female 13·5–15·5 mm. long. The buccal capsule opens antero-dorsally, and is relatively shallow. It is followed by a very large oesophageal funnel which contains two small sub-ventral lancets. The oral margin is provided with four pairs of large teeth and a rudimentary leaf-crown. The bursa is well developed; the ventral rays are close together and parallel; the antero-lateral ray is short, thick and divergent from the other laterals; the dorsal bifurcates twice. Spicules equal, 0·83–0·87 mm. long and accompanied by a gubernaculum. The vulva is posterior and eggs measure 125–195 by 60–92 μ.

Life-cycle. Probably direct.

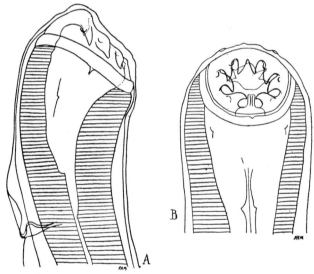

Fig. 97. *Agriostomum vryburgi*: A, anterior end, lateral view; B, anterior end, dorsal view

Pathogenicity. Little is known about this, but the parasites will undoubtedly be harmful blood-suckers and cause clinical signs like other hookworms in heavy infections.

SUBFAMILY: NECATORINAE LANE, 1917

Genus: Necator Stiles, 1903

Species of this genus have one pair of ventral cutting plates and, at the base of the buccal capsule, one pair of ventral teeth and one pair of subdorsal teeth. The termination of the dorsal gutter projects into the buccal capsule as a prominence called the *dorsal cone*.

N. americanus (Stiles, 1902) is a common hookworm of man, occurring in most warm climates, especially in America and Africa. It has also been recorded from the dog and, in Australia, in the pig. Good experimental infections have been achieved in the dog by Miller (1966) using corticosteroid treatment. The parasite is relatively unimportant from the veterinary aspect, but it is a cause of severe hookworm disease in man in India, the Far East, Australia and the southern United States, to which countries it probably spread from Africa. In the United States it is the predominant human hookworm.

N. suillus Ackert & Payne, 1922 has been reported from the pig in Trinidad and possibly from South Brazil. There is some doubt about the identity of the parasite and some authors recognise it as a pig strain of *N. americanus*.

Genus: Bunostomum Railliet, 1902
(syn. Monodontus, Molin, 1861)

B. trigonocephalum (Rudolphi, 1808) is a hookworm which occurs in the small intestine (ileum and jejunum) of sheep and goats in many parts of the world and in Scottish red deer. It has also been recorded from

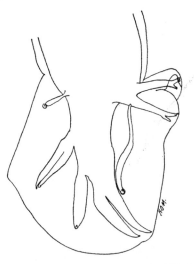
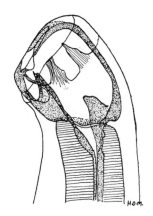

FIG. 98. *Necator americanus*, Hind End of Male, Lateral View (Original)

FIG. 99. *Bunostomum trigonocephalum*, Anterior End, Lateral View (Original)

cattle, but the accuracy of this record seems to be doubtful. Male 12–17 mm., female 19–26 mm. long. The anterior end is bent in a dorsal direction, so that the buccal capsule opens antero-dorsally; it is relatively large and bears at its ventral margin a pair of chitinous plates. Near its base is a pair of small subventral lancets. The dorsal gutter, carrying the duct of the dorsal oesophageal gland, ends in a large dorsal cone, which projects into the buccal cavity. There are no dorsal teeth in the buccal capsule. The bursa is well developed and has an asymmetrical dorsal lobe. The right externo-dorsal ray arises higher up on the dorsal stem and is longer than the left. It arises near the bifurcation of the dorsal ray, which divides into two tridigitate branches. The spicules are slender, alate and 0·6–0·64 mm. long. The vulva opens a short distance in front of the middle of the body. The eggs measure 79–97 by 47–50 μ (usually 92 by 50 μ), the ends are bluntly rounded and the embryonic cells are darkly granulated. The eggs can be differentiated from those of other worms in fresh sheep faeces.

Life-cycle. The development is direct. Infection of the host occurs through the mouth or through the skin. Following skin penetration

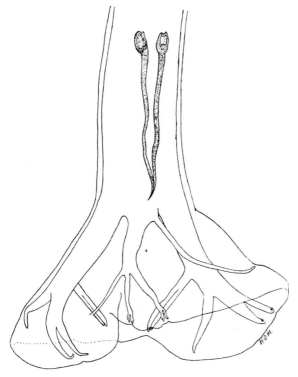

Fig. 100. *Bunostomum trigonocephalum*, Hind End of Male, Dorsal View (Original)

the larvae pass to the lungs, where the third ecdysis occurs. The fourth-stage larvae, which have a buccal capsule, reach the intestine again after 11 days and the first eggs are passed 30–56 days after infection.

Pathogenesis. As in the case of ancylostomiasis (see p. 216) the adult worms attach themselves to the intestinal mucosa and suck blood.

Clinical signs. The main clinical signs are progressive anaemia, with associated changes in the blood picture, hydraemia and oedema, which shows especially in the intermandibular region as a 'bottle-jaw'. The animals become weak and emaciated and the appetite usually decreases. The skin is dry and the wool of sheep falls out in irregular patches. Diarrhoea is not infrequent, and the faeces may be dark in colour on account of the presence of altered blood pigments. Death is frequently preceded by complete prostration, which may last for several days.

Post-mortem. The clinical picture is very similar to that of ancylostomiasis. In addition, hydrothorax and effusion of fluid into the pericardium are commonly seen.

Diagnosis is made partly from the clinical signs, but the infection must be differentiated from other worm-infections that cause anaemia by the identification of the eggs in the faeces or the larvae following culture of the faeces.

Treatment—*Phenothiazine* is moderately to highly effective, especially preparations of small particle size. Dose 20–30 g. per animal. *Piperazine citrate* at a dose of 250–450 mg. per kg. is effective. *Thiabendazole* is highly effective at a dose of 75 mg. per kg. Various organo-phosphorus compounds may also be used (see review by Gibson, 1965).

Prophylaxis. In general, the measures described on page 243 should be applied. The infective larvae cannot resist dryness, so that the infection is found invariably on permanently or occasionally moist pastures and can therefore be readily controlled by avoiding such places, which should be drained if possible. Around watering troughs the ground should be kept hard and dry or treated frequently with liberal applications of salt.

B. phlebotomum (Railliet, 1900) is widely distributed and occurs in the small intestine, mainly in the duodenum, of cattle and the zebu, and has also been recorded from sheep, but the accuracy of this is doubtful. Male 10–18 mm., female 24–28 mm. long. It closely resembles the preceding species, but can be differentiated by its shorter dorsal cone, by the presence of two pairs of sub-ventral lancets in the buccal capsule and the longer male spicules, which measure 3·5–4 mm. The eggs measure about 106 by 46 μ. They have blunt ends and darkly pigmented embryonic cells, so that they can be readily differentiated from other worm eggs in the faeces.

Life-cycle. Similar to that of *B. trigonocephalum.*

Pathogenesis and Clinical signs. This species is a serious pathogen in many parts of the world, e.g. Africa, Australia, southern and mid-west states of U.S.A. However, it may also cause serious ill health in cattle in Europe. In stabled cattle an itching of the legs, probably caused by the entry of the skin-penetrating larvae through the skin, which makes the animals stamp their feet and lick their legs, may occur. Diarrhoea, anaemia and marked weakness, especially in calves are the clinical signs.

Diagnosis has to be confirmed by finding the eggs in the faeces or by the identification of infective larvae cultured in faeces.

Treatment—Phenothiazine is variable in its effect (20-100 per cent); dose 300-450 mg. per kg. Low-level dosage of phenothiazine has a marked effect on the egg output of *B. phlebotomum*. *Piperazine* has a poor action. *Bephenium hydroxynaphthoate* is effective at 225 mg. per kg. *Thiabendazole* at a dose of 50-110 mg. per kg. is very effective. *Trichlorophon* is effective at a dose of 110 mg. per kg. *Ruelene* at a dose of 38·5 mg. per kg. is very effective.

Prophylaxis. As in the case of *B. trigonocephalum*. Stabled cattle should be protected by hygienic measures, especially by frequent removal of faeces, by keeping the floors and bedding dry, and preventing contamination of the food and water.

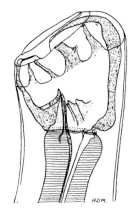

FIG. 101. *Gaigeria pachyscelis*, Anterior End, Lateral View (Original)

Genus: Gaigeria Railliet & Henry, 1910

G. pachyscelis Railliet & Henry, 1910, the only known species of this genus, is a hookworm which occurs in the duodenum of sheep and goats in India and Africa. Male up to 20 mm., female up to 30 mm. long. In general it resembles *Bunostomum trigonocephalum*. The buccal capsule contains a large dorsal cone, but no dorsal tooth, and a pair of subventral lancets which have several cusps each. The male bursa has small lateral lobes joined together ventrally and a voluminous dorsal lobe. The antero-lateral ray is short and blunt and it is separated widely from the other lateral rays. The externo-dorsal rays arise from the main stem of the dorsal ray, which is cleft for about a quarter of its length, the two short branches ending in three very small digitations. The spicules are slender with recurved unbarbed ends; they are 1·25–1·33 mm. long. The eggs measure 105–129 by 50–55 μ and have blunt ends.

Life-cycle. Direct and similar to that of other hookworms. The infective larvae are sheathed and resemble those of *Bunostomum trigonocephalum*. They have no resistance against desiccation. According to Ortlepp (1937) infection occurs only through the skin. The larvae reach the lungs via the blood, where the third ecdysis occurs, and they remain for about 13 days. The fourth-stage larva, which has a globular buccal capsule with a dorsal cone and a pair of sub-ventral lancets, then creeps up the bronchi and trachea to the pharynx and is swallowed down, reaching the intestine, where the fourth ecdysis occurs and the worms grow adult in about 10 weeks from the time of infection.

Pathogenicity and Clinical signs. Similar to *Bunostomum trigonocephalum.*

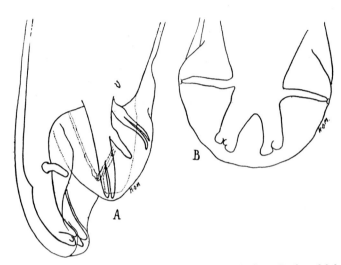

Fig. 102. *Gaigeria pachyscelis*: A, hind end of male, lateral view; B, dorsal lobe of male bursa with dorsal rays (Original)

The worms are exceedingly virulent blood-suckers and about twenty-four are stated to be sufficient to cause death. The parasite is more pathogenic to merinos than to the hairy breeds of sheep, such as Persians. In severe infections death occurs suddenly, the only sign being anaemia. In more chronic cases the usual signs of hookworm infection are seen. The worms are found attached to the mucosa of the first part of the small intestine, frequently in groups of two or three, the groups being surrounded by a quantity of fresh blood. Observations made in South-West Africa indicate that the larvae, penetrating through the skin of the feet of sheep, are instrumental in introducing the organisms of foot-rot.

Diagnosis can be made by finding the characteristic eggs in the faeces.

Treatment. As described for *Bunostomum trigonocephalum.*

Prophylaxis. Moist pastures and all moist ground should be avoided. Since infection occurs via the skin only, it is essential that the surroundings of watering troughs should be kept dry or be treated with salt. In South Africa the distribution of the parasite is closely associated with sandy soil.

Genus: Globocephalus Molin, 1861

Several species of this genus occur in the small intestine of the pig. *G. samoensis* is found especially in Eastern countries (India, Samoa, New Guinea and Java), while *G. urosubulatus* and *G. longemucronatus* have been recorded from Europe, Africa and America. The worms are about 4-8 mm. long and fairly stout. The mouth opens sub-dorsally and the buccal

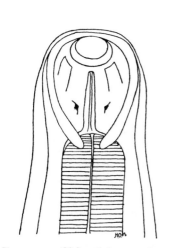

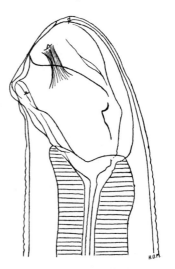

FIG. 103. *Globocephalus urosubulatus*, Dorsal View of Anterior End (Original)

FIG. 104. *Uncinaria stenocephala*, Anterior End, Lateral View (Original)

capsule is globular or funnel-shaped with an external chitinoid ring. There are neither leaf-crowns nor teeth at the oral margin. Near the base of the buccal capsule a pair of subventral teeth are usually present, but they may be small or absent in some specimens. The dorsal gutter is prominent, extending almost to the oral margin. The male bursa is well developed, the spicules are slender and a gubernaculum is present. The vulva is situated posteriorly.

Life-cycle. Probably direct.

Pathogenicity. Very little is known about this.

Genus: Uncinaria Fröhlich, 1789

U. stenocephala (Railliet, 1884) is a hookworm found in the dog, cat and fox in Europe and North America. Male 5-8·5 mm., female 7-12 mm. long. It has a pair of chitinous plates instead of teeth at the ventral border of the large, funnel-shaped buccal capsule. Near the base of the buccal capsule there is a pair of subventral teeth. The dorsal cone does not project into the buccal capsule. There are no dorsal teeth in the buccal capsule. The male bursa is well developed and has a short dorsal lobe and two large and separate lateral lobes. The externo-dorsal rays arise at the base of the dorsal ray, which is cleft for about half its length, the two branches being bidigitate or tridigitate. The antero-lateral ray diverges from the other lateral rays. The spicules are slender and 0·64–0·76 mm. long. The eggs resemble those of *A. caninum* but are slightly longer and decidedly stouter, being 65–80 μ by 40–50 μ.

Life-cycle. Direct, resembling that of *Ancylostoma*.

ANCYLOSTOMIASIS AND UNCINARIASIS IN DOGS CATS AND FOXES

Pathogenesis. In animals that have acquired, after a previous infection, some degree of immunity, the entrance of larvae through the skin may give rise to a marked local reaction in the skin and subcutaneous tissues. Pulmonary lesions due to migrating larvae are usually not as severe as to cause clinical disease. The adult parasites attach themselves to the mucosa of the intestine and suck blood. Wells (1931) observed that the worm (*A. caninum*) fills its intestine with blood and then ejects it through the anus at more or less regular intervals. He calculated that one worm would remove about 0·8 ml. of blood in 24 hours, so that in a severe infection a large proportion of the host's blood will be lost daily. This author was inclined to think that the process of blood-sucking subserved mainly a respiratory function and that the worm further utilised only simple, diffusible substances prepared for assimilation by the host, since erythrocytes in the blood are ejected by the worm. Extensive work in the 1920's (Foster & Landsberg, 1934) and more recently with radio-isotopes (Clarke *et al.*, 1961) has confirmed that the anaemia of hookworm disease is characteristic of an iron deficiency anaemia which results from the excessive blood-letting activities of the hookworms. However, the blood loss is likely to be nearer 0·1 ml. per day per worm than 0·8 ml. Essentially no anaemia results while the iron reserves of the body are adequate but when these are depleted, anaemia quickly results. The rapidity of the drain on the iron reserves is in general a function of the number of worms present, large numbers inducing anaemia quickly and smaller numbers taking a longer time. Where there is a marginal dietary intake of iron even a slight blood loss could result in anaemia.

Other factors which require consideration in the genesis of hookworm anaemia are impaired intestinal absorption and disturbances in erythropoiesis. Impaired intestinal absorption in human hookworm disease has been demonstrated by Sheehy *et al.* (1962). Patients with severe hookworm infection showed abnormalities of the small bowel, the villi were clubbed or fused into large masses and the columnar cells were disoriented. These authors considered the above changes secondary to an inflammatory response in the *lamina propria*. Malabsorption was demonstrated with regard to vitamin A, xylose and fat. Foy & Kondi (1961) also suggested that impaired re-absorption of iron from the intestinal bleeding may be a contributory factor in hookworm anaemia.

There appears to be little depression of haemopoiesis in hookworm disease and in experimental studies Krupp (1961) found that erythropoiesis was either stimulated or remained in the upper limits of normal.

A more general account of the anaemias in helminth infection is given by Baker & Douglas (1966) which should be consulted for its up-to-date consideration of the subject.

Immunity to hookworm infection. It is now well established that dogs become immune to hookworm infection. Graded doses of larvae given subcutaneously or orally may induce this, egg counts rising following the initial infections to reach a maximum about 2 months after infection. Thereafter there is a marked fall in egg counts and large numbers of adult worms are passed in the faeces (McCoy, 1931). McCoy regarded this curative phenomenon as a 'crisis' and it is probably comparable to the phenomenon of 'self cure' seen in *Haemonchus contortus* infection. Where infections are built up too rapidly death occurs before the immune response can control the infection.

More recent work by Dow *et al.* (1961) and Miller (1965a, b) has demonstrated that immunity to *A. caninum* and *U. stenocephala* can be induced by infecting dogs with infective larvae which have been subjected to 40 kiloroentgens of X-rays. Such immunisation can also be carried out in young puppies which have acquired infection prenatally, in that the existing burden is removed by anthelmintic medication and the X-irradiated vaccine applied.

Clinical signs. Ancylostomiasis and uncinariasis occur frequently in summer and especially in animals that are confined on a relatively small area of moist ground, like dogs in kennels and foxes in runs. It is seen in animals of all ages, and prenatal infection may cause a sudden onset of severe anaemia, coma and death about 3 weeks after birth. In foxes it occurs usually when they are 2–6 months old. The disease may be acute and rapidly fatal in susceptible animals, while others may develop a marked degree of resistance to the effects of infection, which may, however, be broken down by an intercurrent disease or adverse conditions. The chief clinical sign is anaemia, accompanied by hydraemia, sometimes oedemas, general weakness and emaciation. In the later stages of the disease the blood changes may include eosinophilia. Growth is stunted and the coat becomes dry and harsh; in foxes the fur is poor. Itching of the skin and areas of dermatitis, caused by penetration of the skin by the larvae of the worms, may be observed. The faeces are often diarrhoeic and contain bloody mucus, or they may be of a tarry nature. Death is as a rule preceded by marked weakness, particularly in the hind-quarters, and extreme paleness of the mucous membranes.

Post-mortem. Anaemia and cachexia are conspicuous, while oedemas and ascites are frequently seen. The liver has a light brown colour and shows fatty changes. The intestinal contents are haemorrhagic. The mucosa is usually swollen, covered with mucus, and shows numerous small red bite-marks of the worms. The latter are found attached to the mucosa, or sometimes free, and their colour is grey or reddish, depending on the amount of blood in their intestines.

Diagnosis is made from the clinical signs and confirmed by finding the eggs of the worms in the faeces. In acute prenatal infection a severe anaemia may develop before eggs are demonstrable in the faeces of the puppy.

Treatment. In addition to the use of the specific anthelmintics mentioned below, severely affected animals may require blood transfusions or at least some form of easily assimilable iron therapy. Further supportive treatment should include protein rich foods.

Tetrachloroethylene was introduced in the mid 1920's and has since been used extensively for the treatment of hookworms. At a dosage rate of 0·2 ml. per kg. it is 99 per cent efficient. Preparative treatment consists of an overnight fast before dosing and is followed by a saline laxative.

Bephenium compounds such as bephenium chloride, bromide, iodide or hydroxynaphthoate in a single dose of more than 20 mg. per kg. show 99·4 per cent efficiency. A related compound, *Thenium* (Thenium *p*-chloro-benzene sulphonate) is highly effective against *A. caninum* and *U. stenocephala* at a rate of 200–250 mg. per kg. twice daily.

Disophenol (2:6-diiodo-4-nitrophenol) is highly effective. A single subcutaneous dose of 7·5 mg. per kg. is highly efficient against adult *A. caninum* and *A. braziliense* but 10 mg. per kg. is necessary for good action against *U. stenocephala*.

Prophylaxis. The pre-infective stages are not resistant to desiccation, so that ground and pens on which susceptible animals are kept should be as dry as possible and faeces should be removed at short intervals. In fox-runs high grass is undesirable, because it helps to keep the ground moist and the infective larvae migrate on to it after dew has fallen if the temperature is not too low; high grass thus increases the chances of infection. The floors of kennels could be treated with common salt or sodium borate which help to kill the larvae.

Cutaneous Larva Migrans. This condition may be compared with *visceral larva migrans* (p. 164). It occurs in man and other hosts and is caused by the larvae of nematodes or parasitic insects which enter the skin and migrate in it, causing papules, inflamed tracks, sometimes with thickening of the skin and pruritus. The larvae of *Ancylostoma braziliense* frequently cause it, but other nematodes whose larvae may cause it are *Uncinaria stenocephala*, *Ancylostoma caninum* (experimentally), *Ancylostoma duodenale*, *Necator americanus*, *Bunostomum phlebotomum*, and species of *Strongyloides* and *Gnathostoma*. Among insect larvae which may cause creeping eruption are those of *Hypoderma bovis* and *Gastrophilus* (especially *G. intestinalis*) and there is one record of creeping eruption ascribed to the larvae of *Echinorhynchus sphaerocephalus*. Further information on larva migrans may be obtained in Beaver (1956, 1966) and Weiner (1960).

FAMILY: AMIDOSTOMIDAE BAYLIS & DAUBNEY, 1926

The only species here described is parasitic in the mucosa of the gizzard, proventriculus and crop of geese and ducks. The shallow, broad buccal capsule has no leaf-crowns. The oesophagus is lined by three longitudinal ridges or plates. The male spicules are short with bifurcate or trifurcate ends. The vulva of the female is in the posterior half of the body.

Genus: Amidostomum Railliet & Henry, 1909

A. anseris (Zeder, 1800) (syn. *A. nodulosum*) occurs in domestic and wild geese and ducks in the mucosa of the gizzard and sometimes also

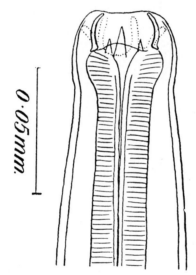

0·05mm.

FIG. 105. *Amidostomum anseris*, Anterior End, Dorsal View (after Baylis)

the proventriculus and the oesophagus. The worms are slender and reddish in colour. Male 10–17 mm., female 12–24 mm. long. The buccal capsule is short, wide and thick-walled, with three pointed teeth at its base. The lateral lobes of the male bursa are longer than the dorsal lobe, the ventro-ventral and latero-ventral rays diverge widely, the three lateral rays are separate, and the short externo-dorsal ray arises separately from the dorsal ray, which divides near its end into two bidigitate branches. The equal spicules are 0·2–0·3 mm. long and each ends in two branches. The vulva is situated at the posterior fifth of the body and may be covered by a flap. The eggs measure 100–110 by 50–60 μ and contain a segmenting embryo when laid.

Life-cycle. Direct like that of other strongyles. Kobulej (1956) stated that development to the infective third larval stage occurs inside the egg. The development of the first larva is very rapid under optimal conditions, being complete in 12 hours at 30°C. The first larva remains in its sheath, as the second larva also does, so that the third larva is enclosed by two sheaths, the three larvae being distinguishable by the shapes of their tails. In water at 0°C the infective larvae were active for 2 months and were not harmed by freezing, unless this was severe; but they were very sensitive to drying and both the eggs and larvae are killed by drying for 30–60 hours. Infection is by ingestion. Third-stage larvae are found in the glands of the *tunica propria*, where they reach maturity in about 40 days (Cowan, 1955).

Pathogenesis. The worms are very pathogenic to young geese, while the adult birds may act as carriers of the infection without showing clinical signs. The parasites burrow into the mucous and submucous tissues of the gizzard and proventriculus, sucking blood and causing marked irritation, inflammatory changes and haemorrhage. In severe cases there is extensive necrosis of the horny lining of the gizzard.

Clinical signs. Heavily infected birds lose their appetite and become emaciated, anaemic, weak and easily tired. Diarrhoea is not unusual. Death is often preceded by prostration.

Post mortem. The feathers around the anus are soiled and matted with faeces. The carcass is anaemic and emaciated. The horny lining of the gizzard forms a necrotic, fragile mass with a brownish colour, probably due to the admixture of blood pigments. The worms are found partly buried in the necrotic mass. The propria mucosa shows haemorrhages and localised infiltrations with mononuclear and poly-nuclear leucocytes.

Diagnosis. A definite diagnosis can be made only by autopsy of a selected case.

Treatment. Two to 3 ml. carbon tetrachloride, administered in a mixture of flour and water as vehicle has been recommended. Drugs such as methyridine and thiabendazole should be tried.

Prophylaxis. General hygienic measures are indicated and special attention should be given to young ducks. Treatment of the adult birds before the breeding season is recommended.

SUPERFAMILY: TRICHOSTRONGYLOIDEA CRAM, 1927

Stoma reduced or rudimentary. Corona radiata absent. Lips six or three or absent. Thin bodied, bursa well developed, rarely reduced. Families of importance include *Trichostrongylidae, Ollulanidae, Dictyo-caulidae*.

FAMILY: TRICHOSTRONGYLIDAE LEIPER, 1912

Mostly small forms in which the buccal capsule is absent or very small and is devoid of leaf-crowns, and usually bears no teeth. The male bursa is well developed, with large lateral lobes and a small dorsal lobe. Adults parasitic in the alimentary canals of sheep, cattle, equines and other vertebrates. Genera of importance include *Trichostrongylus*, *Graphidium*, *Ostertagia*, *Marshallagia*, *Cooperia*, *Nematodirus*, *Haemonchus* and *Mecistocirrus*.

Genus: Trichostrongylus Looss, 1905

The species of this genus are small, slender, pale reddish-brown worms without a specially-developed head-end. There is no buccal capsule. The excretory pore is usually situated in a conspicuous ventral notch near the anterior extremity. The male bursa has long lateral lobes, while the dorsal lobe is not well defined. The ventral rays of the male bursa are separated widely and the ventro-ventral ray is conspicuously thinner than the latero-ventral, which runs parallel with the lateral rays. The postero-lateral ray diverges from the other lateral rays and lies near to the externo-dorsal ray. The dorsal ray is slender and cleft near its tip into two branches which have short digitations. The spicules are stout, ridged and pigmented brown, and a gubernaculum is present. The vulva opens a short distance behind the middle of the body and the uteri are opposed (amphidelph). The eggs are oval, thin-shelled and segmenting when they are laid.

T. colubriformis (Giles, 1892) (syn. *T. instabilis*) occurs in the anterior portion of the small intestine and sometimes also in the abomasum of

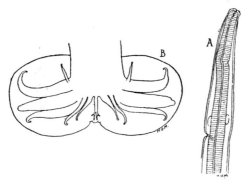

Fɪɢ. 106. *Trichostrongylus colubriformis* (syn. *T. instabilis*): A, anterior end, lateral view; B, bursa of male opened out (Original)

sheep, goat, cattle, camel and various antelopes. It has also been recorded from the rabbit (*Lepus californicus melanotis*), the pig, the dog and man. Male 4–5·5 mm., female 5–7 mm. long. Spicules equal, 0·135–0·156 mm. long. The eggs measure 79–101 by 39–47 μ.

T. falculatus Ransom, 1911 occurs in the small intestine of sheep and goat and some antelopes in South Africa and Australia. Spicules subequal, about 0·1 mm. long.

9

T. vitrinus Looss, 1905 occurs in the small intestine of sheep, goat, rabbit, camel and man. Spicules equal, 0·16–0·17 mm. long. Eggs measure 93–118 by 41–52 μ.

T. capricola Ransom, 1907 occurs in the small intestine of sheep and goat. Spicules equal, 0·13–0·145 mm. long.

T. probolurus (Railliet, 1896) occurs in the small intestine of sheep, camel and man. Spicules equal, 0·126–0·134 mm. long.

T. axei (Cobbold, 1879) (syn. *T. extenuatus*) occurs in the abomasum of sheep, goats, cattle, deer and wild antelopes and in the stomach of the pig, horse, donkey and man. The spicules are unequal and dissimilar, the right is 0·085–0·095 mm. long and the left 0·11–0·15 mm. Eggs measure 79–92 by 31–41 μ.

T. rugatus Mönnig, 1925 occurs in the small intestine of sheep and goat in South Africa and Australia. Spicules unequal and dissimilar, the right is 0·137–0·145 mm. long and the left 0·141–0·152 mm.

T. longispicularis Gordon, 1933 (Fig. 107) occurs in sheep in Australia and cattle in Australia, Europe and North America. The male is 5·5 mm. in length. Spicules sub-equal, right 175–180 μ, left 190 μ. Both spicules end bluntly, are rounded at the tip and have a tongue-like semi-transparent membrane projecting from the tip.

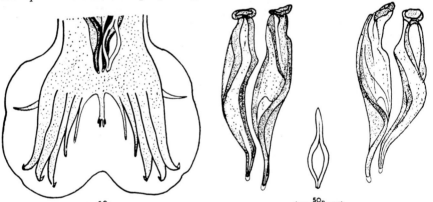

FIG. 107.   *T. longispicularis*, Male   FIG. 108.   *T. longispicularis*, Spicules and
            Bursa-Ventral View   Gubernaculum

T. drepanoformis has been described from sheep in Australia. Spicules are bent near the middle to form an angle of 90°.

Life-cycle of Trichostrongylus spp. The eggs which are passed in the faeces of the host are strongyle-like, being thin shelled and in the eight to thirty-two cell (blastomere) stage. Their development to first stage larvae and subsequently to infective larvae is comparable to that of the horse strongyles (see p. 183). Thus the infective third-stage larva is produced in about 4–6 days under optimal conditions (27°C, O₂, H₂O). Lower temperatures greatly delay development and below 9°C (48·2°F) little or no development occurs.

The bionomics of *Trichostrongylus* spp. larvae are discussed by Levine (1963) and Soulsby (1965). Migration of larvae on blades of grass occurs when the light intensity is about 62 ft-candles, moisture favours migration but more than 0·12 ml. of water per sq. cm. of soil hinders movement. Consequently the greatest number of larvae are on blades of grass in the early morning and early evening when temperature, humidity and light intensity are favourable. Work by Silangwa & Todd (1964) has demonstrated however that only a small proportion (2–3 per cent) of sheep trichostrongyle larvae migrate up grass blades and of those which do only 59 per cent reach as far as the first inch above the soil.

The survival of *Trichostrongylus* spp. infective larvae on pasture has been studied by many workers. (see summaries by Levine, 1963 and Soulsby, 1965). Essentially the infective larvae of this genus behave similarly to those of *Haemonchus*. Thus the most destructive effects are high temperature and dryness and it is unlikely that substantial numbers will survive more than 4–6 months on pasture under any conditions of exposure. *Trichostrongylus* spp. are slightly more resistant to cold than *Haemonchus* spp. and there may be some survival over winter.

Exsheathment. Following ingestion of infective larvae, completing of the second moult, or exsheathment, must occur before the parasitic cycle can begin. This consists of the shedding of the retained sheath of the second stage larva and the physiology of this has been extensively studied by Rogers (1960, 1963, 1966), Rogers & Sommerville (1960) and Sommerville (1960). Essentially the process consists of two stages: the first is a host stimulus which causes larvae to secrete 'exsheathing fluid' and the second is the attack by exsheathing fluid on the sheath so that a break in it occurs and larvae, aided by their own movements, are able to escape from it.

The host stimulus consists of the unionised components of bicarbonate–carbon dioxide buffer, undissociated CO_2 and dissolved gaseous CO_2. Rogers (1960) reported that 70 per cent exsheathment of *Trichostrongylus axei* infective larvae occurred in 3 hours at 37°C at pH 7·3 in 0·02 M sodium dithionite when the total concentration of carbonic acid plus dissolved gaseous CO_2 was about $0·5 \times 10^{-3}$ M. With *H. contortus* larvae $1·5 \times 10^{-3}$ M was necessary to give the same results.

The host stimulus has its main effect on larvae within about 30 minutes and the exsheathing fluid produced attacks an encircling area about 20 μ from the anterior end of the larva. This first appears as a refractile line across the sheath, consisting of a swelling and separation of the sheath in that area. Ultimately the anterior end is detached as a cap and the larva then wriggles out of the sheath.

The mechanism by which exsheathing fluid disrupts the sheath is as yet unknown: it is obviously enzymatic in nature and the substrate attacked is localised to a narrow area on the inside of the sheath. Rogers (1963) has demonstrated that the exsheathing fluid of *H. contortus* contains an enzyme with properties similar to leucine aminopeptidase which acts on the substrate L-leucyl-β-naphthylamide and he (Rogers, 1965) considers this is the enzyme concerned in the reaction. The leucine aminopeptidases produced by *H. contortus* and *T. colubriformis* are highly specific and will attack the substrates in their own sheaths only. In turn leucine aminopeptidase from mammalian tissue has little effect on the sheaths of either species of nematode.

In recent work (Rogers, 1966) it was demonstrated that a low concentration of iodine inhibits exsheathment of larvae of *H. contortus* and *T. colubriformis* and such inhibition can be reversed by subsequent treatment with hydrogen sulphide water.

Parasitic development. Douvres (1957) has described the development of *T. colubriformis* and *T. axei* in cattle. Parasitic third-stage larvae are found in the abomasum or small intestine 2–5 days after infection, fourth-stage larvae occur about 7 days after infection and fifth-stage larvae are found 15 days after infection. The prepatent period is about 20 days. The morphological features of the various developmental stages are described by Douvres.

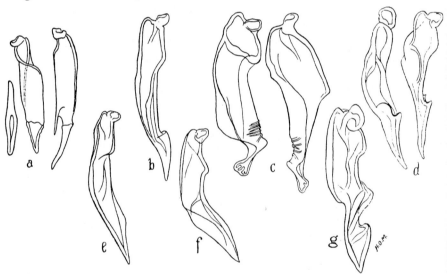

FIG. 109. Spicules of Some Species of *Trichostrongylus*: *a*, spicules and gubernaculum of *T. axei* spicules of *b*, *T. colubriformis*; *c*, *T. rugatus*; *d*, *T. falculatus*; *e*, *T. vitrinus*; *f*, *T. capricola*; *g*, *T. probolurus* (all drawn to same scale; both spicules shown only where they are unequal and dissimilar) (Original)

Pathogenesis. The intestinal forms penetrate into the mucosa underneath the epithelium, rarely deeper, producing desquamation, which may be extensive in heavy infections. The worms are not blood-suckers, nevertheless an anaemia may be associated with heavy infection, this being due to a shortening of the life of the red cell, impaired erythropoiesis or to a reduction of the amino acid pool (see Baker & Douglas, 1966).

It has been estimated that about 2000 worms are necessary to produce marked clinical signs in a year-old sheep, and many more may be needed to produce fatal results, but the effects of the worm vary according to the age and nutrition of the host. *T. axei* penetrates into the mucosa of the absomasum of ruminants or the stomach in equines and produces irregular, circumscribed wart-like thickenings with a finely verrucose surface.

Clinical signs. In horses heavy infections with *T. axei* may cause signs of gastro-intestinal disturbance, but in such cases other worms present in the alimentary canal may be additional causes of the signs observed. The same may be true of cattle. In sheep and goats young animals are especially susceptible. In South Africa trichostrongylosis is a disease of Persian sheep especially, merinos being much less susceptible. When a severe infection is acquired within a short time the disease may be acute and may rapidly lead to death. Such animals usually show neither emaciation nor anaemia, but become weak in the legs, and are unable to stand shortly before they die. In more chronic cases the appetite is variable, emaciation occurs, the skin becomes dry, and there may be alternating constipation and diarrhoea; if anaemia is noticeable, it is mild. In Australia the parasites cause serious losses in young merino sheep which pass dark, diarrhoeic faeces, the worm being for this occasion popularly known as the 'black scours worm'.

Post mortem. In acute cases the carcass shows no other lesions than those in the intestine. The mucosa of this organ is swollen, especially in the duodenum, sometimes slightly haemorrhagic, and it may be covered with mucus. The worms can be found by scraping the mucosa into a glass dish of water or by smearing scrapings over a glass plate, which is held up to the light.

In chronic cases the carcass is emaciated and the liver may show fatty changes. The lesions in the intestine are as described above. In the duodenum the submucous glands are greatly enlarged.

Immunology of Trichostrongylus *spp. infection.* Infection induces immunity to re-infection. Both the intake of infective larvae and the presence of adult worms are concerned with the immune response and the immunity is specific, at least at the generic level, in that sheep immune to *H. contortus* are susceptible to *Trichostrongylus* spp. and *vice versa*. Re-infection of sheep with infective larvae induces self-cure (see p. 238). Jarrett et al. (1960) using X-irradiated larvae of *T. colubriformis* have been able to induce a high degree of resistance to challenge infection, thus double vaccination with irradiated infective larvae reduced the number of worms developing from a challenge infection of 10,000 larvae by approximately 97 per cent. Recently Silverman et al. (1962) have prepared immunising antigens by cultivating *T. colubriformis* in artificial media. Such antigens were highly effective in protecting guinea-pigs against infection and mortality.

Diagnosis must be confined by making faeces cultures and identifying the infective larvae.

Treatment. See pp. 241–243.

Prophylaxis. The general preventive measures described below (p. 243) should be applied.

T. tenuis (Mehlis, 1846) occurs in Europe, Asia and North America in the caeca and small intestine of domestic and wild ducks and geese, fowl, guinea-fowl, turkey, pheasant and partridge. Male 5–6·5 mm., female 7·3–9 mm. long. The spicules are 0·13–0·15 mm. long and curved.

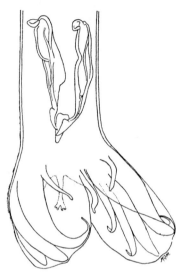

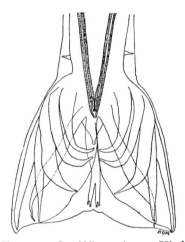

Fig. 110. *Trichostrongylus retortaeformis*, Hind End of Male, Ventral View (Original)

Fig. 111. *Graphidium strigosum*, Hind End of Male, Ventral View (Original)

Life-cycle. The eggs are passed in the faeces of the host, and, under favourable conditions, the larvae develop to the infective stage as those of other strongyles do. The worms mature in the birds in 7 days after infection.

Pathogenicity. Severe infections may cause a haemorrhagic typhlitis with diarrhoea. Later the birds suffer from loss of appetite, emaciation and anaemia.

T. retortaeformis (Zeder, 1800) occurs in the small intestine, rarely the stomach, of the rabbit, hare and goat. Male 5–7 mm., female 6–9 mm. long. The spicules are 0·12–0·14 mm. long. The eggs measure 85–91 by 46–56 μ.

Life-cycle. Direct.

Pathogenicity. The parasites penetrate into the mucosa, causing desquamation, and in heavy infections an inflammation with much mucous exudate may be seen. The affected animals suffer from anaemia and may die.

Genus: Graphidium Railliet & Henry, 1909

G. strigosum (Dujardin, 1845) occurs in the stomach and small intestine of the rabbit and hare in Europe. Male 8–16 mm., female 11–20 mm. long. The body cuticle bears forty to sixty longitudinal ridges. The male bursa has large lateral lobes and a small dorsal lobe. The spicules are 1·1–2·4 mm. long, slender, and each ends distally in several points. The vulva opens 1·14–3·28 mm. from the posterior extremity. The eggs measure 98–106 by 50–58 μ.

Life-cycle. Direct.

Pathogenicity. The worms penetrate deeply into the wall of the stomach or intestine. In some cases no signs are seen even with severe infections, while in other cases anaemia, cachexia and even death may result.

Control. No satisfactory anthelmintic is known but probably thiabendazole would be of value. For prophylaxis hygienic measures are indicated, such as frequent removal of faeces and dryness of quarters.

Genus: Obeliscoides Graybill, 1924

O. cuniculi (Graybill, 1923) occurs in the stomach of rabbits in the U.S.A. Male 10–14 mm., female 15–18 mm. Spicules brown in colour, 440–470 μ long and are bifurcated at the distal end, each bifurcation ending in a hook. Eggs 76–86 μ by 44–45 μ.

Life-cycle. Direct. Prepatent period about 19 days.

Pathogenicity. Except in heavy infections this parasite appears to cause no harm.

Genus: Ostertagia Ransom, 1907

The species of this genus, which occur in the abomasum and rarely the small intestine of sheep, goats, cattle and other ruminants, are usually known as brown stomach-worms, because they have this colour when they are fresh. The worms are slender. The cuticle of the anterior extremity may be slightly inflated, transversely striated, and the 'head' is not more than 0·025 mm. wide. The rest of the body cuticle bears twenty-five to thirty-five longitudinal ridges and has no transverse striations. The male bursa has lateral and dorsal lobes and an accessory bursal membrane situated anteriorly on the dorsal side. The spicules are pigmented brown, relatively short, and end posteriorly in two or three processes. The vulva of the female may be covered by a small anterior flap.

O. ostertagi (Stiles, 1892) occurs in the abomasum of cattle and sheep, rarely the horse. Male 6·5–7·5 mm., female 8·3–9·2 mm. long. The spicules are 0·22–0·23 mm. long, and each ends in three bluntly-hooked processes. The vulva opens in the posterior fifth of the body and is covered by a flap. The eggs measure 80–85 by 40–45 μ.

O. circumcincta (Stadelmann, 1894) occurs in the abomasum of sheep and goats. Male 7·5–8·5 mm., female 9·8–12·2 mm. long. The spicules are slender, 0·28–0·32 mm. long. Each ends in a large knobbed and a small, acute process. The vulva is usually covered by a flap, and opens in the last fifth of the body. The eggs measure 80–100 by 40–50 μ. Near the tip of the female tail there is a thickened band which bears four to five transverse striations. A similar band is also seen in some other species of this genus.

O. trifurcata Ransom, 1907 occurs in the abomasum of sheep and goats. Male 6·5–7 mm. long. The spicules are about 0·18 mm. long and each ends in a stout, knobbed tip, while just behind the middle two sharp spurs are given off medially.

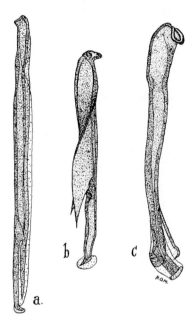

FIG. 112. Spicules of Common *Ostertagia* Species: a, *O. circumcincta*; b, *O. trifurcata*; c, *O. ostertagi* (All same magnification) (Original)

O. lyrata Sjöberg, 1926 occurs in cattle in Europe, Africa and North America. It may also occur in sheep and deer. It is very similar to *O. ostertagi*.

Several other species of *Ostertagia* may occur in sheep or cattle and these include *O. pinnata* (sheep in India, Kenya, Britain), *O. mentulata* (sheep and camel in Western Australia), *O. occidentalis* (sheep in France and Rocky Mountain Region of U.S.A.), *O. crimensis* (cattle and deer in Crimea and Britain), *O. podjapolskyi* (cattle in Britain; moufflon in Crimea) and *Teladorsagia dantiani* (sheep and goats in U.S.S.R., Britain, other parts of Europe and U.S.A.).

Life-cycles. Direct and essentially similar to those of the other members of the Trichostrongylidae. However many species of the genus have a tendency to undergo a histotropic phase of development in the abomasal mucosa and a proportion of an infection may show an extended prepatent period. Some larvae may mature by the twenty-third day after infection but others may remain in the mucosa for up to 3 months without becoming mature. On repeated infection the abomasal mucosa become studded with many small nodules, which can become confluent to give a nodular appearance. In such cases large numbers of retarded larval stages are found in the mucosa.

The infective larvae of *Ostertagia* spp. can survive on pasture for relatively long periods. The forms in cattle are especially important in this respect since the faecal pad may serve as a reservoir for larvae during dry weather. Durie (1961) reported that such larvae, as well as those of *Haemonchus placei*, *T. axei*, *Cooperia* spp. and *Oesophagostomum radiatum*, can survive in faecal pads for 4 months or more. When wet conditions return, waves of larvae may migrate from the faecal pad to contaminate the surrounding pasture. Larvae freed from the faecal pad may survive for about 5–7 weeks depending on the environmental conditions. In general the larvae of *Ostertagia* spp. survive better than those of *Trichostrongylus* spp. and *Haemonchus* spp.

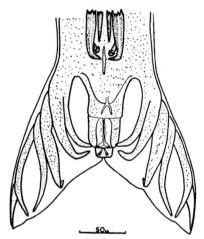

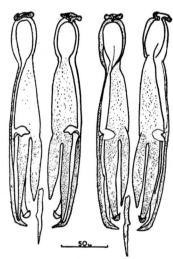

FIG. 113. *Ostertagia lyrata* Male Bursa, Ventral View

FIG. 114. *Ostertagia lyrata*, Spicules and Gubernaculum; Ventral View on the Left, Dorsal View on the Right

Pathogenesis. When the infective larvae of *O. ostertagi* are ingested by the host they penetrate into the mucosa of the abomasum, causing the formation of small, circular, raised areas about 1–2 mm. in diameter. In these nodular lesions the worms develop and the adults may also be found in them, partly projecting through a small opening in the centre, or they may live free on the mucosa. *Ostertagia* spp. infection is chiefly of importance in cattle. Two forms of the disease are seen. One form occurs in calves, being associated with adult parasites, consisting of an abomasitis with oedema and necrosis, decreased albumin levels and a significant reduction in weight gain and often death follows. The other form consists of a severe clinical entity in housed cattle. It is characterised by severe chronic diarrhoea and emaciation and frequently ends fatally (Martin *et al.*, 1957). In some animals more than 200,000 parasites may be found, of which 60 per cent may be immature. The abomasal mucosa is greatly thickened and oedematous, at times there may be superficial necrosis along with an acute inflammatory exudate. There is a marked reduction of serum proteins, levels as low as 4–5 g. per 100 having been observed, this being principally due to a loss of serum albumin. Mulligan *et al.* (1963) have demonstrated that the half life albumin in affected animals is much shortened.

Treatment. See p. 241.

Prophylaxis. The general measures described on p. 243 should be applied. Poorly-fed and young animals are more susceptible than others.

Genus: Marshallagia Orloff, 1933

M. marshalli (Ransom, 1907). Found in the abomasum of sheep in France and the U.S.A. It is similar to the *Ostertagia* spp. Male 10–13 mm.; female 12–20 mm. Characterised by a long, slender dorsal ray, 280–400 μ long, which is bifurcated near the tip. Spicules 250–280 μ long and yellowish-brown in colour: they are split into three processes at the tip. The eggs are large measuring 160–200 μ by 75–100 μ.
This species is not known to be pathogenic.

Genus: Cooperia Ransom, 1907

Species of this genus, which are usually found in the small intestine, rarely in the abomasum, of ruminants, are relatively small worms, of a reddish colour when fresh. The cuticle of the anterior extremity frequently forms a cephalic swelling, and the rest of the body cuticle bears fourteen to sixteen longitudinal ridges which are transversely striated. The male bursa has a small dorsal lobe. The latero-ventral ray is thicker than the ventro-ventral and divergent from it, but its tip again approaches the latter. The postero-lateral is slender and the externo-dorsal usually arises from the base of the dorsal stem. The spicules are stout, relatively short, pigmented brown, and usually have a ridged, wing-like expansion at the middle. An accessory piece is absent. The vulva may be covered by a flap and is situated behind the middle of the body.

C. curticei (Railliet, 1893) occurs in sheep and goats. Male 4·5–5·4 mm., female 5·8–6·2 mm. long. Spicules 0·135–0·145 mm. long.

C. punctata (v. Linstow, 1907) occurs in cattle and rarely in sheep. Male 4·7–5·9 mm., female 5·7–7·5 mm. long. Spicules 0·12–0·15 mm. long.

C. pectinata (Ransom, 1907) occurs in cattle and rarely in sheep. The male is 7 mm. and the female 7·5–9 mm. long. Spicules 0·24–0·28 mm. long.

C. oncophora (Railliet, 1898) occurs in cattle and sheep and rarely the horse. Male 5·5–9 mm., female 6–8 mm. long. Spicules 0·24–0·3 mm. long.

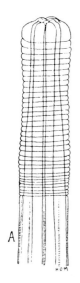
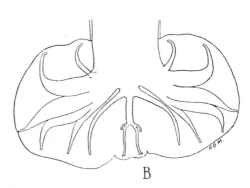

Fig. 115. *Cooperia curticei*: A, anterior end; B, bursa of male, opened out (Original)

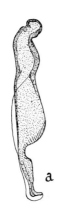
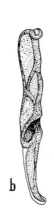
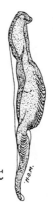

Fig. 116. Spicules of Common *Cooperia* Species: a, *C. curticei*; b, *C. punctata*; c, *C. pectinata* (Not drawn to same scale) (Original)

C. mcmasteri Gordon, 1932 is primarily a parasite of cattle in Britain, Australia and North America. The male measures 6·8 mm. and the female 7·9 mm. In general it resembles *C. oncophora* but the bursa is larger and the rays of the bursa longer and thinner. The spicules are also thinner, 270 μ in length and end in a bifurcation, the external part of which ends in a small conical expansion.

Other species of *Cooperia* include *C. bisonis* (cattle in U.S.A. and U.S.S.R.), *C. spatulata* (sheep and cattle in Malaysia), and *Paracooperia nodulosa* (zebra and buffalo in India and Philippines).

Life-cycle. Direct and in general similar to that of *Trichostrongylus* spp. Infection of the host occurs through its mouth. The infective larva has a pointed tail and is surrounded by a sheath with a medium-sized tail.

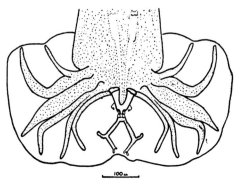

FIG. 117. *Cooperia mcmasteri*, Male Bursa, Ventral View

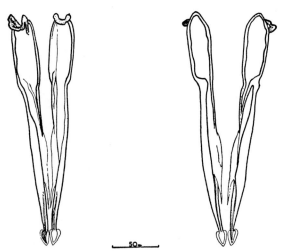

FIG. 118. *Cooperia mcmasteri*, Spicules

Pathogenicity. The worms penetrate into the mucosa of the small intestine and suck blood. A light infection is of no consequence, but young cattle and sheep may be severely affected by heavy infections, which are usually acquired on wet pastures. The clinical signs and lesions are similar to those of trichostrongylosis.

Diagnosis has to be made by faeces culture and the identification of the infective larvae. The eggs of species of the genus *Cooperia* cannot be specifically identified in the faeces.

Treatment and Prophylaxis. See pp. 241–243.

Genus: Nematodirus Ransom, 1907

The species of this genus are relatively long worms with a filiform anterior portion. They have an inflated cuticle around the anterior end and about fourteen to eighteen longitudinal ridges on the body cuticle. The anterior part of the body is thinner than the posterior part. The male bursa has elongate lateral lobes which are covered internally by rounded or oval cuticular bosses, while the dorsal lobe with its supporting rays is split in two and each half is attached to a lateral lobe. The spicules are long and slender and their tips are fused together. The ventral rays are parallel and close together. Except in *N. battus*, the medio-lateral and postero-lateral rays lie close together, except at their tips. The tail of the female is short and truncate, with a slender terminal appendage. The vulva opens at the posterior third of the body. The eggs are so large that their size readily distinguishes them from those of other trichostrongylid species usually found in farm mammals. Eggs passed in the faeces of the host contain about eight cells.

N. spathiger (Railliet, 1896), frequently confused with *N. filicollis* (Rudolph, 1802), is the commonest species and occurs in the small intestine of sheep, cattle and other ruminants. Male 10–15 mm., female 15–23 mm. long. Spicules 0·7–1·21 mm. long, terminating together in a spoon-shaped expansion. The eggs measure 175–260 by 106–110 μ and contain an embryo of about eight cells when passed by the host.

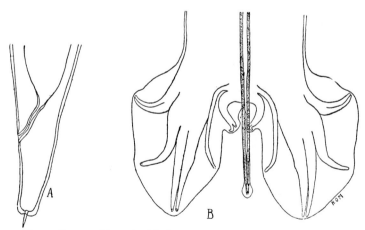

FIG. 119. *Nematodirus spathiger*: A, hind end of female; B, hind end of male, bursa opened out (Original)

Life-cycle. The eggs develop under suitable conditions outside the host, but the larva hatches only when the infective stage has been reached after two ecdyses. When the infective larva leaves the egg-shell it is enclosed in the cuticle of the second stage, which has a very long tail. The tail of the larva itself ends in a dorsal and a ventral lobe, as if a wedge had been cut out between them, and in this notch arises a backwardly pro-jecting finger-like appendage. The infective larvae in the egg are very resistant to desiccation and freezing. Larvae liberated from the egg have an ecology comparable to the infective stages of the *Ostertagia* spp. Larvae develop to maturity in the intestine in about 3 weeks after infection.

Pathogenicity. The pathogenicity of these worms depends on their numbers and on the resistance of the host. In heavy infections severe pathogenic effects are produced by the larval stages. There is destruc-tion of the mucosa, necrosis of villi and the lumen of the bowel contains necrotic material, blood cells and many larval stages.

Treatment and Prophylaxis. See pp. 241–243.

N. battus. This species (Fig. 120) was discovered independently by Crofton & Thomas (1954) in England, and Morgan (unpublished) in Scotland. The male is 10–16, the female 15–24 mm. long. The spicules of the male are 850–950 μ long and meet only at the tips in a flattened, bluntly-pointed projection. The medio-lateral and postero-lateral rays of the male bursa are divergent, not parallel as they are in *N. spathiger* and *N. filicollis*. The eggs measure 152–182 by 67–77 μ and have a brown shell.

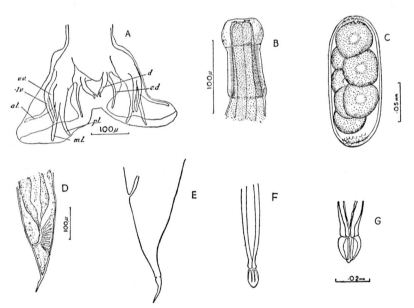

Fig. 120. *Nematodirus battus.* A, bursa; B, anterior end; C, egg; D, E, posterior end of female; F, G, tips of the long spicule of the male. (A, B, E, G, from Crofton & Thomas, 1954; C, D, F, from Morgan, D.O., unpublished)

N. filicollis (Rudolphi, 1802) occurs in the small intestine of sheep, cattle, goats and deer and is cosmopolitan in distribution. It is essen-tially similar to *N. spathiger* from which it can be differentiated by the spicules which end in a narrow, pointed enlargement, this being distinct from the spoon shaped arrangement seen in *N. spathiger*. The eggs measure 130–200 by 70–90 μ.

N. helvetianus May, 1920, is chiefly a parasite of cattle in Europe (Switzerland, Great Britain) and the U.S.A. It also occurs in sheep in these areas. The male is 11–17 mm. and the female 18–25 mm. The dorsal lobe of the bursa is not separated from the lateral lobes, the spicules measure 0·9–1·25 mm. and at the distal end they form a point, the enclosing membrane being lanceolate. The eggs measure 160–230 by 85–121 μ.

Other species of *Nematodirus* which occur include *N. abnormalis* (in sheep, goats, camels in North America, Europe and the U.S.S.R.) and *N. rufaevastitatis* (sheep, Wyoming, U.S.A.).

Life-cycles. The preparasitic development of *N. helvetianus* is similar to that of *N. spathiger*, development to the infective stage occurring within the egg and hatching occurring when this stage is reached. A similar development also occurs in the host.

The preparasitic developments of *N. battus* and *N. filicollis*, however, differ somewhat in that although infective larvae are developed in the egg hatching does not occur promptly as with the other two species. Under natural conditions a period of exposure to low temperature followed by exposure to a higher temperature is necessary for hatching. Thomas & Stevens (1960) found that when larvae of *N. battus* in eggs were exposed to temperatures of −2–3°C the number of larvae which hatched when the larvae were returned to 21°C increased as the exposure to the low temperature increased, a maximum hatching occurring after 7 months' exposure to low temperature. Similar results were obtained with eggs of *N. filicollis*. Consequently it is clear that the infective larvae can remain inactive in the egg for considerable periods of time, hatching occurring only when adequate temperature and moisture are available. In Great Britain a definite gradation of hatching occurs; thus with *N. spathiger* hatching occurs normally when the third stage larva is reached, with *N. filicollis* hatching is erratic in late winter to spring but with *N. battus* hatching is constantly and uniformly delayed until the spring.

Pathogenesis. The clinical effects of *Nematodirus* spp. infection are comparable to acute trichostrongylosis. However in Great Britain a specific disease entity in lambs due to *N. battus* occurs, associated with a mortality of about 10 per cent. The clinical signs are an acute diarrhoea with dehydration and prostration. Such disease is associated with mass hatching of *N. battus* larvae on pasture in the spring. The major clinical effect is due to the larval stages of the parasite.

Genus: Haemonchus Cobb, 1898

H. contortus (Rudolphi, 1803) occurs in the abomasum of sheep, goats, cattle and numerous other ruminants in most parts of the world.

It is commonly known as the 'stomach-worm' or 'wireworm' of ruminants, and is one of their most pathogenic parasites. Male 10–20 mm., female 18–30 mm. long. The male has an even reddish colour, while in the female the white ovaries are spirally wound around the red intestine, producing the appearance of a barber's pole. The cuticle is in parts transversely striated and also bears a number of longitudinal ridges.

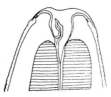

FIG. 121. *Haemonchus contortus*, Anterior End, Lateral View

The cervical papillae are prominent and spine-like. A small buccal cavity is present, containing a dorsal lancet. The male bursa has elongate lateral lobes supported by long, slender rays, while the small dorsal lobe is asymmetrically situated against the left lateral lobe and supported by a Y-shaped dorsal ray. The spicules are 0·46–0·506 mm. long, each

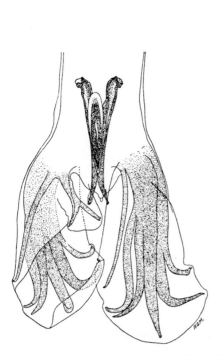
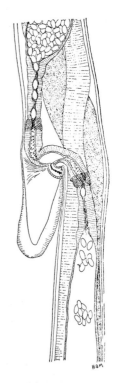

FIG. 122. *Haemonchus contortus*, Hind End of Male, Dorsal View (Original)

FIG. 123. *Haemonchus contortus*, Vulvar Region of Female (Original)

provided with a small barb near its extremity. The vulva of the female is covered by an anterior flap, which is usually large and very prominent, but may be reduced to a small knob-like structure in some specimens. The eggs measure 70–85 by 41–48 μ, and those passed in the faeces of the host contain an embryo divided into sixteen to thirty-two cells.

Das & Whitlock (1960) have studied the comparative morphology of *Haemonchus* spp. from various geographic regions. In view of the consistent morphological differences which were found they suggested that two new sub-species and a new variety of *Haemonchus contortus* be created namely *Haemonchus contortus contortus* (Australia), *H. contortus cayugensis* (New York State, U.S.A.) and *H. contortus* var *utkalensis* (Orissa, India).

Haemonchus placei (Place, 1893) Ransom, 1911. For many years it has been common to refer to the *Haemonchus* species of cattle as *H. contortus*. Studies in Australia by Roberts *et al.* (1954) led them to conclude that the cattle and sheep forms were distinct and represented two species, *H. contortus* in sheep and *H. placei* in cattle. Studies by Bremner (1955) on the chromosomes (2N = 11 male; 12 female) indicated differences in the X chromosome in the two species, in the cattle species it measured 8 μ whereas in the sheep form it was similar to the autosomes and measured 3 μ. Subsequently, the conclusion of the Australian workers was generally accepted and Herlich *et al.* (1958) demonstrated the occurrence of the two species in the U.S.A.

The major differences are based on mean spicule lengths, the distance between the barbs and the tip of the spicules and differences in size and activity of infective larvae. Thus mean spicule lengths are *H. contortus* 398–431 μ; *H. placei* 454–470 μ; barb to tip of spicule left *H. contortus* 41–46 μ, *H. placei* 52–54 μ; right *H. contortus* 21–40 μ, *H. placei* 27–37 μ.

H. similis Travassos, 1914. This species has been reported from cattle and deer in Florida, Louisiana and Texas, and also occurs in cattle in Europe and Brazil. It differs from *H. contortus* in that the terminal processes of dorsal ray are longer and the spicules are shorter being 139–334 μ long.

H. longistipes Railliet & Henry, 1909 occurs in the camel and dromedary in North Africa and India. The spicules are much longer than those of the other species, being a mean of 625 μ.

Life-cycles of Haemonchus *spp.* The preparasitic development of *H. contortus* and *H. placei* are very similar to that of other strongyles. Detailed studies of the embryonation of eggs and the development of larvae of *H. contortus* have been carried out by Dinaburg (1944), Silverman & Campbell (1959) and Dinnik & Dinnik (1958) and the ecology of larvae on pasture has been reviewed by Crofton (1963) and Levine (1963).

Essentially, under satisfactory environmental conditions infective larvae are reached in 4–6 days. Low temperatures retard development and below 9°C little or no development takes place. Eggs which have reached the 'prehatch' stage are more resistant to adverse conditions and can survive freezing and desiccation more readily than other stages.

Infective larvae of *H. contortus* are not highly resistant to adverse conditions and regardless of conditions of exposure it is unlikely that larvae will survive for more than 6 months and in fact the majority will have been destroyed much earlier than this. The most destructive effects are dryness and high temperatures. There is little survival of *H. contortus* larvae over winter, though a few may do so (Kates, 1950).

The larvae of *H. placei* behave similarly to those of *H. contortus* except that the faecal pad of cattle may serve as a reservoir for larvae. Durie (1961) has reported that larvae may survive here for several months and ultimately be released when the faecal pad is sufficiently moistened by rain.

Following ingestion of infective larvae exsheathment (see p. 223) occurs in the rumen and parasitic larval stages migrate to the abomasum where they reach maturity in 19 days in the case of *H. contortus* and in 26–28 days in the case of *H. placei*. The parasitic development of *H. contortus* is detailed in the classic work of Veglia (1915) and that of *H. placei* is described by Bremner (1956).

Pathogenesis. The principal feature of *Haemonchus* spp. infection is anaemia, due to the blood-letting activities of the parasite. There is a reduced erythrocyte level, a decreased haemoglobin level and reduced packed cell volume. A detailed consideration of the kinetics of the blood changes in haemonchosis is given by Baker & Douglas (1966). In heavy infections the anaemia is frequently fatal and may be so before eggs are produced by the worms since the loss of blood commences with the fourth-stage larvae.

Clinical signs. In acute cases—that is, when lambs or young sheep, which are the most susceptible, acquire a sudden, severe infection—anaemia develops rapidly and the animals die without showing much more than signs of anaemia and hydraemia. In more chronic cases anaemia is also the main sign, and oedematous swellings (called bottle-jaw or watery poke) are frequently seen under the jaw and others may develop along the ventral aspect of the abdomen. The animals become progressively weak and later walk with a swaying gait. The skin becomes pale, and in sheep the wool falls out in patches. Occasionally diarrhoea or constipation may occur and the appetite is variable. Shortly before death great weakness may lead to prostration.

Immunology of Haemonchus *infections.* Probably one of the best known phenomena of immunity to helminths is the 'self cure' reaction which occurs in *H. contortus* infection. This reaction which results in the loss of a burden of parasites can be induced in suitably infected and sensitised sheep by a challenge dose of infective larvae, the reaction apparently being initiated when the challenge larvae moult from the third to the fourth larval stage. The self cure reaction is more likely to occur in sheep which have experienced several suitably spaced doses of larvae rather than those which carry an initial infection. The reaction is accompanied by a rise in circulating antibody but this rise occurs after the self cure reaction has taken place. Further studies of this reaction by Stewart (1953) indicated that it was essentially a reaction associated with hypersensitivity of the abomasal mucosa and indeed the reaction was associated with a significant rise in blood histamine between the second and fourth days following the administration of the larvae. Sheep failing to show self cure of the infection showed no rise in circulating histamine. The self cure reaction could be induced by the injection of exsheathed *H. contortus* larvae into the abomasum as well as by the administration of ensheathed larvae by mouth. The reaction is dependent on antigens associated with living larvae and which act locally since the intraperitoneal injection of living larvae, while producing a good antibody response fails to induce self cure. Similarly dead infective larvae given by mouth fail to induce it and the addition of heated *H. contortus* antigen to strips of the abomasum of sheep which had regularly exhibited the self cure reaction, failed to induce contraction.

The association of 'self cure' with the moulting period of the challenge dose of larvae was demonstrated by Soulsby & Stewart (1960), directly by examining the abomasal population of parasites at the time of self cure, and indirectly by obtaining serological evidence of a marked reaction to exsheathing fluid at the time of self cure. A more detailed consideration of the self cure reaction is given by Soulsby (1966).

The reaction is not entirely specific since challenge with *H. contortus* larvae will induce self cure of a *Trichostrongylus* spp. infection: however the reverse, namely challenge with *Trichostrongylus* larvae, does not induce self cure of a *H. contortus* infection. The self cure reaction is not solely an experimental entity. It is an important mechanism for terminating natural gastro-intestinal parasitism in sheep in Great Britain (Soulsby, 1957) and in Australia natural burdens of *H. contortus* are terminated by the process, especially after rain when the intake of infective larvae provides the stimulus for the reaction.

A substantial degree of immunity to *H. contortus* has been produced under experimental conditions by the use of X-irradiated infective larvae. In Australia, Mulligan *et al.* (1961) showed that sheep immunised with two doses of *H. contortus* larvae irradiated at the 60 kiloroentgen level produced very significant resistance to challenge. However such results have been obtained with sheep aged 6–9 months. Animals younger than this respond poorly or not at all to immunisation against *H. contortus* (Manton *et al.*, 1962).

The immune response to *H. placei* infection differs from that induced by *H. contortus*. Roberts (1957) was unable to induce self cure. He demonstrated that a marked resistance to re-infection was acquired quite rapidly, even after a single dose of larvae. The immunity is manifested by

a marked inhibition of development of fourth-stage larvae in the abomasal mucosa. Such inhibited larvae can persist for a considerable time
and are apparently inhibited by the presence of a population of adult
worms. The removal of such adult worms by anthelmintic treatment
may allow the inhibited larvae to develop to maturity and this new
population may be seriously pathogenic.

Post mortem. The mucous membranes and the skin are pale, while
the blood has a watery appearance. The internal organs are also markedly
pale. Hydrothorax, fluid in the pericardium, and ascites are usually
conspicuous and an extreme cachexia is present, the fat being replaced
by a gelatinous tissue. The liver has a light-brown colour; it is fragile
and shows fatty changes. The abomasum contains reddish-brown, fluid
ingesta and a large number of worms that are readily seen and that swim
about actively if the carcass is still warm. The mucosa is swollen and
covered with small red bite-marks of the parasites. Occasionally shallow
ulcers with ragged edges are found, and a number of the worms may be
firmly attached with their anterior extremities in these ulcers. The
intestine may contain a few worms which are being passed out by the
host.

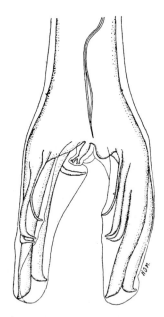

Fig. 124. *Mecistocirrus digitatus*, Hind End of Male, Dorsal View (Original)

Diagnosis. The clinical signs alone may lead to a suspicion of haemonchosis, but a definite diagnosis can only be made by autopsy of selected
cases or by faeces culture and the identification of the infective larvae.

Treatment. See p. 241.

Genus: Mecistocirrus Railliet & Henry, 1912

M. digitatus (von Linstow, 1906) occurs in the abomasum of sheep, cattle, zebu, buffalo and the stomach of the pig and rarely man in eastern countries and in Central America. Male up to 31 mm., female up to 43 mm. long. The cuticle bears about thirty longitudinal ridges. The cervical papillae are prominent and the small buccal capsule contains a lancet as in *Haemonchus*. The female resembles that of the latter species in having the ovaries wound spirally around the intestine, but is readily distinguished from it by the position of the vulva which is situated about 0·6–0·9 mm. from the tip of the tail. The male bursa has a small, symmetrical dorsal lobe; the ventro-ventral ray is small, while the latero-ventral and antero-lateral rays are conspicuously longer than the other rays. The spicules are slender, 3·8–7 mm. long, and united together for almost their whole length. The eggs measure 95–120 by 56–60 μ.

Life-cycle. This is direct, the prepatent period being about 60 days (Fernando, 1962). In this infection the fourth larval stage is of long duration, lasting from the ninth to the twenty-eighth day of infection.

Pathogenicity, etc.. Very similar to *Haemonchus*.

TREATMENT OF GASTRO–INTESTINAL NEMATODES OF RUMINANTS

An extensive literature exists on this subject and no attempt will be made to give other than a brief indication of the present compounds which are most in use. Those wishing further information are referred to Gibson (1965) who thoroughly reviews veterinary anthelmintic medication.

Phenothiazine

Sheep. Dose 600–700 mg. per kg. Highly efficient against abomasal worms and *O. columbianum*. Fine particle form more efficient. Low level dosage has been used extensively, chiefly U.S.A., and in one area has led to a partially resistant strain of *H. contortus*. Little effect on larval stages.

Cattle. Dose 50–80 g. per animal. Efficient against abomasal parasites, though effect variable against *Ostertagia*. Lack of effect on larval stages a drawback in cattle, especially for *H. placei* and *O. ostertagi*.

Toxicity in cattle more important than in sheep. Photosensitisation may occur in tropical and subtropical areas.

Organo-phosphorus Compounds

Neguvon (Bayer L 13/59). In sheep a dose of 110 mg. per kg. effective against *H. contortus*, variable against *Trichostrongylus* spp. In cattle 44 mg. per kg. highly active against *H. placei* and *O. radiatum*; 110 mg. per kg. effective against *Cooperia* spp., *O. ostertagi*, *T. axei*.

Ruelene. In sheep a dose of 100–200 mg. per kg. effective against *Ostertagia* spp., *Trichostrongylus* spp. and *Nematodirus*.

In cattle a dose of 39 mg. per kg. highly effective against *Cooperia* spp.

Asuntol (Bayer 21/199: Co-Ral). In sheep doses of 10–25 mg. per kg. have good action against abomasal worms and *Cooperia* spp., *Strongyloides papillosus* and *O. columbianum*.

In cattle a rate of 25 mg. per kg. highly effective against *Haemonchus*, *Ostertagia*, *Trichostrongylus*, *Cooperia* but erratic against *Nematodirus* and *Bunostomum*.

Haloxon. In sheep at dose of 30–55 mg. per kg. highly effective against both abomasal and intestinal nematodes. Also has activity against the larval stages of *Haemonchus*, *Trichostrongylus* and *Ostertagia*.

Bephenium Compounds

In sheep bephenium embonate at dose of 250 mg. per kg. highly effective against adults and larvae of *Nematodirus* spp. Bephenium hydroxynaphthoate at dose of 250 mg. per kg. shows high activity against *Haemonchus*, *Ostertagia*, *Trichostrongylus*, *Cooperia* and *Nematodirus* spp.

In cattle doses of 125–225 mg. per kg. of bephenium hydroxynaphthoate have high efficiency against *Cooperia*, *Oesophagostomum*, *Ostertagia*, *Haemonchus*, *Nematodirus* spp.

Methyridine (2-(β-methoxyethyl) pyridine = Promintic)

The recommended dose is 1 ml. of a 90 per cent solution per 10 lb. bodyweight (= 200 mg. per kg. bodyweight) given subcutaneously at any convenient site, but preferably not near to a joint. The usual dose is 200 mg. per kg. There may be transient swelling at the site of injection, especially in cattle, but the drug is otherwise well tolerated. It is rapidly absorbed and preferentially excreted into anterior part of the small intestine. Drug causes irreversible depolymerisation of neuromuscular junction of the worm and is active against both mature and immature worms. High efficiency is reported against intestinal *Trichostrongylus*, *Cooperia*, and *Nematodirus* spp; also highly effective against *Strongyloides*, *Trichuris*, *Chabertia*, and *Oesophagostomum* spp. Variable effects may be seen against *Osteragia* and *Haemonchus* spp. of abomasum and possibly this is associated with the acid environment and passage of the drug through the cuticle of the worm.

Tetramisole [d1, 2, 3, 5, 6-*tetrahydro-6-phenyl-imidazo* (2, 1-b) *thiazole hydrochloride*]

Dose of 15 mg. per kg., has high efficiency against all stages of all nematodes, except *Trichuris*, in alimentary canal of sheep and cattle; also effective against *Dictyocaulus* spp. in cattle and sheep. Walley (1966) states it to be safe administered by any route, having a 4- to 6-fold safety margin.

Pyrantel tartrate [*trans*-1-*methyl*-2 [2-(*a-thienylvinyl*)] 1, 4, 5, 6-*tetrahydropyri-mindine tartrate*]

Conwell (1966) has reported that a single oral dose of 25 mg. per kg. as a 5 per cent aqueous solution to sheep is highly effective against *Ostertagia, Trichostrongylus, Nematodirus, Cooperia,* and *Chabertia* species and their larval stages. It is safe for pregnant animals.

Thiabendazole (2-(4'-*thiazolyl*)-*benzimidazole*)

A single oral dose of 50 mg. per kg. to sheep and 100 mg. per kg. to cattle removes more than 95 per cent of species of *Trichostrongylus, Cooperia, Nematodirus, Ostertagia, Haemonchus, Oesophagostomum, Bunostomum, Chabertia, Strongyloides* and *Trichuris* and also inhibits the egg production and development of the larvae of these species.

PROPHYLAXIS AGAINST NEMATODES PARASITIC IN RUMINANTS

Experience has shown that the following measures are of the utmost importance in the control of nematode parasites, including the lung-worms next to be described, of ruminants:

1. The animals should be well fed and supplied with licks containing those minerals in which the pasture is deficient. Well-nourished animals are usually much less susceptible to infection than others, and even if some worms do establish themselves, their effects are hardly noticed and a spontaneous cure soon occurs. If, however, the pasture is heavily infected, the worm burden may be too severe even for the well-fed.

2. The animals should be regularly treated in order to keep them free of the most harmful worms, like *Haemonchus contortus,* so that they will be able themselves to overcome the other parasites.

3. Overstocking tends to concentrate worm infection and should there-fore be avoided. On the other hand, pasture rotation allows the animals to graze on clean pastures at intervals while the infected paddocks can be left to become clean. It is most important however that pasture which has been vacated be left a sufficient time for the major part of the population of infective larvae to die.

4. Because calves, lambs and young sheep are the most susceptible to worms, they should be separated from their mothers as early as possible and graze in a clean paddock. In countries where a dry season occurs the beginning of the dry season is the best lambing time if provision for green fodder can be made. The lambs then arrive at a fairly safe period, while the dry conditions also assist in cleansing a paddock into which the lambs can be put after weaning. The use of various grazing techniques for the control of gastro-intestinal parasites of sheep is discussed by Spedding (1962).

5. Wet or moist pastures as well as other wet places like the edges of pools of water or dams, which present very suitable conditions for the development and maintenance of worm larvae, should be avoided. The

animals are best watered from troughs surrounded by gravelled areas, in order to prevent moisture from accumulating. If the water of a dam has to be used, it should be fenced in and the water led to a trough through pipes which do not catch the mud at the bottom of the dam.

6. Stabled animals should be fed from raised troughs and hay-racks, and great care must be taken that the food is not contaminated by bedding or faeces and that infective larvae do not migrate into it from the floor.

More detailed accounts of the measures for control can be obtained from Gordon (1958) and Soulsby (1965).

Genus: Hyostrongylus Hall, 1921

H. rubidus (Hassall & Stiles, 1892) occurs in the stomach of the pig in many countries. Male 4–7 mm., female 5–10 mm. long. The worms are slender and reddish when they are fresh. The body cuticle is transversely striated and also bears forty to forty-five longitudinal striations. The bursa is well developed, but the dorsal lobe is small. The spicules

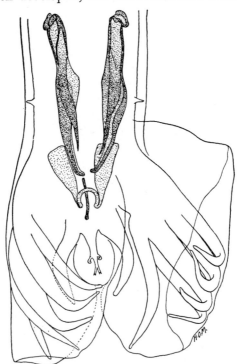

FIG. 125. *Hyostrongylus rubidus*, Hind End of Male, Ventral View (Original)

are 0·13 mm. long. There is a narrow gubernaculum and a well-developed telamon. The vulva is situated 1·3–1·7 mm. anterior to the anus. The eggs measure 71–78 by 35–42 μ.

Life-cycle. The eggs hatch, at ordinary temperatures, in 39 hours and the larvae develop to the infective stage in 7 days. They are not very resistant to drying or low temperatures. Infection occurs per os and not through the skin. The worms reach maturity in 17–19 days. Kotlán (1949, 1960) studied the histotropic larval phases in the stomachs of pigs and rabbits and found that the larvae penetrate into the pits of the gastric glands, moving about in these until they become adults, this histotropic phase requiring 13–14 days. Some adults then return to the lumen of the stomach, but others may remain in the gastric glands for several months, causing the formation of nodules the size of a lentil.

Pathogenicity. The parasites burrow into the gastric mucosa and suck blood. They appear to be comparatively harmless in the absence of other factors that would affect the general health of the host or the gastric mucosa in particular. They may be found in apparently healthy pigs without causing any ill effects, but in others are associated with a marked gastritis and in some cases marked ulceration. The animals lose condition rapidly and become weak, showing incoordination and a tendency to lie down frequently. The appetite may vary, but the animals are usually thirsty. Diarrhoea occurs and the faeces may be dark in colour.

Post-mortem. The degree of emaciation of the carcass depends on the severity of the case. The main lesions are found in the stomach, varying from hyperaemia and a catarrh in mild cases to a croupous gastritis. In the latter case the mucosa is thickened and shows areas covered with yellow, corrugated pseudo-membranes. The worms are found in these membranes as well as in the mucosa.

Diagnosis. A tentative diagnosis can be made by finding the eggs of the worm in the faeces, but it can be definitely confirmed only by autopsy of a selected case.

Treatment. Carbon disulphide has been used with success at a dose of 0·027–0·22 ml. per kg. A general dose is 0·1 ml. per kg. after starvation for 36–48 hours.

Thiabendazole has been reported to be highly effective (Shanks, 1963).

Prophylaxis. Hygienic measures, particularly frequent removal of faeces from sites and effective drainage in the runs or paddocks, are indicated.

Genus: Ornithostrongylus Travassos, 1914

O. quadriradiatus (Stevenson, 1904) occurs in the crop, proventriculus and small intestine of the pigeon in North America, South Africa, Australia. It has also been reported in pigeons in Great Britain. Male 9–12 mm., female 18–24 mm. long. The fresh worms are red. The cuticle of the head is slightly inflated and the body cuticle has a number of longitudinal striations. In the male bursa the ventral rays are close together and the dorsal is fairly short. The spicules are 0·15–0·16 mm. long, each ending in three pointed processes. A telamon is present; it is roughly cross-shaped, the two arms forming an incomplete ring through which the spicules pass. The vulva opens about 5 mm. from the posterior extremity. The eggs measure 70–75 by 38–40 μ.

Life-cycle. Direct, like that of other Trichostrongylidae.

Pathogenicity. The worms burrow into the intestinal mucosa and severe infections cause a catarrhal enteritis. They are also blood-suckers and in severe infections a haemorrhagic enteritis with ulceration and necrosis may be seen. The parasite may be reponsible for heavy losses in breeding establishments.

Treatment. Phenothiazine at the rate of 0·4 g. per kg. has been used with success, but it is likely that thiabendazole will also be useful.

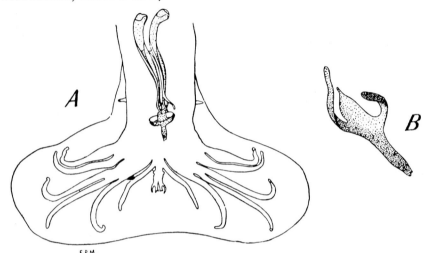

FIG. 126. *Ornithostrongylus quadriradiatus*: *A*, bursa, ventral view; *B*, 'telamon', ventral view (from Baylis, after Stevenson)

Prophylaxis. A general improvement in hygiene is indicated. Pigeon lofts should be cleaned out regularly. Where ornamental pigeons and doves are hand fed, the place of feeding should be changed regularly to avoid an accumulation of eggs and infective larvae.

Genus: Libyostrongylus Lane, 1923

L. douglassii (Cobbold, 1882) occurs in the proventriculus of the ostrich in South Africa. Male about 4–6 mm., female 5–6 mm. long. The colour of fresh specimens is yellowish-red. The male bursa is well developed and the dorsal ray is long and cleft in its distal half, forming three small branches on either side. The spicules are 0·14–0·158 mm. long, each ending in a large and a small spine. The vulva opens 0·8 mm. from the posterior extremity. ·The eggs measure 59–74 by 36–44 μ.

Life-cycle. The eggs are passed in the faeces of the host and the development and bionomics of the free-living stages resemble those of other strongyle species. The infective larval stage is reached under optimal conditions in 60 hours. The infective larva is about 0·745 mm. long, including the sheath, and morphologically closely resembles the larvae of *Trichostrongylus* spp. Eggs containing fully formed embryos can resist desiccation as long as 3 years, and the infective larvae remain viable under dry conditions for 9 months or longer. Infection of the host occurs per os. The worms develop to maturity in the ostrich in about 33 days, the first eggs being passed in the faeces on the thirty-sixth day.

Pathogenesis. The young parasites penetrate deeply into the lumina of the glands in the proventriculus. The adults live in the surface epithelium of the organ, sucking blood and causing severe irritation.

Clinical signs. Chicks are most susceptible to infection, and adult birds, although susceptible, suffer much less from the parasite, especially when they are well fed. The birds become anaemic, weak, emaciated and stunted in growth. Severe losses of chicks may be experienced.

Post-mortem. Apart from emaciation and anaemia the characteristic lesions are found in the proventriculus. The mucosa is swollen and covered with an excessive amount of tough mucus. The mucosa is desquamated in patches and pseudo-membranes may be present, covering haemorrhagic areas. The worms are found in and underneath the mucus and the pseudo-membranes.

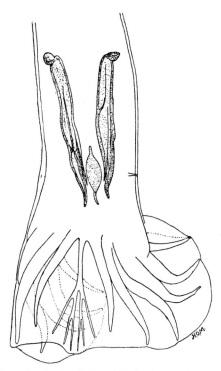

Fig. 127. *Libyostrongylus douglassii*, Hind End of Male, Dorsal View (Original)

Diagnosis. The signs would lead to a tentative diagnosis, which must be confirmed by finding the infective larvae in faeces cultures or by autopsy of a selected bird. The eggs cannot be differentiated readily from those of *Codiostomum struthionis*.

No satisfactory treatment is known.

Prophylaxis. Since birds and runs may remain infected for long periods, the chicks should be kept away from the adult birds in clean runs and fed with crops grown on clean lands. If hens and chicks are kept together, the droppings of the adult birds should be removed every 24–48 hours. Infected adult birds suffer little effect from the parasites when they are well fed.

FAMILY: OLLULANIDAE SKRJABIN & SCHIKHOBALOVA, 1952

Trichostrongyloidea in which the female has two, three or more caudal processes (mucrones). Parasites oviparous or viviparous. Genus of importance *Ollulanus.*

Genus: Ollulanus Leuckart, 1865

O. tricuspis Leuckart, 1865 occurs in the stomach of the cat, fox, wild *Felidae* and the pig. Male 0·7–0·8 mm., female 0·8–1 mm. long. A small buccal cavity is present. The male bursa is well developed, and the spicules, which are 0·046–0·057 mm. long and stout, are each split

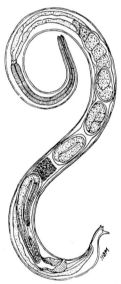

FIG. 128. *Ollulanus tricuspis,* Female (Original)

into two for a considerable distance. The tail of the female ends in three or more short cusps. The vulva is situated in the posterior part of the body, and there is only one uterus and ovary.

Life-cycle. The worms are viviparous and the larvae develop in the uterus of the female to the third larval stage. The infection is spread through the vomit of an infected animal which is eaten by another susceptible one.

Pathogenicity. This parasite is considered to be comparatively harmless to cats, although the worms burrow into the gastric mucosa, causing slight erosions and increased secretion of mucus. A chronic catarrhal hypertrophic gastritis and emaciation in the pig has been ascribed to this parasite.

There is no satisfactory treatment and control is dependent on hygiene.

FAMILY: DICTYOCAULIDAE SKRJABIN, 1941

It has been common to classify nematodes in this group in the family Metastrongylidae and thus include it along with the other nematodes which are found in the air passages or blood vessels of the lungs. The placing of the genus *Dictyocaulus* in the superfamily Trichostrongyloidea rather than the Metastrongyloidea (see later) is based on the consideration that it does not require intermediate hosts and is thus a 'geohelminth' whereas members of the Metastrongyloidea, as far as is known, require intermediate hosts and are 'biohelminths', according to Russian workers.

Trichostrongyloidea: occur in the respiratory passages of the lungs; the bursa is well formed and bursal rays well developed, some may be fused at the distal part. Spicules short and reticulated. Life-cycle direct. Genus of importance: *Dictyocaulus.*

Genus: Dictyocaulus Railliet & Henry, 1907

D. filaria (Rudolphi, 1809) occurs in the bronchi of sheep, goats and some wild ruminants. It has a world-wide distribution and causes serious losses. Male 3–8 cm., female 5–10 cm. long. The worms have a milk-white colour and the intestine shows as a dark line. There are four very small lips and a very small, shallow buccal capsule. In the male bursa the medio- and postero-lateral rays are fused together except at their tips; the externo-dorsals arise separately and the dorsal ray is cleft right from its base. The spicules are stout, dark-brown, boot-shaped and 0·4–0·64 mm. long. The vulva is situated not far behind the middle of the body. The eggs measure 112–138 by 69–90 μ and contain fully formed larvae when laid.

Life-cycle. The eggs may hatch in the lungs, but are usually coughed up and swallowed, and hatch while they pass through the alimentary tract of the host. Some eggs may be expelled in the nasal discharge or sputum. The first-stage larva passed in the faeces is 0·55–0·58 mm. long and can be easily recognised by the presence of a small cuticular knob at the anterior extremity and numerous brownish food granules in the intestinal cells. The free stages do not feed, but exist on these food granules. After 1–2 days the larva reaches the second stage, but does not cast the old cuticle until the third or infective stage is reached, so that the latter is for some time enclosed in two sheaths. The first is then cast while the second is retained for protection. The larvae require moisture for their development and, at a temperature of about 27°C, reach the infective stage in 6–7 days. The infective larvae are not very active and have a weak negative geotropism. They can withstand moderately dry conditions for a few days, but are able to live in moist conditions for several months and are fairly resistant to low temperatures.

Infection of the host occurs per os. Larvae penetrate into the intestinal wall within 3 days and pass via the lymph vessels to the mesenteric lymph glands, where they develop and perform the third ecdysis about 4 days after infection. In the fourth stage males and females can be distinguished. The worms now pass via the lymph and blood vessels to the lungs, where they are arrested in the capillaries and break through into the air passages. Development to maturity in the host takes about 4 weeks.

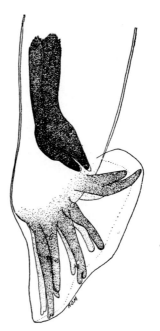

FIG. 129. *Dictyocaulus filaria*, Hind End of Male, Lateral View (Original)

Pathogenesis. The worms live in the small bronchi, producing a catarrhal parasitic bronchitis. The inflammatory process spreads to the surrounding peribronchial tissues and the exudate frequently passes back into the bronchioles and alveoli, causing atelectasis and catarrh, or pneumonia. Secondary bacterial infection may lead to more extensive areas of pneumonia.

Clinical signs. Young animals are chiefly affected, but the disease may occur at all ages and is usually chronic. The animals may cough and a tenacious mucus exudes from the nostrils, but cough is not always present and it is not a reliable guide to the severity of the infection. Dyspnoea is usually obvious, the respiration is more rapid than normal and abnormal lung sounds can be heard on auscultation. Diarrhoea is not infrequent but this is due to co-existing infection with other Trichostrongylidae. The temperature is not elevated unless pneumonia develops.

Post-mortem. The lungs show atelectatic areas of variable size. The bronchi in the affected parts contain the worms and a large amount of mucus which is mixed with blood, and is slightly opaque on account of the presence of desquamated epithelial cells, leucocytes and the eggs of the worms. The bronchial mucosa and the peribronchial tissues are inflamed and infiltrated with leucocytes. Localised and often cone-shaped areas of pneumonia, accompanied by atelectasis and compensatory emphysema, may be present. In some cases proliferation of the bronchial epithelium has occurred.

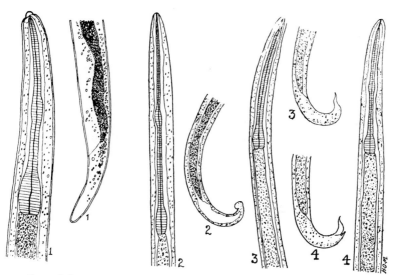

FIG. 130. Larval Stages of Lungworms as found in Fresh Faeces of Hosts. Anterior and posterior ends of 1, *Dictyocaulus filaria*; 2, *Metastrongylus apri*; 3, *Protostrongylus rufescens*; 4, *Muellerius capillaris* (Original)

Diagnosis is made by finding the larvae in the fresh faeces. Eggs may be found in the sputum or nasal discharge, but their absence is not significant.

Treatment. See p. 254.

Prophylaxis. The animals must be removed from infected ground, placed on dry pastures and supplied with clean drinking water. Moist pastures must be avoided, while dry pastures are fairly safe, because the infective larvae are not very resistant to dryness. The general prophylactic measures described on p. 254 are also important. The larvae may live through the winter in cold climates, and the infection is acquired either from overwintered larvae or from those shed by older animals, which show no clinical signs. They should therefore not be grazed together with the young stock.

D. viviparus (Bloch, 1782) occurs in the bronchi of cattle and deer and has a cosmopolitan distribution. Male 4–5·5 cm., female 6–8 cm. long. The worm closely resembles the preceding species, but the medio- and postero-lateral rays are completely fused and the spicules are only 0·195–0·215 mm. long. The eggs measure 82–88 by 33–38 μ.

Life-cycle. Similar to that of *D. filaria.* The infective stage is reached in about 4 days. The first-stage larva found in the fresh faeces of the host is 0·3–0·36 mm. long and has no anterior knob, but the intestinal cells also contain numerous brownish granules. The infective larvae of *D. viviparus* are relatively inactive and are frequently found coiled up, showing very little movement. Consequently there is little migration of larvae from the faecal pads onto herbage, except during heavy rainfall, and larvae which do reach the herbage are capable of limited vertical migration only. In view of this relative inactivity some other mechan- ism(s) must be operative in the 'translation' of larvae from the faecal pad to infective larvae on the herbage. Michel & Rose (1954) conclude that in order for larvae to get onto the herbage in meaningful numbers, it is necessary for faeces to get onto the herbage. Consequently condi- tions which lead to loose faeces or diarrhoea will be expected to be conducive to 'translation', and long lush herbage is one of such factors. Associated gastro-intestinal parasitism may be another. A further method of 'translation' may be by fungi since Robinson (1962) has reported that the fungus *Pilobus* may accumulate larvae of *D. viviparus* on the upper surface of the sporangium, which when it explodes may propel the larvae as far as 10 ft.! The fungus is very common in cattle faeces; surveys in Britain having shown it to be present in 95 per cent of samples examined.

The developmental cycle in the bovine is essentially the same as that of *D. filaria* of sheep. Thus infective larvae exsheath in the small intestine, penetrate the bowel wall and are carried to the local mesenteric lymph nodes. Here they moult to fourth-stage larvae and then continue their migration to the lungs via the thoracic duct and right heart. Jarrett & Sharp (1963) were unable to recover larvae from the lungs earlier than the seventh day of infection and under 'normal circumstances' fourth- stage larvae did not appear in the lungs until the thirteenth to fifteenth day of infection. Fifth-stage larvae are produced in the lungs by the fifteenth day and sexual maturity is reached on the twenty-second day of infection.

In massive infections (240,000 larvae) third-stage larvae may be found in the lungs as early as 24 hours after infection (Poynter *et al.,* 1960), however it would appear that this is a feature of massive infections only, either in the bovine or the guinea-pig, which may also serve as a host for the parasite.

The longevity of the parasite in the lungs may be prolonged in the case of a few worms; however, the majority of the burden is expelled within 50–70 days of infection. A further factor of importance, particulary from the point of view of the persistence of infection in a herd is the persistence of the parasite in an inhibited form in the lungs for several months.

Pathogenesis. Extensive accounts of the pathology and pathogenesis of bovine parasitic bronchitis have been published by Jarrett *et al.* (1957, 1960a) which should be consulted in their entirety for full appreciation. A summary of the major points of the pathogenesis is given by Soulsby (1965) which are further summarised below. The major pathogenic phases are the prepatent phase in the lungs, the patent phase and the post-patent phase. The prepatent phase is associated with blockage of many respiratory bronchioles with an eosinophilic exudate and collapse of alveoli. This, clinically, is associated with the onset of tachypnoea and coughing. Emphysema may develop. The patent phase is associated with adult parasites in the bronchi and trachea. There is severe damage to the epithelium of these organs, marked exudation into the bronchi and blockage of air passages. In addition, aspiration of eggs and larvae into the bronchioles and alveoli occurs leading to consolidation of lobules. Lesions which become obvious in the late prepatent stage of the infection, namely epithelialisation of the alveolar epithelium and 'hyaline membrane' formation remain and may become more marked.

By 50 days, if the animals survive, the post-patent phase commences, this being a process of recovery. Clinically the respiratory rate decreases, coughing is less frequent and weight gain is resumed. Severe epithelialisation may persist in some animals for some time but by 90 days worms are usually no longer present and the lesions remaining consist of peribronchial fibrosis and epithelialisation of a few alveoli surrounding some of the bronchi.

A possible complication of *D. viviparus* infection is acute pulmonary emphysema. This is possibly closely related to a similar condition known as 'fog fever'. Where it has been associated with *D. viviparus* the animals affected are often adult and it would appear that a heavy infection has been acquired by a partially immune animal. The relationship of other manifestations of acute pulmonary oedema and emphysema to *D. viviparus* infection has yet to be fully clarified.

Immunity. The immunology of *D. viviparus* infection is reviewed by Soulsby (1965). In summary, essentially an initial infection may lead to the fairly rapid acquisition of immunity, so much so that Michel (1962) found a considerable measure of immunity as early as 10 days after an initial infection.

Artificial immunisation has been markedly successful using X-irradiated infective larvae and a commercial vaccine is now available, having been developed from the work of Jarrett *et al.* (1960b). This vaccine which consists of two doses of 1000 irradiated larvae given at an interval of a month has been used in hundreds of thousands of animals in Great Britain and various countries in Europe and the U.S.A. with outstanding success.

Diagnosis. This is based on the clinical signs of bronchitis, rapid

10

breathing, coughing, etc., and the demonstration of larvae in the faeces. Usually parasitic bronchitis, Husk or Hoose, is a herd problem, seen especially in young calves and the first indication of it may be an increased incidence of coughing in animals which have recently been placed on pasture. Other pneumonic conditions may be confused with it, e.g. epizootic bronchitis or 'virus pneumonia', *Pasteurella* infection, and 'cuffing pneumonia'.

Treatment. Aerosol therapy using 'ascaridole' (oil of chenopodium plus santonin) has been used in Germany (Enigk, 1957), a good recovery being achieved in 78 per cent of 5000 treated cattle.

Cyanacethydrazide is recommended at a dose of 15 mg. per kg. subcutaneously or 17·5 mg. per kg. orally by Walley (1957). It is stated to 'stupefy' the worms which are then passed out by the ciliary action of the trachea and bronchi. Despite the acclaim for this compound various independent workers have stated it to be of little value in animals with clinical infections. In light infections it would appear to have value.

Diethylcarbamazine is effective only against the larval stages of the parasite. Given at the rate of 55 mg. per kg. daily for 5 days on the fourteenth to eighteenth day after infection it will suppress infection, but if given later it will not suppress patency of the infection or prevent death. Despite this limitation the drug can be used when the first indication of parasitic bronchitis is evident and it will be effective against a good proportion of a naturally acquired infection.

Methyridine given subcutaneously at a dose of 200 mg. per kg. shows good activity. It is also effective against gastro-intestinal nematodes which are frequently present as a concomitant infection.

Tetramisole is effective in both cattle and sheep at a dose of 15 mg. per kg. (see p. 242). It is also highly effective against intestinal worms.

Prophylaxis. Grazing management should be improved, especially to provide clean pasture for young calves. Animals continuously exposed to infection are at little risk provided the rate of acquisition of the infection is sufficient to stimulate a satisfactory immunity and not too large to cause clinical illness.

By far the most satisfactory control measure is immunisation by the X-irradiated larval vaccine mentioned previously.

D. arnfieldi (Cobbold, 1884) occurs in the bronchi of the horse, donkey and tapir and is found in most countries. Male up to 36 mm., female up to 60 mm. long. The medio- and postero-lateral rays of the male bursa are fused for about half their length. The spicules are 0·2–0·24 mm. long. The eggs measure 80–100 by 50–60 μ.

Life-cycle. Similar to that of *D. filaria*, but most eggs do not hatch before being passed in the faeces. The fourth-stage larvae are found in the lung parenchyma during their passage from the lymph-vessels to the bronchi. The worms grow adult in 39 days after infection.

Pathogenicity. As a rule this parasite is not very pathogenic, although some authors state that it is able to produce clinical signs and lesions like other species of this genus. The donkey appears to be the most natural host of this parasite and may harbour a large number of the worms

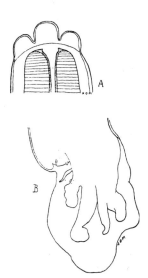

FIG. 131. *Metastrongylus apri.* A, anterior end, lateral view; B, bursa of male, lateral view (Original)

without showing appreciable signs. With regard to treatment, little is known. Symptomatic and prophylactic treatment should be applied as for other lung-worm diseases.

SUPERFAMILY: METASTRONGYLOIDEA LANE, 1917

Stoma reduced or rudimentary, frequently six lips around mouth. Usually thin bodied. Bursa more or less reduced or even absent, bursal rays fused to varying degrees. Parasites of the respiratory passages and blood vessels of the lungs. Where life-cycle is known, intermediate hosts are required. Families of importance include *Metastrongylidae, Protostrongylidae, Crenosomatidae, Filaroididae.*

FAMILY: METASTRONGYLIDAE LEIPER, 1908

Dorsal ray much reduced. Spicules long and filiform. Genus of importance: *Metastrongylus.*

Genus: Metastrongylus Molin, 1861

M. apri (Gmelin, 1790) (syn. *M. elongatus*) occurs in the bronchi and bronchioles of the pig, and wild pigs, and has also been recorded from the

sheep, deer, ox and other ruminants and accidentally in man. Its distribution is cosmopolitan. Male up to 25 mm., female up to 58 mm. long.
The worms are white and have six small lips or papillae around the oral
aperture. The male bursa is relatively small; the antero-lateral ray is
large and has a swollen tip; the medio-lateral and postero-lateral rays
are fused and the dorsal rays are much reduced. The spicules are filiform,
4–4·2 mm. long, and end in a single hook each. The posterior end of
the female is flexed ventrad. The vulva opens near the anus and the
vagina is 2 mm. long. The eggs measure 45–57 by 38–41 μ and contain
a fully developed embryo when laid.

   Life-cycle. The eggs are passed in the faeces of the host and may hatch
soon thereafter or only after they have been swallowed by the intermediate
host. The first-stage larva is 0·25–0·3 mm. long; its intestinal cells are
filled with opaque granules, the hind end is strongly curved and the tip
of the tail is bluntly rounded or swollen. The larvae may live up to 3
months in moist surroundings, but are not infective and can proceed
with their development only after they have been ingested by a suitable
species of earthworm. The following species are concerned in various
countries: *Lumbricus terrestris, L. rubellus, Diplocardia* sp., *Eisenia austriaca,
E. lönnbergi, Dendrobaena rubida, Helodrilus foetidus,* and *H. caliginosus.*
Rose (1959) studied the development and resistance of the eggs in the
soil and their development in the intermediate hosts. The larvae develop
in the blood vessels in the walls of the oesophagus and proventriculus of
the intermediate host and in blood spaces outside these organs and reach
the infective stage in about 10 days, after performing two ecdyses and
retaining the second skin as a sheath. They grow to about 0·52 mm.,
and when they are infective, they concentrate in the blood vessels of
the earthworm. The latter does not suffer from even very severe infections and the larvae can pass the winter in the earthworm. They
do not escape spontaneously from the intermediate host, but if the
earthworm is hurt or dies, the liberated larvae are able to live in moist
soil for about 2 weeks. Pigs become infected by ingesting infected earthworms or accidentally liberated infective larvae. In the pig the development is similar to that of *D. filaria* in the sheep, the larvae passing through
the mesenteric lymphatic glands, where they moult once and then reach
the lungs, where they grow adult after a further moult. The first eggs
are laid after about 24 days.

   M. pudendotectus (Wostokow, 1905) (syn. *M. brevivaginatus, Choero-
strongylus pudendotectus*) also occurs in the pig in most parts of the world.
Male 16–18 mm., female 19–37 mm. long. It differs from the preceding
species mainly in having a larger bursa, spicules only 1·2–1·4 mm. long
and provided with double hooks, and the vagina 0·5 mm. long. The
tail of the female is straight and a swelling covers the vulva and anus.
The eggs measure 57–63 by 39–42 μ.

   Life-cycle. Similar to that of *M. apri.*

M. salmi Gedoelst, 1923 occurs in the pig in the Congo, Indo-China and the United States. The spicules are 2–2·1 mm. long and the vagina of the female 1·5 mm.

Pathogenicity. In general the disease entity is similar to that caused by *D. filaria*, but the pig lungworms are not as pathogenic as those which occur in ruminants. In young pigs a marked verminous bronchitis and pneumonia may sometimes be seen, which are possibly due to secondary bacterial infection. As a rule, however, the parasites cause mainly loss of condition and retarded growth, which is rather important in pigs. The parasites may sometimes die in the small bronchioles and give rise to the formation of nodules, which must be differentiated from tuberculous nodules at autopsy or at meat inspection.

Shope (1941, 1943) found that the virus of swine influenza is carried by the larvae of pig lungworms and persists in them, when they are carried by earthworms, for 32 months. Pigs infected with such larvae acquire influenza from them, and he showed (1958) that the larvae can carry the virus of swine fever to pigs in a form which requires some form of stress to provoke this virus to pathogenicity. Mackenzie (1958) found that *M. apri* had a negligible effect on pigs experimentally infected with it, but that lesions resembling those of virus pneumonia could be produced. In a later report Mackenzie (1963) reported that the clinical signs and

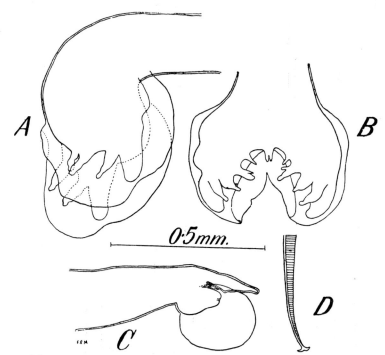

FIG. 132. *Metastrongylus pudendotectus.* A, lateral view of bursa; B, dorsal view of bursa; C, posterior end of female; D, tip of spicule. The scale refers to the figures above it. (from Baylis, after Gedoelst)

lesions of virus pneumonia (epizootic pneumonia) were enhanced by *Metastrongylus* infection.

Diagnosis is made by demonstrating the larvae in the fresh faeces.

Treatment. Comparable to that for *Dictyocaulus viviparus* (see p. 254).

Prophylaxis. Infected pigs should be kept on dry ground or in sties with concrete floors and their faeces should be disposed of in such a way that they do not spread the infection. Clean and young pigs should be run on clean fields, preferably where there are no earthworms. Infected paddocks and fields may remain infected for a considerable time, since the intermediate stage can live in the earthworm for an unknown period.

FAMILY: PROTOSTRONGYLIDAE LEIPER, 1926

Hair-like forms occurring in the alveoli, bronchioles and parenchyma of the lungs of various species of mammals. Bursa much reduced or absent. Rays of bursa reduced. Spicules marked often with membranous expansions. Gubernaculum and telamon well developed. Genera of importance include *Protostrongylus, Müllerius, Cystocaulus, Spiculocaulus, Bicaulus* etc.

Genus: Protostrongylus Kamensky, 1905

The taxonomy of this genus is discussed by Schulz *et al.* (1933) and Dougherty (1944, 1951).

P. rufescens (Leuckart, 1865) occurs in the small bronchioles of sheep, goats and deer in Europe, Africa, Australia and North America. Male 16–28 mm., female 25–35 mm. long. The worms are slender and reddish in colour. The bursa is short and strengthened dorso-laterally by a chitinous plate on either side. The ventral, lateral and externo-dorsal rays are present, but the dorsal is a very thick trunk which bears six papillae on its ventral surface. The spicules are about 0·26 mm. long, tubular, with broad, membranous expansions. A gubernaculum is present as well as a strongly developed telamon. The latter is pigmented brown in its posterior portion, where it forms two arms, each provided distally with a number of teeth. The vulva opens near the anus. The eggs are unsegmented when they are laid and measure 75–120 by 45–82 μ. Several other members of the genus may occur in sheep and goats and these include *Protostrongylus hobmaieri* (Schulz, Orlov & Kutass, 1933); *P. davtiani* (Sawina, 1940); *P. brevispiculum* Mikacic, 1939; *P. stilesi* Dikmans, 1931. These forms are possibly cosmopolitan in distribution, but a detailed survey of their incidence has yet to be made in many countries.

Life-cycle. The eggs develop in the lungs of the host and the first-stage larva which is passed in the faeces is 0·25–0·32 mm. long. The tip of its tail has a wavy outline, but is devoid of a dorsal spine (cf. *Muellerius*). For its further development the larva requires an intermediate host, which may be one of several species of snail of the genera *Helicella*, *Theba*, *Abida*, *Zebrina*, *Arianta* etc. First-stage larvae penetrate the foot of the snail. The development to the infective stage requires 12–14 days and two ecdyses are performed. The final host becomes infected by swallowing the snail with its food and the larvae pass to the lungs of the host via the mesenteric lymphatic glands, in which the third ecdysis takes place.

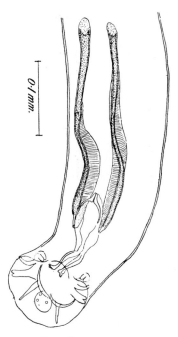

0·1 mm.

FIG. 133. *Cystocaulus ?Nigrescens*, Posterior End of Male, Ventral View (after Baylis)

Pathogenesis. The worms live in the small bronchioles, where they produce an irritation and local areas of inflammation develop. The resulting exudate fills those alveoli which are situated distally to the seat of the parasites, and the inflammatory process spreads to the peribronchial tissues. The affected alveolar and bronchial epithelium is desquamated, blood-vessels are occluded and an infiltration with round cells and proliferation of connective tissue takes place in the area. The result is a small focus of lobular pneumonia, roughly conical in shape and yellowish-grey in colour. The pleura at the base of the focus may be involved in a fibrinous pleuritis. The number of such foci in the lungs depends on the number of parasites present. As a rule the animals show no definite clinical signs, although severe infections would undoubtedly affect the general health, and the weakened lungs are susceptible to bacterial invasion which may produce acute pneumonia.

Diagnosis can be made by finding the larvae in the faeces.

Treatment. Emetine hydrochloride has been used extensively for the Protostrongylidae in the U.S.S.R. A dose of a 1 per cent solution at the rate of 8–9 mg. per kg. divided into three doses has been reported to have 97–98 per cent efficacy on *Muellerius capillaris* (Shumakovich, 1948). Comparable results for *M. capillaris* and *P. rufescens* have been obtained with emetine hydrochloride by Durbin (1954).

Cyanacethydrazide has been reported to have good effect against *P. rufescens* (Walley, 1957), and Kassai (1958) found diethylcarbamazine phosphate active against *Protostrongylus* spp.

Prophylaxis. Where the extermination of the snail intermediate host is possible this should be carried out. Special attention must be paid to the lambs; they should not be run on pastures previously used for infected animals. Pastures may remain infected for a considerable period, as the worm larvae are protected in the snails. The snails creep up plants in the early morning and evening and in rainy weather and the animals should therefore not be allowed to graze at such times, particularly in the autumn, when the infection most frequently occurs.

Genus: Cystocaulus Schulz, Orloff & Kutass, 1933

C. nigrescens (Jerke, 1911). This species occurs in the lung parenchyma and in sub-pleural nodules of sheep and goats. It is common in sheep in Eastern Europe and the U.S.S.R., it has been reported from Great Britain, the Middle East and probably occurs elsewhere in sheep raising areas of the world. Both sexes are threadlike, the male 8–9 cm. and the female 13–16 cm. The spicules measure 275–379 μ and the gubernaculum is 120–174 μ in length and the crura are dark brown in colour.

The developmental cycle includes land snails of the genera *Helix*, *Helicella*, *Theba*, *Cepaea* and *Monacha*.

The pathogenic effects of *C. nigrescens* infection are similar to those of the *Prostostrongylus* spp.

No effective treatment is known.

Genus: Muellerius Cameron, 1927

M. capillaris (Muller, 1889) occurs in the lungs of sheep, goats and chamois in Europe, Australia, South Africa, and the United States. It is probably the commonest lungworm of sheep in Europe. Male 12–14 mm., female 19–23 mm. long. The posterior end of the male is spirally coiled and there is no bursa, but a number of papillae surround the cloacal opening. The spicules are 0·15 mm. long; they are curved and each consists of a proximal half which is alate and two distal serrated arms ending in sharp points. The vulva opens close to the anus and has a small cuticular swelling on its posterior border. The eggs measure about 100 by 20 μ and are unsegmented when laid.

Life-cycle. The eggs develop in the lungs of the host and the first-stage larvae are passed in the faeces. They are 0·23–0·3 mm. long. The oeso-phagus has two swellings, one near the middle and the other at the distal extremity. The tail of the larva has an undulating tip and a dorsal spine (cf. *Protostrongylus*). These larvae can resist a fair amount of drying, are most active at relatively low temperatures (17°–27°C) and are not killed by freezing. For further development they require a snail inter-mediate host, into which they penetrate through the foot or by which they are swallowed. A large number of species are known to be suitable inter-mediate hosts; for instance, species of the nude slugs *Limax*, *Agriolimax* and *Arion*, and the snails *Helix* and *Succinea*. The development in the snail and in the sheep is very similar to that of *Protostrongylus*. The in-fective larvae can live in the snail probably for as long as the snail lives, and for up to a week after the death of the snail.

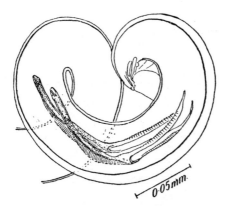

FIG. 134. *Muellerius capillaris*, Posterior End of Male, Lateral View (after Baylis)

Pathogenesis. This parasite is usually not found in lambs under 6 months of age. The adult worms live in the alveoli and the pulmonary paren-chyma, especially in the sub-pleural tissue. The worms produce greyish nodules up to 2 cm. in diameter. These consist of necrotic masses, result-ing from the degeneration of accumulated leucocytes and pulmonary tissues, and they are surrounded by a wall of connective tissue and a few giant cells. These nodules may calcify. Smaller separate foci are formed by the eggs which are surrounded by leucocytes and epithelioid cells, while the adjoining pulmonary tissue is hyperaemic and the alveoli become filled with round cells. After the egg has hatched the reaction subsides and the lesion may heal. An adenoma-like proliferation of the bronchial epithelium is seen in some cases.

The infected animal as a rule shows no clinical signs, but heavy in-fections weaken the lungs and assist in reducing the general health and resistance of the host. Secondary bacterial infection of the nodules is not uncommon and at times these may colaesce to form localised septic lesions.

Diagnosis can be made by finding the larvae in the fresh faeces.

Prophylaxis. As in the case of *Protostrongylus.* The nude slugs can be more easily controlled than shelled snails, and spreading of lime has been recommended for this purpose.

Treatment. The only satisfactory treatment appears to be emetine hydrochloride at the rate of 8–9 mg. per kg. (in a 1 per cent solution) given subcutaneously or intramuscularly.

Genus: Bicaulus Schulz & Boev, 1940

Dougherty considers the genus synonymous with *Varestrongylus* Bhalerao, 1932.

B. schulzi (Boev & Wolf, 1938) (syn. *Varestrongylus sinicus,* Dikmans, 1945, *V. schulzi* Dougherty & Goble, 1946). Thread-like forms in the lung parenchyma of sheep and goats. Male 12–15 mm., female 22–25 mm. Spicules 333–378 μ; gubernaculum 190–210 μ. Developmental cycle similar to *Protostrongylus* spp.

B. sagittatus (Müller, 1891). In *Cervus elaphus* in Europe.

Genus: Neostrongylus Gebauer, 1932

N. linearis (Marotel, 1913). A small worm, male 5–8 mm., female 13–15 mm. Spicules unequal in size, one 320–360 μ, the other 160–180 μ. In sheep and goats in Central Europe and Middle East.

Genus: Elaphostrongylus Cameron, 1931

Protostrongylidae occurring in deer. Several species have previously been included in this genus and other genera, e.g. *Pneumostrongylus* and *Parelaphostrongylus* have been regarded by some authors as congeneric with *Elaphostrongylus.* Members of these various genera occur in the lungs and blood vessels of the central nervous system of deer and at times are associated with neurological disorders. The present consideration of the various genera is based on the conclusions of Skrjabin *et al.* (1952) who restrict the species in the genus *Elaphostrongylus* to two forms *E. cervi* and *E. panticola.*

E. cervi Cameron, 1931 has been recorded from the muscles of the red deer in Scotland. As far as is known this species does not enter the central nervous system.

E. panticola Labimow, 1945 occurs in the brain of *Cervus elaphus* and *Cervus nippon* in the U.S.S.R. It may be responsible for ataxia and paresis in these animals. A further species *E. rangiferi* occurs in reindeer in Sweden and may cause similar neurological disorders as *E. panticola* (see reviews by Anderson, 1963, 1964).

Genus: Parelaphostrongylus Boev & Schulz, 1950

Similar to *Elaphostrongylus*, but differs in that the gubernaculum consists of a paired corpus and a paired crura, instead of being simple and single. In addition the genus possesses two dorsal rays instead of one. *P. odocoilei* (A. & M. Hobmaier, 1934) Boev & Schulz, 1950 is the sole species of this genus. It is synonymous with *Elaphostrongylus odocoilei* A. & M. Hobmaier, 1934, and occurs in the blood vessels of the spinal cord, in the muscles adjacent to the abdominal cavity and the vessels of the upper part of the hind legs of the black tailed deer (*Odocoileus columbianus*) in California. The developmental cycle includes land snails of the genera *Helix*, *Agriolimax* and *Epigramophora*.

Genus: Odocoileostrongylus Schulz, 1951

O. tenuis (Dougherty, 1945) Schulz, 1951. It is the sole species in this genus. It is filiform with an undivided bursa in the male, the dorsal ray is large and the spicules are massive and short. It measures 48–65 mm. in length. The parasite occurs in deer, being found in the small bronchi and in the blood vessels of the central nervous system. It has been described from a paralysed sheep under the name *Neurofilaria cornellensis*, but this name was discarded when it was realised that the parasite was a metastrongyle and not a filarid. It has also been referred to as *Pneumostrongylus tenuis* Dougherty, 1945.

O. tenuis is a common parasite of the white-tailed deer (*Odocoileus virginianus borealis*) in North America. Mature parasites occur in the central nervous system and eggs are carried by the blood stream to the lungs where they form small emboli. Larvae hatch from such eggs, enter the alveoli and pass out in the faeces. Snails of the genera *Discus*, *Zonitoides*, *Deroceras*, *Stenotrema* and *Limnaea* serve as intermediate hosts (Anderson, 1963). Infection of fawns with infected snails results in fourth and fifth-stage larvae in the brain and spinal cord 25 days after infection; by 50 days immature adults are found in the duramater of the spinal cord and cerebral hemispheres and patency of the infection occurs about 90 days after infection.

Pathogenesis. In the white-tailed deer the parasite appears to cause relatively little clinical effect however the parasite has been incriminated as the cause of moose disease in Canada. This is a neurological disorder of moose (*Alces alces americana*) and usually occurs only where moose and white-tailed deer share the same range. Moose disease is thus a cerebrospinal-nematodiasis (see also *Setaria digitata*) with deer as the normal, reservoir host (see Anderson, 1963, 1964).

FAMILY: FILAROIDIDAE SCHULZ, 1951

Metastrongyloidea with a small or rudimentary bursa, bursa sometimes absent. Lateral and ventral rays short or digitiform. Parasites of the respiratory system of mammals. Genera of importance: *Filaroides, Aelurostrongylus, Angiostrongylus.*

Genus: Filaroides v. Beneden, 1858 (syn. Oslerus)

F. osleri (Cobbold, 1879) occurs in nodules in the trachea and bronchi and rarely in the lungs of the dog. The worm is not frequently seen, although it has been found in America, England, India, South Africa and New Zealand. Male 5 mm. long and slender, female 9–15 mm. long and stouter. The hind end of the male is rounded and bears a few papillae. The spicules are short and slightly unequal. The vulva is close to the anus and the worms lay eggs with thin shells, containing larvae and measuring about 80 by 50 μ. The larva has a short S-shaped tail.

Life-cycle—unknown but probably entails development in a snail.

Pathogenesis. The worms live in or under the mucosa of the trachea or bronchi and cause the development of small tumours. These are greyish-white or pink in colour, usually less than 1 cm. in diameter, polypoid or sessile and of the nature of a granuloma, with cavities in which the worms are lodged. In severe infections many haemorrhagic wart-like lesions may cover the area of the bifurcation of the trachea. The clinical signs depend on the severity of the infection and the size and number of the tumours. Young dogs are chiefly affected and the disease is chronic but occasionally may be fatal. The most marked clinical sign is a rasping persistent cough. Loss of appetite and emaciation may be noted.

Diagnosis can be made by bronchoscopy or by finding the eggs in the sputum. Larvae may be found in the faeces, however they are neither plentiful nor highly active and must be looked for very carefully.

Treatment. Malherbe (1954) obtained good results with 5 ml. of either lithium or antimony thiomalate or Stibophen given to dogs for 9–22 weeks, which was not toxic, and also with a combination of either of these with diethylcarbamazine given daily for 7 days, the latter being not effective by itself. Dorrington (1959) found that Dictycide relieved the cough and restored dogs to show condition, though it did not apparently eradicate the worms. Le Roux (1959) also recorded successful results with Dictycide.

Prophylaxis. Until the life-history is known, reliance must be placed on general hygienic measures.

Other species of the genus include *Filaroides milski* (dogs in U.S.A.: in lung parenchyma), *Filaroides bronchialis* (mink and polecats) and *Filaroides* (*Anafilaroides*) *rostratus* (cats in Ceylon). *F. milski* and *F. rostratus* use terrestrial gastropods such as *Helix, Succinea, Zonitoides* and *Agriolimax* spp. as intermediate hosts, the infective stage being reached in these in 16–18 days.

Genus: Aelurostrongylus Cameron, 1927

A. abstrusus (Railliet, 1898) occurs in the lungs of the cat in Europe and the United States. The male measures up to 7·5 mm. and the female is 9·86 mm. long. The male bursa is short and the lobes are not distinct. All the bursal rays can be distinguished; the dorsal forms two stout branches. The spicules are simple and 0·13–0·15 mm. long. The vulva opens near the posterior extremity and the eggs measure about 80 by 70 μ.

Life-cycle. The adult worms live in the terminal respiratory bronchioles and alveolar ducts. Eggs are forced into the alveolar ducts and into the adjacent alveoli, forming small nodules. Eggs on the periphery of the lesion hatch first and larvae escape into the air passages, which they ascend, and they are passed out in the faeces of the host. They are about 0·36 mm. long and the tail has an undulating appendage of variable shape and usually a dorsal projection. The larvae live only about two weeks in the free state. For further development they require snails and slugs—mainly *Epiphragmophora* spp. and also *Agriolimax agrestis, A. columbianus, Helix asperus, Helminthoglypta californiensis, H. nickliniana, H. arrosa*—as intermediate hosts in which two ecdyses occur.

Various auxiliary or transport hosts, such as rodents, frogs, lizards and birds, which eat infected snails and in which the worm larvae encyst, may aid in infecting cats. The larvae penetrate the mucosa of the oesophagus, stomach or intestine of the cat. They are transported via the blood and finally reach the lungs, where they grow adult in about 6 weeks.

Pathogenesis. The typical lesions are sub-pleural nodules which are firm, raised and greyish in colour. These vary in diameter from 1 to 10 mm. and they may become confluent forming larger lesions. In heavy infections, which tend to be fatal, there may be creamy yellow areas on the lungs and the pleural cavity may be filled with a thick milky fluid rich in eggs and larvae. Incision of the lungs produces a milky exudate in acute cases but in the chronic infection calcification is common (Hamilton, 1963).

Clinical signs consist of a chronic cough with gradual wasting. Hamilton (1963) reports prolonged respiratory trouble with coughing, sneezing and a nasal discharge.

In heavy infections the animal may cough and suffer from diarrhoea and emaciation, which may be followed by death, or recovery may take place. In very severe infections the simultaneous deposition of a large number of eggs in the lungs may cause sudden death.

Diagnosis can be made by finding the larvae in the faeces.

Treatment. Symptomatic treatment can be given. Sudduth (1955) obtained prompt clinical improvement and absence of larvae from the faeces 5 months after administration of three intravenous doses of a 20 per cent solution of sodium iodide or diethylcarbamazine at intervals of 5 days.

Prophylaxis is in most cases impracticable, since it would imply preventing cats from catching mice, lizards etc.

Genus: Bronchostrongylus Cameron, 1931

B. subcrenatus (Railliet & Henry, 1913). This species, formerly known only from the leopard and tiger, was found in a domestic cat in Nyasaland by Fitzsimmons (1961), who described it and gave the literature about it. The adult worm superificially resembles *Aelurostrongylus abstrusus* and Fitzsimmons gives the differential features by which these two species may be distinguished. Its molluscan intermediate hosts are species of the genera *Helicella, Chondrula, Monacla, Retinella* and *Limax* and mice may act as transport hosts of the infective larvae. The mice eat the molluscs and may carry viable infective larvae in cysts on the surface of their lungs for at least 120 days. Cats infect themselves by eating the mice.

Genus: Angiostrongylus Kamensky, 1905

A. vasorum (Baillet, 1866) (syn. *Haemostrongylus vasorum*) occurs in the pulmonary artery and rarely in the right ventricle of the dog and fox. Male 14–18 mm., female 18–25 mm. long and relatively stout. The bursa is small, but all the rays can be distinguished; the ventrals are fused for most of their length and the dorsal ray is stout with short terminal branches. The vulva is situated in the posterior half of the body. The eggs measure 70–80 by 40–50 μ and are unsegmented when laid.

Life-cycle. The eggs are arrested in the lung capillaries, where they develop and hatch. The larvae escape into the air passages and are passed in the faeces of the host. They are 0·36 mm. long and have a pointed tail with a small, wavy appendage. The rest of the life-cycle is unknown, but it is likely a snail serves as an intermediate host. Guilhon (1960) has created infection in dogs with this species by feeding snails of the genus *Arion* taken from an area of endemic infection.

Pathogenesis. The parasites and their eggs cause obliteration of the small pulmonary arterial branches through irritation of the vascular walls. This later leads to perivascular sclerosis and pulmonary emphysema. Nodules of various sizes, consisting of partly organised thrombi, may be present in the lungs. Hypertrophy of the heart and congestion of the liver with consequent ascites follow on the lung disturbances. Affected animals suffer from dyspnoea and may die of cardiac insufficiency.

Diagnosis. The worms are usually found at autopsy, but in cases of dyspnoea a diagnosis might be made by finding the larvae in the sputum or fresh faeces. The larva is about 330 μ in length, it has a small cephalic button, the tail is pointed and possesses an undulation with a dorsal appendage.

Treatment. No treatment is known.

Prophylaxis. Since the life-cycle is unknown, nothing beyond hygienic measures can be recommended, except that snail control would be a wise policy.

A. cantonensis (Chen, 1935) Dougherty, 1946. This is the rat lung-worm. It is a relatively common parasite of the lungs of rats in Australia, various Pacific Islands, Malaya, Taiwan etc. Its importance lies in the fact that in the human it may be the cause of eosinophilic meningitis, which may be serious and also, at times, fatal.

The parasite is filiform, 17–25 mm. in length and in the rat development occurs in the brain and later in the lungs.

Eosinophilic meningitis due to this parasite was reported by Rosen *et al.* (1962), who found a number of young adults of *A. cantonensis* in the brain and meninges of a patient who died in a mental hospital in Hawaii. Since then it has become clear that *A. cantonensis* is an important zoonosis in the Pacific area.

The life-cycle of *A. cantonensis* involves land snails such as *Agriolimax laevis*, *Limax arborum*, *L. maximus*, *Derocercas reticulatum* etc. Human infection may arise from the consumption of improperly cooked vegetables contaminated with these snails. In more detailed studies in Tahiti, Alicata & Brown (1962) suggested that the eating of raw fresh-water prawns (*Macrobrachium* spp.) taioro etc., may be a major source of human infection.

Genus: Gurltia Wolffhügel, 1933

G. paralysans Wolffhügel, 1933 occurs in thigh veins of *Felidae* in South America. Male 12 mm., female 20–23 mm. May cause lameness of the posterior extremity.

Genus: Vogeloides Orlov, Davtian, Lubimov, 1933

V. massinoi (Davtian, 1933) Dougherty, 1952 occurs in cats in U.S.S.R. and U.S.A.

Genus: Pneumospirura Wu & Hu, 1938

P. capsulata Gerichter, 1948 occurs in *Meles meles*.

Genus: Metathelazia Skinker, 1931

Several species occur, including *M. californica* Skinker, 1931, from various *Felidae*, *M. felis* (Vogel, 1928), from *Felis pardalis* and *M. multipapillata* Gerichter, 1948, from *Erinaceus europaeus*.

Genus: Skrjabingylus Petrov, 1927

S. nasicola (Leuckart, 1842). This species occurs in the nasal sinuses of mink, polecat, and fox and may cause decalcification and atrophy of the walls of these cavities. The parasite is 7–10 mm. in the male and 18–22 mm. in the female. The spicules are similar being 220–230 μ in length and the gubernaculum is marked.

FAMILY: CRENOSOMATIDAE SCHULZ, 1951

Fairly short worms, cuticle at the anterior end thrown into ring formation. Bursa well developed. Parasites of lungs are carnivors and insectivors. Genus of importance: *Crenosoma*.

Genus: Crenosoma Molin, 1861

C. vulpis (Dujardin, 1845) occurs in the bronchi and sometimes also the trachea of the fox. Male 3·5–8 mm., female 12–15 mm. long. The cuticle of the anterior end of both sexes has eighteen to twenty-six overlapping circular folds, which bear small spines. The ventral rays are partly fused and also the medio- and postero-laterals; the externo-dorsals arise separately; the dorsal is stout and bears two small processes distally. The spicules are about 0·37 mm. long and each has a slender dorsal spur in the posterior third. A gubernaculum is present. The vulva is situated near the middle of the body. The worms are viviparous and produce larvae which are 0·265–0·33 mm. long. The oesophagus of the larva is 0·105–0·113 mm. long and the tail 0·035–0·036 mm. There is a fairly transparent vestibulum, and the intestine consists of fourteen to sixteen cells.

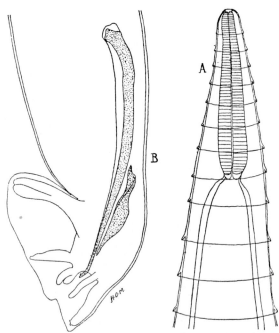

FIG. 135. *Crenosoma vulpis*: A, anterior end, dorsal view; B, hind end of male, lateral view (Original)

Life-cycle. Wetzel (1940) found that the larvae penetrate into the foot of land snails or slugs (*Helix pomatia, Cepea hortensis, C. nemoralis, Arianta arbustorum, Agriolimax agrestis, Arion hortensis, A. circumscriptus*) in which they reach the infective stage in 16–17 days. When such snails are eaten by the final host the larvae pass via the lymphatic glands to the blood and lungs, where they grow adult in 21 days.

Pathogenicity. A similar disease entity is produced to that seen with *Capillaria aerophila*, consisting of a rhino-tracheitis, bronchitis and a nasal discharge. In heavy infections a broncho-pneumonia may be a complication.

Diagnosis. The disease should be suspected on silver fox farms when the prevalence of chronic tracheo-bronchitis is substantial. Larvae may be found in the faeces or nasal discharge and the condition should be differentiated from that caused by *Capillaria aerophila*, though the two frequently occur together.

Treatment. Fouadin and anthiomaline have been reported to give satisfactory results.

Prophylaxis. The runs of foxes should be kept dry and free of grass in order to produce conditions which are unsuitable for the intermediate host. Molluscicides may be applied to soil, or animals may be kept on wire floors to avoid contact with the earth.

SUBCLASS: PHASMIDIA Chitwood & Chitwood, 1933

ORDER: SPIRURIDA CHITWOOD, 1933

Oseophagus essentially divided into two regions, an anterior muscular and a posterior glandular region; ventro-lateral cephalic papillae absent. Parasites of vertebrates, development of larval stages in arthropods. Suborders of importance: Spirurata, Filariata, Camallanata.

SUBORDER: SPIRURATA RAILLIET, 1913

Oesophageal glands multinucleate. Well developed labial structures. Frequently parasites of the digestive tract. Ovovipiparous. Super-families of importance: Spiruroidea, Physalopteroidea.

SUPERFAMILY: SPIRUROIDEA RAILLIET & HENRY, 1915

Nematodes with two lateral lips which may be further subdivided. A pharynx or cylindrical buccal capsule is usually present. The oeso-phagus consists of a short, anterior, muscular portion followed by a longer, wide, glandular portion. The hind end of the male is usually spirally coiled and bears lateral alae and papillae. The spicules are, as a rule, unequal and dissimilar. The vulva opens near the middle of the body in most cases, but its position is variable. The eggs are usually thick-shelled and contain larvae when laid. The adults are parasites of vertebrates, frequently living in the lumen or the wall of the stomach. The life-cycle as a rule includes an intermediate host which is an arthro-pod. Families of importance: *Spiruridae*, *Thelaziidae*, *Tetrameridae*, *Acuariidae*.

FAMILY: SPIRURIDAE OERLEY, 1885

With the typical characteristics of the sub order. Genera of importance: *Habronema* and *Hartertia*.

Genus: Habronema Diesing, 1861

H. muscae Carter, 1861 occurs in the stomach of equines. Male 8–14 mm., female 13–22 mm. long. There are two lateral lips, each being trilobed. The pharynx is cylindrical and provided with a thick cuticular lining. The male has wide caudal alae, four pairs of precloacal papillae and one or two papillae behind the cloaca. The cloacal region of the body is covered with small cuticular bosses or ridges. The left spicule is slender and 2·5 mm. long, the right stouter and only 0·5 mm. long. The vulva is situated near the middle of the body and opens dorso-laterally, the vagina running for some distance in the body wall. The eggs have thin shells and measure 40–50 by 10–12 μ.

H. microstoma (Schneider, 1866), also a parasite in the stomach of equines, closely resembles the preceding species. It is larger, the male being 16–22 mm. long and the female 15–25 mm. The pharynx contains a dorsal and a ventral tooth in its anterior part. The male has four pairs of precloacal papillae. The left spicule measures 0·76–0·8 mm. and the right 0·35–0·38 mm. The eggs measure 45–49 by 16 μ and hatch in the uterus of the female.

H. megastoma (Rudolphi, 1819) occurs in tumours of the stomach wall, rarely free in the stomach of equines. Male 7–10 mm., female 10–13 mm. long. It can easily be recognised by its 'head', which is constricted off from the body. The pharynx is funnel-shaped. The male has four pairs of precloacal papillae. The left spicule is 0·46 mm. long and the right 0·24 mm. The worms are viviparous.

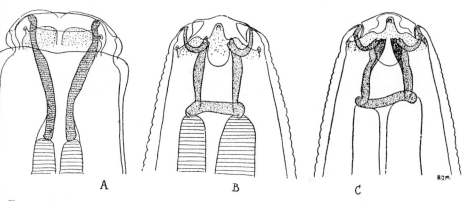

A   B   C

FIG. 136. *Habronema* Species of Equines, Heads in Lateral View: A, *H. megastoma*; B, *H. muscae*; C, *H. microstoma* (Original)

Life-cycle. The larvae are passed in the faeces of the host and are ingested by the maggots of flies which develop in the manure. *H. muscae* and *H. megastoma* develop in the house fly, *Musca domestica*, while *H. microstoma* develops in the stable fly, *Stomoxys calcitrans*. The worms reach the infective stage in the maggot at about the time when the latter pupates. In the adult fly the larvae occur free in the haemocoele and pass forward into the proboscis. Larvae are deposited on the lips, nostrils and wounds of the horse when the fly feeds. In the case of *H. microstoma* in *S. calcitrans* the infective larvae interfere with the ability of the fly to penetrate the skin with the proboscis and it reverts to an imbibing method of feeding, obtaining nourishment from moist surfaces such as the lips, nostrils and wounds of horses. It is also possible that equines may become infected by swallowing flies that fall into food or water. The larvae are liberated in the stomach, where they grow to maturity.

Pathogenesis. *H. megastoma* produces large tumours of the stomach wall which have one or more openings and a number of cavities in which the worms are located. These tumours may interfere mechanically with the function of the stomach, but are otherwise not particularly harmful. The other two species occur free in the stomach and may penetrate into the mucosa. They produce an irritation which leads to a chronic catarrhal gastritis with the formation of much mucus. *H. microstoma* may produce ulcers of the stomach.

Cutaneous habronemiasis, also known as 'summer sores', 'bursati', 'granular dermatitis' etc., is caused by *Habronema* larvae which are deposited in existing wounds by infected flies. The condition is seen in Australia, Africa, the East, North America and the U.S.S.R.

All three species of *Habronema* may be concerned in the condition: generally larvae are deposited by flies on wounds, however larvae may also penetrate the apparently intact skin (Nishiyama, 1958).

Habronema spp. larvae may also be associated with a granular conjunctivitis, this being seen in areas where cutaneous habronemiasis is prevalent. The lesion is seen on the inner canthus of the eye and is in the form of a wart-like lesion. Rarely the whole conjunctiva is a mass of granulation tissue.

Habronema spp. may also be found in the lungs, being associated with fibrotic nodules 0·5–2·0 cm. in diameter which develop around the finer bronchioles, being essentially a nodular peribronchitis.

Clinical signs. Gastric habronemiasis is not known to cause marked clinical signs, but it is probably the cause of some cases of chronic gastritis. If the tumours of *H. megastoma* occur near the pylorus they may interfere with the closing of the sphincter and cause digestive disorders.

The lesions of cutaneous habronemiasis occur mainly in warm countries and during the summer. They are seen on those parts of the body that are liable to be injured, such as the legs, withers, sometimes the sheath and the canthus of the eye. They vary in size and have an uneven surface which consists of a soft, brownish-red material and which covers a mass of firmer granulations. The wounds show a tendency to increase in size and do not respond to ordinary treatment until the following winter, when they often heal up spontaneously. In some cases chronic lesions develop in the form of granulomata which may reach a considerable size.

Diagnosis. The gastric infection is difficult to diagnose because the larvae are not readily found in the faeces. Some worms or larvae may be found by gastric lavage through a stomach tube.

Treatment. The animal should be starved overnight and in the morning 8–10 litres of a 2 per cent solution of sodium bicarbonate at body temperature are administered into the stomach by means of a stomach tube, in order to loosen the mucus in which the worms lie. The fluid should be withdrawn if possible, but usually it passes into the intestine. Carbon bisulphide is then administered through the tube at the rate of 5 ml. per 100 kg. bodyweight, followed by a small quantity of water to wash down the drug. This treatment is effective for *H. muscae* and

H. microstoma. The worms in the tumours generally cannot be reached. Neither phenothiazine nor piperazine is effective.

For cutaneous habronemiasis surgical removal may be useful especially when the lesion has become pedunculated. The operation site should be adequately covered to prevent further deposition of larvae by flies.

Various compounds have been used in treatment, these include repeated hypotonic saline, 1 per cent potassium permanganate, 3 per cent neoarsphenamine, tartar emetic etc. French workers have recommended chromic acid in a 10 per cent solution: this is applied two or three times and apart from killing the larvae, it forms a thick crust which protects the lesion from further attack. Radiotherapy has also been used in France, a course of 200–400 roentgens is applied weekly for 4 or more weeks.

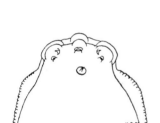
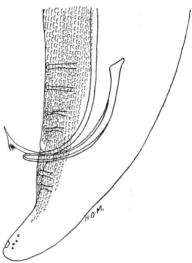

FIG. 137. *Hartertia gallinarum*, Anterior End, Lateral View (Original)

FIG. 138. *Hartertia gallinarum*, Hind End of Male, Lateral View (Original)

Prophylaxis. Habronemiasis can be controlled effectively by hygienic manure disposal, which controls flies and kills the worm larvae by the heat of the fermenting manure. Further measures should be taken against flies in stables and against the contamination of food and water by flies. The cutaneous infection can be prevented by suitable protection of all wounds.

Genus: Hartertia Seurat, 1915

H. gallinarum (Theiler, 1919) occurs in the small intestine of the fowl and wild bustards in Africa. Male 28–40 mm., female 60–110 mm. long. Macroscopically the worms closely resemble *Ascaridia galli*. They have two lateral lips, each divided medially into three lobes. The male hind end has lateral alae, ventral cuticular bosses, four pairs of pre-cloacal and two pairs of post-cloacal papillae. The anterior lip of the cloaca bears a cuticular thickening, which may resemble a papilla. The left spicule is 2·3 mm. long, acutely pointed and provided with four large barbs, while the right is 0·63 mm. long and ends bluntly. The vulva opens in the anterior third of the body. The eggs have thick shells; they measure 45–53 by 27–33 μ and contain fully developed embryos when laid.

Life-cycle. The eggs are passed in the faeces of the host and for further development have to be ingested by certain termites (*Macrohodothermes mossambicus transvaalensis*). Only the workers become infected. The larvae develop in the body cavity of the termite and reach a length of 1 cm. or more. The termites do not appear to suffer from the parasites. Fowls become infected by ingesting such termites and the worms grow to maturity in the bird in 3 weeks.

Pathogenicity. Depending on the severity of the infection, the parasites produce various degrees of emaciation, weakness, diarrhoea, decrease of egg production or death.

Diagnosis can be made by finding the eggs in the faeces, but it may not always be possible to distinguish them from eggs of other spirurids occurring in fowls. Diagnosis should therefore be confirmed by autopsy of a selected case.

Treatment. As in the case of *Ascaridia galli.*

Prophylaxis. All termites in the vicinity of the fowl runs should be destroyed.

FAMILY: THELAZIIDAE RAILLIET, 1916

Spiruroidea with no pseudolabia; mouth capsule present. Hind end of male with many pre- and post-anal papillae. Spicules unequal. Parasites of the conjunctival sac, lacrimal duct and digestive tract of birds and mammals. Genera of importance include *Thelazia, Oxyspirura, Spirocerca, Ascarops, Physocephalus, Simondsia* and *Gongylonema.*

Genus: Thelazia Bosc, 1819

T. rhodesii (Desmarest, 1828) occurs in cattle, sheep, goats and buffaloes in Europe, Asia and Africa. Milky-white worms, male 8–12 mm., female 12–18 mm. long. The cuticle bears prominent transverse striations. The male has about fourteen pairs of precloacal and three pairs of post-cloacal papillae. The spicules are 0·75–0·85 and 0·115–0·13 mm. long.

T. gulosa Railliet & Henry, 1910 occurs in cattle in France and Sumatra.

T. alfortensis Railliet & Henry, 1910 occurs in cattle in France.

T. lacrymalis (Gurlt, 1831) occurs in the horse.

T. callipaeda Railliet & Henry, 1910 occurs under the nictitating membrane of the dog in the Far East and has also been reported from the rabbit and man. Male 7–11·5 mm., female 7–17 mm. long. The cuticle has fine transverse striations. The male has five pairs and one single pre-cloacal papilla and two pairs of post-cloacals. The left spicule is about twelve times as long as the right. The vulva is situated in the oesophageal region. The eggs when laid contain fully developed larvae which, soon after laying, extend themselves as well as the shells and so become sheathed larvae.

T. californiensis Price, 1930 occurs in sheep, deer, cat and dog in the United States.

T. skrjabini Ershov, 1928 occurs in calves.

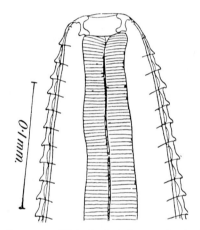 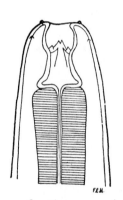

FIG. 139. *Thelazia rhodesii,* Anterior End of Female, Lateral View (after Baylis)

FIG. 140. *Oxyspirura mansoni,* Anterior End, Ventral View (from Baylis, after Yorke & Maplestone)

Life-cycle. Klesov (1950) and Krastin (1950, 1952) have shown that the intermediate hosts of *T. rhodesii* are *Musca larvipara* and *M. convexifrons*, that those of *T. gulosa* are *Musca larvipara* and *M. amica* and that that of *T. skrjabini* is possibly *M. amica*. Klesov found that the first larvae of *T. rhodesii* enter the gut of the fly from the eye secretions of the definitive host and penetrate to the ovarian follicles of the fly, where they develop, becoming second larvae 3·6–4 mm. long, which grow and moult to become third, infective larvae. The third larvae leave the ovarian follicles and migrate to the mouth parts of the fly, from which they are transferred to cattle. The infective larvae are 5·06–7·9 mm. long and their development in the fly requires 15–30 days. When infected flies were allowed access to calves, and when infective larvae were experimentally introduced into calves, adult *T. rhodesii* appeared in 20–25 days. The infective larvae of *T. gulosa* are smaller; when they were put on the conjunctiva of a calf, adult *T. gulosa* appeared 7 days later. Krastin obtained infective larvae of *T. gulosa* from *Musca amica* and placed them on the eye region of a calf; 6 weeks later he obtained one adult *T. gulosa*.

Genus: Oxyspirura v. Drasche in Stossich, 1897

O. mansoni (Cobbold, 1879) occurs under the nictitating membrane of the fowl, turkey and pea-fowl in many countries. Male 10–16 mm., female 12–19 mm. long. The cuticle is smooth and the pharynx roughly resembles an hourglass in shape. The male tail is curved ventrad and bears no alae. There are four pairs of pre-cloacal and two pairs of post-cloacal papillae. The left spicule is slender, 3–3·5 mm. long, and the right 0·2–0·22 mm. long and stout. The vulva is situated in the posterior part of the body and the eggs measure 50–65 by 45 μ.

O. parvorum Sweet, 1910 described from the fowl in Australia, is possibly identical with the preceding species.

Life-cycle. The eggs of the parasite pass down the lacrimal ducts and out in the faeces of the bird. The intermediate stages develop in the cockroach *Pycnoscelus surinamensis*, and the fowls acquire the parasite by ingesting infected cockroaches. The larvae escape from the intermediate host after it has been ingested and apparently wander up the oseophagus, pharynx and lacrimal duct to the eye, as they have been found there 20 minutes after cockroaches were fed to the chicks.

Pathogenesis. In many cases eyeworms have practically no pathogenic effect on the host, especially in the larger animals. In South Africa, *T. rhodesii* is found frequently in calves without causing any lesions. In some cases lesions of keratitis, ophthalmia etc. ascribed to these parasites are probably due to other causes, however there can be no doubt that the parasites do cause disease of the eye. Lesions may occur in one or both eyes; initially there is a mild conjunctivitis which may progress to congestion of the conjunctiva and the cornea. As the condition becomes more serious the cornea becomes cloudy, there is marked lacrimation and the affected eye becomes markedly swollen and covered with exudate and pus.

Without treatment a progressive keratitis occurs, there is ulceration of the cornea leading to protusion of the contents of the anterior chamber.

Diagnosis. A definitive diagnosis is made by the detection of the parasites in the conjunctival sac. It may be necessary to instil local anaesthetic to allow manipulation. Examination of the lacrimal secretions may reveal eggs or first-stage larvae.

Treatment. Removal of the adult parasites with fine forceps, using local anaesthesia is helpful. Halpin & Kirkly (1962) have reported that a subcutaneous dose of 20 ml. of methyridine produces rapid recovery from *Thelazia* infection. Local application of 2–3 per cent boric acid, 0·05 per cent mercuric chloride, 0·05 per cent iodine, 0·5 per cent lysol or 0·5 per cent diethylcarbamazine, have been shown effective.

Prophylaxis. In accordance with the life-cycles given above, prophylaxis should include general hygiene measures and control of the cockroaches, beetles and species of *Musca* mentioned above. In the case of poultry cockroaches should be exterminated.

Genus: Spirocerca Railliet & Henry, 1911

S. lupi (Rudolphi, 1809) (syn. *S. sanguinolenta*) occurs in the walls of the oesophagus, stomach and aorta, and more rarely free in the stomach and in other organs of the dog, fox, wolf and jackal. It is common in most warm countries. The worms are usually coiled in a spiral and have a blood-red colour. Male 30–54 mm., female 54–80 mm. long and rather stout. The lips are trilobed and the pharynx is short. The male tail bears lateral alae, four pairs and one unpaired median pre-cloacal papilla and two pairs of post-cloacal papillae, while a group of minute papillae is situated near to the tip of the tail. The left spicule is 2·45–2·8 mm. long, the right 0·475–0·75 mm. The eggs have thick shells; they measure 30–37 by 11–15 μ and contain larvae when laid.

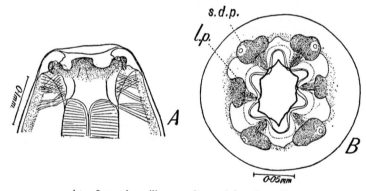

l.p. Lateral papilla   *s.d.p.* subdorsal papilla

FIG. 141. *Spirocerca lupi*, Anterior End of Female: A, lateral view; B, *en face* view (after Baylis)

Life-cycle. The eggs are passed in the faeces of the host and hatch only after they have been ingested by a suitable coprophagous beetle (*Scarabeus sacer, Akis, Atenchus, Geotrupes, Gymnopleurus, Cauthon* spp. and others). The larvae develop to the infective stage and become encysted in the beetle, chiefly on the tracheal tubes. If such beetles are swallowed by an unsuitable host, the larval worms become encysted again in the oesophagus, mesentery or other organ of this host. Such cysts have been found in numerous amphibia, reptiles, birds and small mammals. The final host may become infected by ingesting either beetles that contain infective larvae or other animals in which the encysted forms occur. On being liberated in the stomach the larvae penetrate into the stomach wall and, reaching the arteries, migrate in the walls of the gastric and gastro-epiploic arteries to the coeliac artery and thence to the aorta, reaching the upper thoracic aorta in about 3 weeks. From this siste the majority migrate to the oesophagus, traversing the connective tissue of the thoracic cavity in this area. Some may enter veins and reach other organs.

Pathogenesis. The migrating larvae produce haemorrhages, inflammatory reactions and necrosis, as well as purulent streaks or abscesses in the tissues in which they penetrate. These lesions heal rapidly after the larvae have passed on, but stenosis of the vessels may remain. The adult parasites produce nodules in the oesophagus, stomach and aorta, which contain cavities that harbour one or more of the worms. The nodules in the wall of the aorta may lead to stenosis, formation of aneurysms or rupture of the vessel, followed by fatal haemorrhage. In severe infections the nodular mass in the oesophageal wall may become large and peduncu-

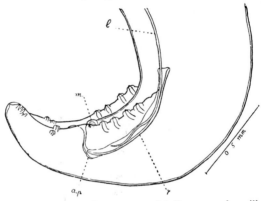

a.p. Accessory piece   m. Median preanal papilla
 l.   Left spicule   r. Right spicule

FIG. 142. *Spirocerca lupi*, Posterior End of Male, Lateral View (after Baylis)

lated and protrude into the lumen of the oesophagus. If marked this mass leads to an interference with digestion and occasionally persistent vomiting and emaciation.

A serious complication of *S. lupi* infection is that it may be an important factor in the development of a malignant tumor in the oesophagus (see Bailey, 1963). All cases of oesophageal sarcoma have so far been associated with *S. lupi* infection. The neoplasm may be extensive and may metastasise to the lungs and elsewhere. The neoplasm has been found mainly in hounds, setters and pointers, but its general incidence in other breeds has yet to be determined.

A long-standing complication is hypertrophic pulmonary osteoarthropathy of the long bones.

Other complications of *S. lupi* infection include pyaemic nephritis, derived from septic foci in the oesophageal lesions, spondylitis of the adjacent thoracic vertebrae and aplastic anaemia.

Clinical signs. The oesophageal lesions may cause interference with deglutition, respiration and circulation. Those in the stomach produce vomiting which is at times so persistent that the animal is unable to retain its food and loses condition rapidly. Sometimes worms may be passed in the vomit. In less serious cases the lesions cause difficulty in swallowing or interfere mechanically with the action of the stomach. Aortic infection is usually not observed until sudden death is caused by rupture. Where a neoplasm has developed there is general wasting and emaciation, perhaps thickening of the long bones in long standing cases, and more specific signs depending on the site of the metastises of the tumour.

Diagnosis. Infections in the alimentary canal can be diagnosed by finding the eggs in the faeces or the vomit, but eggs are not passed unless the tumour has acquired an opening into the lumen of the organ. It may be difficult to differentiate this infection from one with *Physaloptera* in the stomach. Aortic infection will only be diagnosed tentatively on account of the presence of stenosis or aneurysm. Contrast radiography is useful to demonstrate abnormalities in the thoracic region.

Treatment. McGaughey (1950) and Rao (1953) found that 10 mg. of the piperazine derivative, diethylcarbamazine (Hetrazan, Banocide, Caricide), per lb. bodyweight given daily, caused the signs to disappear in 4–10 days. However, this treatment may only cause suppression of the egg production and not elimination of the worms (Vaidyanathan, 1952). Darne & Webb (1964) found Disophenol (2,6-di-iodo-4-nitrophenol) effective in doses of 1 ml. per 10 lb. bodyweight.

Prophylaxis. Infected animals should be isolated and their vomit and faeces disposed of, so that the infection is not allowed to spread. Healthy animals should be prevented as far as possible from eating dung beetles, frogs, mice, hedgehogs, lizards etc., which may carry the encysted larvae.

S. arctica Petrow, 1927 occurs in the dog, fox and wolf (*Vulpes lagopus*) in Northern Russia.

Genus: Ascarops v. Beneden, 1873 (syn. Arduenna)

A. strongylina (Rudolphi, 1819) occurs in the stomach of the pig and wild boar in most parts of the world. Male 10–15 mm., female 16–22 mm. long. A cervical ala is present only on the left side of the body. The pharynx is 0·083–0·098 mm. long and its wall is strengthened by thickenings in the form of a triple or quadruple spiral. The right caudal ala of the male is about twice as large as the left and there are four pairs of pre-cloacal papillae and one pair of post-cloacals, all situated asymmetrically. The left spicule is 2·24–2·95 mm. long and the right 0·46–0·62 mm. The eggs measure 34–39 by 20 μ and have thick shells surrounded by a thin membrane which produces an irregular outline. They contain larvae when laid.

Life-cycle. The eggs are passed in the faeces of the host, and when they are swallowed by coprophagous beetles (species of *Aphodius*, *Onthophagus* and *Gymnopleurus*), the larvae develop in these to the infective stage. Pigs become infected by ingesting such beetles.

A. dentata (von Linstow, 1904) is a larger species than the preceding one, the male being 25 mm. and the female 55 mm. long. It occurs in pigs in Indo-China and the Malay region. The buccal capsule is provided with a pair of teeth anteriorly.

Genus: Physocephalus Diesing, 1861

P. sexalatus (Molin, 1860) occurs in the stomach of the pig and has also been recorded from some other animals; for instance, hares and rabbits. The male is 6–13 mm. and the female 13–22·5 mm. long. The

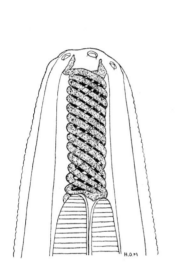

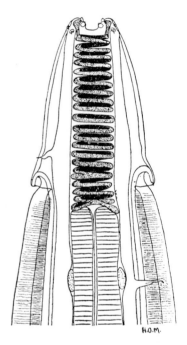

Fig. 143. *Ascarops strongylina,* Anterior End, Lateral View (Original)

Fig. 144. *Physocephalus sexalatus,* Anterior End, Dorsal View (Original)

cuticle of the anterior extremity is slightly inflated in the region of the pharynx. This inflation is followed by three cervical alae on either side. The cervical papillae are very asymmetrically situated. The mouth is small and toothless. The pharynx is 0·263–0·315 mm. long and its walls are strengthened by a single spiral thickening which breaks up into complete rings in the middle portion. The caudal alae of the male are narrow and symmetrical, and there are four pairs of pre-cloacal papillae and the same number of post-cloacal papillae. The left spicule measures 2·1–2·25 mm. and the right 0·3–0·4 mm. The eggs have thick shells, contain larvae when laid and measure 34–39 by 15–17 μ.

Life-cycle. Similar to that of *Ascarops.* A large number of beetles are known to act as intermediate hosts, including species of *Scarabeus, Phanaeus, Gymnopleurus, Geotrupes* and *Onthophagus.* As in the case of *Spirocerca* the larvae become encysted, chiefly in the walls of the alimentary canal, in unsuitable hosts which swallow infected beetles. Cram (1936) found that birds which had eaten beetles on a field used for pigs harboured numerous cysts containing these larvae, but their health was not affected. In the pig the larvae penetrate deeply into the mucosa of the stomach and grow adult in about 6 weeks.

Pathogenesis. *Ascarops* and *Physocephalus* are common stomach worms of pigs, but cause no marked disturbance unless they occur in fairly large numbers or the resistance of the animal is weakened by another factor. The worms then irritate the mucosa and produce an inflammation.

Clinical signs. Affected animals, especially young ones, show signs of a chronic or acute gastritis. They lose their appetite, but usually have a marked thirst. Growth is retarded or emaciation and even death may occur.

Post mortem. The gastric contents are small in quantity and there is much mucus. The mucosa, particularly in the fundus region, is reddened and swollen, or it may be covered with pseudo-membranes, underneath which the tissues are markedly reddened and ulcerated. The worms are found free or partly embedded in the mucosa.

Diagnosis can be made by finding the eggs of the worms in the faeces.

Treatment. Carbon disulphide at a dose of 0·1 ml. per kg. given after 36–48 hours starvation is 83–100 per cent effective. *Sodium fluoride* is effective against *A. strongylina* and *P. sexalatus* as a 1 per cent mixture in food.

Prophylaxis. Infected pigs should not be allowed to disseminate the eggs with their faeces and the latter should therefore be disposed of in a suitable way. Healthy pigs should be prevented as far as possible from ingesting dung beetles. The measures advocated for the prevention of *Ascaris* will be effective against the spirurids of pigs to a certain extent, but dung beetles may fly a fair distance.

Genus: Simondsia Cobbold, 1864

Simondsia paradoxa (Cobbold, 1864) occurs in the stomach of pigs in Europe. The worm is peculiar in that the posterior parts of the bodies of the females, which are globular in shape, are lodged in small cysts in the stomach wall, while the anterior, slender portions protrude. The gravid female is 15 mm. long and has lateral cervical alae and a large dorsal and a large ventral tooth. The eggs are oval or ellipsoidal and are 20–29 μ long. The male has a spirally-coiled tail and a cylindrical body, 12–15 mm. long, and occurs free or partly embedded in the mucosa.

Genus: Gongylonema Molin, 1857

G. pulchrum Molin, 1857 (syn. *G. scutatum*), occurs in the sheep, goat, cattle, pig, zebu, buffalo and less frequently the horse, camel, donkey and wild boar. It also occurs in man. It is found in most parts of the world. The worm inhabits the oesophagus, where it lies in zigzag fashion embedded in the mucosa or submucosa. In ruminants it may also occur in the rumen. Male up to 62 mm., female up to 145 mm. long. The cuticle of the anterior end bears a number of round or oval thickenings of various sizes. The cervical alae are well developed. The lips are small and there is a short pharynx with simple walls. The tail of the male is alate, somewhat asymmetrical, and bears a number of papillae which are also asymmetrically arranged. The left spicule is slender and 4–23 mm. long. The right is 0·084–0·18 mm. long and stout. A gubernaculum is present. The vulva opens posteriorly and the eggs measure 50–70 by 25–37 μ.

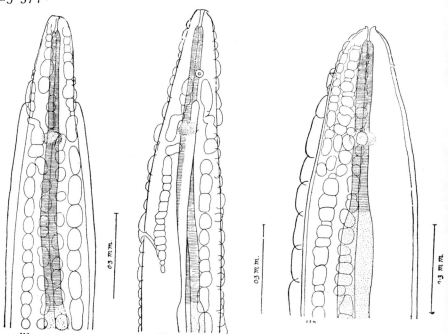

Fig. 145. A, *Gongylonema pulchrum*, Anterior End, Dorsal View; B, The Same, Lateral View; C, *Gongylonema verrucosum*, Anterior End, Dorsal View (after Baylis)

Life-cycle. The eggs of the parasite are passed in the faeces of the host and hatch after they have been swallowed by coprophagous beetles of the genera *Aphodius*, *Onthophagus*, *Blaps*, *Caccobius*, *Onthophagus* and others, in which the larvae develop to the infective stage. The small cockroach *Blatella germanica* can be infected experimentally. Infection of the final host takes place by ingestion of the infected beetles. Larvae will emerge spontaneously from cockroaches which fall into water, but it is improbable that such larvae would be important as a source of infection. The route of migration is not known in all animals but in the guinea-pig, Alicata (1935) found larvae embedded in the wall of the gastro-oesophageal region. He suggested that larvae excysted in the stomach and then migrated anteriorly to the oral cavity, finally migrating to the wall of the oesophagus.

G. verrucosum (Giles, 1892) occurs in the rumen of sheep, goat, cattle, deer and zebu in India, the United States and South Africa. The worms have a reddish colour when fresh. Male 32–41 mm., female 70–95 mm. long. This species has a festooned cervical ala as well as cuticular bosses on the left side only. The left spicule is 9·5–10·5 mm. long and the right 0·26–0·32 mm.

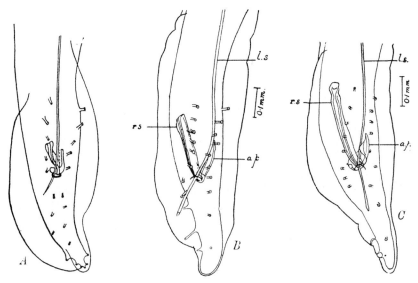

a.p. Accessory piece   *l.s.* Left spicule   *r.s.* Right spicule

FIG. 146. Posterior End of Male, Ventral View, of A, *Gongylonema pulchrum*; B, *G. mönnigi*; C, *G. verrucosum* (after Baylis)

G. mönnig Baylis, 1926 occurs in the rumen of the sheep and goat in South Africa. Male 42 mm., female 102–113 mm. long. It resembles *G. verrucosum*, but the cervical ala is not festooned. The left spicule is about 15 mm. long and the right 0·26 mm. The gubernaculum also differs from that of the preceding species.

G. ingluvicola Ransom, 1904 and **G. crami** Smit, 1927 occur in the crop of the fowl. The eggs measure about 58 by 35 μ. *Blatella germanica* may be infected with this worm.

Pathogenicity—None.

FAMILY: ACUARIIDAE SEURAT, 1913

The cuticle of the anterior part of the body is ornamented with 'cordons' —cuticular ridges or grooves—or epaulette-like thickenings. The cordons may be either recurrent, i.e. they run down the body and turn back forwards again, or non-recurrent, i.e. they do not do this; and they may or may not anastomose. For further details see Cram (1927). The lips are usually small and triangular in shape and the pharynx is cylindrical. Parasites in the walls of the gizzard, proventriculus, oesophagus or crop of birds.

Genus: Acuaria Bremser, 1811

The species of this genus are characterised by the presence of four non-recurrent cordons on the anterior end of the body, which usually do not anastomose. They are grouped in a number of subgenera which are considered as separate genera by some authors.

A. (Cheilospirura) hamulosa (Diesing, 1851) occurs in the gizzard of the fowl and turkey in most countries. Male 10–14 mm., female 16–29 mm. long. The cordons are double cuticular ridges with an irregular outline and extend far back along the body. The male has four pairs of pre-cloacal and six pairs of post-cloacal papillae. The left spicule is slender and 1·63–1·8 mm. long, the right flattened and 0·23–0·25 mm. long. The vulva is situated just behind the middle and the eggs measure 40–45 by 24–27 μ.

Life-cycle. The eggs pass out in the faeces of the host and hatch after they have been swallowed by the intermediate hosts, which are grasshoppers *Melanoplus*, various beetles and weevils. In these hosts the infective larva develops and the final host acquires the infection by ingesting such insects.

Pathogenesis. The parasites live underneath the horny lining of the gizzard, producing soft nodules in the musculature and thus weakening it.

Clinical signs. Mild infections are usually not noticed, nor does the location of the worms allow them to be seen at autopsy. Severe infections produce emaciation, droopiness, weakness and anaemia. Cases have been described in which the gizzard was weakened to such a degree that a rupture in the form of a large sac developed.

Post mortem. In mild infections the worms are noticed only if the horny lining of the gizzard is removed. They are found in soft, yellowish-red nodules which are most frequently seen in the thinner parts of the wall. In severe cases the horny lining may be partly destroyed, and the worms are found below the necrotic material in the altered musculature.

Diagnosis. Several species of *Acuaria* may occur in fowls and turkeys and their eggs are difficult to distinguish from one another. Spirurid eggs in the faeces would lead to a tentative diagnosis, which has to be confirmed at autopsy of a selected case.

Treatment. No satisfactory remedy is known, but carbon tetrachloride, tetrachloroethylene and oil of chenopodium have been recommended.

Prophylaxis is difficult in the case of birds that run free, since they cannot be prevented from eating the intermediate hosts. When the infection is troublesome the birds have to be kept confined on bare ground and the entrance of insects into the runs, as well as meal beetles and weevils into the food, must be prevented.

A. (**Dispharynx**) **spiralis** (Molin, 1858) occurs in the walls of the proventriculus and oesophagus, more rarely in the intestine, of the fowl, turkey, pigeon, guinea-fowl, pheasant and other birds in many countries. Male 7–8·3 mm., female 9–10·2 mm. long. The cordons have a sinuous course and are recurrent, but do not anastomose. The male has four pairs of pre-cloacal and five pairs of post-cloacal papillae. The left spicule is

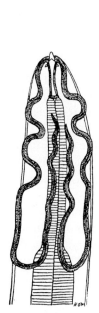
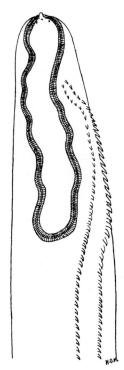

FIG. 147. *Acuaria* (*Dispharynx*) *spiralis*, Anterior End, Lateral View (Original)

FIG. 148. *Acuaria* (*Echinuria*) *uncinata*, Anterior End, Lateral View (Original)

slender and 0·4–0·52 mm. long, the right 0·15–0·2 mm. long and boat-shaped. The vulva is situated in the posterior part of the body. The eggs measure 33–40 by 18–25 μ; they have thick shells and contain larvae when laid.

Life-cycle. The eggs hatch after having been swallowed by the inter-mediate host, which is an isopod (*Porcellio laevis, P. scaber* and *Armadillidum vulgare*). The larvae develop in the body cavity of the isopod, and when the latter is eaten by a suitable bird the parasite grows to maturity in it.

Pathogenesis. The effects of the parasites vary with the severity of the infection. If few are present they apparently do not penetrate into the mucosa, which may then show inflammation and thickening only; but in severe infections deep ulcers, in which the anterior extremities of the

II

worms are embedded, may be seen in the proventriculus. There is an extensive destruction of the glands of this organ and a marked cellular infiltration of the underlying tissues. The affected birds, particularly young ones, rapidly lose weight in spite of a voracious appetite and become very weak and anaemic. This parasite may cause severe losses.

Diagnosis. As in the case of *A. hamulosa.*

Treatment. No satisfactory remedy is known. Tetrachloroethylene or carbon tetrachloride may be useful.

Prophylaxis. Where this parasite is troublesome the birds should be confined on bare ground and measures taken to combat the intermediate hosts.

A. (Echinuria) uncinata (Rudolphi, 1819) occurs in the oesophagus, proventriculus, gizzard and small intestine of the duck, goose, swan and wild aquatic birds. Male 8–10 mm., female 12–18·5 mm. long. The cordons are non-recurrent and they anastomose in pairs. The cuticle bears also four longitudinal rows of spines. The left spicule is 0·706 mm. long and the right 0·208 mm. There are four pairs of pre-cloacal and four pairs of post-cloacal papillae; the pre-cloacal papillae stand in two groups of two on either side. The vulva is situated near the posterior extremity and the eggs measure 37 by 20 μ.

Life-cycle. The eggs are passed in the faeces of the bird and are swallowed by water fleas (*Daphnia pulex*), in which they hatch and the infective larvae develop. When suitable aquatic birds ingest the infected intermediate hosts the parasites develop to maturity.

Pathogenesis. The worms penetrate into the wall of the alimentary canal, causing a marked inflammation and the formation of nodules which have a caseous content. In the proventriculus and the gizzard the nodules may become so large that they cause mechanical interference and even obstruction to the passage of food. The birds become dull, the feathers are ruffled and feeding may stop completely. Sudden death is known to occur.

Diagnosis. As in the case of *A. hamulosa.*

Treatment—unknown.

Prophylaxis will obviously be difficult, however exclusion of wild water fowl from breeding areas, drainage of stagnant pools or treatment of the water with insecticides to kill the *Daphnia* are appropriate control measures.

Several other species of *Acuaria* and related parasites occur in poultry and occasionally produce disease. Those described above are the commonest and most important.

FAMILY: TETRAMERIDAE TRAVASSOS, 1924

Species of this family are related to the *Acuariidae*, but have no cordons. They show marked sexual dimorphism, the male being white and filiform, with or without spines on the cuticle and tail end and the female globular (*Tetrameres*) or coiled (*Microtetrameres*).

Genus: Tetrameres Creplin, 1846

This genus is remarkable for the fact that the mature female is almost spherical in shape, blood-red in colour and lies embedded in the proventricular glands of birds. The male is slender and its body cuticle is usually armed with four rows of spines; it is mostly found free in the lumen of the proventriculus, but it may follow the female into the gland temporarily for copulation.

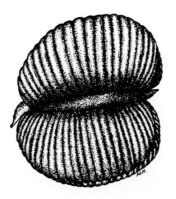

FIG. 149. *Tetrameres americana*, Female, Lateral View (Original)

T. americana Cram, 1927 occurs in the proventriculus of the fowl and turkey, and has been recorded from the United States and South Africa. Male 5–5·5 mm. long, female 3·5–4·5 by 3 mm. The latter is sub-spherical and has four deep grooves in the regions of the longitudinal lines, while the anterior and posterior extremities project as conical appendages.

Life-cycle. The eggs are passed in the faeces of the bird and hatch after they have been swallowed by a suitable orthopteran insect (*Melanoplus femurrubrum, M. differentialis* and *Blattella germanica*). Infection of the final host occurs through ingestion of the infected intermediate host and, according to Cram, the males and females migrate into the proventricular glands, where they copulate. The males then leave the glands and die. The females contain eggs 35 days after infection, but reach their full size only after 3 months.

Pathogenicity. The worms suck blood, but the greatest damage is done when the young worms migrate into the wall of the proventriculus, causing marked irritation and inflammation, which may kill chicks. At autopsy the adult females can be seen from the outside of the proventriculus as dark objects in the depth of the tissues.

Treatment. No suitable remedy is known.

Prophylaxis. Birds confined on bare ground will be less liable to acquire the parasites than those running free. Young chicks particularly should be prevented from eating the intermediate hosts and can be reared on wire floors for this purpose.

T. fissispina (Diesing, 1861) occurs in the duck, pigeon, fowl, turkey and wild aquatic birds and has a wide distribution. Male 3–6 mm. long, female 2·5–6 by 1–3·5 mm. The intermediate hosts are the water crustacea *Daphnia pulex* and *Gammarus pulex*, and in the final host the sexes are stated to copulate before the females migrate into the glands.

T. crami Swales, 1933 occurs in domestic and wild ducks in North America. Male up to 4·1 mm. long, females 1·5–3·5 by 1·2–2·2 mm. The intermediate hosts are amphipods: *Gammarus fasciatus* and *Hyalella knickerbockeri*. Severely infected birds are poor in condition.

SUPERFAMILY: PHYSALOPTEROIDEA SOBOLEV, 1949

Spirurata with pseudolabia well developed; pseudolabia armed with one or more teeth. Families of importance: *Physalopteridae, Gnathostomatidae*.

FAMILY: PHYSALOPTERIDAE LEIPER, 1909

The cuticle usually forms a collar-like projection around the anterior extremity. The lips are simple and bear small teeth on their medial surfaces. A pharynx is absent. Genus of importance: *Physaloptera*.

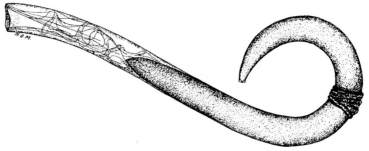

FIG. 150. *Physaloptera praeputialis*, Female, Lateral View (after Mönnig)

Genus: Physaloptera Rudolphi, 1819

P. praeputialis von Linstow, 1889 occurs in the stomach of the cat and wild *Felidae* in China, the East Indies, Africa and South America. Male 13–40 mm., female 15–48 mm. long. The worms are stout, and the cuticle in both sexes is posteriorly extended to form a sheath which projects beyond the caudal end of the body. In the fertilised female the vulva is covered by a conspicuous ring of brown cement material. Each lip bears at the middle of its free edge a set of three flattened, internal teeth, and externally to these a single conical external tooth of about the same height as the internals. The male tail bears large lateral alae, joined together anteriorly across the ventral surface. There are four pairs of pedunculated papillae, three sessile papillae on the anterior lip of the cloaca and five pairs of sessile post-cloacal papillae. The left spicule is 1–1·2 mm. long and the right 0·84–0·9 mm. The eggs measure 49–58 by 30–34 μ.

Several other species of *Physaloptera* have been described from domestic animals. The following may be particularly noted:

P. rara Hall & Wigdor, 1918, known from the duodenum of a dog in the United States. *P. canis* Mönnig, 1928 occurs in the stomach of the dog and cat in South Africa. The eggs measure about 40 by 34 μ. *P. felidis* Ackert, 1936 occurs in the stomach and duodenum of cats in the United States, producing erosions at the points of attachment and sometimes a severe catarrhal gastritis with vomition and loss of condition. *P. caucasica* von Linstow, 1902, normally a parasite of monkeys in Africa, may also be found in humans.

Life-cycle. It is now known that Orthoptera and beetles may be intermediate hosts of *P. rara* and *P. praeputialis*. Petri & Ameel (1950) found that the third stage larvae of *P. rara* will develop in the cockroach, *Blatta germanica*, in the field cricket, *Gryllus animilis*, in the flour beetle, *Tribolium confusum*, and in ground beetles, *Harpatalus* spp., and that the third-stage larvae of *P. praeputialis* will develop in *Blatella germanica*, *Gryllus animilis* and *Centophilus* spp.

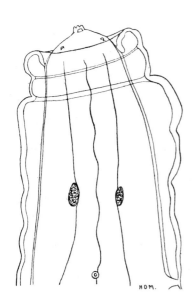

FIG. 151. *Physaloptera canis*, Anterior End, Lateral View (Original)

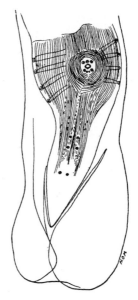

FIG. 152. *Physaloptera canis*, Hind End of Male, Ventral View (Original)

Pathogenesis. The parasites, which occur in the stomach, are usually firmly attached to the mucosa, on which they feed, or they may also suck blood. Apparently they occasionally change their site of attachment and leave numerous small wounds which may continue to bleed. In this way the mucosa becomes eroded and highly inflamed. A *Physaloptera* sp. in badgers in the U.S.A. (Ehlers, 1931) has been reported to cause loss of weight, shaggy fur, a quarrelsome nature and tarry faeces. Advanced clinical signs included paresis.

Diagnosis may be made from the clinical signs and the presence of spirurid eggs in the faeces, which must be differentiated from those of *Spirocerca lupi*.

Treatment. Ehlers (1931) was successful in expelling the worms from badgers by the administration of about 0·75 ml. carbon disulphide after fasting for 18–24 hours.

Prophylaxis. No definite recommendation can be made but, because the intermediate hosts are the beetles and Orthoptera mentioned above, steps should be taken to prevent the hosts from ingesting these insects.

FAMILY: GNATHOSTOMATIDAE RAILLIET, 1895

The lips are large and trilobed, and on their medial surfaces the cuticle forms toothlike ridges which interlock with those of the opposite lip. Genus of importance: *Gnathostoma*.

Genus: Gnathostoma Owen, 1836

G. spinigerum Owen, 1836 occurs in the stomach of the cat, dog, mink, polecat and several wild Carnivora and as an erratic parasite under the skin of man. Male 10–25 mm., female 9–31 mm. long. There is a large head-bulb, containing four submedian cavities or 'ballonets' which each communicate with a cervical sac. These cavities contain a fluid and apparently serve to fix the head in the tissues of the host by contraction of the cervical sacs and consequent swelling of the head-bulb. The cuticle of the head-bulb is armed with six to eleven transverse rows of hooks, while the anterior two-thirds of the body bears large, flat, cuticular spines with denticulate posterior edges. The ventral, caudal region of the male bears small spines and four pairs of large pedunculate papillae as well as several smaller sessile ones. The left spicule is 1·1–2·63 mm. long and the right 0·4–0·8 mm. The vulva opens 4–8 mm. from the posterior end. The eggs are oval with a thin cap at one pole; they have a greenish shell ornamented with fine granulations, are passed in the one-cell or morula stage and measure about 69 by 37 μ.

Life-cycle. The eggs hatch in the water in 4 days or longer. The larvae are sheathed and motile and die in a few days unless they are ingested by a *Cyclops*. In the latter they grow to 0·372 mm. long in 7 days or more, developing a definite cephalic bulb with four transverse rows of single-pointed spines, a pair of trilobate lips and two pairs of contractile cervical sacs. When the *Cyclops* is eaten by a fresh-water fish (*Clarias batrachus*, *Ophiocephalus striatus*, *Glossogobius giurus*, *Thereapon argenteus*), or by several species of frogs and reptiles, the parasites grow further to about 4·5 mm. long and become encysted. Such encysted forms, when fed to cats, become mature in the stomach wall in about 6 months. The young worms apparently sometimes migrate in the body of the final host, reaching the liver and other organs.

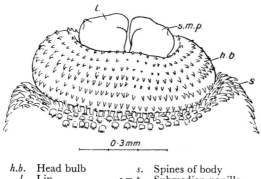

h.b.	Head bulb	s.	Spines of body
l.	Lip	s.m.p.	Submedian papilla

FIG. 153. *Gnathostoma spinigerum*, Anterior End, Dorsal View (after Baylis & Lane, in *Proc. Zool. Soc.*)

Pathogenesis. The young worms which pass through the liver cause much destruction of the tissues of this organ, leaving behind them characteristic yellow mosaic markings on the surface and burrows filled with necrotic material in the parenchyma. They also wander through other organs, including the mesentery and diaphragm, and they may enter the pleural cavity. Severe infections may therefore cause various disturbances in these organs. The adult worms penetrate into the wall of the stomach, producing cavities filled with a sanguino-purulent fluid. These cavities later develop into thick-walled cysts, each containing up to nine worms. The connection of the cysts with the stomach lumen may be very small and a similar minute canal may lead into the peritoneal cavity, providing the possibility for the development of peritonitis. Chandler (1925) considers this to be a very pathogenic and fatal parasite of cats, consistently killing its host. Cats with gastric tumours were found only at certain seasons, and they seemed to die out, so that none were found at other times.

Diagnosis. The eggs of the parasites are not always found in the faeces, so that diagnosis may be a difficult matter.

Treatment and Prophylaxis—unknown.

G. hispidum Fedtchenko, 1872 occurs in the stomach of the pig in Europe and Asia. Male 15–25 mm., female 22–45 mm. long. The whole body is covered with spines. The left spicule is 0·88–1·29 mm. long and the right 0·32–0·4 mm. The eggs measure 72–74 by 39–42 μ.

The young worms migrate in the abdominal organs of the host, particularly the liver, where they may cause a hepatitis. The adults are found deeply embedded in the gastric mucosa, producing cavities which contain a reddish fluid and are surrounded by an inflamed area. Severe infections may produce a marked gastritis.

Gnathostomiasis in humans is caused by the morphologically, but not sexually, mature stages of *G. spinigerum* and occasionally *G. hispidum*. The parasites do not usually enter the stomach but migrate at random in the body, frequently under the skin but also in the mucous membranes and the eye. In the skin they form abscess pockets or deep cutaneous tunnels. The lesions occur in any periferal part but the digits and the breasts are frequently affected.

Human infection is most probably acquired by eating inadequately cooked frogs or fish. Surveys of fish sold in markets in the East showed in Thailand that 92 per cent of frogs, 80 per cent of eels and 37 per cent of fish were infected with the larval stages while in Japan 60–100 per cent of *Ophiocephalus argus* were infected (Miyazaki, 1954).

ORDER: SPIRURIDA CHITWOOD, 1933

SUBORDER: FILARIATA Skrjabin, 1915

Spirurida with rudimentary stoma, no labial structures. Vulva anterior.
Superfamily of importance Filarioidea.

SUPERFAMILY: FILARIOIDEA WEINLAND, 1858

These are long and relatively thin worms. As a rule the mouth is small
and not surrounded by lips, and there is neither a buccal capsule nor a
pharynx. The oesophagus has anterior muscular and posterior glandular
portions. The male is frequently much smaller than the female and the
spicules are unequal and dissimilar. The vulva is usually situated near the
anterior extremity and fully developed larvae are born. The worms live
in the body cavities, blood or lymph vessels or connective tissues of their
hosts. Families of importance: *Filariidae, Setariidae*.

The larvae are known as microfilariae. They are in some cases enclosed
in a thin membrane or sheath which is apparently the very flexible egg-
shell. They reach the bloodstream or the tissue lymph spaces of the host,
whence they may be taken up by species of mosquitoes, fleas etc. In these
intermediate hosts the larvae develop to the infective stage and, passing
into the body cavity, reach the proboscis of the arthropod. When the
latter again sucks blood the larvae break their way out and enter the
final host, to complete their development.

The microfilariae of certain species of this group appear in the blood
stream of the final host, appearing either only during the day, or only
during the night, this phenomenon being known as diurnal or nocturnal
periodicity. For instance, in *Wuchereria bancrofti* of man, which is transmitted by mosquitoes, the microfilariae are much more numerous in the
peripheral blood vessels at night than during the day and they are said
to have a nocturnal periodicity. In *Loa loa*, also a human parasite, which
is transmitted by the Tabanid fly *Chrysops*, the reverse is the case and the
larvae are said to have a diurnal periodicity. Recent studies by Hawking
(1964) with *Wuchereria bancrofti* indicate that periodicity is a function of
the microfilariae and not the host. Hawking postulates the release of
microfilarial from the lungs, where they accumulate during the day, is
mediated by a 'fixative force' which fixes the microfilariae in the lungs
and a 'switch' mechanism which switches the fixative force off at night.
The fixative force is increased by raising the oxygen tension of the
pulmonary capillaries (e.g. by giving O_2, administration of isoprenaline)
and the switch mechanism is postulated to be an inherent circadian rhythm
which is also influenced by similar rhythms of the host.

Microfilariae may survive in the host for several weeks, either after the
death of the adult worm or if they are transferred to uninfected animals.

FAMILY: FILARIIDAE COBBOLD, 1864

Head of the adult without a peribuccal chitinous ring or other structures. Genera of importance: *Dirofilaria, Mansonella, Brugia, Wuchereria, Parafilaria, Ornithofilaria, Onchocerca, Elaeophora, Suifilaria, Wehrdikmansia*.

Genus: Dirofilaria Railliet & Henry, 1911

D. immitis (Leidy, 1856) occurs in the dog, cat, fox and wolf in Southern Europe, India, China, Japan, Australia and North and South America. The worms live mainly in the right ventricle and the pulmonary artery, but have also been found in other parts of the body. Male 12–16 cm., female 25–30 cm. long. The worms are slender and white in colour. The oesophagus is 1·25–1·5 mm. long. The hind end of the male is spirally coiled and the tail bears small lateral alae. There are four to

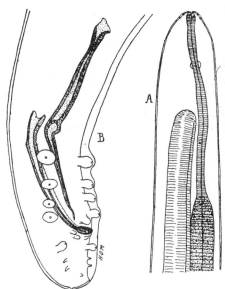

FIG. 154. *Dirofilaria immitis*: A, Anterior end of Female, Lateral View; B, Hind End of Male, Ventro-Lateral View (Original)

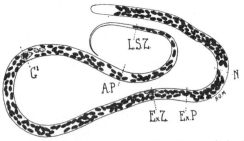

A.P.   Anal pore   G¹   First genital cell
Ex.P. Excretory pore   L.S.Z. Last tail cell
Ex.Z. Excretory cell   N.   Nerve ring

FIG. 155. *Microfilaria immitis*, showing 'Fixed Points' for Measurements (Original)

six, usually five, pairs of ovoid papillae, of which one pair is post-cloacal, two pairs of finger-shaped papillae lateral and posterior to the cloacal opening, and three to four pairs of small conical papillae near the tip of the tail. The left spicule is 0·324–0·375 mm. long and pointed, the right is 0·19–0·229 mm. long and ends bluntly. The vulva is situated just behind the end of the oesophagus.

Microfilariae may be found in the blood at all times but there is a tendency towards periodicity. This appears to vary in different countries. Thus in the U.S.A. Schnelle (1944) observed minimum microfilaraemia at 11.00 a.m. and maximum at 4.30 p.m.; in France, Euzéby & Laine (1951) found the lowest number 8.00 a.m. and the greatest at 8.00 p.m. With a Chinese strain of *D. immitis*, Webber & Hawking (1955) found minimum parasitaemia at 6.00 a.m. and maximum at 6.00 p.m. The larvae have a long, slender tail. Since different methods of fixation cause various degrees of contraction of the microfilariae, it is customary to express the distance of certain fixed points from the anterior extremity as percentages of the total length. In this way accurate descriptions of the larvae are obtained. The fixed points usually used are the position of the nerve ring (N), the excretory pore (Ex.P.), the excretory cell (Ex.Z.), the first genital cell (G.1), second genital cell (G.2), third genital cell (G.3), the anal pore (A.P.) and the last nucleus or last tail cell (L.S.Z.). An elongate 'central body' is seen with some methods of staining. For *D. immitis* microfilariae the mean percentages of the distance of these reference points as given by Newton & Wright (1956) are: nerve ring, 23·8; excretory pore, 32·7; excretory cell, 38·6; first genital cell, 67·9; second genital cell, 74·1; third genital cell, 79·4; anal pore, 82; and last nucleus, 92·7: with a total range in size of 307 to 322 μ and a mean of 313 μ. These figures should be compared with those of other microfilariae of the dog, given in Table 1, page 300.

Life-cycle. The intermediate hosts are mosquitoes of the genera *Culex*, *Aedes*, *Anopheles* and *Myzorhynchus*. This species does not develop, as has been stated, in fleas. Taylor (1960) has described the development in the mosquito. For the first 24 hours after a blood meal the microfilariae are found in the stomach of the insect: during the next 24 hours they migrate to the malpighian tubules where they develop over the next 15–16 days. For the first 6 or 7 days the developing larvae are found inside the cells of the tubules. By the fourth day after infection of the mosquito the 'sausage stage' larva occurs, this being the second-stage larva and it measures 220–240 μ in length by 20–25 μ in diameter. In this stage the excretory and intestinal cells have increased in number and these ultimately produce their respective organs which are evident in the 'elongated sausage form' which occurs on the ninth to tenth day after infection. At this time it measures 500 μ by 20 μ. This latter stage feeds on the cells of the malpighian tubules and enters the body cavity. From here it migrates through the thorax ending up in the cephalic spaces of the head or in the cavity of the labium. The final, infective, stage is produced in the labium and this measures 800–900 μ.

Development takes about 15–17 days in temperate countries while in tropical areas it may be as short as 8–10 days.

Infection of the dog occurs when the infected mosquito takes a blood meal. Initially, migration in the dog occurs adjacent to the site of infection, larvae being found in the submuscular membranes and a few in the sub-cutaneous tissue (Kume & Itagaki, 1955). From 85 to 120 days after infection developmental stages are found in the heart or pulmonary artery being 3·2–11 cm. in length at this time. In a further 2 months maturity is reached and microfilariae are shed into the blood.

Pathogenesis. Many dogs may be infected with *D. immitis* without show-ing any clinical signs of infection other than microfilariae in the blood. In heavy infections however the worms cause circulatory distress, due to mechanical interference and a progressive endarteritis. In large numbers they interfere with the function of the heart valves, masses of worms being found in the right atrium, right ventricle and the upper pulmonary arterial tree. The right side of the heart is markedly dilated and hypertrophied. This in turn leads to congestion and later cirrhosis of the liver and ascites. Endarteritis takes 9–10 months to become apparent and cause sufficient change to affect the heart (Hennigar & Ferguson, 1957).

Clinically the disease syndrome starts with a phase of ventricular hypertrophy, which is a phase of compensation, but later cardiac dilation occurs, with insufficiency. Associated effects include oedema of the lungs, kidney and liver and later portal hypertension, congestion of the intestines and ultimately ascites, hydrothorax and oedema of the dependent parts of the body occurs.

Cutaneous manifestations have been described by Vaughan (1952), these consisting of an eczematous dermatitis associated with intense irritation. Similar lesions have been reported from France and Japan. However, since parasites of the genus *Dipetalonema* may also occur along with *D. immitis* it is possible that some of the reported skin lesions may be due to these and not *D. immitis*.

The clinical signs depend on the number of worms present in the dog. The most common clinical signs are a chronic cough and a lack of stamina. Later there are signs of cardiac insufficiency such as rapid breathing, a discernible heart murmur and collapse after exercise. The electrocardio-gram may be normal at rest but after exercise the 'T' wave may be inverted. Various other clinical signs occur, these being dependent on the organs affected secondarily.

Diagnosis. This is based on the clinical signs and the demonstration of microfilariae in the blood. It is important to specifically identify the microfilariae of *D. immitis* since other microfilariae may occur in the dog. In the U.S.A. microfilariae of *Dipetalonema reconditum*, which is common in dogs, may readily be confused with those of *D. immitis*. Microfilariae may often be readily detected by a simple blood examination, a drop of blood being placed on a slide, covered with a cover glass and examined directly. The microfilariae will be seen moving actively. Where their numbers are few a better chance of finding them may be achieved by taking a sample of capillary blood or by examining the serum from clotted blood.

D. immitis microfilariae are generally more motile than those of *D. reconditum* and are usually more numerous, however these are guides to identification rather than absolute criteria. A method of differentiation has been described by Newton & Wright (1956) as follows: 1 ml. of blood is mixed with 9 ml. of 2 per cent formalin solution: the mixture is centrifuged for 5 minutes and the sediment placed on a slide with a drop of 1 : 1000 solution of methylene blue. Attention is paid to the tail of the microfilariae which in *D. immitis* is straight and in *Dipetalonema* is curved in the form of a 'button hook'. A further method of differentiating the two species of microfilaria is given by Sawyer *et al.* (1965) as follows: Thick blood films from the marginal ear vein are dehaemoglobinised in tap water for 10 minutes and transferred without drying to a 1 to 50 dilution of 1 per cent brilliant cresyl blue (in 0·8 per cent saline) for about 10 minutes. The slides are then rinsed in saline and mounted in saline. Microfilariae are then examined by both 'high dry' and oil immersion objectives for the presence of a cephalic hook. With this method of staining the hook is readily seen in *D. reconditum* while it is absent in *D. immitis* microfilariae. The method also allows a more satisfactory examination of the internal structure of the microfilariae, the genital cells being especially clear.

Treatment. A detailed review of the treatment of *D. immitis* infection is given by Gibson (1965). Only a brief summary will be given here.

Diethylcarbamazine is effective mainly against microfilariae but has been used extensively against the adults. Dosage 25 mg. per kg., three times daily for 20–30 days. May also be used prophylactically, being given for 5–7 days every 45 days during the period when mosquitoes are active.

Fouadin—a trivalent antimony compound—is given intravenously, intramuscularly or intraperitoneally as a 6·3 per cent aqueous solution: dosage 2·0–2·5 ml. daily rising to 3·5 ml. per day on the twelfth day.

Arsenamide is effective against adult worms. Dose 1·0 mg. per kg. daily for 15 days.

Filarsen (dichlorophenarsine hydrochloride) is effective against adult worms. Dose 1 mg. per kg. three times daily for 10 days.

Dithiazanine iodide is effective against microfilariae only. Given orally at dose of 22 mg. per kg. in food for 10–20 days.

Prophylaxis. Control measures are difficult especially in endemic areas. Insect repellants may have limited benefit. The strategic use of filaricidal drugs may be of value: thus dogs may be treated 2–5 months after exposure to mosquitoes in a heart worm area. Similar dogs may be treated for 5–7 days every 45 days during the season when mosquitoes are active.

D. repens Railliet & Henry, 1911 occurs in the subcutaneous connective tissue of the dog in Italy, India and Indo-China. Nelson (1960) found it in dogs, cats and genet cats (*Genetta tigrina*) in Kenya and found that its microfilariae develop in *Aedes pembaensis, A. aegypti, Mansonia uniformis* and *Mansonia africanus*.

D. corynodes (Linstow, 1899) (syn. *D. aethiops* Webber, 1955). This species occurs in monkeys (*Cercopithecus aethiops, Colobus* sp.) and its vectors are mosquitoes. Nelson (1960) found that its microfilariae develop in *Aedes aegypti* and *A. pembaensis* in Kenya.

D. conjunctivae (Addario, 1885) has been reported from humans, being associated with hazel-nut sized nodules on the head, eyelids and other parts of the body. It closely resembles *D. repeus* and several workers consider it identical with that species.

D. tenuis Chandler, 1942 occurs in the subcutaneous tissues of raccoons in the Southern parts of the U.S.A. Oribel & Beaver (1965) consider this to be the most common species of *Dirofilaria* in the subcutaneous tissues of man in the U.S.A. They also suggest that forms which have previously been reported as *D. conjunctivae* are probably *D. tenuis*.

Genus: Suifilaria Ortlepp, 1937

S. suis Ortlepp, 1937 was described from the pig in South Africa. The adult parasites live in the subcutaneous and intermuscular connective tissue and are not easily seen. The males are 17–25 mm. long, the females 32–40 mm. long and 0·15–17 mm. thick. The hind end of the male is spirally coiled; the spicules are unequal, the right measuring about 0·1 mm., the left 0·655–0·87 mm. long. The tail of the female ends abruptly and bears on its end a number of small tubercles. Eggs 51–61 by 28–32 μ.

Life-cycle. Unknown. The females appear to lay their eggs in the skin of the pig, because the skin of infected pigs shows numerous small, vesicular eruptions which contain the eggs of the worm.

Pathogenicity. The worms may produce small, whitish nodules in the connective tissues which may be taken for young *Cysticercus cellulosae* until they are more closely examined. Otherwise they do not affect the health of the pig, except for the fact that the skin vesicles containing the eggs eventually burst and may then become secondarily infected and develop into abscesses.

Genus: Mansonella Faust, 1929

M. ozzardi (Manson, 1897) Faust, 1929 occurs in the peritoneal membranes of man in South America only from the Guianas up to, and along, the north coast. Its microfilariae are not sheathed and its intermediate host is *Culicoides furens*.

Genus: Brugia Buckley, 1960

This genus was established by Buckley (1960) to include the species of *Wuchereria* which belong to what is called the *'malayi'* group of this genus, that is to say, *W. malayi* (Brug, 1927), *W. pahangi* (Buckley & Edeson, 1956) and *W. patei* (Buckley, Nelson & Heisch, 1958). Buckley *et al.* (1958) explain that the microfilariae of all these species are alike and are distinguished from the microfilariae of *W. bancrofti*, which infects man, by the facts that the microfilariae of species of the genus *Brugia* have two distinct tail nuclei, one terminal and the other sub-terminal, while the adult male has only five pairs of adanal papillae and there is, in the centre of the left spicule, a section of complex structure instead of the simple centre section in the left spicule of *W. bancrofti*. A further difference is that the species of *Wuchereria* are larger (female up to 100 mm. long and 300 μ broad; male up to 40 mm. long and 190 μ broad), while species of the genus *Brugia* are small (female up to 60 mm. long and 190 μ broad; male up to 25 mm. long and less than 100 μ broad).

The genotype of this new genus is *Brugia (Wuchereria) malayi* (Brug, 1927). All the species of the genus are parasitic in the lymphatic systems of primates, carnivores and insectivores.

B. malayi Buckley, 1960 (syn. *Wuchereria malayi*, Brug., 1927; Rao & Maplestone, 1940) occurs in man, monkeys (*Macaca irus* and *M. rhesus*), the slow loris (*Nycticebus coucang*), the civet cat (*Viverra tangalunga*) and the cat in India and Malaya. Its vectors are several species of *Mansonia* and *Anopheles*. Its pathogenesis and control are discussed in textbooks of medical parasitology.

B. patei Buckley, 1960 (syn. *Wuchereria patei*, Buckley, Nelson & Heisch, 1958) occurs in dogs, cats, the genet cat (*Viverra tigrina*) and the bush baby (*Galago crassicaudatus*) in Africa (see Nelson, 1960; Buckley *et al.*, 1958). Nelson (1960) did not find it in man. He studied the development of its microfilarial larvae in *Mansonia uniformis* and found these larvae in Kenya in this species of mosquito and also in *Mansonia africanus* and *Aedes pembaensis*.

B. pahangi Buckley, 1960 (syn. *Wuchereria pahangi*, Buckley & Edeson, 1958) occurs in the dog, cat, tiger (*Panthera tigris*), civet cat (*Viverra tangalunga*), slow loris (*Nycticebus coucang*) and wild cat (*Felis planiceps*). Its intermediate hosts are mosquitoes, members of the genera *Mansonia* transmitting it in the East and *Armigeres obturbans* in Kenya (Nelson, 1959).

Genus: Wuchereria da Silva Aranjo, 1877

This genus contains the well-known species *W. bancrofti* (Cobbold, 1877) Seurat, 1921, which infects the lymphatic system of man in the warmer parts of both the eastern and western hemispheres and causes Bancroft's filariasis of man, one feature of which is elephantiasis of the infected tissues. The generic and specific names of this species commemorate the names of its discoverer O. Wucher and the subsequent work of Bancroft on it. The worm and the disease it causes are fully described in textbooks of medical parasitology.

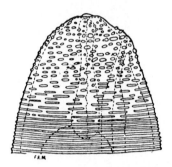

Fig. 156. *Parafilaria multipapilosa*, Anterior End of Female, Lateral View (from Baylis, after Yorke & Maplestone)

Genus: Parafilaria Yorke & Maplestone, 1926

P. multipapillosa (Condamine & Drouilly, 1878) (syn. *Filari haemorrhagica*) occurs in equines in eastern countries. It has been reported in Great Britain, being imported in horses from eastern Europe. Male 28 mm., female 40–70 mm. long. The anterior end of the body bears a large number of papilliform thickenings. The worms live in the subcutaneous and intermuscular connective tissue and produce subcutaneous nodules which appear suddenly, break open, bleed and then heal up. The

TABLE 1. COMPARATIVE SIZES OF MICROFILARIAE FOUND IN DOGS
(Percentage distance from the anterior end)

Species	NR	EP	EC	G.1	G.2	G.3	G.4	AP	LTC	Range (μ)	Mea
Dirofilaria immitis	23·8	32·7	38·6	67·9	74·1	75·4	79·4	82·0	92·9	307–322	3
Dipetalonema reconditum	20·8	21·0	34·5	70·1	75·7	77·2	78·6	80·7	89·0	246–293	2
Dirofilia repens	23·0	30·0	33·0	62·5	—	—	66·0	70·0	—	—	290
Dipetalonema grassii	—	—	—	—	—	—	—	—	—	—	5
Brugia malayi	24·5	35·0	40·0	64·0	—	—	80·0	83·0	—	—	220
Brugia patei	Similar to *B. malayi* except cephalic space 4·8 μ instead of 6·9 μ										
Brugia pahangi	22·0	31·0	33·0	68·0	73·0	74·0	78·0	80·0	—	—	2
Dipetalonema dracumculoides	45 μ*	66–70 μ*	—	—	—	—	—	53–55 μ†	20 μ†	195–230	

* Measurements in microns from anterior end.
† Measurements in microns from posterior end.
NR, nerve ring; EP, excretory pore; EC, excretory cell; G.1, first genital cell; G.2, se genital cell; G.3, third genital cell; G.4, fourth genital cell; AP, anal pore; LTC, last tail ce

PLATE IX

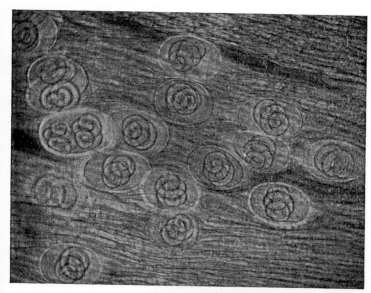

A. *Trichinella spiralis* cysts in skeletal muscle of rat. The cysts are about 3 months old, and calcification, which begins at the poles, has not yet commenced. One of the cysts to the middle left of the illustration contains two larvae, though this is uncommon. × 45. (Crown copyright)

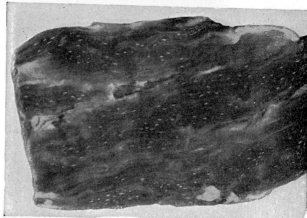

B. Trichiniasis of muscle of pig. The trichinellae have become encapsulated and the cysts have undergone well-marked calcification. (H. Thornton)

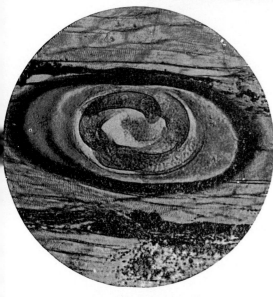

C. Larva of *Trichinella spiralis* in human muscle showing calcification of cyst wall. Some of the adjacent muscle fibres are degenerating and have lost their typical cross-striation. × 240. (Dr. J. F. Brailsford)

PLATE X

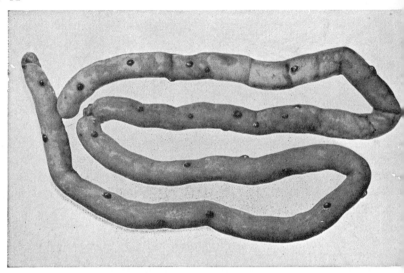

A. Small intestine of ox (everted) showing lesions of pimply gut caused *Oesophagostomum radiatum*. (H. Thornton)

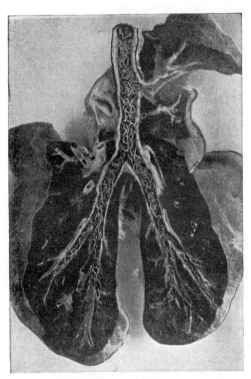

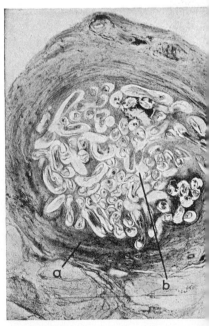

B. Lungs of a sheep affected with parasitic bronchitis. Numerous specimens of *Dictyocaulus filaria* are present in the trachea and bronchi. (Crown copyright)

C. Section through an *Onchocerca* nod showing (a) fibrous capsule and (b) cen spongy portion with sections of the par: in many of the reticular spaces. ×3 (H. Thornton)

condition is seen during the summer and disappears in winter, but may re-appear the next summer. The intermediate host in the U.S.S.R. is the blood sucking fly *Haematobia atripalpis*. In experimental infections the infective stage was produced in 10–15 days at air temperatures of 20–36°C (Gnedina & Osipov, 1960).

P. **bovicola** de Jesus, 1934 causes haemorrhagic nodules on the skin of cattle in the Philippines, Morocco, parts of the Mediterranean basin and it may also occur in India. The life-cycle is unknown but it is probably similar to that of *P. multipapillosa*. The disease in cattle is similar to that in horses, nodules on the skin developing rapidly and exuding blood within a few hours. Injections of 100 ml. per cent tartar emetic are reported to give goods results and sometimes one injection suffices.

Genus: Ornithofilaria Gönnert, 1937

O. **fallisensis** Anderson, 1954. This species occurs in anatid birds (see Lapage, 1961) and may be transmitted to the domesticated duck. Its life history and transmission by black flies (Simuliidae) have been described by Anderson (1954, 1955).

Genus: Onchocerca Diesing, 1841

The species of this genus are elongate, filariform worms. They live in the connective tissue of their hosts, often giving rise to the formation of firm nodules in which they lie coiled up. The cuticle is transversely striated and, in addition, bears characteristic spiral thickenings which are usually interrupted in the lateral fields.

O. **gibsoni** Cleland & Johnston, 1910 occurs in cattle and the zebu in Australia, India, Ceylon, the Malay region and Southern Africa. The worms are usually found in nodules which occur especially on the brisket and the external surfaces of the hind-limbs and it is difficult to extricate complete specimens. The male is 30–53 mm. long, the female 140–190 mm., but it is stated that she may be 500 mm. or more long. The tail of the male is curved ventrad; it bears small lateral alae and six to nine papillae on either side. The spicules measure 0·14–0·22 mm. and 0·047–0·094 mm. respectively. The microfilariae are 240–280 μ in length (mean 266 μ); they are not sheathed; the nerve ring is situated about 60–70 μ from the anterior end; the anterior and posterior portions of the larvae which contain no nuclei are respectively 2·5–5 μ and 9–13 μ long; the body cuticle bears rather pronounced transverse striations.

Life-cycle. The intermediate host is the midge *Culicoides pungens*.

Pathogenesis and Lesions. The parasites at first wander about in the connective tissue and later, when they come to rest, a nodule is formed around them. The head of the worm becomes fixed and surrounded by fibroblasts and then successive portions of the body are drawn into the nodule, where they eventually lie coiled up and surrounded by fibrous tissue in different stages of development. The 'worm nest' proper is surrounded by a fibrous tissue capsule which increases in thickness as the lesion grows older. The whole nodule may be up to 5 cm. in diameter, and it is ovoid or flattened in shape. Microfilariae are not frequent in the worm nests. In older nodules degeneration of the tissues and calcification of the worms frequently take place. The surrounding capsule consists of dense fibrous tissue which contains blood vessels, clusters of leucocytes and lymph spaces. The walls of the vessels are much thickened and their lumina often obliterated. The microfilariae are more frequent here and appear to wander out along the lymph spaces. Local thickenings of the skin, caused by the microfilariae, have been described. Infected animals show no clinical signs except the nodular swellings under the skin. The importance of the parasites is mainly that infected carcasses are not suitable for sale on most markets.

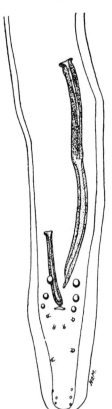

FIG. 157. *Onchocerca gibsoni*, Hind End of Male, Ventral View (Original)

Diagnosis. The microfilariae are very rarely found in the blood, but they can be found in the subcutaneous lymph spaces. It is recommended that a piece of the skin be pinched up above the nodule, the surface epidermis shaved off with a sharp knife, and that the fluid which exudes be examined. Microfiliarae may be found even though no nodules are present.

Treatment. No method of treatment is known.

Prophylaxis. It is advisable to protect the animals as far as possible against the bites of blood-sucking insects. Control of flies and insecticide treatment of their breeding places will help.

O. gutturosa Neumann, 1910 occurs in the ligamentum nuchae and other parts of the body of cattle. Male 2·9–3·9 cm., female 60 cm. or more. The microfilariae are found in the skin of the host and, according to Steward (1937), are transmitted by *Simulium ornatum*, in which they develop to the infective stage in about 3 weeks.

Bremner (1955) described the morphological differences between *O. gutturosa* and *O. gibsoni*.

The adult parasite causes nodular lesions in the ligamentum nuchae, especially at its insertion into the spinous processes of the thoracic vertebrae. These eventually become fibrotic and later calcified but there is no evidence that the lesions cause any clinical condition.

The microfilariae of *O. gutturosa* have been incriminated as the cause of a dermatitis of cattle in the Far East, especially Japan. 'Kose' or 'Wahi', as it is called, is seasonal in incidence, occurring in the summer and disappearing during the winter. Native black oxen are particularly prone to the disease. Lesions occur on the head, withers, neck and shoulders, a marked pruritus leading to thickening of the skin with loss of hair. Microscopic examination shows large numbers of microfilariae (Ishihara, 1958).

The most satisfactory treatment is diethylcarbamazine at a dose of 80 mg. per kg. given for two consecutive days.

O. cervicalis Railliet & Henry, 1910 occurs in the ligamentum nuchae of the horse and mule in many countries of the world. The male is 6–7 cm. in length and the female up to 30 cm. The microfilariae are 200–240 μ in length by 4–5 μ in diameter, unsheathed and have a short tail.

Life-cycle. Development occurs in the biting midge *Culicoides nubeculosus*, the larval stages developing in the thoracic muscles of the insect. Infective forms 600–700 μ in length are present in the proboscis of the fly 24–25 days after infection. In addition to *C. nubeculosus*, *C. obsoletus* and *C. parroti* may act as intermediate host and also the mosquitoes *Anopheles maculipennis* and *A. sacharovi* have been reported as intermediate hosts (Yoeli *et al.*, 1948).

Pathogenesis. For many years this species was assumed to be the cause of fistulous withers or poll evil in the horse. There is now no adequate evidence to sustain this belief. The parasites do produce lesions in the cervical ligament which initially are dark and show necrosis and later show fibrosis and cellular infiltration. Eventually caseation and calcification occur. No marked clinical entity can be ascribed to the adult worms (Supperer, 1953).

The microfilariae of *O. cervicalis* have been incriminated as the cause of equine periodic ophthalmia of horses (Lagraulet, 1962; Roberts, 1963). The lesions consist of a keratitis or iriditis and numerous microfilariae are found in the cornea. The iris, ciliary body and choroid show inflammatory foci.

O. reticulata Diesing, 1841 occurs in the connective tissue of the flexor tendons and the suspensory ligament of the fetlock, chiefly in the foreleg, of the horse, mule and donkey. The microfilariae occur in the skin and measure 330–370 μ and possess a long whiplash-like tail. Development is similar to *O. cervicalis* occurring in *Culicoides nabeculosus*.

Pathogenesis. Many horses may be infected; Supperer (1953) found 86 per cent infected in Austria, but the parasites appear to cause little clinical effect generally. In heavy infections there are many parasitic nodules in the tendons which may reach twice their normal thickness. After an initial oedematous reaction which may lead to lameness the nodules become fibrosed and can be felt as irregular masses on the flexor tendon and suspensory ligament.

The microfilariae of *O. reticulata* and to a lesser extent those of *O. cervicalis* are reported to be the cause of a chronic dermatitis of horses in Japan, the Philippines and the Indian subcontinent. A similar condition has been seen in horses in the U.S.A. by Dikmans (1948), scrapings of the lesions showing microfilariae of *O. reticulata*. In the East the condition is known as 'Kasen' summer mange or equine dhobie itch and is seasonal, being severe in summer and disappearing during the winter (Ishihara, 1958). A more detailed account of the condition is given by Soulsby (1965).

O. armillata Railliet & Henry, 1909. This species is common in cattle in Africa. Its vector is as yet unknown. Chodnik (1958) has described it and the histopathology of the lesions of the aorta which it causes.

Several other species of this genus are occasionally found in bovines and other domestic animals. None of the life-cycles are known and the parasites have little significance.

Genus: Elaeophora Railliet & Henry, 1912

E. poeli (Vryburg, 1897) occurs in the aorta of cattle and the zebu in Indo-China, the Malay Peninsula, Sumatra and the Philippines. Male 45–70 mm., female 40–300 mm. long. There are no lips and the oesophagus is very long. The tail of the male bears five to seven pairs of papillae, two pairs being pre-cloacal. The spicules measure 0·192–0·25 mm. and 0·12–0·132 mm. respectively. The uterus has four branches. The embryos are 0·34–0·36 mm. long, thick anteriorly and tapering posteriorly.

Life-cycle—unknown. The male occurs in nodules in the wall of the aorta, while the female is fixed in the nodules with its anterior extremity, and the rest of its body hangs free in the lumen of the vessel. The site of the parasites is the thoracic portion of the aorta, often along the dorsal aspects near the openings of the vertebral arteries. The affected vessel is diffusely swollen. Its wall is thickened and less elastic than normal on account of the development of connective tissue. The intima is uneven, it contains fibrous tracks, and is raised by the nodules which lie between the intima and the media. The nodules measure 8–13 mm. in diameter and contain thrombi in process of organisation and the worms. There is no evidence that the parasites produce clinical disease.

E. schneideri Wehr & Dikmans, 1935, occurs in the arteries of sheep in the states of New Mexico, Arizona and possibly Colorado and Utah in the U.S.A. The adult worms measure 6–12 cm. in length. The oesophagus is very long, the tail of the male is tightly coiled and the spicules are unequal, the larger being 1·11 mm. long, the smaller 0·4 mm. The worms are frequently found lying together in pairs in the arteries. Microfilariae 270 μ in length by 17 μ in thickness, bluntly rounded anteriorly, tapering posteriorly, occur in the skin.

The life-cycle is unknown.

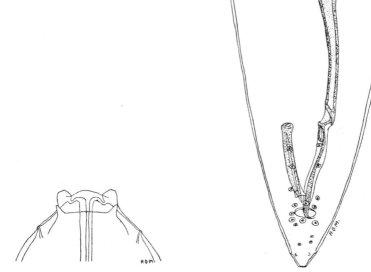

FIG. 158. *Setaria equina*, Anterior End, Lateral View (Original)

FIG. 159. *Setaria equina*, Hind End of Male, Ventral View (Original)

E. schneideri produces filarial dermatitis or elaeophoriasis, this being a circumscribed dermatitis involving the poll region but may extend to the face, nostrils or hind feet. It occurs in sheep grazed in summer at altitudes about 6000 ft. The adult worms are usually found in the arteries supplying the areas where the lesions occur, thus the carotid, maxillary and brachial are affected anteriorly and the iliac, tibial and digital posteriorly.

Pathogenesis. The adult worms cause little serious damage though thrombus formation may occur. The microfilariae are caught up in the skin and cause an intense dermatitis, the intense itching causes animals to rub and scratch and hence laceration of the tissues is common. The usual lesion is a circumscribed area 5–10 cm. in diameter on the poll though this may extend to other parts as stated above. Lesions on the coronary band may produce a club foot appearance (Kemper, 1957).

The lesions show periods of quiescence alternating with periods of activity. During the former, the lesions may become encrusted and the crusts may be dislodged during the active period producing a haemorrhagic lesion. The onset of the period of activity is probably due to a new generation of microfilariae reaching the skin.

After prolonged activity the lesions ultimately resolve, healing occurs with growth of new wool and the animal appears normal.

Adult worms have been found in deer, as have the cutaneous lesions, though these are not common. It is possible that the deer is the normal host for the parasite.

Diagnosis. The lesions are fairly characteristic and microfilariae can be demonstrated in the skin. The most satisfactory method of diagnosis is to macerate a piece of skin in warm saline and examine the material for microfilariae after about 2 hours.

Treatment. Piperazine hexahydrate at a dose of 180 g. per animal or 120 g. per gallon of drinking water for 3 days.

Trolene (Dow ET–57) at a dose of 300 mg. per kg.

Other treatments include Fouadin (4 ml. daily until 88 ml. given); diethylcarbamazine (100 mg. per kg.); sodium antimonyl tartrate in trypan blue with 1 per cent phenol (Trichicide) (15–40 ml. for six injections).

Prophylaxis. The intermediate host is probably a biting fly which occurs at altitudes above 6000 ft. Consequently fly control may be practised if practicable, or the pastures avoided.

E. böhmi Supperer, 1953 occurs in the arteries and veins of the extremities of horses in Austria. Male 4·5–6 cm., female 4–20 cm. Microfilariae resemble those of *Onchocerca reticulata*, 230–290 μ. Life-cycle unknown.

The parasites cause thickening of the blood vessel walls and there may be nodules formed containing disintegrated or calcified worms. Usually no clinical signs are associated with the infection.

Genus: Wehrdikmansia Caballero, 1945 (syn. Acanthospiculum, Skrjabin & Schikhobalova, 1946)

W. cervipedis (Wehr & Dikmans, 1935) occurs in the subcutaneous tissues of deer, frequently of the neck and fore and hind legs. It has been reported in Europe and the U.S.A. Male 5·5–6 cm., female 18–20 cm. Anterior end rounded, body finely striated, posterior end of male coiled, no caudal alae, spicules unequal. The life-cycle is unknown. A local fibrous lesion may be caused and the parasites are seen as thick, threadlike objects when the animal is skinned.

W. rugosicauda Böhm & Supperer, 1953 occurs in the subcutaneous fascia of the forequarters of *Capreolus capreolus* in Austria. A small form 2·2–2·5 cm. in length.

W. flexuosa (Wedl, 1856) occurs in deer in Eastern Europe and the U.S.S.R. Male 5·4–7·5 cm. g. female up to 10 cm.

FAMILY SETARIIDAE SKRJABIN & SCHIKHOBALOVA, 1945

Head of adult with a peribuccal chitinous ring, with lateral epaulette-like structure or with small teeth. Genera of importance: *Setaria*, *Dipetalonema*, *Stephanofilaria*.

Genus: Setaria Viborg, 1795

The worms of this genus are commonly found in the peritoneal cavity of ungulates. They are several centimetres long, milk-white in colour and taper especially towards the hind end, which is spirally coiled. The mouth is surrounded by a cuticular ring which bears dorsal and ventral and frequently also lateral prominences, giving a characteristic appearance to the worm. The tail of the male bears four pairs of pre-cloacal and usually also four pairs of post-cloacal papillae. The spicules are unequal and dissimilar. The tail of the female may bear spines or a few large, conical projections, while in both sexes there is a pair of small appendages near the tip of the tail. The sheathed microfilariae occur in the blood of the host. Yeh-Liang-Sheng (1959) has provided a revision of the genus, in which there is a deal of confusion. Yeh considers that the generic name *Setaria* should be reserved for forms which occur in equines and the genus *Artionema* applied to those forms which occur in the Bovidae and Cervidae.

S. equina (Abildgaard, 1789) is a common parasite of equines in all parts of the world. Male 40–80 mm., female 70–150 mm. long. There are large lateral and smaller, simple, dorsal and ventral peribuccal prominences. The left spicule is 0·63–0·66 mm. long and the right 0·14–0·23 mm. The tail of the female ends in a simple point. This worm is found in the peritoneal cavity and sometimes in the scrotum. It has also been recorded from the pleural cavity and the lungs of the horse and from the eye of cattle.

Life-cycle. There tends to be a slight periodicity, the microfilariae reaching their maximum number in the evening. Microfilariae develop in the thoracic muscles of culicine mosquitoes such as *Aedes aegypti, A. pembaensis* and *Culex* spp. (Heisch *et al.*, 1959). Infective larvae are produced in 12–16 days, depending on the environmental temperatures and in the horse adult parasites occur 8–10 months after infection.

Pathogenesis. Generally non-pathogenic. A slight fibrinous peritonitis may occur but this is of no consequence.

S. labiato-papillosa (Alissandrini, 1838) occurs in the peritoneal cavity of cattle, deer and antelope and is probably cosmopolitan in distribution. This species has frequently been referred to as *S. cervi*, however there is some confusion in the allocation of specific names in this genus (see Yeh-Liang-Sheng, 1959), and Skrjabin & Schikhobalova (1948) give *S. cervi* Maplestone, 1931, as a parasite of *Cervus axis*. Shoho (1958) has proposed that *S. cervi* should be referred to as *S. axis*. Böhm & Supperer (1955) consider *S. labiato-papillosa* and *S. digitata* identical since they were able to find intermediate forms between the two, indicating that a range of characters occur. However Yeh-Liang-Sheng (1959) reported distinct differences between *S. labiato-papillosa* and *S. digitata* and recommended the species be retained as valid.

Male 40–60 mm., female 60–120 mm. Peribuccal ring distinct, the dorsal and ventral prominences are distinct and are 120–150 μ apart. The mouth opening is elongated. The spicules are unequal and measure 120–150 μ and 300–370 μ. The tail of the female terminates in a marked button which is divided into a number of papillae. The microfilariae are sheathed and measure 240–260 μ.

Life-cycle. For many years it was considered that this parasite was transmitted by the stable fly, *Stomoxys calcitrans* (Noe, 1903), but there is little evidence for this and the work has never been verified. It is more likely that it is transmitted by culicine mosquitoes.

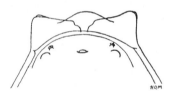

FIG. 160. *Setaria cervi*, Anterior End, Lateral View (Original)

No pathogenic entity has been ascribed to the presence of the parasite in the peritoneal cavity. Erratic migrations may occur and occlusion of the oviduct in a cow has been reported.

S. digitata von Linstow, 1906 occurs in the peritoneal cavity of cattle, buffalo and zebu in the Far East. It is similar to *S. labiato-papillosa*, the male being 40–50 mm. and the female 60–80 mm. in length. The distance between the dorsal and ventral prominences of the peribuccal ring is 60–75 μ and the mouth opening is round. The tail of the female ends in a simple button and the spicules of the male are 130–140 μ and 250–270 μ. The microfilariae are similar to those of *S. labiato-papillosa*.

Life-cycle. Development occurs in mosquitoes such as *Armigeres obturbans*, *Aedes togoi*, *Anopheles Lyrcanus*, and in *Culex pipiens* (Ochi, 1953).

Pathogenicity. The adult parasites cause little or no harm in the peritoneal cavity, however, immature forms of the parasite occur in the central nervous system of sheep, goats and horses in the Far East, causing the entity epizootic cerebrospinal nematodiasis. The condition has been extensively studied by Japanese workers and described in detail by Innes & Shoho (1952, 1953) whose work should be consulted for further information. The condition has been produced experimentally (Shoho, 1960). The disease caused by *S. digitata* occurs in the summer and autumn, when the mosquito intermediate hosts of *S. digitata* are active. The affected animals suffer from acute focal encephalomyelomalacia, which causes acute or subacute paralysis of all four limbs, or of the hind limbs only, without constitutional symptoms, but the signs vary according to the sites of the lesions and may be slight if relatively unimportant nervous areas are affected. The lesions are microscopic and may be overlooked. They are usually single tracks left by migrating young worms and may be found in any part of the central nervous system. Acute malacia occurs in the track of the worm, with disintegration of all tissues at the centre of the lesion and secondary degeneration of the nerve tracts with gigantic swellings of the axis cylinders and eosinophilic infiltration. Occasionally cavities are seen and the lesions are only rarely disseminated. Sugawa *et al.* (1949) found a malacic lesion with and without the presence of *S. digitata* in horses suffering from Japanese B. encephalitis. It is possible that the virus of Japanese B. encephalitis may be transmitted to human children and horses by *S. digitata*.

Treatment. For the treatment of epizootic cerebrospinal nematodiasis Shoho (1952) has recommended 40 mg. per kg. bodyweight of diethylcarbamazine given for 1–3 days.

Several other species of *Setaria* are found in domestic animals, deer and antelope, these include *S. congolensis* Railliet & Henry, 1911, in the peritoneal cavity of pigs in Africa (Congo), *S. altaica* Rajewskaya, 1928, in *Cervus canadensis asiaticus* in U.S.S.R., *S. cornuta* (von Linstow, 1899), in antelopes in Africa etc.

Genus: Dipetalonema Diesing, 1861 (syn. Acanthocheilonema, Cobbold, 1870)

Dipetalonema dracunculoides (Cobbold, 1870). This species occurs in the peritoneal membranes of dogs and hyaenas in Africa. Nelson (1960) found it in these hosts in Kenya and discussed the incidence of this and other species of this genus in Kenya. He stated that its microfilariae are very like those of *Dirofilaria immitis*, but differ in having a short, blunt tail. The male measures 24–30 mm. long and 100–200 μ broad and has unequal spicules, the female measuring 32–60 mm. long by 260–300 μ broad. The microfilariae are not sheathed.

D. reconditum (Grassi, 1890). This species has been reported from the body cavity, connective tissues and kidney of dogs in Italy, Africa and the U.S.A. Lindsey (1962) obtained 175 intact adults from fifteen of twenty dogs in the U.S.A., the parasites occurring in the subcutaneous tissues. Lindsey recorded the average length of females as 23·4 mm. with a range of 17–32 mm. Males had an average length of 13 mm. The spicules are unequal. Microfilariae from gravid uteri examined by Lindsey were 263·9–278·2 μ (mean 270·6 μ) with a width of 4·7–5·8 μ (mean 5·2 μ): one microfilaria possessed a button-hook tail. Microfilariae from the gravid uterus of two *D. immitis* worms were 298·6–313·6 μ (mean 308·9 μ) for one worm and 291·2–309·8 μ (mean 298·8 μ) for the other.

Development of *D. recondilum* occurs in fleas, *Ctenocephalides felis*, *C. canis* and *Pulex irritans*, and in ticks *Rhipiciphalus sanguineus* and *Heterodoxus spiniger*. Chabaud (1954) considers the tick the principal intermediate host.

No pathogenic effects have been ascribed to the parasite but its microfilariae must be differentiated from those of *D. immitis* in the diagnosis of heartworm infection.

D. grassi Noe, 1907, occurs in the subcutaneous tissues of dogs in Italy and Kenya. It is a small form, the female measuring 25 mm. in length. The microfilariae are large, 570 μ in length, with a hook-shaped tail. Development occurs in the tick *Rhipicephalus sanguineus*. No pathology is associated with the infection.

D. evansi (Lewis, 1882) occurs in the pulmonary and spermatic arteries and lymph nodes of camels in Egypt, the Far East and Eastern U.S.S.R. This is a fairly large filarid, the male being 75–90 mm. and the female 170–215 mm. The microfilariae measure 250–300 μ.

Up to 80 per cent of camels may be infected in the Eastern Republics of the U.S.S.R. and it is suspected that the mosquito *Aedes detritus* is an intermediate host. Infected camels suffer arteriosclerosis and heart insufficiency. A parasitic orchitis may occur or aneurysms in the spermatic vessels. The treatment recommended by Soviet workers is fouadin at a dose of 0·5 ml. per kg.

D. perstans (Manson, 1891) Railliet, Henry & Langeron, 1912. Manson-Bahr (1960) records this species under the generic name *Tetrapetalonema* (Faust, 1935). Its adults occur in the peritoneal or pleural cavities (rarely in the pericardium) of man and apes in tropical Africa generally and in Algiers and Tunis, and in South America from Venezuela down to the Argentine. Its intermediate hosts are *Culicoides austeni* and *C. grahami*. The worm is not very pathogenic. Its microfilariae are not sheathed and they show no periodicity in the blood.

D. streptocerca (Macfie & Corson, 1922), the adult and microfilariae of which have been found in the skin of man in Central Africa and in Ghana. They may cause oedema and elephantiasis of the skin. The intermediate hosts are *Culicoides austeni* and probably also *C. grahami*.

Genus: Stephanofilaria Ihle & Ihle-Landenberg, 1933

S. dedoesi Ihle & Ihle-Landenberg, 1933, occurs in the skin of cattle in Celebes, Sumatra and Java. Male 2·3–3·2 mm., female 6·1–8·5 mm. long. The oral aperture is surrounded by a protruding cuticular rim which has a denticulate edge. Near to the anterior extremity there is a circular thickening which bears a number of small cuticular spines. Male spicules unequal. Female without an anus.

Life-cycle—unknown. It is suspected that the parasites are transmitted by blood-sucking arthropods.

Pathogenicity and Lesions. Bubberman & Kraneveld (1933) describe a verminous dermatitis, commonly known as 'cascado', which is produced by these parasites. Poor condition and high rainfall are predisposing factors and the incidence may be 90 per cent in cattle. The lesions occur particularly on the sides of the neck, the withers, dewlap, shoulders and around the eyes. A number of small papules develop and coalesce to form a larger lesion covered with crusts; the hair falls out and the skin thickens, but it is rich in blood and lymph which can be squeezed out readily. The lesion extends outwards while the centre becomes hard and covered with a thick, dry crust and may reach a size of 25 cm. diameter. Itching leads to rubbing, which may aggravate the lesion. The worms live in the epithelial layers of the skin and cause an inflammation of the rete Malpighii with proliferation and destruction of epithelial cells, destruction of hair follicles and skin glands and infiltration with small cells. Dikmans (1948) found that skin lesions in cattle in America contained both the microfilarial larvae and adult worms.

Diagnosis. After removal of the crusts deep skin scrapings are made and the microfilariae can be found in this material.

Treatment. No remedy is known. Spontaneous recovery may occur.

S. stilesi Chitwood, 1934, is found in the United States and causes lesions resembling 'cascado' mostly on the underside of the abdomen of cattle.

S. kaeli Buckley, 1937, causes lesions on the legs of cattle in the Malay Peninsula.

S. assamensis Pande, 1936, causes 'hump sore' of cattle in India.

ORDER: SPIRURIDA CHITWOOD 1933

SUBORDER: CAMALLANATA Chitwood, 1936; Skrjabin & Schulz, 1940

Oesophageal glands uninucleate. No well-developed labial structures (sometimes with lateral jaws). Larvae with large pocket-like phasmids. Superfamily of importance Dracunculoidea.

Superfamily: Dracunculoidea Cameron, 1934

Stoma rudimentary; internal circle of cephalic papillae well developed. Family of importance *Dracunculidae*.

Family: Dracunculidae Leiper, 1912

Anterior end with helmet. Females very much larger than the male. Anus and vulva atrophied in the gravid female. Genera of importance: *Dracunculus, Avioserpens*.

Genus: Dracunculus Reichard, 1759

D. medinensis (Linnaeus, 1758), the 'guinea-worm', is a parasite of man which occurs especially in Southern Asia and Africa. It has also been found in the horse, dog, cattle and other animals in these areas. The male is 12–29 mm. long. The female may be 100–400 cm. long and 1·7 mm. thick and has no vulva. The adult female lives in the subcutaneous connective tissue, and cutaneous swellings, which later become ulcers, develop around its anterior extremity. When these lesions come in contact with water the uterus prolapses through the anterior end of the worm or through its mouth and ruptures, discharging a mass of larvae which are 500–750 μ long, into the water. These larvae have to develop in a species of *Cyclops* to become infective for the final host. Infection of the latter takes place through drinking water which contains the infected *Cyclops* and the worms develop to maturity in about 1 year. Shortly before the parasite comes to the surface of the body the host may show symptoms such as urticaria, itching and a rise of temperature.

The classical method of treatment is to remove the worm, which must be done carefully without breaking it. It is usually tied to a small stick and gradually rolled up in the course of a few days or weeks. Diethylcarbamazine in large doses is stated to kill the adult worms and the developing larval stages.

D. insignis (Leidy, 1858) Chandler, 1942 is a form which occurs in wild carnivors and the dog in North America. It may be separated from

D. medinensis on the basis of length of gubernaculum and number of preanal papillae. Ewing and Hibbs (1966) have listed the guinea worm infections reported in North American carnivores and it is likely that the infection occurs in all states of the U.S.A. The parasite is commonly found in the subcutaneous tissues of the limbs but occasionally it may be found elsewhere, such as the conjunctiva, heart, vertebral column, scrotum, etc. It is associated with swellings on the tiba and tarsus which progress to non-healing ulcers. It is presumed that the life cycle of *D. insignis* is similar to that of *D. medinensis*.

Genus: Avioserpens Wehr & Chitwood, 1934

A. taiwana (Sugimoto, 1919, 1934), is a species found in domesticated ducks in China, mainly in the dry season (January to April), and in Formosa, where disease caused by it may also occur in September to October. It affects ducks 3 weeks to 2 months old. The male is unknown. The female is up to 25 cm. long by 0·8 mm. in width. The anterior end is rounded, the mouth being surrounded by a chitinous rim bearing two prominent lateral papillae. There are four smaller papillae further back on the head. The uterus is large and filled with larvae. The vagina and vulva and anus are atrophied. The tail ends in a conical papilla.

Life-cycle. The larvae of this species occur in *Cyclops* sp. in Formosa.

Pathogenicity. The worms cause the formation of swellings under the mandible, which are at first soft and movable and after about 1 month hard and painful. They may reach the size of a large nut. They interfere with swallowing and respiration and may cause death from inanition or asphyxia. Occasionally the swellings occur on the shoulders and legs and interfere with the bird's movements. Numerous microfilariae are found in the blood. Usually the adult worms escape by piercing the swelling and healing occurs, the disease lasting about 1½ months. Sometimes the worms die in the swellings, which may then become abscesses. The general effect on birds that survive is unthriftiness and retardation of growth.

Treatment. Removal of the worms through an incision into the most prominent part of the swelling and antiseptic treatment of the swelling results in cure in a week or so.

Prophylaxis. Arrangements should be made for rearing ducklings in the rainy season and to provide them with water free from *Cyclops*. They should not be allowed access to marshland.

The Aphasmid Nematodes

SUBCLASS APHASMIDIA CHITWOOD & CHITWOOD, 1933

Nematodes with phasmids absent. Caudal glands present or absent. Caudal alae usually absent.

ORDER TRICHOCEPHALIDA (SKRJABIN & SCHULZ, 1928) SPASSKY, 1954

SUBORDER TRICHURATA NEVEAU–LEMAIRE, 1936 (syn. *Trichocephalata*, Skrjabin & Schulz, 1928)

Nematodes in which the muscular tissue of the oesophagus is much reduced, oesophageal glands outside the contour of the oesophagus in the form of a single row of cells. Males with one or no spicules. Families of importance, *Trichinellidae*, *Trichuridae* and *Capillariidae*.

FAMILY: TRICHINELLIDAE WARD, 1907

The adults of the single species of this family are small, the posterior part of the body being only slightly thicker than the anterior part. The male has neither a copulatory spicule nor a spicule sheath. The female is larviparous.

Genus: Trichinella Railliet, 1895

T. spiralis (Owen, 1833) (syn. *Trichina spiralis*) occurs in the small intestine of man, pig, rat and many other mammals. Even birds have been infected experimentally. It is probably cosmopolitan in distribution, but has not been found in some countries. The male is 1·4–1·6 mm. long and the female 3–4 mm. The body is slender and the oesophageal portion is not markedly narrower than the posterior part. The hind end of the male bears a pair of lateral flaps on either side of the cloacal opening, with two pairs of papillae between them. There is neither a spicule nor a sheath. The vulva is situated near the middle of the oesophageal region. The eggs measure 40 by 30 μ and contain fully-developed embryos when in the uterus of the female.

Life-cycle. The life-cycle is initiated when encysted muscle larvae are ingested. These are liberated within a few hours by the digestive processes and development to the adult stage is rapid, being complete in 4 days. Copulation occurs about 40 hours after infection. After copulation has taken place in the intestine the males die and the females penetrate into the mucosa via Lieberkühn's glands and some may reach the lymph spaces. Here they produce, over a period of several weeks, eggs that hatch inside the uterus of the worm. The longevity of the female worm is not known with certainty but probably few are left in the bowel after 5–6 weeks. In experimental infections a marked loss of adults occurs about the twelfth day of infection, however this depends on the animal used. The loss of adult worms is greatly accelerated in previously

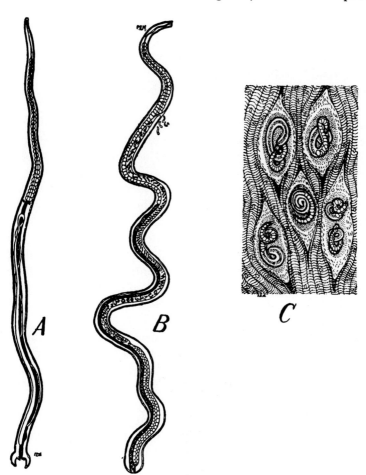

Fig. 161. *Trichinella spiralis*: A, adult male; B, adult female; C, larvae encapsuled in muscle (from Baylis, after Fiebiger)

sensitised animals. The first larvae, which are about 0·1 mm. long, enter the lymph and pass in it by way of the thoracic duct to the left superior vena cava and thus reach the blood, by which they are distributed all over the body. They develop further, especially in the voluntary muscles, especially those of the diaphragm, tongue, larynx, eye and the masticatory and intercostal muscles. They have also been found in the liver, pancreas and kidney. The larvae enter the sarcolemma of the striated muscle fibres and grow rapidly; after 30 days they measure 0·8–1 mm. in length and have begun to coil inside a cyst which arises from tissue histiocytes in the area. The cyst wall is fully formed after about 3 months and measures 0·4–0·6 by 0·25 mm. The affected muscle fibres degenerate and the cysts usually begin to calcify after 6–9 months, but the larvae in them may live for several years. Cases in which the larvae lived for 11 and even 24 years have been recorded. In the cysts the larvae cannot develop further, but must await ingestion of the infected meat by another host. In this other host the larvae are liberated from their cysts in the stomach and grow adult in the intestine, beginning to deposit larvae within 6–7 days. Prenatal infection with this parasite appears to be rare, but it has been produced experimentally following heavy infections.

Pathogenesis and Clinical signs. The parasite is of principal importance in human medicine and it is unusual for any obvious clinical entity to be associated with the infection in domestic or wild animals. The intestinal forms may produce a certain amount of irritation and cause a marked enteritis in heavy infections. The most important pathogenic effects are produced by the larvae in the muscles. Heavy infections may lead to death, especially through paralysis of the respiratory muscles. The clinical signs which accompany trichinosis are very variable and may simulate those of a variety of other diseases; they include diarrhoea, fever, stiffness and pain in the affected muscles, dyspnoea, hoarseness, sometimes an oedema of the face and deafness. A marked eosinophilia is usually present. A crisis is usually reached after about 4 weeks, when the egg-production of the females begins to decline and the larvae become encapsulated.

Epidemics of trichinosis occasionally occur in human beings when a number of people partake of insufficiently-cooked trichinous meat of a pig, bear or other host. Further information on the subject of trichinosis may be obtained from Gould (1945), Madsen (1961), Kozar (1962) and Larsh (1963).

Diagnosis. In the human a provisional diagnosis may be made on the clinical signs of muscular pain, oedema of the eyelid and face etc., such being pathognominic when trichinosis exists in an area. The adult worms may, on occasion, be found in the faeces but this is more accidental than the rule. Larvae may be demonstrated in muscle taken by biopsy, the sample either being examined pressed between two pieces of glass or after digestion in an acid pepsin (1 per cent) solution. A circulating eosinophilia may be present, possibly reaching 25 per cent in the more active stages of the disease. It is good supportive evidence for a diagnosis of trichinosis.

A number of immunodiagnostic tests have been used in diagnosis. These include complement fixation, haemagglutination, flocculation and intradermal techniques. With symptomatic cases of trichinosis there is usually a good correlation between the immunodiagnostic test and the presence of the infection, however with asymptomic cases there may be considerable difficulty in assessing the results. This is especially so with the intradermal test in which sensitivity persists for many years. Possibly the most satisfactory immunodiagnostic test in human medicine is the bentonite flocculation technique. Details of the preparation of antigens are given by Kagan (1960). For reviews of the immunology and diagnostic tests in trichinosis see Kagan (1960), Larsh (1963) and Soulsby (1963).

The diagnosis of *T. spiralis* infection in animals depends mainly on the detection of the infection at meat inspection. Various diagnostic tests have been studied, especially in pigs, and though they will adequately detect experimental infections their level of usefulness is much lower in natural infections.

In Germany, pig muscle samples are routinely examined at slaughter houses by 'trichinoscopes'. These consist of a compressorium to press the muscle and the image of the muscle is projected on a screen. A more adequate, but more laborious and time-consuming method, is digestion of muscle samples with an acid pepsin mixture for several hours. This is best carried out in a Baermann apparatus and the resulting sediment is examined for larvae. A further method is to infect experimental animals with the suspected muscle and later to examine the carcase for infection.

Treatment. Thiabendazole has been demonstrated to be effective against both the adult intestinal phase and the larval muscle phase. It has also been used successfully in human infection.

Methyridine is effective against the muscle stage of the infection in experimental animals.

Control and Prevention. Human trichinosis is disseminated chiefly by the pig. This animal is most usually infected from raw garbage which contains scraps of trichinous meat. Grain fed pigs usually show a low incidence of infection and when regulations are in force requiring that garbage be cooked before being fed to pigs, the incidence is also low. Though rats were at one time thought to play a major part in the epidemiology, there is little critical evidence to support this idea. It is certain they become infected, but so do at least forty-nine other species of mammals (Madsen, 1961), but there is no strong evidence that they are responsible for any large number of swine infections.

Infection of various wild animals, including wild boar, polar bear, walrus, seal and certain fur bearing animals, may be responsible for human infection in certain areas of the world, e.g. Arctic, Central Europe etc.

Man usually acquires the infection mainly from pork and sausages which are eaten raw or partly cooked. In arctic regions the consumption of bear, fox, walrus etc., which are considered delicacies by the Eskimaux, frequently leads to trichinosis. Cameron (1962) has suggested that whole communities may be wiped out by trichinosis in the Arctic regions of Canada. Prophylaxis should therefore aim at the elimination of uncooked garbage in the feed of pigs and, as far as man is concerned, the thorough cooking of all pork products. Ordinary roasting of household joints of pork cannot, however, be relied upon to kill larvae in the deeper parts of such joints and there are records of the infection of man by eating roasted joints of pork. To be sure that heat kills the larvae, it is necessary to ensure that all parts of the meat, including the deepest portions, reach a temperature of 137°F. Salting and other methods of curing are not reliable, unless the preserving process is thorough. The larvae are killed by rapidly lowering the temperature of pork to −35°C for a short period or to −18°C for 24 hours. Curing for 40 days at a temperature of not less than 36°F followed by smoking at 113°F for 10 days is necessary for certain destruction of the cysts. The United States Government Regulations require that the meat should be stored at a temperature not higher than 5°F for 20 days or that all parts of it should be heated to 137°F.

Gould *et al.* (1962) have demonstrated the feasibility of using gamma irradiation to sterilise meat. They maintain the method is simple and rapid and meat so treated still retains its flavour.

FAMILY: TRICHURIDAE RAILLIET, 1915
(TRICHOCEPHALIDAE BAIRD, 1853)

The name of the important genus in this family, *Trichuris*, represents an error, in that it literally means 'hair-tail' and not 'hair-head' as is presumed was intended. Consequently the substitute name *Trichocephalus* was proposed, but under the rules of priority of the International Code of Zoological Nomenclature it is, strictly, not acceptable. It has, however, been adopted by many European and Soviet parasitologists.

Members of the family are medium to large worms, the posterior part of the body being much thicker than the anterior. Genus of importance: *Trichuris*.

Genus: Trichuris Roederer, 1761 (syn. Trichocephalus)

The worms belonging to this genus are generally known as 'whipworms', since the anterior part of the body is long and slender, while the posterior part is much thicker. The hind end of the male is curled and there is one spicule surrounded by a protrusible sheath which is usually armed with fine cuticular spines. The vulva is situated at the beginning of the wide part of the body.

T. ovis (Abildgaard, 1795) has been recorded from the caecum of the goat, sheep, cattle and many other ruminants. The male of *T. ovis* is 50–80 mm. long; the anterior end constitutes three-quarters of the length. The female is 35–70 mm. long, of which the anterior end forms two-thirds to four-fifths. The fully-evaginated spicule is 5–6 mm. long. The sheath bears an oblong swelling a short distance from its distal extremity and is covered with minute spines which decrease in size towards the distal extremity. The eggs are brown, barrel-shaped, with a transparent plug at either pole, and measure 70–80 by 30–42 μ, including the plugs. They contain an unsegmented embryo when laid.

T. globulosa (v. Linstow, 1901) occurs in the caecum of the camel, sheep, goats, cattle and other ruminants, and is the common form found in these animals in South Africa and possibly also in some other parts of the world. The male is 40–70 mm. long and the female 42–60 mm., the anterior part constituting about two-thirds to three-quarters of the length. The spicule measures 4·2–4·8 mm. and its sheath bears a terminal, spherical expansion on which the spines are larger than on the remaining portion. The eggs measure 68 by 36 μ and are similar to those of *T. ovis*.

T. vulpis (Fröhlich, 1789) occurs in the caecum and other parts of the intestine of the dog and fox. The worms are 45–75 mm. long, about three-quarters of this being made up by the anterior portion. The spicule is 9–11 mm. long and the sheath bears small spines only on the proximal portion. The eggs measure 70–89 by 37–40 μ and have a brown colour.

T. suis (Schrank, 1788) occurs in pig, wild pig and wild boar. It is cosmopolitan in distribution. Morphologically it is identical to *T. trichiura* (Linnaeus, 1771) of man and other primates and some workers believe the two to be identical. However, there is no critical evidence to show that the two parasites are interchangeable between the two hosts. The male is 30–50 mm. long and the female 35–50 mm. The anterior portion forms about two-thirds of the total length. The spicule is 2–3·35 mm. long, with a blunt tip, and its sheath is variable in shape and in the extent of its spinous armature. The eggs measure 50–60 by 21–25 μ.

Life-cycle. The eggs reach the infective stage after about 3 weeks under favourable conditions, however development may be much more prolonged at lower temperatures (e.g. 6–20°C). Infective eggs may remain viable for several years. The host acquires the infection by ingesting the eggs, and the larvae reach the caecum, where they grow adult in 1–3 months, depending on the species.

Pathogenicity. Opinion about the pathogenicity of these species varies, but there is little doubt that they can produce an acute or chronic inflammation, especially in the caecum of the dog and man.

In sheep, cattle and swine naturally acquired infections are seldom severe enough to cause clinical disease. In a study of experimental infection of *T. suis*, Powers *et al.* (1960) reported a haemorrhagic necrosis and oedema of the caecal mucosa. Later nodule formation occurred. In acute infections there was a profuse watery haemorrhagic diarrhoea associated with a marked retardation of growth which continued until death. Such effects were seen with burdens of 6000–13,000 worms.

Many dogs are infected but the burdens seem to have little clinical effect. Nevertheless severe infections are not uncommon and several hundred or thousand worms may cause a profuse diarrhoea, loss of weight and unthriftiness. In severe cases the faeces may be markedly haemorrhagic or even frank blood. Then there is evidence of anaemia, sometimes jaundice, the infection terminating in death.

Diagnosis is made by demonstration of the characteristic barrel-shaped eggs in the faeces.

Treatment

Dogs: N-butyl chloride (0·1–10 ml. per kg.) has been reported effective, especially if given hourly for 5 hours. The effect, however, may be very variable (0–100 per cent). The compound is well tolerated.

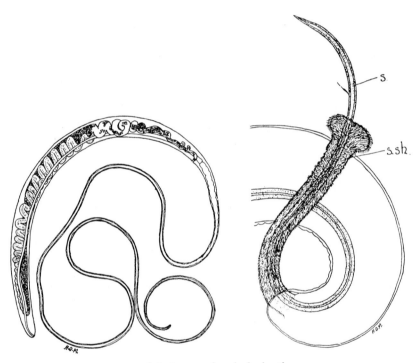

s. Spicule   s.sh. spicule sheath

Fig. 162.   *Trichuris globulosa*, Female   Fig. 163.   *Trichuris globulosa*, Male, Hind
(Original)   End (Original)

Whipcide (Phthalofyne) (3-methyl-1-pentyn-3-yl sodium phthalate), at a dose of 250 mg. per kg. either orally or by i.v. injection is generally highly effective and usually without severe side effects.

Diathiazane iodide has been used successfully in human medicine but it is not well-tolerated by dogs. Dosage rate is 10–20 mg. per kg. for 6–10 days.

Glycobiarsol (p-glycolylamino-phenyl-arsonic-bismuth). A single dose of 1000 mg. per kg. or five to ten daily doses of 200 mg. per kg. is reported to be quite effective and well tolerated.

Methyridine [2(β-methoxyethyl) pyridine]. McGregor *et al.* (1962) gave 44 mg. per kg. subcutaneously and reported good effects, eggs disappearing from the faeces in 5–7 days and in those dogs examined at *post mortem*, no worms were found. The injections caused pain, vomition.

Swine: *Hygromycin* 80 million units per tons of feed highly effective.

Trichlorophon, 75 mg. per kg. intramuscularly has been reported highly effective (Balconi & Todd, 1962).

Sheep and Cattle: *Methyridine*, 200 mg. per kg. orally or subcutaneously is highly effective.

Prophylaxis. Improved hygiene is necessary. Dog kennels and exercise yards etc. should be regularly cleaned. Heavily infected soil should be avoided for several months to allow the natural agencies of sunlight and dryness to kill the eggs.

FAMILY CAPILLARIIDAE NEVEU–LEMAIRE, 1936

Trichurata in which the oesophageal part of the body is shorter than the posterior part and more or less equal in thickness. Genus of importance: *Capillaria*.

Genus: Capillaria Zeder, 1800

The worms of this genus are closely related to *Trichuris*, but they are small and slender and the posterior part of the body is not conspicuously thicker than the anterior part. The life histories of species occurring in mammals are, so far as we know, direct, but those of some species occurring in birds (e.g. *C. annulata* and *C. caudinflata*) are indirect, earthworms being the intermediate hosts. The eggs have polar plugs. The genus contains numerous species, among which the following may be encountered by the veterinarian:

SPECIES FOUND IN BIRDS

The complex taxonomy of these species here given is that of Madsen (1952).

(*a*) *Species found in the intestine*

C. caudinflata (Molin, 1858) Wawilowa, 1926 (syn. *C. caudinflatum* (Molin, 1858), *C. longicollis* (Mehlis, 1831)). This species occurs in the small intestine of the fowl, pigeon and related wild birds. Male 9–14 mm., female 14–25 mm. long. The oesophagus is almost half as long as the body in the male and one-third as long in the female. The tail of the female is cylindrical up to the end. The vulva has a conspicuous projecting appendage. The eggs measure 60–65 by 23 μ. The life history of this species is indirect. The eggs, like those of *C. annulata*, are swallowed by earthworms (*Eisenia foetida*, *Allolobophora caliginosa*) and birds infect themselves by eating these. Morehouse (1944), however, concluded that no larval development occurs in the earthworm, although passage through the earthworm and hatching of the larvae in it appear to be necessary.

C. obsignata (Holger Madsen, 1945) (syn. *C. columbae*). This species occurs in the small intestine of the pigeon, fowl, turkey and related wild birds. Male 9·5–11·5 mm., female 10·5-14·5 mm. long. In the male the oesophagus is more than half as long as the body; in the female it is shorter. The tail of the female tapers posteriorly. The eggs measure 48–53 by 24 μ.

C. anatis (Schrank, 1790) Travassos, 1915 (syn. *C. retusa, C. collaris, C. anseris* H. Madsen, 1945, *C. mergi* H. Madsen, 1945). This species occurs in the caeca of domesticated gallinaceous and anatine birds and the caeca of gallinaceous game birds in Europe.

(b) Species found in the crop and oesophagus

C. annulata (Molin, 1958). This species occurs in the crop and the oesophagus of the fowl, turkey and related birds. Male 15–25 mm., female 37–80 mm. long. The cuticle of the anterior end forms a characteristic swelling. The eggs measure 60–65 by 25–28 μ. The life history of this species resembles that of *C. caudinflata*, earthworms being the intermediate hosts. The earthworms *Eisenia foetida, Allolobophora caliginosa* and some of the genera *Lumbricus* and *Dendrobaena* are concerned, the infective larvae being reached in them in ˙14–21 days (Allen, 1949). However, Morehouse (1944) states that no development occurs in the earthworm, rather passage through it to induce hatching of the eggs is the essential requirement. Madsen (1952) regards this species as being synonymous with *C. contorta* (see below).

C. contorta (Creplin, 1839) Travassos, 1915. This species occurs in the crop, oesophagus and mouth of the turkey, duck and many wild birds. The males are 12–17 mm. long and the females 27–38 mm. The eggs measure 48–56 by 21–24 μ. The life history of this species is, so far as we know, direct, but Madsen (1952) concluded that *C. contorta* is synonymous with *C. annulata*, the correct name for both these species being *C. contorta*. He suggests that the life history of the species here described as *C. contorta* may sometimes require the passage of the eggs through earthworms, so that it may be either direct or indirect.

Pathogenicity. Small numbers of the worms produce no lesions, but large numbers produce an inflammation varying in degree from a simple catarrh to a croupous inflammation with the formation of diphtheritic pseudo-membranes.

Within recent years *Capillaria* spp. have become important parasites in the deep litter and broiler methods of rearing poultry. Apart from causing death they also are responsible for lower growth rates, decreased egg production, and decreased fertility of the flock (Geevaerts, 1962).

Clinical signs consist of diarrhoea, emaciation, the feathers round the vent are matted together and the birds have an unkempt appearance.

Heavy burdens of *C. caudinflata* may occur in turkeys kept in straw yards, the straw providing good cover for earthworms. Similarly this parasite may be responsible for heavy mortality in pheasant chicks especially where they are reared intensively. *Capillaria obsignata* may be troublesome in pigeons when they are kept on a large scale for commercial purposes.

Diagnosis. This is usually made at *post mortem* when large numbers of parasites can be found. The eggs may also be detected in large numbers in the faeces.

Treatment. The most effective compound is methyridine. It is most satisfactory given in the drinking water at the rate of 200–400 mg. per 100 ml. for 24 hours (Friedhoff, 1963): it may also be injected subcutaneously at the rate of 150 mg. per kg. and this dose affects all developmental stages of the parasite (Broome, 1963).

Prophylaxis. This is a matter of hygiene, but presents many difficulties. The animals should be fed and watered in such a way that contamination with eggs of the worms is eliminated as far as possible.

SPECIES FOUND IN MAMMALS

C. entomelas (Dujardin, 1845) occurs in the small intestine of the mink, beech marten and polecat, and may cause a haemorrhagic enteritis, particularly in mink. The infection is acquired chiefly by animals kept in boxes and can be prevented only by hygienic measures. The eggs measure 56–63 by 23–27 μ.

C. plica (Rudolphi, 1819) occurs in the urinary bladder and sometimes the pelvis of the kidney of dogs, cats and foxes. It is apparently relatively harmless and no treatment except sanitation is known. The male is 13–30 mm. and the female 30–60 mm. long. It has been stated that the life history of this species is direct, but Enigk (1950) recorded that it may be indirect, the larvae entering the connective tissue of earthworms and foxes infecting themselves by eating infected earthworms; adult parasites are found about 60 days after infection. The eggs are passed in the urine and are colourless; they measure 63–68 by 24–27 μ. Other species of urinary bladder capillarids include *Capillaria felis cati* which has been recorded from the cat in Egypt and elsewhere. It is possible that this species is identical to *C. plica*. *Capillaria mucronata* is found in the urinary bladder of mink.

C. cutanea. According to Moroshita & Tani (1960), this species causes the formation of subcutaneous nodules, oedema and blisters in monkeys and they thought that it was the cause of cutaneous creeping eruption in the finger and ankle of a Japanese adult male.

C. hepatica (Bancroft, 1893) (syn. *Hepaticola hepatica*) occurs in the liver of numerous rodents and other animals, including the rat, mouse, squirrel, muskrat, rabbit and dog. The worms are very thin and cannot easily be removed from the tissue, so that it is difficult to measure their length. Lengths of 4–12 cm. have been reported. Their eggs are laid in the liver and can be seen in the form of irregular yellow streaks and patches on the surface and in sections. The life-cycle is more or less direct, though eggs trapped in the liver of the infected host must be liberated by the digestive processes of a 'transport' host, the eggs then passing to the soil where they become infective. In the early stages of infection of the initial host a few eggs may be passed in the faeces but subsequently eggs are trapped in the liver. Infection of another host is by ingestion of the embryonated egg in food or water. Infection can take place by the ingestion of food contaminated from a decomposing infected carcase.

Human infections have been recorded, these being associated with a subacute hepatitis with eosinophilia (see Otto *et al.*, 1954).

C. bovis (Schnyder, 1906) occurs in the small intestine of cattle, being cosmopolitan in distribution. The male is 8–9 mm. and the female 12–20 mm. in length. The eggs measure 50 by 25 μ. There is no evidence that this species is responsible for any ill effects.

C. longipes Ransom, 1911 occurs in the small intestine of sheep and is cosmopolitan in distribution. The male is 11–13 mm. in length and the female up to 20 mm. The eggs measure 45–50 μ by 22–25 μ. The life-cycle is direct. No well-defined pathological entity has been associated with infection by this species.

C. aerophila (Creplin, 1839) (syn. *Eucoleus aerophilus*) occurs in the trachea, bronchi and rarely the nasal cavities of dogs and foxes. It has also been recorded from the cat, pine marten, beech marten, wolf (*Lupus lupus*) and the badger. The male is 24·5 mm. long and the female 32 mm. There is one spicule and a spicule sheath armed with spines. The eggs measure 59–80 by 30–40 μ, including the polar plugs. They have a slight greenish tinge, and the thick shells have a 'netted' surface.

Life-cycle. This is direct. The eggs are laid in the lungs, coughed up and swallowed, and are therefore passed in the faeces. They develop in the open, reaching the infective stage after 5–7 weeks, and may remain viable for over a year under favourable conditions. The infective larva does not hatch out of the egg until the infective egg is swallowed by a suitable host. The eggs then hatch in the intestine and the larvae migrate to the lungs in 7–10 days, reaching maturity 40 days after infection.

Pathogenesis. Animals with mild infections show no clinical signs. Severe infections cause a chronic tracheitis and bronchitis. The affected animals are susceptible to secondary infections by bacteria which may cause broncho-pneumonia. There is a whistling noise while the animal breathes and a deep, wheezing cough, especially at night. A nasal discharge is frequently seen. The mouth may be held open on account of dyspnoea. The animals become emaciated and anaemic, while the fur grows harsh.

Diagnosis is made by finding the eggs in the faeces, in the sputum or nasal discharge. These should be differentiated from those of *C. plica* and *T. vulpis*.

Treatment. None is known at present. Mechanical removal of worms with a tracheal brush has been suggested.

Prophylaxis. The disease occurs chiefly in young foxes up to 18 months old. The parasite is most troublesome where the soil of the pens is shaded or not properly drained. The infection is also acquired in breeding boxes, where the eggs are allowed to accumulate. Dry pens and clean boxes should therefore be the object of preventive measures.

SUBCLASS: APHASMIDIA CHITWOOD & CHITWOOD, 1933

SUBORDER: DIOCTOPHYMATA SKRJABIN, 1927

Oesophageal glands multinucleate, caudal glands absent, vagina tubular, reproductive system highly developed. Male with one spicule, muscular caudal sucker present. Families of importance *Dioctophymidae* and *Soboliphymidae*.

FAMILY: DIOCTOPHYMIDAE RAILLIET, 1915

This group contains three genera (*Dioctophyma*, *Hystrichis* and *Eustrongylides*) in which the alimentary canal is attached to the abdominal wall by four longitudinal bands of suspensory muscles. The tail of the male bears a terminal, cup-shaped 'bursa' without rays and there is a single spicule. The female has a single genital tube and the eggs have thick, pitted shells.

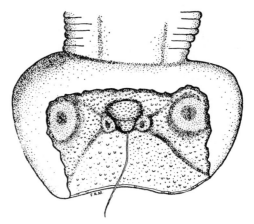

FIG. 164. *Dioctophyma renale*, Posterior End of Male, Ventral View (from Baylis, after Stefanski)

Genus: Dioctophyma Collet–Meygret, 1802 (syn. Dioctophyme)

D. renale (Goeze, 1782) (syn. *Eustrongylus gigas*) is the largest nematode known and occurs in various countries in the kidneys and other organs of the dog, fox, otter, beech marten, pine marten, polecat, mink, weasel, other wild carnivores and the seal, and it has also occasionally been found in the pig, horse, cattle and man. The male measures up to 35 cm. by 3–4 mm., and the female up to 103 cm. by 5–12 mm. The worms have a blood-red colour. The spicule is 5–6 mm. long, but it may reach up to 12–14·5 mm. long. The eggs are barrel-shaped and the shells are pitted except at the poles. They measure 71–84 by 46–52 μ and are not segmented when laid.

Life-cycle. The eggs are passed in the urine of the host and develop slowly in water, requiring 1–7 months according to the temperature. They do not hatch until they have been swallowed by the intermediate host, but they may remain viable for 2 years. Woodhead (1950) found that eggs derived from wild mink in Michigan hatched when they were swallowed by the branchiobdellid oligochaete annelid worm, *Cambarincola chirocephala*, which is parasitic on crayfish, and that the first larvae of *D. renale* encysted in the tissues of the crayfish. When infected crayfish were eaten by the bullhead fish, *Ameirus melas*, the larvae encysted in the liver and mesentery of this fish and became third and then fourth larvae. Mink infected themselves by eating infected fish. More recent work by Karmanova (1960) in the U.S.S.R. has indicated a different life-cycle to that proposed by Woodhead. Karmanova reported hatching of the first-stage larva in the annelid *Lumbriculus variegatus* and development to fourth-stage larvae in the blood vessels of the annelid. Infection of the final host is by ingestion of the infected annelid. This life-cycle shows more relationships to that of other members of this group (e.g. *Hystrichis*) and would allow an explanation of the occurrences of infection in non-fish-eating animals such as horses and cattle.

In the final host the infective larvae penetrate the bowel wall and initially develop in the body cavity and then penetrate the kidney. Blood migration does not appear to occur (Haelberg, 1953).

Pathogenesis and Lesions. The right kidney appears to be invaded much more frequently than the left. The worms apparently enter the pelvis and destroy the parenchyma. Eventually only the capsule is left as a much-distended bladder, containing one or more worms and a haemorrhagic fluid. If some of the kidney parenchyma is left, it may be partly calcified. Often a worm projects into the ureter. They may also wander down into the bladder and pass out through the urethra. In the abdominal cavity the worms may be found free or encapsulated, causing a chronic peritonitis with adhesions in various places. Frequently they lie between the lobes of the liver and destroy the surface of this organ. Small nodules containing eggs of the parasite may be found in the liver and the omentum. The worms have also been found in the pleural cavity.

Clinical signs. Frequently no signs are shown, since the normal kidney can serve the needs of the body. In other cases the infected animals grow thin and they may show signs of kidney trouble together with nervous signs. Retention of urine and death from uraemia may occur.

Diagnosis can be made by finding the eggs in the urine if the parasites occur in the kidneys.

Treatment. The worms may be removed surgically.

Genus: Hystrichis Dujardin, 1845

The species of this genus occur in aquatic birds. The anterior extremity is somewhat swollen and bears several rows of small spines.

H. tricolor Dujardin, 1845, occurs in the glands of the proventriculus of domestic and wild ducks, where it produces nodules and destruction of the tissues. The male is about 25 mm. long and the female up to 40 mm.

Life-cycle. The eggs measure 85–88 μ by 36–40 μ, they have truncated poles and are covered with tubercles. They develop slowly in water, reaching the embryonated stage in about 60 days. Further development occurs in oligochaetes such as *Criodrilis lacuum* (Glossoscolecidae) and *Allolobophora dubiosa* (Lumbricidae) (Karmanov, 1956). The first-stage larva hatches in the digestive tract of the annelid and migrates to the supraneural blood vessel where three ecdyses occur producing a fourth-stage larva. Birds became infected by eating infected earthworms and the mature parasite is produced in 1 month, the longevity being about 45–50 days.

Pathogenesis. Nodules are produced in the wall of the proventriculus: these may perforate to the pleural cavity and cause adhesion of the organs in that area. Suppuration of the nodule and the local area is not uncommon. The parasite is intricately sewn in the lesion and difficult to extract in a complete state.

Genus: Eustrongylides Jägerskiöld, 1909

E. tubifex (Nitzsch, 1819) occurs in the intestine of anatine birds in Europe. Head not spiny, mouth small, cuticle markedly annulated, oesophagus very long, without dilation. Male up to 34 mm. by 2 mm. in thickness, bursal cup trumpet-shaped. Spicule long and slender. Female 35–45 mm., vulva near anus, eggs 70 μ by 44 μ, an operculum at either pole and markedly pitted.

The developmental cycle is unknown but fish have been incriminated.

E. papillosus (Rudolphi, 1802) is similar to *E. tubifex* and is found sewn into the mucosa of the oesophagus and proventriculus of ducks and geese. The species measures up to 30 mm. in length, the bursal cup has a fringed margin and the eggs measure 68 by 38 μ. The life-cycle is unknown but fish probably serve as intermediate hosts.

Marked nodule formation occurs in the wall of the anterior digestive tract.

FAMILY: SOBOLIPHYMIDAE PETROV, 1930

Possessing a muscular cephalic sucker. Mouth feebly developed. Bursal cup campanulate. Genus of importance *Soboliphyme.*

Genus: Soboliphyme Petrov, 1930

S. baturini Petrov, 1930 occurs in the intestines of foxes, sable and cats in the Soviet Union (Siberia) and has been found in the wolverine in North America.

SUPERFAMILY: MERMITHOIDEA

Species of this superfamily belong to the Class Nematoda. They are not parasitic in domesticated animals, but may be swallowed with drinking water or otherwise found in the neighbourhood of farm stock, and they may be mistaken for parasitic nematodes. They are smooth, hair-like worms, whitish or brownish in colour, and the adults are free-living in soil or water. The pharynx may extend along half the length or more of the body and it is not connected with the intestine, which becomes a double row of cells packed with reserve food materials. The males are much smaller than the females. Parthenogenesis may occur. The larvae are parasitic in terrestrial invertebrates, which they may kill.

FAMILY: MERMITHIDAE

The larvae are economically important because they are parasitic inside the bodies of the nymphs or larvae of insects (grasshoppers, earwigs, ants), whose viscera they destroy, so that these insects may fail to develop or may die. The larvae of *Mermis subnigrescens* are parasitic in grasshoppers and earwigs, those of *Paramermis* in grasshoppers and those of *Allomermis* in ants. *Mermis subnigrescens* has been called the rain-worm, because the adults appear out of the soil after rain in the summer in thundery weather and climb up plants to lay their eggs.

FAMILY: TETRADONEMATIDAE

The larvae of the relatively few species of this family are parasitic in the larvae of the Diptera *Sepsis* and *Sciara*.

CLASS: NEMATOMORPHA (GORDIACEA, HAIRWORMS)

Species of this class are not parasitic in domesticated animals. They are cylindrical, relatively very long worms, with a smooth cuticle devoid of rings. The anterior end is clear with a dark ring behind the clear area. The posterior end of the male ends in two broad processes and the posterior end of the female in three similar processes. The nervous system consists of cerebral ganglia and a mid-ventral nerve cord. There is no pharynx and the end of the alimentary canal tends to degenerate. The sexes are in separate individuals and the sexual ducts of both sexes open into the intestine. The adults are not parasitic, but the larval phases are.

ORDER: GORDIOIDEA (HAIRWORMS)

The adults live in fresh water and the larvae are parasitic in insects (grasshoppers, crickets, cockroaches, beetles) that live near fresh water, or in centipedes or millipedes.

ORDER: NECTONEMATOIDEA

There is only one genus of this order, *Nectonema*, the species of which are pelagic and marine. They are up to 20 cm. long and their larvae are parasitic in the crab and hermit-crab.

Phylum: Acanthocephala Rudolphi, 1808

The Acanthocephala are a group of parasitic worms usually considered as being closely allied to the Nematoda. They are commonly called 'thorny-headed worms'.

Morphology. The body is in most cases cylindrical and is covered with a thick cuticle. Underneath this is a matrix without definite cell walls, but containing a number of nuclei and fine, branching vessels, of which the function is not known. Next follow circular and longitudinal muscles which line the body cavity.

An alimentary canal is absent. The worms feed like cestodes, by absorbing their nourishment through the body wall. Anteriorly the body bears an evaginable proboscis, which is a hollow, cylindrical or oval structure armed with transverse or longitudinal rows of recurved hooks and lies in a proboscis sac. Next to the proboscis sac a pair of elongate, hollow organs, the 'lemnisci', project into the body cavity. The proboscis is retracted by special muscles which are inserted in the body wall and it is evaginated by the contraction of the proboscis sac. The lemnisci are connected with the proboscis and probably secrete or store the proboscis fluid.

The excretory system consists of a pair of nephridia which discharge into the genital ducts.

From the proboscis sac a 'suspensory ligament' runs backwards through the body cavity and provides attachment for the genital organs. The male has two testes which lie in a tandem position. The vasa deferentia unite to form an ejaculatory duct, and this opens through a 'penis' which projects into an evaginable sac or 'bursa' at the posterior extremity of the body. A group of cement glands or prostate glands are connected with the ejaculatory duct. They appear to secrete a substance which protects the vulva of the female after copulation.

In the female the ovary discharges its ova into the body cavity, where they appear to be fertilised and the embryo develops for some time, forming around itself a shell of three layers. The 'uterine bell' is a special organ which swallows the eggs through an anterior opening and passes the mature eggs through into the vagina, while the immature ones are returned to the body cavity through a small pore situated posteriorly. The eggs contain larvae which are provided with an anterior circlet of hooks.

331

Development. As far as the life-cycles are known the eggs require to be ingested by an intermediate host, which is usually an arthropod. Whether vertebrates can act as intermediate hosts is uncertain. In some cases larval forms are found encapsulated in vertebrates, but these are probably secondary intermediate hosts or wrong hosts in which the immature parasites have become encysted, as in the case of some spirurid nematodes. The adult parasites occur chiefly in aquatic vertebrates, mainly fishes and birds.

ORDER PALAEACANTHOCEPHALA MEYER, 1931

FAMILY: POLYMORPHIDAE MEYER, 1931

Usually small worms with a cylindrical body. Genera of importance:
Polymorphus, Filicollis.

Genus: Polymorphus Lühe, 1911

P. boschadis (Schrank, 1788) (syn. *Echinorhynchus polymorphus* Bremser,
E. minutus Zeder) occurs in the small intestine of the duck, swan, fowl,
goose and various wild aquatic birds. Male about 3 mm. long, female
up to 10 mm. long. The worms have an orange colour when fresh. The
cuticle is spiny anteriorly, and behind this region the body is constricted.
The proboscis has sixteen longitudinal rows of seven to ten hooks each,

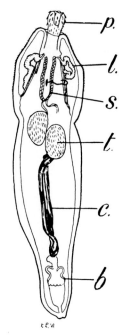

b. Bursa copulatrix	*c.* Cement glands
l. Lemniscus	*p.* Proboscis
s. Proboscis sac	*t.* Testis

FIG. 165. *Polymorphus boschadis*, Male (from Baylis, after Lühe)

which decrease in size posteriorly. The testes are oval, situated diagonally,
and the cement glands are elongate. The eggs are spindle-shaped and
measure about 110 by 19 μ. Their outer shell is thin, while the middle
shell is thick and irregularly constricted at the poles. The embryo has a
yellowish-red colour.

Life-cycle. The embryo develops in the crustacean *Gammarus pulex*, and possibly also in the crayfish *Potamobius astacus*. The final host acquires the infection by ingesting the infected intermediate host.

Pathogenesis. The worms are located in the posterior part of the small intestine, where they penetrate deeply into the mucosa with their probosces. At the points of attachment small nodules can be seen from the peritoneal surface. The parasites produce cachexia, and heavy infections can cause severe losses of ducks.

Diagnosis can be made by finding the eggs in the faeces.

Treatment. Little is known about the treatment of *Polymorphus* infections. Petrochencho (1949) has reported that carbon tetrachloride at a dose of 0.5 ml. per kg. is up to 98 per cent effective.

Prophylaxis. The birds have to be kept away from water harbouring infected intermediate hosts.

Genus: Filicollis Lühe, 1911

F. anatis (Schrank, 1788) occurs in the small intestine of the duck, goose, swan and wild aquatic birds. Male 6–8 mm. long and white in colour, female 10–25 mm. long and yellowish. The male has an ovoid

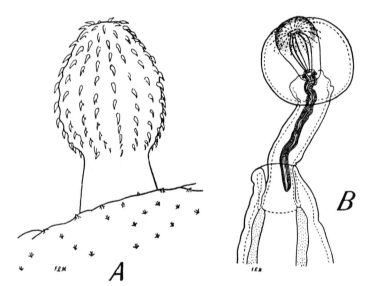

FIG. 166. *Filicollis anatis*: *A*, anterior end of male; *B*, anterior end of female, less highly magnified (from Baylis, after Lühe)

proboscis with eighteen longitudinal rows of ten to eleven hooks each and the anterior part of the body is armed with small spines. The lemnisci are long in both sexes. The female has a long, slender neck, while the proboscis is globular in shape and about 2–3 mm. in diameter. There are eighteen rows of ten to eleven hooks each arranged in a star-shaped pattern at the apex of the proboscis. The eggs are oval and measure 62-70 by 19-23 μ.

Life-cycle. The eggs are passed in the faeces of the host and the larval stage develops in the crustacean *Asellus aquaticus* (Isopoda). The final host acquires the infection by ingesting such isopods and the worms grow adult in about 4 weeks.

Pathogenesis. The parasites are situated in the middle portion of the small intestine and also further back in severe infections. While the male attaches its proboscis in the mucosa, the female worm pierces through the mucous and muscular layers of the wall, so that its proboscis comes to lie directly underneath the peritoneum. In some cases the peritoneum may even be ruptured. The parasites are obviously harmful; they cause emaciation and frequently the death of their hosts.

Diagnosis can be made by finding the eggs in the faeces.

Treatment and Prophylaxis. As in the case of *P. boschadis.*

Several other related species occur in wild water fowl. Thus *Profilicollis botulus* has been reported to be responsible for seasonal high mortality in the eider duck in Scotland (Rayski & Garden, 1961). Development occurs in the common shore crab *Carcinus moenas*. *Polymorphus magnus* occurs in the intestines of wild anseniforms in Eastern Europe and the Soviet Union. Development occurs in *Gammarus lacustris*.

ORDER: ARCHIACANTHOCEPHALA MEYER, 1931

FAMILY: OLIGACANTHORHYNCHIDAE MEYER, 1931

Usually large to medium sized worms. Proboscis not retractile. Genus of importance *Macracanthorhynchus*.

Genus: Macracanthorhynchus Travassos, 1916

M. hirudinaceus (Pallas, 1781) (syn. *Echinorhynchus gigas*) occurs in the small intestine of the pig and is widely distributed. The worms are usually more or less curved and have a pale reddish colour. The male is up to 10 cm. long and the female up to 35 cm. or even more and 4–10 mm. thick. The cuticle is transversely wrinkled. The proboscis is relatively small and bears about six transverse rows of six hooks each, which decrease in size backwards. The eggs measure 67–110 by 40–65 μ and have four shells, of which the second is dark brown and pitted.

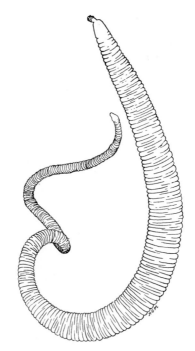

FIG. 167. *Macracanthorhynchus hirudinaceus.* × 1½ (Original)

Life-cycle. The eggs are passed in the faeces of the pig and are very resistant to cold and dryness, being able to live for several years in the open. They hatch when they have been ingested by the larvae of certain beetles feeding in the manure or infected soil (*Melolontha vulgaris*, a number of dung beetles and the water beetle, *Tropisternus collaris*). The young worm eventually becomes encysted in the body cavity of the insect. Pigs become infected by ingesting either the grubs or the adult beetles which harbour the infective stage of the worm. Development in the pig takes 2-3 months. A female lays about 260,000 eggs per day and lays for about 10 months.

Pathogenesis. The parasites penetrate with their probosces deeply into the intestinal wall and may produce perforation and death from peritonitis. Apart from this possibility mild infections are not very harmful, but severe infections may cause slow growth or emaciation, which are very important in pigs.

Diagnosis can be made by finding the eggs in the faeces.

Treatment. No satisfactory remedy is known. Nicotine sulphate and carbon tetrachloride, especially mixtures of both have given satisfactory results.

Prophylaxis. The pigs would have to be prevented from ingesting the larvae or adults of the intermediate hosts. Where pigs are kept in sties or small runs regular removal and suitable disposal of faeces will assist in reducing the infection.

FAMILY: PACHYSENTIDAE MEYER, 1931

Genus: Oncicola Travassos, 1916

O. canis (Kaupp, 1919) is a small parasite which occurs in the intestine of the dog in the United States. It has been suggested that the parasite may also occur in the coyote. The male is 6–13 mm. long and the female 7–14 mm., both sexes being 2–4 mm. thick. The shape of the body is roughly conical, tapering backwards, and it has a dark grey colour. The proboscis bears six transverse rows of six hooks each. The anterior hooks have the shape of a taenioid hook, while the posterior ones resemble rose thorns. The lemnisci are very long and slender. The testes are oval, tandem and situated in the anterior half of the body. The eggs are oval, brown in colour and measure 59–71 by 40–50 μ.

Life-cycle. Immature forms, about 4 mm. long, which are believed to belong to this species, have been found encysted in the connective tissue and muscles of the armadillo (*Dasypus novemcinctus*). Whether this animal is the only or a secondary intermediate host or a false final host is uncertain. Probably dogs could acquire the parasite by ingesting the immature forms which occur in the armadillo.

Pathogenicity. The worms lie with their probosces deeply embedded in the intestinal wall, penetrating right through to the peritoneum. The parasite may possibly cause rabiform signs in dogs. Such were observed in a dog which harboured about 300 of the worms.

Diagnosis can be made by finding the eggs in the faeces.

Treatment and Prophylaxis—unknown.

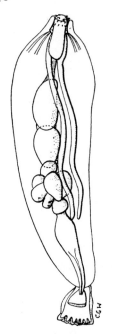

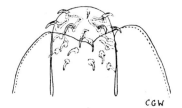

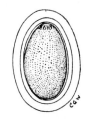

FIG. 168.   *Oncicola canis*,
Male (after Prince)

FIG. 169.   *Oncicola canis*,
Anterior End (after Price)

FIG. 170.   *Oncicola canis*,
Egg (after Price)

Phylum: Annelida

CLASS: HIRUDINEA

The Hirudinea or leeches, are not usually considered as 'helminths', but are included here as parasitic worms in the wide sense of the term. They are soft-bodied and usually dorso-ventrally flattened worms with a true metameric segmentation, but this has become obscured by specialisation. The annulations visible externally are more numerous than the metameric segments, the number of which, according to different authorities, is thirty-three or thirty-four and these segments are externally subdivided by transverse lines into two to fourteen rings each. The anterior region is differentiated to form a head which bears a triangular anteroventral sucker. The posterior seven segments form a large sucker except in one genus, and the anus is situated on the dorsal aspect of the hind end. The ninth, tenth and eleventh segments form the clitellar organ which serves to secrete the cocoon in which the eggs are deposited.

In the Gnathobdellidae the anterior sucker contains the oral aperture, which is provided with three strong toothed jaws, while the Rhynchobdellidae have a protrusible proboscis, but no jaws. There is a short oesophagus and a stomach (crop), which is usually provided with paired, segmentally-arranged, blind sacs for storage of ingested blood, followed by an intestine and a rectum. The body cavity is filled with a lacunar tissue. The excretory organs are segmentally arranged nephridia.

The worms are hermaphrodite. There are several to many testes which have a common duct on either side, and one pair of ovaries. The median male genital opening is on the tenth segment and the median female genital opening on the eleventh segment. The eggs are laid in cocoons secreted by the clitellum.

The leeches are occasional parasites. They feed on blood of various animals to which they attach themselves and drop off after having engorged. They have pharyngeal glands which secrete an anticoagulatory substance; this is injected into the wound made by the leech, and bleeding may continue for some time after the leech has dropped off. Leeches are vectors of certain trypanosomes and their relatives are parasitic in marine and freshwater fish.

The species of medical and veterinary interest belong to the Gnathobdellidae.

Genus: Hirudo Linnaeus, 1758

H. medicinalis Linnaeus, 1758, is the leech formerly used for medicinal purposes. It is 8–12 cm. long and 1–2 cm. wide. The dorsal surface is greyish-green with six longitudinal reddish bands; the ventral surface is olive-green with a black band on either side. It occurs in Europe and North Africa and lives in marshes, small streams and pools of water. It is of little interest as a possible parasite, but occasionally animals may become infected.

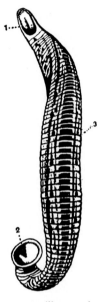

1, Mouth; 2, posterior sucker; 3, sensory papillae on the anterior annulus of each segment. The remaining four annuli which make up each true segment are indicated by the markings on the dorsal surface

FIG. 171. *Hirudo medicinalis* (from Shipley, A. E. & McBride, E. W., *Zoology*, 1901. Cambridge University Press)

Genus: Limnatis Moquin-Tandon, 1826

L. nilotica (Savigny, 1820) occurs in Europe and North Africa in pools of water which contain plants. It is 8–12 cm. long and its body is soft. The dorsal surface is fairly dark brown or greenish and usually has several longitudinal rows of black spots. The ventral surface is darker than the dorsal and there is frequently an orange band on either side. The anterior lip has a longitudinal groove on its inner surface. The adult worms live at the bottom in the mud; the young leeches, however, occur near the surface and are very easily attracted by steps at the water's edge.

The young leeches can readily be swallowed by animals drinking in such ponds, and infection occurs chiefly in dry years when water is scarce. This leech is very troublesome in Bulgaria; cattle, buffaloes, equines, sheep, dogs, pigs and man may become infected.

Pathogenesis. The parasites attach themselves in the pharynx and nasal cavities, where they may stay for days or even weeks. They suck blood, so that in severe infections anaemia and loss of condition may be produced. More serious is the frequent occurrence of oedemas in the affected areas. Blood or bloody froth may often be seen exuding from the mouth or nostrils of the animals. There is dyspnoea, and in severe cases the neck is extended and the mouth is held open. Oedematous swellings may be seen in the parotid and intermandibular regions. Death may be caused by asphyxia, and it may occur suddenly as a result of oedema of the glottis.

Diagnosis is made from the clinical signs and by finding the parasites in the pharynx.

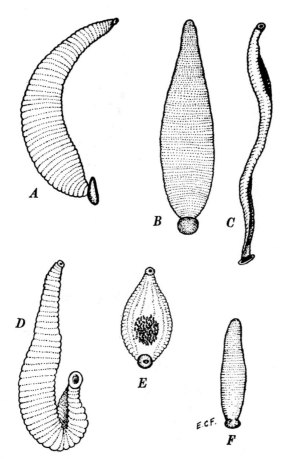

A, *Limnatis nilotica* (adapted from Brumpt); B, dorsal view and C, lateral view of extended specimen of *Hirudo medicinalis* (adapted from Schmidt); D, *Haemopis sanguisuga* (adapted from Blanchard); E, *Placobdella parasitica*, ventral view, with brood of attached young (adapted from Hemingway in Nachtrieb); F, *Haemadipsa zeylanica*, dorsal view (adapted from Brumpt)

FIG. 172. Habit Sketches of Leeches. × 1 (from Faust, E. C., *Animal Agents and Vectors of Human Disease*, 1955, Henry Kimpton, London, by courtesy of the Publisher)

Treatment. The injection of chloroform water gives very successful results. An elastic catheter is passed through the inferior nasal meatus and to the free end a 60 ml. syringe containing the solution is attached. The solution is injected slowly while the catheter is revolved, the head of the animal being held in a horizontal position. In extreme cases tracheotomy may be necessary.

Prophylaxis. The animals should be watered from clean troughs. Leeches in water can be killed by means of copper sulphate as applied for snails.

L. africana occurs in West Africa. It is about 12 cm. long when fully extended. According to Sambor. it is found attached in the nasal cavities of man, dogs and monkeys and frequently protrudes through the nostril. The leech is taken in while drinking infected water, and it may cause debility and marked local disturbances. It may enter, and cause bleeding from, the vagina or urethra of people bathing.

Genus: Haemadipsa Tennant, 1861

The species of this genus are small leeches, measuring about 2–3 cm. in length. They occur in tropical forests of Asia and South America and live on trees, shrubs and rocks, attaching themselves to passing animals and human beings. These leeches are very active and creep in even under tight-fitting clothing. Their bite is not painful, but the wounds may bleed for a long time. When groups of these leeches attach themselves to the ankles of human beings or the legs of horses and other animals, severe irritation and anaemia may result. Death has been attributed to them, but they are not usually fatal.

Species found in aquatic birds. Aquatic birds belonging to the family Anatidae may harbour in their nasal cavities leeches belonging to various genera, among which are: *Dina parva, Protoclepsis tesselata, Placobdella rugosa* and *Theromyzon* spp. Roberts (1955) described severe kerato-conjunctivitis in domesticated geese in Shropshire, England, caused by numerous individuals of the small species *Theromyzon tessulatum*, normally an inhabitant of the nasal sinuses, which had attacked the eyes of the geese. For species recorded from these and other Anatidae see Lapage (1961).

REFERENCES

NEMATODES, GENERAL

BAYLIS, H. A. & DAUBNEY, R. (1926). *A Synopsis of the Families and Genera of the Nematoda.* London: British Museum

BIRD, A. F. (1957). Chemical composition of the Nematode cuticle. Observations on individual layers and extracts from these layers in *Ascaris lumbricoides* cuticle. *Exp. Parasit.,* **6**, 383–403

CHITWOOD, B. G. (1933). A revised classification of the Nematoda. *J. Parasit.,* **20**, 131

CHITWOOD, B. G. & CHITWOOD, M. B. (1937). *An Introduction to Nematology,* sect. I, part I. Baltimore, Maryland: Monumental Printing Co.

HINZ, E. (1963). Elektronenmikroskopische Untersuchungen an *Parascaris equorum. Protopolasma,* **56**, 202–241

LEE, D. L. (1965). The cuticle of adult *Nippostrongylus brasiliensis. Parasitology,* **55**, 173–181

READ, C. P. (1966). Nutrition of intestinal helminths. *The Biology of Parasites* (Ed. by E. J. L. Soulsby). New York and London: Academic Press.

TANAKA, Y. (1961). Histochemical study on tissues of *Ascaris lumbricoides*, with special reference to the digestive organ. *J. Tokyo med. Coll.*, **19**, 1499–1510 (English summary)

ASCAROIDEA

ACKERT, J. E., EDGAR, S. A. & FRICK, L. P. (1939). Goblet cells and age resistance of animals to parasitism. *Trans. Am. microscop. Soc.*, **58**, 81–89
BEAVER, P. C. (1956). Larva migrans. *Exp. Parasit.*, **5**, 587–621
BEAVER, P. C. (1966). Zoonoses, with particular reference to parasites of veterinary importance. *Biology of Parasites* (Ed. by E. J. L. Soulsby). New York: Academic Press
BERGER, H., WOOD, I. B. & WILLEY, C. H. (1961). Observations on the development and egg production of *Ascaris suum* in rabbits. *J. Parasit.* (suppl.), **47**, 15
DE BOER, E. (1935). Experimenteel onderzoek betreffend *Ascaris lumbricoides* van mensch en varken. *Tijdschr. Diergeneesk.*, **62**, 965–973
CAMPBELL, D. H. (1937). The immunological specificity of a polysacchaside fraction from some common parasitic helminths. *J. Parasit.* **23**, 348–353
DONE, J. T., RICHARDSON, M. D. & GIBSON, T. E. (1960). Experimental visceral larva migrans in the pig. *Res. vet. Sci.*, **1**, 133–151
DOUGLAS, J. R. & BAKER, N. R. (1959). The chronology of experimental intrautine infections with *Toxocara canis* (Werner, 1782) in the dog. *J. Parasit.*, **45**, (Suppl.) 43–44
EGERTON, J. R. (1961). The effect of thiabendazole upon *Ascaris* and *Stephanurus* infections. *J. Parasit.*, **47** (Suppl.) 37
FAIRBAIRN, D. (1961). The in vitro hatching of *Ascaris lumbricoides* eggs. *Can. J. Zool.*, **39**, 153–162
LEE, R. P. (1956). Stategic medication against *Neoascaris vitulorum*. *Bull. Epizoot. Dis. Afr.*, **4**, 61–63
LEE, R. P. (1959). *Symposium on Helminthiasis in Domestic Animals*. Publication No. 49. I.A.C.E.D. C.C.T.A. p. 131
PETTER, C. (1960). Etude zoologique de la larva migrans. *Ann. Parasit. hum. comp.*, **35**, 118–137
ROBERTS, F. H. S. (1934). *The Large Roundworm of Pigs, Ascaris lumbricoides L. 1758. Its Life History in Queensland, Economic Influence and Control*. Queensland Dept. Agric. and Stock Animal Hlth Stat. Yeerongpilly, Bull. No. 1, 1–81
ROGERS, W. P. (1960). The physiology of infective processes of Nematode parasites. The stimulus from the animal host. *Proc. R. Soc.* (B), **152**, 367–386
RONEUS, O. (1963). Parasitic liver lesions in swine experimentally produced by visceral larva migrans of *Toxocara cati*. *Acta vet. scand.*, **4**, 170–196
SOULSBY, E. J. L. (1961). Unpublished observations
SOULSBY, E. J. L. (1965). *Textbook of Veterinary Clinical Parasitology*. Vol. I. *Helminths*. Oxford: Blackwell Scientific Publications
SPRENT, J. F. A. (1952). Anatomical distinction between human and pig strains of *Ascaris Nature, Lond.*, **170**, 627–628
SPRENT, J. F. A. (1955). On the invasion of the central nervous system in ascariasis. *Parasitology*, **45**, 41–55
SPRENT, J. F. A. (1956). The life history and development of *Toxocara cati*. *Parasitology*, **46**, 54–78
SPRENT, J. F. A. (1958). Observations on the development of *Toxocara canis* (Werner, 1782) in the dog. *Parasitology*, **48**, 184–209
SPRENT, J. F. A. (1959). The life history and development of *Toxascaris leonina* (von Linstow, 1902) in dog and cat. *Parasitology*, **49**, 330–371
SPRENT, J. F. A. (1961). Post-parturient infection of the bitch with *Toxocara canis*. *J. Parasit.*, **47**, 284
TAFFS, L. F. (1961). Immunological studies on experimental infection of pigs with *Ascaris suum* (Goeze 1782). An introduction with a review of the literature and the demonstration of complement-fixing antibodies in the serum. *J. Helminth.*, **35**, 319–344
TUGWELL, R. L. & ACKERT, J. E. (1952). On the tissue phase of the life cycle of the fowl Nematode *Ascaridia galli* (Schrank). *J. Parasit.*, **38**, 277–288

OXYURATA—SUBULUROIDEA

BAKER, A. D. (1933). Some observations on the development of the caecal worm *Heterakis gallinae* (Gmelin, 1790; Freeborn, 1923), in the domestic fowl. *Sci. Agric*, **13**, 356–363
OSIPOV, A N. (1957). Survival of *Heterakis gallinarum* ova in winter. *Trudy Moskovsk. Vet. Akad.*, **19**, 350–355

RHABDITOIDEA

BEVERIDGE, W. I. B. (1934). Foot-rot in sheep. Skin penetration by Strongyloides larvae as a predisposing factor. *Aust. vet. J.*, **10**, 43–51
CHANG, P. C. H. & Graham, G. L. (1957). Parasitism, parthenogenesis and polyploidy; the life cycle of *Strongyloides papillosus*. *J. Parasit.*, **43** (Suppl.), 13
CHITWOOD, B. G. (1932). The association of *Rhabditis strongyloides* with dermatitis in dogs. *N. Am. Vet.*, **13**, 35–40

IPPEN, R. (1953). Zur Pathogenitat des *Strongyloides ransomi* unter besonderer Berücksuchtigung seines Sitzes in der Schleimhaut der Darmwand. *Arch. exp. vet. Med.*, **7**, 36–57

LITTLE, M. D. (1962). Experimental studies on the life cycle of Strongyloides. *J. Parasit.*, **48**, 41

MONOCOE, D. J. & BATTLE, E. G. (1966). Transcolostral infection of newborn pigs with *Strongyloides ransomi*. *Vet. Med. small Anim. Clin.*, June, 583–586

PANDE, B. P. and RAO, P. (1960). The nematode genus *Strongyloides grassi* 1879 in Indian livestock. I. Observations on natural infections in the donkey (*Equus asinus*). *Br. vet. J.*, **116**, 281

PREMVATI (1958). Studies on Strongyloides of primates. III. Observations on the free-living generations of *S. fülleborni*. *Can. J. Zool.*, **36**, 447–457

SOULSBY, E. J. L. (1965). *Textbook of Veterinary Clinical Parasitology*. Vol. I. Helminths. Oxford: Blackwell Scientific Publications

SUPPERER, R. & PFEIFFER, H. (1960). Ueber die Strongyloidose der Kalber. *Wien tierärztl. Mschr.*, **47**, 361—368

TURNER, J. H. (1959). Experimental strongyloidiasis in sheep and goats. I. Single infections. *Am. J. vet. Res.*, **20**, 102–110

STRONGYLOIDEA—STRONGYLIDAE

DRUDGE, J. H., LYONS, E. T. & SZANTO, J. (1966). Pathogenesis of migrating stages of helminths with special reference to *Strongylus* species. *Biology of Parasites* (Ed. by E. J. L. Soulsby), New York: Academic Press

ENIGK, K. (1952). Zur Entwicklung von *Strongylus vulgaris* (Nematoden) In Wirtstier. *Z. Tropenmed. Parasit,*. **2**, 287–306

ERSHOV, V. S. (1949). Cycle of development of *Delafondia vulgaris* (Loos, 1900) in the horse. *Veterinariya*, **26**, 26–28

FARRELLY, B. T. (1954). The pathogenesis and significance of parasitic endoarteritis and thrombosis in the ascending aorta of the horse. *Vet. Rec.*, **66**, 53–61

LEVINE, N. D. (1963). Weather, climate and bionomics of ruminant nematode larvae. *Advances in Veterinary Science*. Vol. 8, pp. 215–261 (Ed. by C. A. Brandly & E. L. Jungherr). New York: Academic Press.

OLT, A. (1932). Das Aneurysma Verminosum des Pferdes und seine unbekannten Beziehungen zur Kolik. *Dt. tierärztl. Wschr.*, **40**, 326–332

OTTAWAY, C. W. & BINGHAM, M. L. '(1946). Further observation on the incidence of parasitic aneurysm in the horse. *Vet. Rec.*, **58**, 155–159

POYNTER, D. (1956). Effect of a coliform organism (*Escherichia*) on the second ecdysis of nematode larvae parasitic in the horse. *Nature, Lond.*, **177**, 481–482

POYNTER, D. (1960). The arterial lesions produced by *Strongylus vulgaris* and their relationship to the migratory route of the parasite in its host. *Res. Vet. Sci.*, **1**, 205–217

SOULSBY, E. J. L. (1965). *Textbook of Veterinary Clinical Parasitology*. Vol. I. Helminths. Oxford: Blackwell Scientific Publications

THRELKELD, W. (1948). The life history and pathogenicity of *Chabertia ovina*. *Va. agric. exp. St. Tech. Bull. No. II*

WETZEL, R. (1941). Zur Entwicklung des grossen Palisadenwurmes (*Strongylus equinus*) im Pferd. *Arch. wiss. prakt. Tierheilk.*, **76**, 81–118

WETZEL, R. (1952). Die Entwicklungsdauer (Prepatent periode) von *Strongylus endentatus* in Pferd. *Dt. tierärztl. Wschr.*, **59**, 129–130

WETZEL, R. & DERSTEN, W. (1956). Die Leberphase der Entwicklung von *Strongylus edentatus*. *Wien. tierärztl. Mschr.*, **43**, 664–672

WETZEL, R. & ENIGK, K. (1938). Wandern die Larven der Palisadenwurmer (*Strongylus* spec.) der Pferde durch die Lungen. *Arch. wiss. prakt. Tierheilk.*, **73**, 83–93

WETZEL, R. & VOGELSANG, E. G. (1954). Helmintiasis intestinal del equino. *Rev. med. vet. parasit. Caracas*, **13**, 17–25

STRONGYLOIDEA—TRICHONEMATIDAE

ANANTARAMAN, M. (1942). The life history of *Oesophagostomum radiatum*, the bovine nodular worm. *Ind. J. vet. Sci.*, **12**, 87–132

EGERTON, J. R., CUCKLER, A. C., AMES, E. R., BRAMEL, R. G., BRIGHTENBACK, G. E. & WASHKO, F. N. (1962). Anthelmintic effect of thiabendazole on intestinal nematodes in horses. *J. Parasit.* **48** (Suppl.) 29

ENIGK, K. & STOYE, M. (1963). Versuche zur Behandlung des Strongyliden befalls der Pferde mit Thiabendazol. *Dt. tierärztl. Wschr.*, **70**, 257–261

GIBSON, T. E. (1960). Some experiences with small daily doses of phenothiazine as a means of control of strongylid worms in the horse. *Vet. Rec.*, **72**, 37–41

GIBSON, T. E. (1965). *Veterinary Anthelmintic Medication*, 2nd edn. Tech. Comm. No. 33 Commonwealth Bureau of Helminthology. Farnham Royal, England: Commonwealth Agricultural Bureaux

GOLDBERG, A. (1952). Effects of the nematode *Oesophagostomum venulosum* on sheep and goats. *J. Parasit.*, **38**, 35–47

GORDON, H. McL. (1950). Some aspects of parasitic gastro-enteritis of sheep. *Aust. vet. J.* **26**, 14–28, 46–52, 65–72, 93–98

SOULSBY, E. J. L. (1965). *Textbook of Veterinary Clinical Parasitology*. Vol. I. *Helminths*. Oxford: Blackwell Scientific Publications

WETZEL, R. & VOGELSANG, E. G. (1954). Helmintiasis intestinal del equino. *Rev. med. vet. parasit.* Caracas, **13**, 17–25

STRONGYLOIDEA—STEPHANURIDAE

ALICATA, J. E. (1953). Observations on the lethal action of polyborate on swine kidney worm (*Stephanurus dentatus*) larvae in soil. *Am. J. vet. Res.*, **14**, 563–570

ALICATA, J. E. (1961). On the ineffectiveness of thiabendazole against the migrating larval stages of the swine kidney worm (*Stephanurus dentatus*) in rabbits. *J. Parasit.*, **47** (Suppl.) 38

BATTE, E. G., HARKEMA, R. & OSBORNE, J. C. (1960). Observations on the life cycle and pathogenicity of the swine kidney worm (*Stephanurus dentatus*). *J. Am. vet. Med. Ass.*, **136**, 622–625

EGERTON, J. R. (1961). The effect of thiabendazole upon *Ascaris* and *Stephanurus* infections. *J. Parasit.*, **47** (suppl.) 37

TROMBA, E. G. and BAISDON, L. A. (1960) Diagnosis of experimental stephanuriasis in swine by a double diffusion agar precipitin technique. *J. Parasit.*, **46** (Suppl.) 29

STRONGYLOIDEA—SYNGAMIDAE

CLAPHAM, P. A. (1935). The treatment of gapeworm disease. *J. Helminth.* **13**, 3–8

HORTON-SMITH, C., LONG, P. L. & ROWEL, J. G. (1963). Effects of thiabendazole on experimental infestations of *Syngamus trachea*. *Br. Poult. Sci.*, **4**, 217

MORGAN, D. O. & CLAPHAM, P. A. (1934). Some observations on gapeworm in poultry and game birds. *J. Helminth.*, **12**, 63–70

STRONGYLOIDEA—ANCYLOSTOMATIDAE

BAKER, N. R. & DOUGLAS, J. R. (1966). Blood alterations in helminth infections. *Biology of Parasites* (Ed. by E. J. L. Soulsby). New York: Academic Press

BEAVER, P. C. (1956). Parasitological reviews. Larva migrans. *Exp. Parasit.*, **5**, 587–621

BEAVER, P. C. (1966). Zoonoses, with particular reference to parasites of veterinary importance. *Biology of Parasites* (Ed. by E. J. L. Soulsby). New York: Academic Press

BIOCCA, E. (1954). Ridescrizione di *Ancylostoma tubaeforme* (Zeder, 1800) parassita del gatto, considerato erroneamente sinonimo di *Ancylostoma caninum* (Ercolani, 1859) Parassita del cane. *Riv. Parassit.*, **15**, 267–278

BURROWS, R. B. (1962). Comparative morphology of *Ancylostoma tubaeforme* (Zeder, 1800) and *Ancylostoma caninum* (Erocolani, 1859). *J. Parasit.*, **48**, 715–718

CLARKE, C. H., KLING, J. M., WOODLEY, C. H. & SHARP, N. (1961). A quantitative measurement of the blood loss caused by ancytostomiasis in dogs. *Am. J. vet. Res.*, **22**, 370

DOW, C., JARRETT, W. F. H., JENNINGS, F. W., McINTYRE, W. I. M. & MULLIGAN, W. (1961). Studies on immunity to *Uncinaria stenocephala* infection in the dog. Double vaccination with irradiated larvae. *Am. J. vet. Res.*, **22**, 352–354

FOSTER, A. O. & LANSBERG, J. W. (1934). The nature and cause of hookworm anemia. *Am. J. Hyg.*, **20**, 259–290

FOY, H. and KONDI, A. (1961). Symposium on hookworm disease. III. The relation of hookworm loads and species to intestinal blood loss and the genesis of iron deficiency anaemia. *Trans. R. Soc. trop. Med. Hyg.*, **55**, 26–99

GIBSON, T. E. (1965). *Veterinary Anthelmintic Medication*. 2nd edn. Tech. Comm. No. 33, Commonwealth Bureau of Helminthology. Farnham Royal, England: Commonwealth Agricultural Bureaux

KRUPP, I. M. (1961). The effect of *Ancylostoma caninum* infection on erythropoieses in dogs. *Am. J. trop. Med. Hyg.*, **10**, 510–514

McCOY, O. R. (1931). Immunity reactions of the dog against hookworm (*Ancylostoma caninum*) under conditions of repeated infection. *Am. J. Hyg.*, **14**, 268–303

MILLER, T. A. (1965a). Studies on canine ancylostomiasis. Double vaccination with X-irradiated *Ancylostoma caninum* larvae. *J. Am. vet. med. Ass.*, **146**, 41–44

MILLER, T. A. (1965b). Persistence of immunity following double vaccination of pups with X-irradiated *Ancylostoma caninum* larvae. *J. Parasit.*, **51**, 705–711

MILLER, T. A. (1966). Comparison of the immunogenic efficiencies of normal and X-irradiated *Ancylostoma caninum* larvae in dogs. *J. Parasit.*, **52**, 512–519

ORTLEPP, R. J. (1937). Observations on the morphology and life-history of *Gaigeria pachyscelis* (Raill. and Henry, 1910): A hookworm parasite of sheep and goats. *Onderstepoort J. vet. Sci.*, **8**, 183–212

SHEEHY, T. W., MERONEY, W. H., COX, R. S. & SOLER, J. E. (1962). Hookworm disease and malabsorption. *Gastroenterology*, **42**, 148–156

STONE, W. M. & GIRARDEAU, M. H. (1966). *Ancylostoma caninum* larvae present in the colostrum of a bitch. *Vet. Rec.*, **79**, 773

WEINER, D. (1960). Larva migrans. *Vet. Med.*, **55**, 38–40, 45–50

WELLS, H. S. (1931). Observations on the blood sucking activities of the hookworm *Ancylostoma caninum*. *J. Parasit.*, **17**, 167–182

STRONGYLOIDEA—AMIDOSTOMIDAE

COWAN, A. B. (1955). Some preliminary observations on the life history of *Amidostomum anseris* Zeder, 1800. *J. Parasit.*, **41** (Suppl.) 43–44

KOBULEJ, T. (1956). Beiträge zur Biologie des *Amidostomum anseris* (Zeder, 1800). *Acta vet. Hung.*, **6**, 429–449

TRICHOSTRONGYLOIDEA—TRICHOSTRONGYLIDAE

BAKER, N. F. & DOUGLAS, J. R. (1966). Blood alterations in helminths infection. *Biology of Parasites* (Ed. by E. J. L. Soulsby). New York: Academic Press

BREMNER, K. C. (1955). Cytological polymorphism in the nematode *Haemonchus contortus* (Rudolphi, 1803) Cobb, 1898. *Nature, Lond.*, **174**, 704–705

BREMNER, K. C. (1956). The parasitic life cycle of *Haemonchus placei* (Place) Ransom (Nematoda: Trichostrongylidae). *Aust. J. Zool.*, **4**, 146–151

CORNWELL, R. L. (1966). Controlled laboratory trials in sheep with the anthelmintic Pyrantel tartrate. *Vet. Rec.*, **79**, 590–595

CROFTON, H. D. (1963). *Nematode Parasite Population in Sheep and on Pasture*. St. Albans, England: Commonwealth Bureau of Helminthology

CROFTON, H. D. & THOMAS, R. J. (1954). A further description of *Nematodirus battus* Crofton and Thomas, 1951. *J. Helminth.*, **28**, 119–122

DAS, K. M. & WHITLOCK, J. H. (1960). Subspeciation in *Haemonchus contortus* (Rudolphi 1803) Nematoda, Trichostrongyloidea. *Cornell Vet.*, **50**, 182–197

DINABURG, A. G. (1944). Development and survival under outdoor conditions of eggs and larvae of the common ruminant stomach worm *Haemonchus contortus*. *J. agric. Res.*, **69**, 421–433

DINNIK, J. A. & DINNIK, N. N. (1958). Observations on the development of *Haemonchus contortus* larvae under field conditions in the Kenya highlands. *Bull. epizoot. Dis. Afr.*, **6**, 11–21

DOUVRES, F. W. (1957). The morphogenesis of the parasitic stages of *Trichostrongylus axei* and *Trichostrongylus colubriformis*, nematode parasites of cattle. *Proc. helminth. Soc. Wash.*, **24**, 4–11

DURIE, P. H. (1961). Parasitic gastro-interitis of cattle: The distribution and survival of infective strongyle larvae on pasture. *Aust. J. agric. Res.*, **12**, 1200–1211

FERNANDO, S. T. (1962). Ph.D. Thesis, University of Cambridge

GIBSON, T. E. (1965). *Veterinary Anthelmintic Medication*. 2nd. Ed. Tech. Comm. No. 33. Commonwealth Bureau of Helminthology, Farnham Royal, England: Commonwealth Agricultural Bureaux

GORDON, H. McL. (1958). Studies on anthelmintics for sheep. Some organic phosphorus compounds. *Aust. vet. J.*, **34**, 104–110

HERLICH, H., PORTER, D. A. & KNIGHT, R. A. (1958). A study of *Haemonchus* in cattle and sheep. *Am. J. vet. Res.*, **19**, 866–872

JARRETT, W. F. H., JENNINGS, F. W., McINTYRE, W. I. M. & SHARP, N. C. C. (1960). Resistance to *Trichostrongylus colubriformis* produced by X-irradiated Larvae. *Vet. Rec.*, **72**, 884.

KATES, K. C. (1950). Survival on pasture of free-living stages of some common gastro-intestinal nematodes of sheep. *Proc. Helminth. Soc. Wash.*, **17**, 39–58

KOTLAN, A. (1949). On the histotropic phase of the parasitic larvae of *Hyostrongylus rubidus*. *Acat. vet. Hung.*, **1**, 76–82

KOTLAN, A. (1960). *Helminthologie*. Budapest: Akademiai Kiado

LEVINE, N. D. (1963). Weather climate and bionomics of ruminant nematode larvae. *Advances in Veterinary Science* (Ed. by C. A. Brandly & E. L. Jungherr), Vol. 8, pp. 215–261. New York: Academic Press

MANTON, V. J. A., PEACOCK, R., POYNTER, D., SILVERMAN, P. H. & TERRY, R. J. (1962). The influence of age on naturally acquired resistance to *Haemonchus contortus*. *Res. vet. Sci.* **3**, 308–313

MARTIN, W. B., THOMAS, B. A. C. & URQUHART, G. M. (1957). Chronic diarrhoea in housed cattle due to atpical parasitic gastritis. *Vet. Rec.*, **69**, 736–739

MULLIGAN, W., GORDON, H. McL., STEWART, D. F. & WAGLAND, B. M. (1961) The use of irradiated larvae as immunizing agents in *Haemonchus controtus* and *Trichostrongylus colubriformis* infections of sheep. *Aust. J. agric. Res.*, **12**, 1175–1187

MULLIGAN, W., DALTON, R. G. & ANDERSON, N. (1963). Ostertagiasis in cattle. *Vet. Rec.*, **75**, 1014

ROBERTS, F. H. S. (1957). Reactions of calves to infestation with the stomach worm *Haemonchus placei* (Place, 1893) Ransom, 1911. *Aust. J. agric. Res.*, **8**, 740–767

ROBERTS, F. H. S., TURNER, H. N. & McKEVETT, M. (1954). On the specific distinctness of the ovine and bovine 'strains' of *Haemonchus contortus* (Rudolphi) Cobb (Nematoda: Trichostrongylidae). *Aust. J. Zool.*, **2**, 275–295

ROGERS, W. P. (1960). The physiology of infective processes of nematode parasites. The stimulus from the animal host. *Proc. R. Soc.* (B), **152**, 367–386

ROGERS, W. P. (1963). Physiology of infection with nematodes: Some effects of the host stimulus on infective stages. *Ann. N. Y. Acad. Sci.*, **113**, 208–216

ROGERS, W. P. (1965). The role of leucine aminopeptidase in the moulting of nematode parasites. *Comp. Biochem. Physiol.*, **14**, 311–321

ROGERS, W. P. (1966). Exsheathment and hatching mechanisms in helminths. *Biology of Parasites* (Ed. by E. J. L. Soulsby). New York: Academic Press

ROGERS, W. P. & SOMMERVILLE, R. I. (1960). The physiology of the second ecdysis of parasitic nematodes. *Parasitology*, **50**, 329–348

SHANKS, P. L. (1963). Treatment of *Hyostrongylus rubidus* in Sows. *Vet. Rec.*, **75**, 287
SILANGWA, S. M. & TODD, A. C. (1964). Vertical migration of trichostrongylid larvae on grasses. *J. Parasit.*, **50**, 278–285
SILVERMAN, P. H. & CAMPBELL, J. A. (1959). Studies on parasitic worms of sheep in Scotland. I. Embryonic and larval development of *Haemonchus controtus* at constant conditions. *Parasitology*, **49**, 23–38
SILVERMAN, P. H., POYNTER, D. & PODGER, R. R. (1962). Studies on larval antigens derived by cultivation of some parasitic nematodes in simple media. Protection tests in laboratory animals. *J. Parasit.*, **48**, 562–571
SOMMERVILLE, R. I. (1960). The growth of *Cooperia curticei* (Giles, 1892) a nematode parasite of sheep. *Parasitology*, **50**, 261–267
SOULSBY, E. J. L. (1957). Studies on the serological response in sheep to naturally acquired gastro-intestinal nematodes. II. Responses in a low ground flock. *J. Helminth.*, **31**, 145–160
SOULSBY, E. J. L. (1965). *Textbook of Veterinary Clinical Parasitology.* Vol. I. *Helminths.* Oxford: Blackwell Scientific Publications
SOULSBY, E. J. L. (1966). The mechanisms of immunity to gastro-intestinal nematodes. *Biology of Parasites* (Ed. by E. J. L. Soulsby). New York: Academic Press
SOULSBY, E. J. L. & STEWART, D. F. (1960). Serological studies of the self cure reaction in sheep infected with *Haemonchus contortus*. *Aust. J. agric. Res.*, **11**, 595–603
SPEDDING, C. R. W. (1962). Modern trends in animal health and husbandry. The agricultural ecology of sheep grazing. *Br. vet. J.*, **118**, 461–481
STEWART, D. F. (1953). Studies on resistance to sheep to infestation with *Haemonchus contortus* and *Trichostrongylus* spp. and on the immunological reactions of sheep exposed to infestation. V. The nature of the self cure phenomenon. *Aust. J. agric. Res.*, **4**, 100–117
THOMAS, R. J. & STEVENS, A. J. (1960). Ecological studies on the development of the pasture stages of *Nematodirus battus* and *N. filicollis*, nematode parasites of sheep. *Parasitology*, **50**, 31–49
WALLEY, J. K. (1966). Tetramisole (dl 2, 3, 5, 6-tetrahydro-6-phenyl-imidazo(2, 1-b)thiazole hydrochloride-Nilverm) in the treatment of gastro-intestinal and lungworms in domestic animals. I. Sheep and goats. *Vet. Rec.*, **78**, 406–414

TRICHOSTRONGYLOIDEA—DICTYOCAULIDAE

ENIGK, K. (1957). Erfahrungen mit der Aerosolbehandlung beim Lungenwurmbefall des Rindes. *Z. tropenmed. Parasit.*, **8**, 54–59
JARRETT, W. F. H., McINTYRE, W. I. M. & URQUHART, G. M. (1957). Husk in cattle. A review of a year's work. *Vet. Rec.*, **66**, 665–676
JARRETT, W. R. H., JENNINGS, F. W., McINTYRE, W. I. M., MULLIGAN. W., SHARP, N. C. C. & URQUHART, G. M. (1960a). Symposium on husk. I. The disease process. *Vet. Rec.*, **72**, 1066–1067, 1068, 1086–1087
JARRETT, W. F. H., JENNINGS, F. W., McINTYRE, W. I. M., MULLIGAN, W. & URQUHART, G. M. (1960b). Immunological studies on *Dictyocaulus viviparus* infection. Immunity produced by the administration of irradiated larvae. *Immunology*, **3**, 145–151
JARRETT, W. F. H. & SHARP, N. C. C. (1963). Vaccination against parasitic disease. Reactions in vaccinated and immune hosts in *Dictyocaulus viviparus* infection. *J. Parasit.*, **49**, 177–189
MICHEL, J. F. & ROSE, J. H. (1954). Some observations on the free-living stages of the cattle lungworm in relation to their natural environment. *J. comp. path.*, **64**, 195–205
MICHEL, J. F. (1962). Studies on resistance to *Dictyocaulus* infection. IV. The rate of acquisition of protective immunity in infection of *D. viviparus*. *J. comp. Path.*, **72**, 281–285
POYNTER, D., JONES, B. V., NELSON, A. M. R., PEACOCK, R., ROBINSON, J., SILVERMAN, P. H. & TERRY, R. J. (1960). Recent experiences with vaccination. *Vet. Rec.*, **72**, 1078–1090
ROBINSON, J. (1962). *Pilobolus* spp. and the translation of the infective larvae of *Dictyocaulus viviparus* from faeces to pastures. *Nature, Lond.*, **193**, 353–354
SOULSBY, E. J. L. (1965). *Textbook of Veterinary Clinical Parasitology.* Vol. I. *Helminths.* Oxford: Blackwell Scientific Publications
WALLEY, J. K. (1957). A new drug for the treatment of lungworms in domestic animals. *Vet. Rec.*, **69**, 815–824, 850–853

METASTRONGYLOIDEA

ALICATA, J. E. & BROWN, R. W. (1962). On the method of human infection with *Angiostrongylus contonensis* in Tahiti. *J. Parasit.*, **48**, 52
ANDERSON, R. I. (1963). The Incidence, development and experimental transmission of *Pneumostrongylus tenuis* (Dougherty) (Metastrongyloidea: Protostrongylidae) of the meninges of the white-tail deer (*Odocoileus virginianus borealis*) in Ontario. *Can. J. Zool.*, **41**, 775–792
ANDERSON, R. I. (1964). Neurologic disease in moose infected experimentally with *Pneumostrongylus tenuis* from white-tailed deer. *Path. Vet.*, **1**, 289–322
DORRINGTON, J. E. (1959). The treatment of *Filaroides osleri* infestation with dictycide. *Jl. S. Afr. vet. med. Ass.*, **30**, 27
DOUGHERTY, E. C. (1944). The genus *Metastrongylus* (Molin, 1861) (Nematoda: Metastrongylidae). *Proc. Helminth. Soc. Wash.*, **11**, 66
DOUGHERTY, E. C. (1951). A further revision in the classification of the family Metastrongylidae (Leiper, 1909) (Phylum Nematoda). *Parasitology*, **41**, 91–96

DURBIN, C. G. (1954). Emetine hydrochloride for the treatment of sheep and goats infested with protostrongyline lungworms. *Vet. Ext. Q. Univ. Pa.*, No. 133, 49–52

FITZSIMMONS, W. M. (1961). *Bronchostrongylus subcrenatus* (Railliet & Henry, 1913) a new parasite recorded from the domestic cat. *Vet. Rec.*, **73**, 101–102

GUILHON, J. (1960). Role des limacides dans le cycle evolutif d'*Angiostrongylus vasorum* (Baillet, 1866). *C. r. Acad. Sci. Paris*, **251**, 2252–2253

HAMILTON, J. M. (1963). *Aelurostrongylus abstrusus* infestation of the cat. *Vet. Rec.*, **75**, 417–422

KASSAI, T. (1958). A juhod tudofergessegeinek orvoslasa ditrazinfosafattal. *Magyar Allot. Lapja*, **13**, 9–13

LE ROUX, P. H. (1959). 'Dictycide' as moontlike behandeling vir *Filaroides osleri*. *J. S. Afr. vet. med. Ass.*, **30**, 40

MACKENZIE, A. (1958). Studies on lungworm infection of pigs. II. Lesions in experimental infections. *Vet. Rec.*, **70**, 903–906

MACKENZIE, A. (1963). Experimental observations on lungworm infection together with virus pneumonia in pigs. *Vet. Rec.*, **75**, 114–116

MALHERBE, N. D. (1954). The chemotheropy of *Filaroides osleri* (Cobbold 1879) infestation in dogs. A progress report. *Jl. S. Afr. vet. med. Ass.*, **25**, 9–12

ROSE, J. H. (1959). *Metastrongylus apri*, the pig lungworm. Observations on the free-living embryonated egg and the larvae in the intermediate host. *Parasitology*, **49**, 439–447

ROSEN, L., CHAPPELL, R., LAQUEUR, G. L., WALLACE, G. D. & WEINSTEIN, P. P. (1962). Eosinophilic meningitis caused by a metastrongylid lungworm of the rat. *J. Am. med. Ass.*, **179**, 620–624

SCHUL'Z, R. S., ORLOFF, I. W. & KUTASS, A. J. (1933). Zur Systematik der SUBFAMILIE *Synthetocaulinae* Skrj. 1932 nebst Beschreibung einiger neuer Gattungen and Arten. *Zool. Anz.*, **102**, 303–310

SHOPE, R. E. (1941). The swine lungworm as a reservoir and intermediate host for swine influenza virus. I. The presence of swine influenza virus in healthy and susceptible pigs. II. The transmission of swine influenza virus by the swine lungworm, *J. Exp. Med.*, **74**, 41–68

SHOPE, R. E. (1943). The swine lungworm as a reservoir and intermediate host for swine influenza virus. III. Factors influencing transmission of the virus and the provocation of influenza. *J. Exp. Med.*, **77**, 111–138

SHOPE, R. E. (1958). The swine lungworm as a reservoir and intermediate host for hog cholera virus. I. The provocation of masked hog cholera virus in lungworm-infested swine by *Ascaris* larvae, *J. exp. Med.*, **107**, 609–622

SHUMAKOVICH, E. E. (1948). Treatment of lung disease in sheep caused by *Mellerius capillaris*. *Proc. Lenin Acad. agric. Sci.*, **13**, 40–43

SKRJABIN, K. I., SHICKHOBALOVA, N. P., SCHULZ, R. S., POPOVA, T. I., BOEV, S. N. & DELYAMURE, S. L. (1952). *Strongylata*. Vol. III. *Key to Parasitic Nematodes*. Academy of Sciences, U.S.S.R. (English edition by Israel Program for Scientific Translations. Jerusalem, 1961.)

SUDDUTH, W. H. (1955). Lungworm infection in cats and its possible treatment. *J. Am. vet. med. Ass.*, **126**, 211–214

WALLEY, J. K. (1957). A new drug for the treatment of lungworms in domestic animals. *Vet. Rec.*, **69**, 818–824, 850–853

WETZEL, R. (1940). Zur Biologie des Fuchslungenwurmes *Crenosoma vulpis* I. Mitteilung. *Arch. wiss., prakt. Tierheilk.*, **75**, 445–460

SPIRUROIDEA

ALICATA, J. E. (1935). Early developmental stages of nematodes occurring in swine. *U.S. Dept. Agric. Tech. Bull. No.* **489**

BAILEY, W. S. (1963). Parasites and cancer: sarcoma in dogs associated with *Spirocerca lupi*. *Ann. N.Y. Acad. Sci.*, **108**, 890–923

CHANDLER, A. C. (1925). A contribution to the life-history of a Gnathostome. *Parasitology* **17**, 237–244

CRAM, E. B. (1927). Bird Parasites of the Nematode Suborders Strongylata, Ascaridata and Spirurata. *U.S. Nat. Mus. Bull.*, **140**

CRAM, E. B. (1936). Species of *Capillaria* parasitic in the upper digestive tract of birds. *U.S. Dept. Agric. Tech. Bull. No.* **516**

DARNE, A. & WEBB, J. L. (1964). The treatment of ankylostomiasis and of spirocercosis in dogs by the new compound, 2,6-diiodo-4-nitrophenol. *Vet. Rec.*, **76**, 171–172

EHLERS, G. H. (1931). The anthelmintic treatment of infestations of the badger with spirurids (*Physaloptera* sp.). *J. Am. vet. med. Ass.*, **31**, 79–87

HALPIN, R. B. & KIRKLY, W. W. (1962). Experience with an anthelmintic *Vet. Rec.*, **74**, 495

KLESOV, M. D. (1950). The biology of two nematodes of the genus *Thelazia* Bose, 1819, parasites of the eye of cattle. *Dokl. Akad. Nauk S.S.S.R.*, **75**, 591–594

KRASTIN, N. I. (1950). Determination of the cycle of development of *Thelazia gulosa*, parasite of the eye of cattle. *Dokl. Akad. Nauk S.S.S.R*, **70**, 549–551

KRASTIN, N. I. (1952). Determination of the cycle of development of *Thelazia skrjabini* (Erschow, 1928), parasite of the eye of cattle. *Dokl. Akad. Nauk S.S.S.R*, **82**, 829–831

McGAUGHEY, C. A. (1950). Preliminary note on the treatment of spirocercosis in dogs with a piperazine compound, Caricide (Lederle). *Vet. Rec.*, **62**, 814–815

MIYAZAKI, I. (1954). Studies on *Gnathostoma* occurring in Japan (Nematoda: *Gnathostomidae*). II. Life history of *Gnathostoma* and morphological comparison of its larval forms. *Kyusu Mem. Med. Sci.*, **5**, 123–140

NISHIYAMA, S. (1958). Studies on habronemiasis in horses. *Bull. Fac. Agric. Kagoshima. Univ.*, No. 7

PETRI, L. H. & AMEEL, D. J. (1950). Studies on the life cycle of *Physaloptera rara* (Hall and Wigdor, 1918), and *Physaloptera praeputialis* Linstow, 1889. *J. Parasit.*, **36**, (Suppl.) 40

RAO, D. S. P. (1953). Spirocercosis in a dog. *Indian vet. J.*, **29**, 548

VAIDYANATHAN, S. N. (1952). *Spirocera lupi* infection in dogs. A few cases treated with Hetrazan (Lederle). *Indian vet. J.*, **29**, 243–247

FILAROIDEA AND DRACUNCULOIDEA

ANDERSON, R. C. (1954). The development of *Ornithofilaria fallisensis* Anderson, 1954, in *Simulium venustum* Sag. *J. Parasit.*, **40**, 12

ANDERSON, R. C. (1955). Black flies (Simuliidae) as vectors of *Ornithofilaria fallisensis* Anderson, 1954. *J. Parasit.*, **41**, 45

BÖHM, L. K. & SUPPERER, R. (1955). Untersuchungen über Setarien (Nematoda) bei heimischen Wiederkäuern und deren Beziehung zur 'Epizootischen cerebrospinalen Nematodiasis' (Setariosis). *Z. Parasitk.*, **17**, 165–174

BREMNER, K. C. (1955). Morphological studies on the microfilariae of *Onchocera gibsoni* (Cleland & Johnston), and *Onchocera gutturosa* (Neumann) (Nematoda: Filaroidea). *Aust. J. Zool.*, **3**, 324–330

BUBBERMAN, C. & KRANEVELD, F. C. (1933). Over een dermatitis squamosa et crustosa circums-cripta by het rund in Nederlandsch Indie genaamd, cascado. III. Het voorkommen van cascado by de geit. *Ned. Ind. Diergeneesk*, **46**, 67–73

BUCKLEY, J. J. C., NELSON, G. S. & NEISCH, R. B. (1958). On *Wuchereria patei* n. sp. from the lymphatics of cats, dogs and genet cats on Pate Island, Kenya. *J. Helminth.*, **32**, 73–80

BUCKLEY, J. J. C. (1960). On *Brugia* gen. nov. for *Wuchereria* spp. of the 'malayi' group, i.e. *W. malayi* (Brug. 1927), *W. pahangi* (Vuckley and Edeson, 1956), and *W. patei* (Buckley, Nelson and Heisch, 1958). *Ann. prop. Med. Parasit.* **54**, 75–77

CHABAUD, A. G. (1954). Sur le cycle evolutif des spirurides et de nematodes des ayant une biologie comparable, valeur systematique des characteres biologiques. *Annls Parasit. hum. Comp.* **29**, 206–249, 358–425

CHODNIK, K. S. (1958). Histopathology of the aortic lesions in cattle infected with *Onchocera armillata* (Filariidae). *Ann. trop. Med. Parasit.* **52**, 145–148

DIKMANS, G. (1948). Skin lesions of domestic animals in the United States due to nematode infestation. *Cornell Vet.*, **38**, 3–23

EUZÉBY, J. & LAINE, B. (1951). Sur la periodicite des microfilaires de *Dirofilaria immitis*. Ses variations sous l'influence de divers facteurs. *Rev. Ved. vet. Toulouse*, **102**, 231–238

EWING, S. A. & HIBBS, C. M. (1966). *Dracunculus insignis* (Leidy, 1858) in dogs and wild carnivors in the Great Plains. *Amer. Mid. Nat.*, **12**, 87–132

GIBSON, T. E. (1965). *Veterinary Anthelmintic Medications*. 2nd edn. Commonwealth Bureau of Helminthology. Farnham Royal, England: Commonwealth Agricultural Bureaux

GNEDINI, M. P. & OSIPOV, A. N. (1960). Contribution to the biology of the nematode *Parafilaria multipapillosa* (Condamine et Drouilly, 1878) parasitic in the horse. *Helminthologia*, **2**, 13–16

HAWKING, F. (1964). The periodicity of microfilariae. VII. The effect of parasympathetic stimulants upon the distribution of microfilariae. *Trans. R. Soc. trop. Med. Hyg.*, **58**, 178–194

HEISCH, R. B., NELSON, G. S. & FURLONG, M. (1959). Studies in filariasis in East Africa. I. Filariasis on the Island of Pate, Kenya. *Trans. R. Soc. trop. Med. Hyg.*, **53**, 41–53

HENNIGAR, G. R. & FERGUSON, R. W. (1957). Pulmonary vascular sclerosis as a result of *Dirofilaria immitis* infection in dogs. *J. Am. vet. med. Ass.*, **131**, 336–340

INNES, J. R. M. & SHOHO, C. (1952). Nematodes, nervous disease, and neurotropic virus infection. Observations in animal pathology of probable significance in medical neurology. *Br. med. J.*, August 366–368

INNES, J. R. M. & SHOHO, C. (1953). Cerebrospinal nematodiasis. Focal encephalomyelo-malacia of animals caused by nematodes (*Setaria digitata*); a disease which may occur in man. *Archs. Neurol. Psychiat.*, **70**, 325–349

ISHIHARA, T. (1958). La filaroise chez les animaux domestiques au Japon. II. La gale d'été ('Kason disease') du Cheval. III. Le Kase ou 'Wahi' maladie du betail. *Bull. Off. Int. Epizoot.*, **49**, 531–535, 536–537

KEMPER, H. E. (1957). Filarial dermatosis of sheep. *J. Am. vet. med. Ass.*, **130**, 220–224

KUME, S. & ITAGAKI, S. (1955). On the life-cycle of *Dirofilaria immitis* in the dog as the final host. *Br. vet. J.*, **111**, 16–24

LAGRAULET, J. (1962). Clinical and histopathological study of ocular lesions encountered during cervical onchocerciasis in horses. *Bull. Soc. Fr. Ophtal.*, **74**, 486–493

LAPAGE, G. (1961). A list of the parasitic Protozoa, Helminths and Arthropoda recorded from species of the family Anatidae (ducks, geese and swans). *Parasitology*, **51**, 1–109

LINDSEY, J. R. (1962). Diagnosis of filarial infections in dogs. II. Confirmation of microfilarial identifications. *J. Parasit.*, **48**, 321–326

MANSON-BAHR, P. (1966). *Manson's Tropical Diseases*. 16th Ed. London: Baillière

13

NELSON, G. S. (1959). The identification of infective filariae larvae in mosquitoes; with a note on the species found in 'wild' mosquitoes on the Kenya Coast. *J. Helminth.*, **33**, 233–256
NELSON, G. S. (1960). Schistosome infections as zoonoses in Africa. *Trans. R. Soc. trop. Med. Hyg.*, **54**, 301–316
NEWTON, W. L. & WRIGHT, W. H. (1956). The occurrence of a dog filariid other than *Dirofilaria immitis* in the United States. *J. Parasit.*, **42**, 246–258
NOE, G. (1903). Studi sul ciclo evolutovo della *Filaria labiato-papillosa*, Alessandrini. Nota preliminarie. *Atti. R. Accad. Lincei Roma*, **12**, 387–393
OCHI, Y. (1953). *Studies on Lumber Paralysis of Sheep.* Tokyo: Bureau of Animal Industry
ORIHEL, T. C. & BEAVER, P. C. (1965). Human infection with filariae of animals in the United States. *Am. J. trop. Med. Hyg.*, **14**, 1010–1029
ROBERTS, S. R. (1963). Etiology of equine periodic ophthalmia, *Am. J. Ophthal.*, **55**, 1049–1055
SAWYER, T. K., RUBIN, F. F. & JACKSON, R. F. (1965). The cephalic hook in microfilariae of *Dipetalonema reconditum* in the differentiation of canine microfilariae. *Proc. Helminth. Soc. Wash.* **32**, 15–20
SCHNELLE, G. B. & YOUNG, R. M. (1944). Clinical studies on microfilarial periodicity in war dogs. *Bull. U.S. Army med. Dept.*, **80**, 52
SHOHO, C. (1952). Further observations on epizootic cerebrospinal nematodiasis. I. Chemotherapeutic control of the disease by 1-diethyl-carbomyl-4-methylpoperazine citrate: Preliminary field trial. *Br. vet. J.*, **108**, 134–141
SHOHO, C. (1958). Studies of cerebro-spinal nematodiasis in Ceylon. V. On the identity of *Setaria* spp. from the abdominal cavity of Ceylon spotted deer *Axis axis ceylonensis.Ceylon vet.J.*, **6**, 15–20
SHOHO, C. (1960). Studies of cerebrospinal nematodiasis in Ceylon. VII. Experimental production of cerebrospinal nematodiasis by the inoculation of infective larvae of *Setaria digitata* into susceptible goats. *Ceylon vet. J.*, **8**, 2–12
SKJABIN, D. I. & SCHIKBOBALOVA, N. I. (1948). *Filariata. Akad. Nauk SSSR. Moscow*
SOULSBY, E. J. L. (1965). *Textbook of Veterinary Clinical Parasitology.* Vol. I. Helminths. Oxford: Blackwell Scientific Publications
STEWARD, J. S. (1937). The occurrence of *Onchocerca gutturosa* Neumann in cattle in England, with an account of its life history and development in *Simulium ornatum* Mg. *Parasitology*, **29**, 212–219
SUGAWA, Y., MOCHIZUKI, H. & YAMAMOTO, S. (1949). *First Report on Japanese Equine Encephalitis.* Government Experimental Station for Animal Hygiene, 9
SUPPERER, R. (1953). Filariosen der Pferde in Oesterreich. *Wien. tierärztl. Mschr.*, **40**, 193–220
TAYLOR, A. E. R. (1960). Studies on the microfilariae of *Loa loa, Wuchereria bancrotti, Brugia malayi, Dirofilaria immitis, D. repens* and *D. aethiops. J. Helminth.* **34**, 13–26
VAUGHAN, A. W. (1952). A report on canine filariasis. *Vet. Rec.*, **64**, 454–455
WEBBER, W. A. F. & HAWKING, F. (1955). Experimental maintenance of *Dirofilaria repens* and *D. immitis* in dogs. *Exp. Parasit.* **4**, 143–164
YEH-LIANG SHENG (1959). A revision of the nematode genus Setaria Viborg, 1795, its host–parasite relationship speciation and evolution. *J. Helminth.* **33**, 1–98
YOELI, M., RODEN, A. T. & ABBOTT, J. D. (1948). Smears from subcutaneous nodules of a mule showing microfilariae *Onchocerca* sp. 2. Developmental forms of same species in *Anopheles Sacharovi* and *A. maculipennis typicus. Trans. R. Soc. trop. Med. Hyg.*, **41**, 444

TRICHURATA—TRICHINELLIDAE

CAMERON, T. W. M. (1962). Trichinellosis in Canada. *Trichinellosis. Proc.* 1st Int. Conf. Trichinellosis (Ed. by Z. Kozar). Warszawa: Polish Scientific Publishers
GOULD, S. E. (1945). *Trichinosis.* Springfield, Illinois: Charles C. Thomas
GOULD, S. E., GOMBERG, H. J. & VILLELLA, J. B. (1962). Effects of different energies of ionizing radiation on *Trichinella spiralis. Trichinellosis. Proc.* 1st Int. Conf. Trichinellosis (Ed. by Z. Kozar). Warszawa: Polish Scientific Publishers
KAGAN, I. G. (1960). Trichinosis: A review of biologic, serologic and immunologic aspects. *J. infect. Dic.*, **107**, 65–93
KOZAR, Z. (1962). Incidence of *Trichinella spiralis* in the world and actual problems connected with trichinellosis. *Trichinellosis. Proc.* 1st Int. Conf. Trichinellosis (Ed. by Z. Kozar). Warszawa: Polish Scientific Publication
LARSH, J. E. (1963). Experimental trichiniasis. *Advances in Parasitology*, Vol. 1, pp. 213–286 (Ed. by B. Dawes). New York: Academic Press
MADSEN, H. (1961). *Meddelelsen om Grønland Kommissioner for Videnskalbelge undersogelser i Grønland.* **159**, 1–124
SOULSBY, E. J. L. (1963). Diagnosis of helminth infections. *Clinical Aspects of Immunology* (Ed. by P. G. H. Gell & R. R. A. Coombs). Oxford: Blackwell Scientific Publications

TRICHURATA—TRICHURIDAE

ALLEN, R. W. (1949). Studies on the life history of *Capillaria annulata* (Molin, 1858) Cram 1926. *J. Parasit.*, **35** (Suppl.) 35
BALCONI, I. R. & TODD, A. C. (1962). A new treatment for trichuriasis in swine. *Vet. Med.* **57**, 798–799

BROOME, A. W. J. (1963). The anthelmintic activity of methyridine (2 (*p*-methoxyethyl) pyridine) against *Capillaria obsignata* in chickens. *Vet. Rec.*, **75**, 1326–1328
ENIGK, K. (1950). Die Biologie von *Capillaria plica* (Trichuroidea, Nematoda). *Z. tropenmed. Parasit.*, **1**, 560–571
FRIEDHOFF, K. (1963). Therapie des capillaria befalles beim Gefflugel. *Berl. Much. tierärztl. Wschr.*, **76**, 151–155
GEEVAERTS, J. (1962). Bestrying van capillariose bij duiven en kippern door methyridine. *Vlaam. diergeneesk. Tijdschr.*, **31**, 105–113
MADSEN, H. (1951). Notes on the species of *Capillaria* (Zeder, 1800), known from gallinaceous birds. *J. Parasit.*, **37**, 257–265
MADSEN, H. (1952). The species of *Capillaria* (Nematoda: Trichinelloidea) parasitic in the digestive tract of Danish gallinaceous and anatine game birds, with a revised list of species of Capillaria in birds.
MCGREGOR, J. K., LARD, L. H. & KINGSCOTE, A. A. (1962). Observations on the anthelmintic effect of methyridine in dogs. *Can. vet J.*, **3**, 67–68
MOREHOUSE, N. F. (1944). Life cycle of *Capillaria caudinflata*, a nematode parasite of the common fowl. *Iowa State Coll. agric. Sci.*, **18**, 217–253
MORISHITA, K. & TANI, T. (1960). A case of *Capillaria* infection causing cutaneous creeping eruption in man. *J. Parasit.*, **46**, 79–93
OTTO, G. F., BERGTHRONG, M., APPLEBY, R. E., RAWLINS, J. C. & WILBUR, O. (1954). Eosinoppilia and hepatomegaly due to *Capillaria hepatica*. *Bull. Johns Hopkins Hosp.*, **94**, 319–336
POWERS, K. G., TODD, A. C., HEZEKIAH, S. & McNUTT, S. H. (1960). Experimental infections of swine with *Trichuris suis*. *Am. J. vet Res.*, **21**, 262–268

DIOCTOPHYMATA

HAELBERG, C. W. (1953). *Dictophyma Renale* (Goeze, 1782). A study of the migration routes to the kidneys of mammals and resultant pathology. *Trans. Am. microscop. Soc.*, **72**, 351–363
KARMANOVA, E. M. (1960). The life cycle of the nematode *Dioctophyme renale* (Goeze 1782). *Dokl. Akad. Nauk SSSR*, **127**, 700–702
WOODHEAD, A. E. (1950). Life history cycle of the giant kidney worm *Dioctophyma renale* (Nematoda) of man and many other mammals. *Trans. Am. Microscop. Soc.*, **70**, 21–46

ACANTHOCEPHALA

PETROCHENKO, V. T. (1949). Cycle of development of *Polymorphus magnus* (Dkthsnin 1913), parasite of domestic and wild ducks. *Dokl. Akad. Nauk SSSR*, **66**, 137–140
RAYSKI, C. & GARDEN, E. A. (1961). Life-cycle of an acnathocephalan parasite of the eider duck. *Nature, Lond.*, **192**, 185–196

ANNELIDA

LAPAGE, G. (1961). A list of the parasitic Protozoa, Helminths and Arthropoda recorded from species of the family Anatidae (ducks, geese and swans). *Parasitology*, **51**, 1–109
ROBERS, H. E. (1955). Leech infestation of the eyes in geese. *Vet. Rec.*, **67**, 203–204

ARTHROPOD PARASITES

Phylum: Arthropoda

THE name of this phylum, derived from the Greek words *arthros*, a joint, and *podos*, a foot, refers to the fact that the members of the phylum have jointed limbs like those of a lobster or crab. The primitive limb of arthropods was biramous, consisting of an unbranched basal piece, called the protopodite, which branched into an inner *endopodite* and an outer *exopodite*. Some of the limbs of some species of arthropod are still of this type.

Arthropods have probably descended from ancestors which also gave origin to the soft-skinned annelid worms, an example of which is the earthworm; but the arthropods have developed an outer covering of *chitin*, which forms an *exoskeleton* in which the whole body is enclosed. This chitinous covering is secreted by chitogenous cells beneath it and it not only covers the external surface of the body, but also passes through the mouth into the anterior part of the alimentary canal called the *stomodaeum* and also through the anus into the posterior part of the alimentary canal called the *proctodaeum*, both of which arise as invaginations from the exterior into the body. The exoskeleton is usually present in the form of chitinous plates, called *sclerites*, a typical segment of the body having a dorsal sclerite, called a *tergum*, a ventral sclerite, called a *sternum* and a lateral plate between the tergum and sternum, which is called a *pleuron*. The tergum, sternum and pleuron of each segment are united by more flexible portions of the chitinous exoskeleton. As the arthropod grows it becomes too big for its chitinous covering and periodically this is cast off and a new exoskeleton is formed. Each casting of the exoskeleton is called an *ecdysis*. The muscles of the body are inserted into the exoskeleton.

Arthropods are metamerically-segmented animals. The segments of arthropods show a tendency to become associated in groups, the anterior segments forming the head, the middle ones the thorax and the posterior ones the abdomen.

The appendages found on the body of an arthropod are typically paired, one pair being usually found on each segment. The appendages on the head are typically one or two pairs of sensory antennae and, behind these, paired appendages modified for feeding. Commonly there is one pair of mandibles and behind these two pairs of maxillae. Behind these again there may be maxillipedes, which are walking legs adapted for feeding. The next group of appendages belongs to the thorax and they are walking legs. Behind them there are, in aquatic species, such as the Crustacea, a variable number of abdominal appendages, some or all of which are used for swimming; but terrestrial species usually lose these or some of them may become modified to perform other functions.

A dominant feature of the internal anatomy of the Arthropoda is the fact that the general body cavity is not a coelom. It is a space full of blood, which is called the *haemocoele*. The blood in it bathes all the organs of the body. The *heart* is an enlarged dorsal blood vessel, which is enclosed in a compartment of the haemocoele full of blood called the *pericardium*. As the heart pulsates, it sucks in blood from the pericardium through openings in its walls called *ostia*. It then pumps the blood into the haemocoele through short arteries, which are usually the only blood vessels in the body.

The respiratory organs of arthropods are also characteristic of the phylum. They are:

(a) *Gills* (branchiae) of various kinds found in larvae, nymphs and adults of species that are aquatic.

(b) *Tracheae*, which are fine, elastic tubes, with a thin, chitinous lining, which are held open by rings or spiral thickenings of the chitinous lining; tracheae branch and ramify among the internal organs, to which they take air that enters them through their external openings or *stigmata*; tracheae are especially characteristic of insects.

Other respiratory structures are *lung-books* and *gill-books* of spiders and crabs respectively. In some forms, e.g. the parasitic mites, respiration is through the cuticle.

The alimentary canal varies in the different classes of arthropods. In all, however, it consists of (a) the *stomodaeum* mentioned above, which is lined by chitin and may be divided into a sucking *pharynx*, a *proventriculus* (crop), and a *gizzard*; (b) the *proctodaeum* mentioned above, which is also lined by chitin; (c) a mid-gut, or *mesenteron*, which connects the proctodaeum with the stomodaeum.

The excretory organs of arthropods also vary in the different classes of the phylum. Those of the class Crustacea are a pair of nephridia which open on the bases of the second antennae. The excretory organs of the Insecta are tubules, called Malpighian tubules, which are arranged in a ring round the alimentary canal. Usually they open into the anterior end of the proctodaeum. Arachnida also have Malpighian tubules that open into the anterior end of the proctodaeum, but they have, in addition, *coxal glands*, which open on the coxae of the legs. These latter are true nephridia, homologous with the nephridia of the Crustacea.

The nervous system of arthropods, consists of cerebral ganglia in the head, united by circum-oesophageal commissures to a ventral double nerve cord that runs along the ventral side of the body and has nerve-ganglia on it. Typically there is one ganglion in each segment, but fusions of segments carry with them fusions of the ganglia associated with them. Associated with this central nervous system are eyes, sensory setae and other special sense-organs, some of which are described below.

The sexes of arthropods are usually separate.

The phylum Arthropoda is divided into the following five classes:

CLASS I: CRUSTACEA

This class includes the crayfishes, lobsters, shrimps, crabs, wood-lice and their relatives. Most of the species are aquatic, and breathe by means of gills, but some species, such as the wood-lice, are terrestrial. Crustacea have two pairs of antennae and numerous pairs of limbs on the thorax and abdomen and these limbs are frequently biramous. The class is divided into two subclasses.

SUBCLASS I: ENTOMOSTRACA

Species belonging to this subclass are usually small Crustacea with a variable number of body-segments. The abdomen often ends in a caudal fork. To this subclass belong some species which are intermediate hosts of parasitic helminths, among which are the species of the genus *Cyclops*, which act as intermediate hosts of the tapeworm *Diphyllobothrium latum* and of the nematode *Dracunculus medinensis*, and *Daphnia*, which act as the intermediate hosts of the spiruroid nematode *Acuaria uncinata*.

SUBCLASS 2: MALACOSTRACA

Species belonging to their subclass are usually larger than the Entomostraca and possess a constant number of body-segments. Typically there are eight segments in the thorax and seven in the abdomen. The character of the appendages clearly marks off the thorax and the abdomen. To this subclass belong the shrimps, lobsters, crayfishes and crabs. This subclass also includes important intermediate hosts of parasitic nematodes, among which are the terrestrial wood-lice and their aquatic relatives belonging to the genus *Asellus* and the 'freshwater shrimp' *Gammarus pulex*.

CLASS II: ONYCHOPHORA

This class contains only the species of the genus *Peripatus*, which show many resemblances to the annelid worms. None of them is parasitic.

CLASS III: MYRIAPODA

Species of this Class are the centipedes and millipedes. Their bodies consist of a number of segments which are, with the exception of the head, not grouped into definite body areas. There are two orders: (1) the *Diplopoda* (millipedes), which are chiefly vegetarian species and have two pairs of limbs on each segment of the body behind the head; some of them are serious pests of crops; (2) the *Chilopoda* (centipedes), which are chiefly carnivorous and have one pair of limbs on each segment of the body behind the head; some species of them are useful enemies of other pests of garden and other crops and some are among the poisonous arthropods described below.

CLASS IV: INSECTA

This Class includes all the insects. Their bodies are divided into three parts, namely, a *head*, which bears one pair of antennae only, a *thorax*, consisting of three segments, which bear three pairs of legs and, typically, two pairs of wings, and an *abdomen*, consisting of a variable number of segments which either has no appendages or the appendages on it are modified for various special purposes. Insects breathe by means of tracheae. They are described in greater detail below.

CLASS V: ARACHNIDA

This Class includes the king-crabs, scorpions, spiders, ticks, mites and their relatives. They not only vary much in structure among themselves, but they also differ considerably from other arthropods.

CLASS: INSECTA LINNAEUS, 1758

The distinguishing features of the Class Insecta have already been given above. The Class includes about 70 per cent of all the known species of animals of all kinds. With the majority of these the veterinarian is not concerned, but some species are of great veterinary importance.

A brief description of the anatomy of insects is given below. This is intended as a guide to the recognition of the important parts of an insect, especially those which are used in identification. A more extensive account of the morphology and physiology of the Insecta will be found in textbooks of entomology such as Imms (1948) and Wigglesworth (1950).

Head. The head is an ovoid or globular capsule, composed of a number of plates or sclerites, at the anterior end of the body. Eyes are usually present and are placed laterally, above the cheeks or genae. They are compound eyes and may meet one another in the midline (holoptic) or they may be wide apart (dichoptic). Simple eyes, or ocelli, may be present and are arranged in a triangle on the dorsum or vertex.

Antennae. These are situated between or in front of the compound eyes. Their form varies greatly, some are elongated and many segmented (mosquitoes) some are short and squat (house flies). They are frequently haired or may carry special bristles (e.g. aristae).

Mouth parts. These consist of: *labrum* or upper lip which forms the upper boundary of the mouth; *labium* or low lip which forms the lower boundary

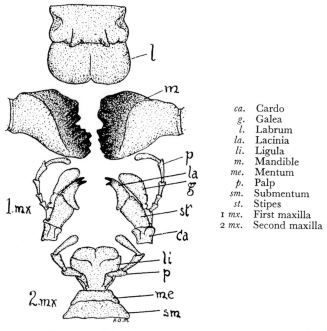

ca.	Cardo
g.	Galea
l.	Labrum
la.	Lacinia
li.	Ligula
m.	Mandible
me.	Mentum
p.	Palp
sm.	Submentum
st.	Stipes
1 *mx.*	First maxilla
2 *mx.*	Second maxilla

Fig. 173. Mouth Parts of Locust (Original)

of the mouth. Between these two structures are two pairs of biting jaws, an upper pair the *mandibles* and a lower pair, the *maxillae*. On the underside of labrum there is a small membranous structure, the *epipharynx* which bears the organ of taste. These two are frequently fused to form the *labrum-epipharynx*. On the upper surface of the *labium* is a further membranous structure, the *hypopharynx* which bears the opening of the salivary duct. Both the maxillae and the labium possess jointed *palps* which are sensory in function.

Great modifications occur in this basic structure. In the chewing insects (e.g. the locust) all the various components can be recognised but in the suctorial forms various structures of the mouth parts may be much modified. Thus the labium may be greatly expanded for imbibing liquid food (house fly) or all parts may be modified into five piercing stylets (mosquitoes).

Thorax. This consists of three segments, the *prothorax, mesothorax* and *metathorax.* These parts may not be distinct in some insects due to fusion. Each segment typically bears a pair of legs and the mesothorax and metathorax typically bear one pair of wings each.

Legs. These consist of a basal coxa by which the leg is attached to the body, this being followed by a trochanter, femur, tibia and tarsus, the latter being composed of a number of joints, usually five. The last tarsal segment is frequently provided with a pair of claws between which is an empodium consisting of a pad, a spine or a bristle. A pair of pads, the pulvilli occur below the claws.

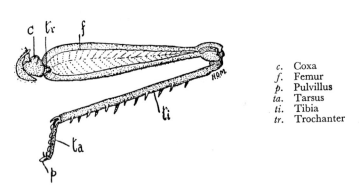

c.	Coxa
f.	Femur
p.	Pulvillus
ta.	Tarsus
ti.	Tibia
tr.	Trochanter

FIG. 174. Leg of a Locust (Original)

Wings. Normally two pairs occur but in the *Diptera* the posterior pair is reduced to a pair of balancers or halteres. Embryonically the wing is sac-like but in the adult insect the two membranes become closely applied to each other. The wings are supported by 'veins' which are breathing tubes or trachea. The arrangement of the veins is a valuable means of identification in many cases.

Abdomen. Usually clearly segmented and soft and membranous. Various structures may be present on the abdomen such as copulatory claspers, an ovipositor and the external genitalia.

The *respiratory system* of insects consists usually of a system of branching tubes, the tracheae, which open through spiracles or stigmata at the sides of the body. The tracheae are composed of a thin layer of chitin strengthened by spiral thickenings secreted by special chitogenous cells. They end in air sacs with very delicate walls. There may be a pair of spiracles to each segment, but they are usually reduced in number, and there are none in the head and the prothorax. The spiracles may be bordered by a thick rim of chitin which bears bristles and they open into a vestibule which contains a valve controlled by muscles. The respiratory movements are produced by muscular contractions and elastic distensions of the body wall.

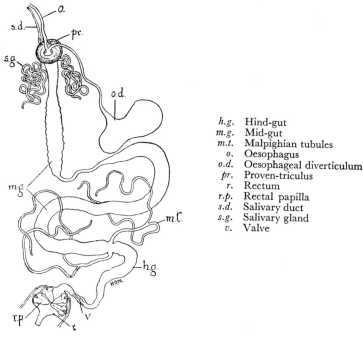

h.g.	Hind-gut
m.g.	Mid-gut
m.t.	Malpighian tubules
o.	Oesophagus
o.d.	Oesophageal diverticulum
pr.	Proven-triculus
r.	Rectum
r.p.	Rectal papilla
s.d.	Salivary duct
s.g.	Salivary gland
v.	Valve

FIG. 175. *Lucilia sericata*, Alimentary Tract (Original)

The *alimentary canal* of insects consists of a stomodaeum, a mesenteron and a proctodaeum. Of stomodaeal origin are the buccal cavity with the salivary glands, the epi- and hypo-pharynx, the pharynx, the proventriculus or gizzard, and the crop, or oesophageal diverticulum or food reservoir. The mesenteron forms the mid-gut. At its posterior end is a ring of Malpighian tubes, which have an excretory function. Proctodaeal are the intestine or hind-gut and the rectum, together with the Malpighian tubes and the papillae of the rectum. A crop is present in most *Diptera* and it is joined to the oesophagus by a narrow tube. In mosquitoes it is represented by three thin bags. The gizzard is present in insects that eat solid food, like the locust, and it contains a complicated set of teeth on its internal surface. The salivary glands are paired and have long ducts, which later join to form a common duct. An oesophageal valve may be present and in the *Cyclorrhapha* the proventriculus is a compact, spherical structure which functions as a valve. In the *Cyclorrhapha* and some other insects there is a delicate, tubular peritrophic membrane within the alimentary canal, extending from the mid-gut to the rectum. Its posterior end is not attached to the intestinal wall. It separates the food from the wall of the intestine, but osmosis takes place through it. In the *Acarina* the mid-gut has several diverticula, which are blind sacs capable of great distension.

The *vascular system* comprises a dorsally situated heart, an aorta and the general body cavity or haemocoele. The heart is a tube surrounded by pericardial cells, and its lumen is divided into a number of compartments by valves which allow the blood to pass forward only. Each compartment opens into the haemocoele through a pair of ostia. Anteriorly there is an aorta which carries the blood to the head, whence it enters the haemocoele and bathes all the organs. The blood is a viscid fluid and contains few cells.

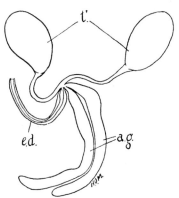

a.g.   Accessory glands
e.d.   Ejaculatory duct
t.   Testes

FIG. 176. *Lucilia sericata*, Male Genital Organs (Original)

The fat-body consists of numerous cells laden with fat and lies in the body wall, lining the haemocoele and surrounding all organs. It is especially large in recently emerged adults, pupae and mature larvae, and may hang into the body cavity in large masses.

The *nervous system* of insects consists of a circumoesophageal commissure with ganglia and a double ventral chain of ganglia from which nerves are given off. This ventral nerve chain originally had a pair of ganglia to each segment, but usually concentration occurs by fusion of the ganglia, especially in the thorax. In some cases the thoracic and abdominal ganglia may all be fused together.

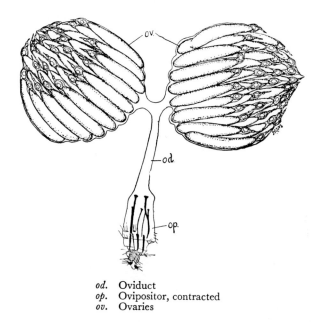

od. Oviduct
op. Ovipositor, contracted
ov. Ovaries

Fig. 177. *Lucilia sericata*, Female Genital Organs (Original)

Reproductive system of insects. The male has two testes, each with a vas deferens forming distally a vesicula seminalis and then fusing to form a common duct. A penis with a sheath and other accessory structures are frequently present. The female has two ovaries, which consist of groups of ovarian tubes, all arising from an apical filament. The ducts unite to form a common duct which bears the receptaculum seminis and ends in the ovipositor. Accessory glands are usually present. Some insects are oviparous, other viviparous or larviparous, and some even pupiparous, like *Glossina* and the *Pipipara*, which give birth to larvae that are ready to pupate. In these latter forms the larvae are nursed in the common portion of the oviduct, the uterus, which is provided with so-called 'milk glands' that secrete a milky fluid through a test to which the mouth of the larva is applied. Only one larva is born at a time. The larva usually lies with its stigmatic plate at the vulva of the fly and is thus able to breathe. Parthenogenesis of various kinds is also found among insects.

Development. As a rule the eggs consist of a large mass of yolk surrounded by the cytoplasm, which undergoes segmentation, and the body of the embryo is formed around the yolk. The rate of development is greatly influenced by the temperature, and sometimes the presence of a fair amount of moisture is absolutely essential, else the eggs may remain dormant. In some cases the young arthropod which hatches from the egg resembles the adult; in other cases it differs from the adult only in size and minor features, or there is a very marked difference, and definite stages, termed the larva, pupa and imago, are seen. Ecdyses always occur, and the different stages separated by ecdyses are called *stadia*, the form of the insect during each stadium being called an *instar*. During its development the insect undergoes a variable degree of change or *metamorphosis*. The only insects that do not undergo some degree of metamorphosis are the primitive bristle-tails and silver-fish and their relatives, which never develop wings and belong to the subclass *Apterygota*. The other insects all undergo a greater or lesser degree of metamorphosis and this fact is expressed in the classification given below. When metamorphosis is complete, as it is, for instance, in the life-history of a butterfly or house fly, the form that leaves the egg is called the *larva*, which feeds and grows and eventually becomes a quiescent phase, called the *pupa* (chrysalis), inside which the adult insect (imago) is formed. When the metamorphosis is simple or slight the form that leaves the egg is more like the adult and it is called the *nymph*, and the nymph merely grows, casting its skin several times, to become the imago. The larvae of species with a complete metamorphosis take various forms. The *polypod larva*, such as the caterpillar of a butterfly, has a well-marked head, a thorax of three segments, each of which bears a pair of clawed legs, and an abdomen of ten segments, which bears five pairs of fleshy hooked legs, called *prolegs*. The *oligopod larvae*, such as that of many beetles, have a well-marked head and three pairs of thoracic legs, but no abdominal legs. The *apodous larva* has no legs either on the thorax or the abdomen and the head is also reduced. The larvae of the house fly and the blow fly and of all Diptera are apodous. Often they are called *maggots*.

The pupae of insects may take three forms. In the most active pupae, such as those of beetles, the wings and legs of the adult insect can be seen externally and they are free from the rest of the body. Pupae of this kind are called *free* or *exarate* pupae. In other pupae, such as those of the butterflies and moths, the horse flies (Brachycera), and the mosquitoes and their relatives (Nematocera), the legs and wings are bound down to the body by moulting fluid, but they can usually be seen externally. Pupae of this kind are called *obtectate* pupae. The pupae of the dipterous *Cyclorrhapha* are, however, enclosed in the cast skin of the last larval phase, which is called the *puparium*. Their skin hardens and the insect inside cannot be seen. Pupae of this kind, such as the pupae of the house flies, are called *coarctate* pupae.

CLASSIFICATION OF INSECTS

The classification of insects used in this book is that adopted by Imms (1948).

CLASS: INSECTA

SUBCLASS: APTERYGOTA

Wingless insects, the wingless condition being primitive. Metamorphosis absent or very slight. One or more pairs of abdominal appendages present other than genitalia and cerci.

Order: Thysanura (silver fish, bristle tails)

Order: Protura (myrientomata)

Order: Collembola (spring-tails)
  (No veterinary importance.)

SUBCLASS: PTERYGOTA

Winged insects, possessing wings in the adult stage or are secondarily wingless, having descended from winged forms. Metamorphosis very varied, rarely slight or absent. No abdominal appendages other than genitalia or cerci.

DIVISION: EXOPTERYGOTA

Wings develop externally as buds. Metamorphosis simple, rarely a pupal stage. The division includes the following orders:

Order: Orthoptera (grasshoppers, cockroaches)

Order: Dermaptera (earwigs)

Order: Plecoptera (stone flies)

Order: Isoptera (termites)

Order: Psocoptera (book lice)

Order: Phthiraptera (lice) (syn. *Anoplura*)

Order: Odonata (dragon-flies)

Order: Thysanoptera (thrips)

Order: Hemiptera (bugs).

DIVISION: ENDOPTERYGOTA

Wings develop internally. Metamorphosis complete. Pupal stage present. The division includes the following orders:

Order: Coleoptera (beetles)

Order: Hymenoptera (bees, wasps)

Order: Lepidoptera (butterflies, moths)

Order: Neuroptera (lace wings)

Order: Aphaniptera (fleas)

Order: Diptera (true flies).

SUBCLASS: PTERYGOTA

DIVISION: EXOPTERYGOTA

ORDER: ORTHOPTERA

Species of this order have two pairs of wings; the anterior (meso-thoracic) pair, which are thickened, act as covers (called *tegmina*) for the hinder (metathoracic) pair, which are membranous. The antennae are usually long and filamentous and many-jointed. The mouth parts are of the type adapted for chewing. Examples of the order are the cock-roaches, locusts, and stick and leaf insects. Grasshoppers belonging to the genus *Melanoplus* are intermediate hosts of the spiruroid nematodes *Tetrameres americana* and *Acuaria hamulosa* etc. Among the cockroaches *Blatella germanica* can be experimentally infected with the spiruroid nematode *Gongylonema pulchrum*, and *Pycnoscelus surinamensis* is an inter-mediate host in Australia of the spiruroid nematode *Oxyspirura parvorum*.

Cockroaches. A cockroach common in many countries is the croton bug, *Blatella (Ectobia) germanica*. The adults measure about 15 mm. in length to the tips of the wings, which are present in both sexes. Their colour is light brown, with two longitudinal dark stripes over the prothorax and wings. Fairly common also is the Oriental roach, *Blatta (Periplaneta) orientalis*, which is almost black, about 25 mm. long, with wings that do not quite reach the tip of the abdomen in the male and are vestigial in the female.

Cockroaches live preferably in warm places and roam about in the dark. At other times they hide in cracks and crevices, behind and along baseboards of walls, around water-pipes and cisterns and in similar places. They feed on starchy or sugary materials, but will eat almost anything if necessary, and are found most frequently in kitchens, bakeries and storerooms in which cereal products are kept. They may be a fre-quent pest in animal quarters. They are not parasites, but may easily spread disease on account of their habits. They have been proved to carry various fungi and protozoa and to act as intermediate hosts of parasitic nematodes.

The eggs are laid in egg-cases which each contain a number of eggs. They may be carried about for some time and may be seen protruding from the abdomen of the female. The egg-cases are deposited in crevices and the rate of development of the eggs and the young cockroaches depends very much on the temperature and the available food supply.

Control of cockroaches is difficult, because they breed rapidly and new infestations readily occur. Traps may catch and reduce the number of *Blatta orientalis*, but they do not exterminate them and they often fail to catch the more active *Blatella germanica*. Poisons may be tried, but cockroaches, and *Blatella germanica* especially, are wary of them. Sodium fluoride kills cockroaches and is not very toxic to animals. It may be mixed with equal parts of flour and sugar. Borax mixed with 3 parts of powdered chocolate, or equal parts of pyrethrum powder and sodium fluoride, or pyrethrum containing 1 per cent of pyrethrins, have been recommended. Fumigation has not succeeded, except with cyanide, which is not often possible.

Among the chlorinated hydrocarbon insecticides, dieldrin or lindane sprayed into the hiding places give effective control, but must be repeated as new infestations occur. Among suggested strengths are 2·5 per cent chlordane emulsion or solution, 0·5 per cent dieldrin solution or 1 per cent dieldrin dust or 2 per cent chlordane. These have been used for the control of *Blatella germanica* in Germany and the United States, but this species has developed resistance to chlordane and lindane and to a less extent to malathion. For strains resistant to chlorinated hydrocarbons organophosphorus insecticides may be tried. Suggested formulae are 1·5 per cent malathion, 1 per cent Dipterex, 0·5 per cent diazinon, or 1·5 per cent chlorthion. Protection for more than a year has been obtained with DDT or dieldrin dissolved in urea-formaldehyde resins.

(For further information, see the periodical publications of WHO, the *Tropical Diseases Bulletin* and the *Journal of Economic Entomology*.)

ORDER: PHTHIRAPTERA (LICE)

Species of this suborder are small and wingless and have dorso-ventrally flattened bodies. Their antennae are short and are composed of three to five segments. The eyes are reduced or absent and the segmentation of the thorax is indistinct. The tarsi consist of one or two segments and each tarsus bears one or two claws. There is 1 pair of spiracles situated on the mesothorax. Typically there are six pairs of abdominal spiracles, but when fusion of abdominal segments occurs there may be fewer than six pairs. The operculated eggs are cemented, without stalks, to the hairs or feathers of the host. There is no metamorphosis. The phase of the life history that leaves the egg resembles the adult and is called the first nymph. There are three ecdyses, the first nymph becoming the second nymph, which becomes the third nymph and this becomes the adult. Thus Scott (1950) found that *Linognathus pedalis*, the foot louse of sheep, passed through three nymphal instars, each of which lasted, under Australian conditions, about 7 days. The eggs required about 17 days to hatch and 5 days were required before the adult female laid eggs, so that the whole period from egg to egg was about 43 days. This species can live off the host for about 18 days, and lambs can be infected from pastures up to 3 days after infected sheep have been removed from the pastures. The whole life history is passed on the host. Uninfected hosts are infected by close contact with infected ones, but lice may also be spread by farm equipment and personnel. Thus lice of horses may be spread by brushes, blankets, harness or other stable equipment.

The lice are divided into two suborders, the characteristics of which are summarised below.

SUBORDER: ANOPLURA (SIPHUNCULATA, SUCKING LICE)

The mouth parts are adapted for sucking the tissue fluids and the blood of the host. The two antennae are visible at the sides of the head and are usually composed of five segments. There is no sexual dimorphism. The thorax is small and its three segments are fused together the abdomen is relatively large, with seven of its nine segments visible the segments often bearing at their sides dark-brown or black areas o thickened chitin, called *paratergal plates*. The eyes are reduced or absent but are present in the human head louse, *Pediculus humanus*, and on the human pubic louse, *Phthirus pubis*. The first pair of legs is usually smaller with weaker claws; the third pair of legs is usually the largest. The two segments of the tarsus are usually not distinguishable. Each tarsus has only one claw. The hair of the host is held between this claw and a thumblike process on the ventral apical angle of the tibia. In the Haema topinidae the hold on the hair is helped by a spiny pad, the *tibial pad* which can be thrust up to lock the grip on the hair. There are thoracic

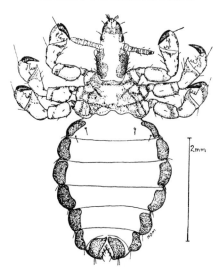

FIG. 178. *Haematopinus suis*, Female (Original)

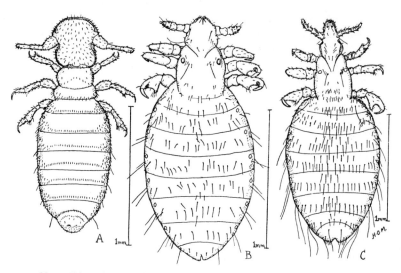

FIG. 179. Sheep Lice: A, *Damalinia ovis*; B, *Linognathus pedalis*; C, *L. africanus* (Original)

spiracles on the dorsal side of the mesothorax and six pairs of abdominal spiracles. The head is usually more or less pointed anteriorly. Three families of veterinary importance occur in this suborder, namely Haematopinidae, Linognathidae and Pediculidae.

FAMILY: HAEMATOPINIDAE

The eyes are absent, the head has forward prolongations (temporal angles) behind the antennae, and the thorax is broad; there are marked

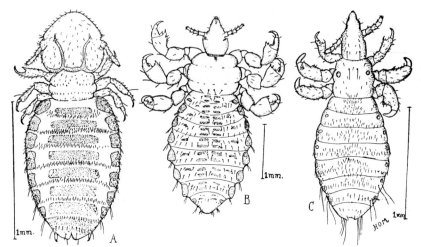

FIG. 180. Cattle Lice: A, *Damalinia bovis;* B, *Haematopinus eurysternus;* C, *Linognathus vituli* (Original)

paratergal plates, and there is one row of spines on each abdominal segment. To this family belong:

Haematopinus asini (Linné, 1755), the sucking louse of equines.

H. suis (Linné, 1758), the very large louse of pigs.

H. eurysternus (Nitzsch, 1818), the 'short-nosed' cattle louse, with a relatively short head and broad thorax and abdomen.

H. quadripertusus (Fahrenhotz, 1916). This species occurs on cattle in Queensland, New Guinea and the Solomon Islands. It was previously thought to be *H. eurysternus.*

FAMILY: LINOGNATHIDAE

The eyes are absent; the abdomen is membranous with numerous hairs on the segments. The first pair of legs are the smallest. Most species are parasitic on ungulates.

To this family belong:

Linognathus ovillus (Neumann, 1907), the body louse or 'blue louse' of sheep, occurs in New Zealand, Australia and Scotland. A better name for it is the 'face-louse', because it occurs chiefly on the face. Its head is much longer than wide and also longer than the thorax.

L. vituli (Linné, 1758), the 'long-nosed' cattle louse, which has an elongate head and body.

L. africanus Kellogg & Paine, 1911, the African 'blue louse' of sheep.

L. pedalis (Osborn, 1896) the 'foot louse' of sheep. This louse occurs on the legs and feet of the sheep where there is no wool.

L. stenopsis (Burmeister, 1838) on goats.

L. setosus (v. Olfers, 1816) (syn. *L. piliferus*) on dogs and foxes.

Solenopotes capillatus Enderlein, 1904, on cattle in Europe, U.S.A. and Australia.

FAMILY: PEDICULIDAE

There are pigmented eyes present; the abdomen has paratergal plates. To this family belong the human head and body lice belonging to the species *Pediculus humanus*, the legs of which are all the same size, the claws being slender; and the human pubic or crab louse, *Phthirus pubis*, which has a very wide thorax and a small abdomen, the first pair of legs being slender with slender claws.

The species of the other families of this suborder are parasitic on seals, walruses and elephant shrews.

SUBORDER: MALLOPHAGA

Species of this suborder are often called biting lice, a name which refers to the fact that many species of this suborder feed on the epithelial debris on the skin of the host, or on the feathers of birds, and have mouth parts adapted for chewing up this material. It is now known, however, that some species of them suck the tissue fluids of their hosts and have mouth parts adapted for this purpose. In species of this suborder the mesothorax and metathorax are fused to form one piece, in front of which the prothorax is a distinct and separate segment. The thoracic spiracles are on the ventral side of the mesothorax. The tarsi of species parasitic on birds have two claws and those of species parasitic on mammals have one claw.

The suborder Mallophaga is divided into three superfamilies:

SUPERFAMILY: ISCHNOCERA

In species of this superfamily the antennae are filiform and visible at the sides of the head and they are composed of three to five segments. The head of an ischnoceran louse may therefore look at first sight somewhat like that of a sucking louse (Anoplura), although it is usually broader. There are no maxillary palps, so that these cannot be mistaken, as the palps of Amblycera (see later) may be, for the antennae. The mandibles bite vertically. In the abdomen segments one and two, and nine and ten, are fused and segment eleven may not be visible. Parasitic on both mammals and birds.

SPECIES OF ISCHNOCERA FOUND ON BIRDS

Cuclotogaster (*Liperus*) **heterographus** Nitzsch, 1866, the 'head louse, of poultry, occurs on the skin and feathers of the head and neck. Male 2·43 mm., female 2·6 mm. long. In the male the first segment of the antenna is long and thick, bearing a posterior process. The abdomen is elongate in the male and barrel-shaped in the female, with dark-brown lateral tergal plates. The eggs are laid singly on the feathers. It occurs on fowls and partridges. It is a dangerous parasite of chicks.

Lipeurus caponis Linné, 1758, the 'wing louse', is a slender, elongate louse which occurs on the under-side of the large wing feathers and moves about very little. It occurs in fowls and pheasants.

Goniodes gigas (Taschenberg, 1879) (syn. *Goniocotes gigas*) is a large louse occurring on the body and feathers of the fowl. Male 3·2 mm., female 5 mm. long.

Goniocotes gallinae (de Geer, 1778) (syn. *Goniocotes hologaster*; *Goniodes hologaster*), the 'fluff louse', occurs in the fluff at the base of the feathers of fowls, pheasants and pigeons. It is a small louse; the male is 1 mm. long and the female 1·6 mm. The body is broad and the head short and wide.

Chelopistes meleagridis (Linné, 1758) (syn. *Goniodes meleagridis*; *Virgula meleagridis*) is a common louse of the turkey, and **Columbicola columbae** (Linné, 1758) (syn. *Lipeurus baculus* Nitzsch) occurs on domestic and wild pigeons. **Anaticola crassicornis** and **A. anseris** may be found on the duck.

SPECIES OF ISCHNOCERA FOUND ON MAMMALS

Damalinia (*Bovicola*) **bovis** (Linné, 1758) (syn. *Trichodectes scalaris*) on cattle.

Damalinia (*Bovicola*) **equi** (Linné, 1758) (syn. *Trichodectes parumpilosus*) on equines.

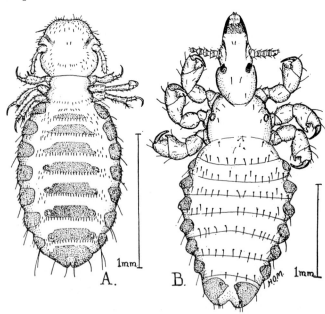

Fig. 181. Lice of the Horse: A, *Damalinia equi*; B, *Haematopinus asini* (Original)

Damalinia (*Bovicola*) **ovis** (Linné, 1758) (syn. *Trichodectes sphaero-cephalus*) on sheep.

Damalinia (*Bovicola*) **caprae** (Gurlt, 1843) (syn. *Trichodectes climax*) on goats.

B. painei (Kellogg & Nakayama, 1914) on goats.

Damalinia limbata (syn. *Tricodectes limbatus*) (Gervais, 1847) on angora goats.

Trichodectes canis (de Geer, 1778) (syn. *T. latus*) on dogs.

Felicola subrostratus (Nitzsch, 1838) (syn. *F. subrostrata*) on cats.

SUPERFAMILY: AMBLYCERA

In species of this superfamily the antennae lie in grooves in the sides of the head and they may not be readily seen. Maxillary palps may, however, be present and these may be visible in mounted specimens and may be confused with the antennae. The antennae, however, may be identified by the fact that usually they consist of four segments and the third segment is stalked, being somewhat the shape of an egg-cup that holds the fourth segment. The palps, when they are present, also have 4 segments, but the third segment is not stalked. The antennae of some species (e.g. those of the genus *Columbicola*) show sexual dimorphism, the antennae of the males being elongate and having a swollen first segment, with an appendage on the third segment. The mandibles bite horizontally. Only nine of the eleven abdominal segments are visible. The head is often broader and more rounded anteriorly than that of the *Anoplura*, but this is not a very reliable character. Parasitic on both mammals and birds. The following species may be encountered by veterinarians:

SPECIES OF AMBLYCERA FOUND ON BIRDS

Menopon gallinae (Linné, 1758) (syn. *M. pallidum*), the 'shaft louse' of poultry, is pale yellow in colour. Male 1·71 mm., female 2·04 mm. long. The thoracic and abdominal segments have each one dorsal row of bristles. This species occurs on fowls and also on ducks and pigeons. It moves about rapidly. The eggs are laid in clusters on the feathers. **M. phaeostomum** (Nitzsch, 1818) occurs on the peacock.

Menacanthus (*Eomenacanthus*) **stramineus** (Nitzsch, 1818) (syn. *Menopon biseriatum*) is the yellow 'body louse' of poultry, occurring on the skin of those parts of the body which are not densely feathered like the breast, thighs and around the anus. It occurs on the fowl, turkey, peacock and Japanese pheasant, and is especially harmful to small chicks. Male 2·8 mm., female 3·3 mm. long. The abdominal segments have each two dorsal rows of bristles. The eggs have characteristic filaments on the anterior half of the shell and on the operculum, and are laid in clusters on the feathers near the skin.

Trinoton anserinum (J. C. Fabricius, 1805) (syn. *Trinoton anseris*) may be found on the duck and the swan.

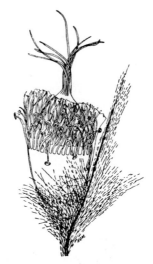

FIG. 182. *Menacanthus stramineus*, Egg attached to Feather (Original)

SPECIES OF AMBLYCERA FOUND ON MAMMALS

Although most of the Amblycera occur on birds, some species are parasitic on mammals, among which **Gyropus ovalis** and **Gliricola porcelli** and **Trimenopon hispidum** may all be found on the guinea-

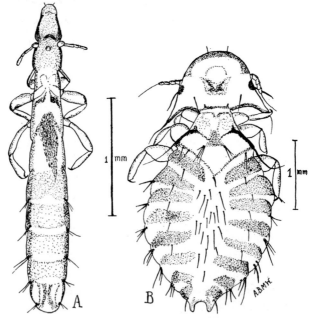

FIG. 183. A, *Columbicola columbae;* B, *Chelopistes meleagridis* (Original)

pig, and the former two species also occur on other rodents. **Hetero-doxus spiniger** is common on the dog in warm countries and **H. longi-tarsus** and **H. macropus** occur on kangaroos and wallabies.

EFFECTS OF LICE ON THEIR HOSTS

The chief effects of lice on their hosts are due to the irritation they cause. They are most numerous in the winter, possibly because of longer hair on the host's coat, closer contact of animals and also lack of general vigour. The hosts become restless and do not feed or sleep well and they may injure themselves or damage their feathers, hair or wool by biting

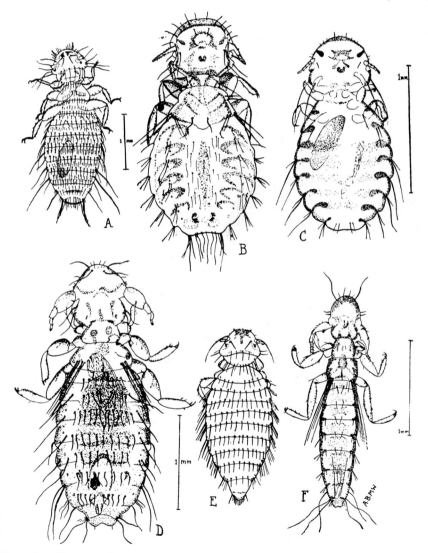

FIG. 184. Common Fowl Lice: A, *Menacanthus stramineus;* B, *Goniocotes gigas;* C, *G. hologaster;* D, *Cuclotogaster heterographus;* E, *Monopon gallinae;* F, *Liperus caponis* (Original)

and scratching the parts of their bodies irritated by the lice. The egg-production of birds and the milk-production of cattle may fall. In mammalian hosts scratching may produce wounds or bruises on the animal, while in sheep the wool is damaged and it is also soiled by the faeces of the lice. The coat becomes rough and shaggy, and, if the irritation is severe, the hair may become matted. Excessive licking of it by calves may lead to the formation of hair-balls in the stomach. The foot louse of sheep is found most frequently around the dew-claws, and severe infections may produce lameness.

Diagnosis is easily made by finding the lice, especially when the animal is standing in the sunlight.

CONTROL AND TREATMENT OF LICE

Poultry. If possible poultry lice should be killed without disturbing the birds, and this is best done by painting the perches in the fowl-house with strong tobacco extract containing 40 per cent nicotine, using about 400 g. for every 50 m. (½ lb. for 100 ft.). The fowl-house should be closed

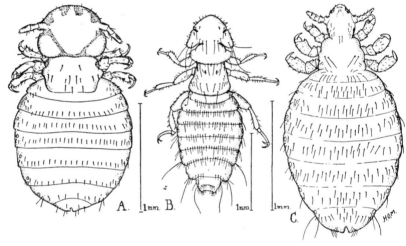

FIG. 185. Dog Lice: A, *Trichodectes canis;* B, *Heterodoxus longitarsus;* C, *Linognathus setosus* (Original)

at the back and sides, but only partly closed in front, so that the fumes will not be too strong for the birds. All the birds should sleep in the building on the following two nights. The warmth of their bodies causes the nicotine to evaporate and to kill the lice. Most or all eggs are also killed, but a second treatment may be necessary 10 days later. BHC has been used as a fumigant applied to the perches at the rate of 3 ml. of 1·5 per cent gamma isomer per linear foot.

Dusts containing sodium fluoride or 1 per cent DDT may be applied as pinches of dust placed between the feathers and near to the skin of the head, neck, back, breast, thighs, wings, tail and below the anus, or they may be shaken on to the bird from a container or applied with a blower. A dust bath containing 0·5 per cent lindane has been found satisfactory. The bath may be made by mixing 1 part of 20 per cent lindane dust with 40 parts of inert powder and it is effective against lice, and also red mite (*Dermanyssus*), the larvae of the soft tick *Argas* and the blood-sucking nematoceran insect *Simulium*, but it may be toxic to young chickens and turkey poults, which must not be allowed access to it. Toxaphene, chlordane, derris, rotenone and pyrethrins have also been used. Kraemer (1959) obtained effective control by spraying the birds with 0·5 per cent Dylox, 0·1 per cent Dow ET-57 or 0·5 per cent Sevin, the 0·5 per cent dust of the last being also effective and the toxicity of these was either nil or negligible. Harrison (1961) reported excellent control of *Menacanthus stramineus*, *Menopon gallinae* and *Haematopinus suis* with 5 per cent Sevin dust. Reports on Dow ET-57 are conflicting, but Hoffman (1960) found sprays of 0·1 per cent malathion or 0·1 per cent Bayer L 21/199 (Co-Ral) effective, as others have also found.

Cattle. DDT, BHC, toxaphene and organophosphorus compounds are effective, but two applications, with an interval of 14 days, must be given. Good control has been obtained with rotenone.

Sheep. For the body louse of sheep (*Damalinia ovis*) dips containing either 0·1 per cent DDT or 0·007 per cent gamma BHC are recommended. The latter remains on the fleece for 2–4 weeks, so that a single dipping covers the life history of the louse and eradicates it. Arsenical dips containing 0·2 per cent arsenic trioxide have also given good results in Australia. Skerman (1959) found that *D. ovis* was eradicated by plunge dipping with 0·01 per cent of aldrin, 0·01 per cent of diazinon and 0·01 per cent of gamma BHC, and that these gave residual protection for 6–20 weeks, diazinon giving the longest protection. Resistance of *D. ovis* to BHC and dieldrin has appeared in the northern part of Great Britain and is possibly widespread in that region. Such resistant strains have been effectively controlled by organophosphorus insecticides. For infestations with the foot louse (*Linognathus pedalis*) foot baths containing DDT or rotenone may be used.

Dogs. For the dog louse (*Trichodectes canis*), washes containing 0·01 per cent gamma BHC should kill all the lice, or a dust containing 0·1 per cent gamma BHC may be used. A dust containing 5 per cent DDT or a wash containing 0·5 to 1 per cent DDT may be tried, but BHC is likely to be better.

Cats. DDT should not be used for the treatment of lice on cats because cats are susceptible to its effects. Roberts *et al.* (1947) reported marked toxic effects on cats, dipping in 1 per cent DDT killing all the cats dipped and serious toxic signs being caused by dips containing 0·5 per cent DDT. The dips were not toxic to the dogs. For cats BHC may also be toxic. Because cats are susceptible to the chlorinated hydrocarbon insecticides a 3 per cent rotenone powder is recommended.

Man. For human body lice the WHO recommends a 10 per cent DDT powder. This does not kill the eggs, but larvae hatching out from them are killed during the long residual action of DDT. Lice resistant to DDT occur in various parts of the world, and for these a 1 per cent lindane powder is used. Pyrethrin or allethrin with a synergist may also be tried, but these have less residual action and must therefore be repeated weekly. For head and crab lice the WHO recommends 1 part in 5 parts of water of a mixture of 68 per cent benzyl benzoate and 6 per cent of DDT, 12 per cent of benzocaine and 14 per cent of Tween 80, sprayed or sponged thoroughly on to the skin, no bath being taken for 24 hours: or weekly applications of the powders mentioned above. Resistance of human lice to the chlorinated hydrocarbon insecticides (DDT, BHC, etc.) has been reported from various parts of the world.

ORDER: HEMIPTERA

This order includes a large number of plant lice and bugs of considerable economic importance. Only a small number of species are blood-suckers and of medical importance.

FAMILY: CIMICIDAE
Genus: Cimex Linné, 1758

C. lectularius Linné, 1758, the bed-bug, which is the best known, and several other species of this genus, attack man and animals to suck blood. The parasites are 4–5 mm. long, flat-bodied, elongate oval in shape

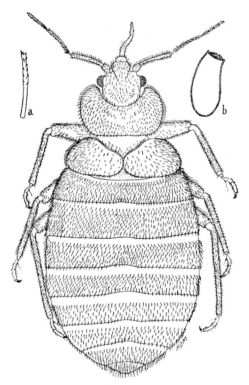

FIG. 186. *Cimex lectularius*, Dorsal View: *a*, a bristle; *b*, egg (Original)

and yellowish-brown to dark brown in colour. The head bears a pair of long antennae with four joints, of which the first is short and the third and fourth are slender. The compound eyes project conspicuously at the sides of the head. The prothorax is large and deeply notched anteriorly where the head is inserted in it. The wings are vestigial. The abdomen has eight visible segments. The whole body is covered with characteristic spinose bristles and some hairs. The tibiae of the legs are long and the tarsi have three joints. The adult has a pair of ventral thoracic stink glands and the young stages have similar dorsal abdominal glands. These glands are responsible for the characteristic odour of the insect. The mouthparts are modified for piercing and sucking. The labrum is small and immovable. The labium forms a tube with four joints and contains the piercing mandibles and maxillae.

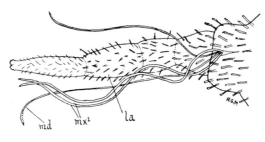

la.   Labium
md.   Mandible
mx¹.   First maxillae

FIG. 187. *Cinex lectularius*, Mouth Parts, Dorsal View (Original)

Life-cycle and habits. The female lays about 150–200 eggs in dark crevices. The egg is creamy white, about 1 mm. long, and has an oper-culum with a thick rim at one pole. The larva hatches after 3–14 days at 23°C or longer at lower temperatures and resembles the adult. There are five nymphal stages. The rate of development depends greatly on the food supply and the temperature. Under favourable conditions the adult stage is reached in 8–13 weeks after hatching.

The bugs live long and can survive long periods of starvation; adults have been kept without food for over a year. The insects live in crevices and cracks of wood near the sleeping-places of their hosts; for instance, in bedsteads or behind picture-rails and skirting-boards, or in the nests or perches of poultry. They are mainly nocturnal insects, but will bite sitting hens also in the daytime. After a meal the bug defaecates and usually turns round in such a way that its faeces fall on or near the wound, thus providing the possibility for transmission of disease through its faeces. Bugs may travel relatively long distances, passing to adjoining houses from an infected one.

Apart from being very annoying insects in human dwellings, several species of bugs at times cause severe irritation and anaemia in poultry, especially fowls, turkeys and pigeons. Besides *C. lectularius*, other species of this genus and *Ornithocoris toledoi* Pinto, 1927, which occurs in Brazil, are known as poultry parasites. *Haematosiphon inodora* is the Mexican chicken bug.

Control. Lindane, chlordane and dieldrin are all powerful killers of bedbugs, and they can be used as sprays, smokes or powders. The WHO recommends, for the control of *Cimex*, application of a 5 per cent emulsion or solution of DDT to baseboards, crevices, beds and mattresses, but resistance to DDT has been recorded in some areas and 0·1–0·9 per cent of gamma BHC may then be used. Where resistance to this also occurs, 0·5–1 per cent malathion or diazinon are suggested, dusts being applied every 2 weeks, but sprays of these organophosphorus compounds are too toxic to human beings.

FAMILY: TRIATOMIDAE

Numerous species of this family are vectors of *Trypanosoma cruzi*, the cause of human trypanosomiasis in South America, natural hosts of this trypanosome being the dog, fox, cat, armadillo, monkey and other animals. Triatomidae are larger than Cimicidae and have well-developed wings, a cone-shaped head and the abdomen is less flattened than that of the Cimicidae.

Control. Because these bugs can fly long distances, control of them is difficult. Houses may be screened and nets may be used to protect beds. For the spraying of dwellings DDT is not so effective. The WHO recommends the application of 50 mg. per sq. ft. of BHC, or 125 mg. per sq. ft. of dieldrin, and elimination of the breeding-places of these bugs.

SUBCLASS: PTERYGOTA

DIVISION: ENDOPTERYGOTA

ORDER: COLEOPTERA

Species of this order are the beetles. They have two pairs of wings. The anterior (mesothoracic) pair are thickened to form hard horny or leathery covers for the posterior (metathoracic) pair. They are called the *elytra*. They usually meet in the mid-dorsal line to form a straight suture there. Beneath them the posterior membranous wings are folded. The mouth parts are adapted for chewing. The metamorphosis is complete. The pupa is free.

The beetles are important as carriers of disease-producing organisms. Some species are intermediate hosts of the spiruroid nematodes *Spirocerca lupi, Ascarops strongylina, Physocephalus sexalatus* and *Gongylonema pulchrum* etc. Scavenger beetles that feed on carcasses have been shown to carry anthrax bacilli, and other pathogenic bacteria may also be spread in this way. Dung beetles may possibly spread bacteria occurring in faeces, but they are especially important as intermediate hosts of numerous tapeworms and nematodes.

ORDER: APHANIPTERA (FLEAS)

The fleas are wingless insects with laterally compressed bodies, about 1·5-4 mm. long. The chitinous covering is thick and dark brown. Compound eyes are absent, but some species have large or small simple eyes. The abdomen has ten segments. The ninth abdominal segment of both the male and the female bears a dorsal plate called the *sensilium* or *pygidium*, which is covered with sensory setae; its function is not known.

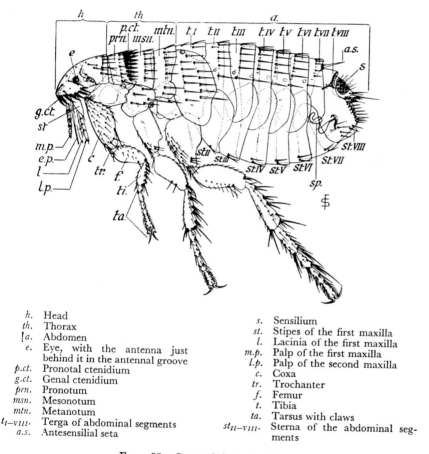

h.	Head	*s.*	Sensilium
th.	Thorax	*st.*	Stipes of the first maxilla
a.	Abdomen	*l.*	Lacinia of the first maxilla
e.	Eye, with the antenna just behind it in the antennal groove	*m.p.*	Palp of the first maxilla
p.ct.	Pronotal ctenidium	*l.p.*	Palp of the second maxilla
g.ct.	Genal ctenidium	*c.*	Coxa
prn.	Pronotum	*tr.*	Trochanter
msn.	Mesonotum	*f.*	Femur
mtn.	Metanotum	*t.*	Tibia
t_{I-VIII}.	Terga of abdominal segments	*ta.*	Tarsus with claws
a.s.	Antesensilial seta	$st_{II-VIII}$.	Sterna of the abdominal segments

FIG. 188. *Ctenocephalides felis felis*

The tergum of the ninth abdominal segment of the male is modified to form the claspers. The penis (*aedeagus*) of the male is chitinous and coiled and its structure is complex. These and other anatomical features used for the classification of fleas are shown in Figs. 188-190. The legs are long, strong and adapted to leaping. In some species, such as the dog flea, *Ctenocephalides canis* (Curtis, 1826), and the cat flea, *C. felis felis* (Bouché, 1835), there are a number of large spines on the head and the thorax known as 'combs' or *ctenidia*. On the cheek (*gena*) there may be a *genal comb* and on the posterior border of the first thoracic segment a *pronotal* comb. Either or both of these combs are absent from some species. The short, clubbed antennae are sunk in antennal grooves on the sides of the head.

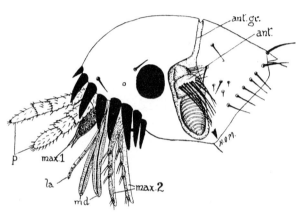

ant.	Antenna	*max.2.*	Palps of second maxillae
ant.gr.	Antennal groove	*md.*	Laciniae of first maxilla
la.	Epipharynx	*p.*	Palps of first maxilla
max.1.	Stipes of first maxilla		

FIG. 189. *Ctenocephalides canis*, Head, Lateral View (Original)

KEY TO THE FLEAS OF VETERINARY IMPORTANCE

1. Thorax reduced, the three thoracic segments together shorter in width than the first abdominal segment (Family: Sarcopsyllidae) . . 2
   Thorax not reduced, the three thoracic segments together much wider than the first abdominal segment (Family: Pulicidae) . . . 3
2. On poultry, no ctenidia, two bristles an occipital lobe
   Echidnophaga gallinacea
   On man and other mammals, frons sharply angled, tropical
   Tunga penetrans
3. General and pronotal ctenidia absent 4
   Genal and/or pronotal ctenidia present 5
4. Mesopleural rod absent, on human . . . . . . *Pulex irritans*
   Mesopleural rod present, on black rats . . . . *Xenopsylla cheopis*
5. Genal and pronotal ctenidia present 6
   Only pronotal ctenidia present 8

6. Genal ctenidium of four elements, vertically placed, on mice

Leptopsylla segnis

Genal ctenidium of four to six elements, obliquely placed, on rabbits

Spilipsyllus cuniculi

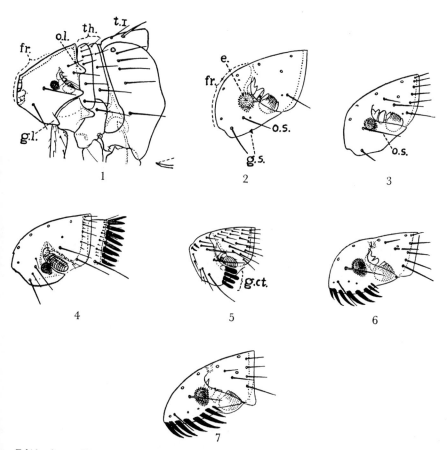

1, *Echidnophaga gallinacea*, the stick-tight flea of poultry, showing the angulate frons (*fr*); the well-developed occipital lobe (*o.l.*) on the occiput; the genal lobe (*g.l.*) directed backwards, the thorax (*th.*) narrower dorsally than the tergum (*t.l.*) of the first abdominal segment, and the absence of ctenidia (cf. *Pulex irritans* and *Xenopsylla cheopis*). 2, *Pulex irritans* of man and other mammals, especially the pig and badger, showing the absence of ctenidia, the smoothly-rounded frons (*fr.*); the position of the ocular seta (*o.s.*) below the eye (contrast its position in the other fleas figured), and the single small spinelet (*g.s.*) on the genal margin; *e*, eye. 3, *Xenopsylla cheopis*, chiefly of the rat, showing the absence of ctenidia. 4, *Ceratophyllus* (*Nosopsyllus*) *fasciatus* of rodents, chiefly rats, which has a pronotal ctenidium, but no genal ctenidium. Note the antenna in its antennal pit behind the eye. 5, *Leptopsylla segnis*, of the house-mouse, showing the vertical genal ctenidium (*g.ct.*) composed of four spines. This flea has a pronotal ctenidium also, but it is not shown in the figure. 6, *Ctenocephalides canis*, chiefly of Canidae, showing the horizontal genal ctenidium (cf. *C. felis felis*), composed of eight to nine spines, the first spine being only about half as long as the second (contrast *C. felis felis*) and the strongly-rounded head (contrast *C. felis felis*). This flea has a pronotal ctenidium also, but it is not shown in the figure. 7, *Ctenocephalides felis* of many mammals, showing the horizontal genal ctenidium, composed of eight to nine spines, the first spine being about as long as the second (contrast *C. canis*) and the elongate head (contrast *C. canis*). This flea has a pronotal ctenidium also, but it is not shown in the figure.

Fig. 190. Heads of Some Common Fleas

Genal ctenidium of eight (sometimes nine) elements, horizontally
    placed 7
7. Frontal spine of genal ctenidium as long as the second spine, head
    with low sloping front about two times as long as high
                                                    Ctenocephalides felis

Frontal spine of genal ctenidium shorter than second spine, head with
    rounded front, about one and a half times as long as high
                                                    Ctenocephalides canis

8. Eighteen to twenty spines in pronotal ctenidium, on rodents
                            Ceratophyllus (Nosopsyllus) fasciatus

More than twenty-four spines in pronotal ctenidium, on poultry
                                        Ceratophyllus gallinae

Life-cycle. The female flea lays up to twenty eggs at a time and some
400–500 during her lifetime. Studies by Mead-Briggs & Rudge (1960)
and Rothschild (1965) using the rabbit flea, *Spilopsyllus cuniculi* have
demonstrated that maturation of the ovaries of the female flea occurred
only on pregnant rabbits. The most effective hormones controlling the
maturation process are the corticosteroids. The oval, glistening eggs
are deposited in dust or dirt, or they may be laid on the host, but soon
drop off, as they are not sticky. The eggs are about 0·5 mm. long, rounded
at the poles and pearly white in colour. The rate of development varies
greatly and depends also on the temperature and humidity. The larvae
may hatch in 2 days, or up to 16 days after the eggs have been laid. The
egg-shell is broken by means of a chitinous spine, which is present on the
head of the first larval instar. The larvae are elongate, slender, maggot-
like creatures, consisting of three thoracic and ten abdominal segments,
each of which bears a few long hairs. The last abdominal segment bears
two hooked processes called the *anal struts*, which are used for holding on
to substrata or for locomotion. The larvae are creamy yellow in colour
and very active, hiding from light. They have masticatory mouth parts
and feed on dry blood, faeces and other organic matter, but apparently
require little food. They are found in crevices in floors, under carpets
and in similar places. A moderate temperature and a high degree of

THE LONGEVITY IN DAYS OF VARIOUS COMMON FLEAS

	Fed	Unfed in air nearly saturated with moisture
Pulex irritans	125	513
Xenopsylla cheopis	38	100
Ceratophyllus fasciatus	95	106
Ctenocephalides felis	58	234
Ceratophyllus gallinae	127	345

humidity are favourable for development, which lasts 7–10 days or longer. The mature maggot is about 6 mm. long. It spins a cocoon which measures about 4 by 2 mm. In this the pupal stage is passed, lasting 10–17 days under average conditions, but it may last several months and a low temperature will cause the imago to stay in the cocoon.

Habits and Significance. Fleas are much less permanent parasites than, for example, lice and frequently leave their hosts. Their longevity varies, with different species of fleas, according to whether they are fed or not, and according to the degree of moisture in their surroundings. Unfed fleas do not live long in dry surroundings, but, in a humid environment, if debris in which they can hide is present, different species may live for 1–4 months. Specimens of the rat flea *Ceratophyllus fasciatus* have been kept without food for 17 months at a temperature of 15·5°C and 70 per cent humidity.

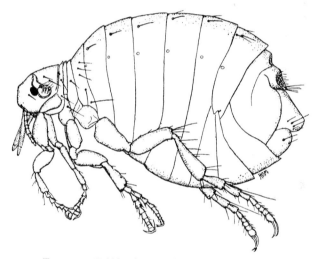

Fig. 191. *Echidnophaga gallinacea* (Original)

Fleas are not markedly specific for their host and may feed on other hosts. In the absence of the normal host they may still feed and they then may be able to survive for longer periods than those indicated in the table on p. 386. Thus *Pulex irritans* may have a maximum life of about 34 months, *Ctenocephalides canis* of 26 months and *Ceratophyllus gallinae* of 17 months.

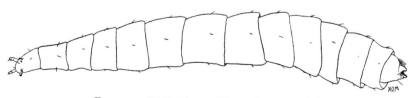

Fig. 192. *Echidnophaga gallinacea*, Larva (Original)

Pathogenesis. Substantial infestations of fleas are especially found on animals which are in poor condition or are suffering from a chronic debilitating disease. Such burdens may be seen in old cats. Infested animals become restless, lose condition and spoil their coats by biting and scratching. A flea bite, initially, is characterised by an area of ischaemia surrounded by an elevated oedematous reddened wheal: this may become indurated and persist for several days especially in hypersensitive animals. The latter may develop a 'flea dermatitis' and this may prove difficult to alleviate. Immunological studies on flea bite hypersensitivity by Young *et al.* (1963) have shown that the saliva of fleas is a hapten which needs to be fixed to the skin of the host before it becomes antigenic.

The 'stick-tight' flea of poultry, *Echidnophaga gallinacea*, may also attack dogs, cats, horses, rabbits, pigeons and ducks. The female flea attaches herself mainly to the comb, wattles and around the eyes of birds. This flea does not jump away when disturbed and large numbers may be seen clustering together. Young birds are quickly killed by these fleas and even adult birds may succumb to heavy infections. The female burrows into the skin, causing the formation of swellings which may ulcerate. The flea lays its eggs in these ulcers. The eggs hatch there and the larvae fall out to develop like the larvae of other fleas, reaching the adult stage in about 4 weeks.

In addition to their direct effects, fleas also are important in the transmission of disease. The classical example is bubonic plague (*Pasteurella pestis*) which is carried by *Xenopsylla cheopis*. Other species may be infected experimentally but are not regarded as important natural vectors. *Xenopsylla astia* and *Xenopsylla braziliensis* are relatively poor transmitters both in nature and artificially. An important factor in plague transmission is the 'blocking' of the chitinous teeth of the proventriculus with blood and plague bacilli. A 'blocked' flea is unable to fill the midgut with blood and wanders from host to host attempting to feed. In so doing it contaminates the new hosts with bacilli.

Enzootic plague (sylvatic plague) exists in wild rodents in China, parts of Africa, South America and in the Western States of the U.S.A. It is considered that the disease became established in the western U.S.A. following the San Francisco earthquake and fire of 1906, rats from the waterfront being driven inland and these infected ground squirrels, which are now the major hosts for the infection.

In addition to the above, the rabbit flea *Spilopsyllus cuniculi* is responsible for the transmission of myxomatosis of rabbits in Europe, *Ctenocephalides canis*, *C. felis* and *Pulex irritans* serve as intermediate hosts for the tapeworm *Dipylidium caninum* and *C. canis* and *C. felis* as intermediate hosts for the filarial worm of dog *Dipetalonema reconditum*.

Control. Pyrethrum and rotenone will kill fleas on their hosts. DDT (5 per cent dust or 1 per cent wash) or BHC (0·01 per cent gamma isomer dust or wash) may also be used. The dangers of intoxication due to

DDT and BHC especially in dogs and cats should be kept in mind. Turk (1959) recommends DDT (5 per cent dust or 0·5 per cent spray or dip) or the same strength of methoxychlor or chlordane, or 0·1–0·2 per cent of lindane dust or 0·06 per cent of lindane as a dip or spray. Fiedler (1958) prefers malathion for the treatment of birds. The environments of the hosts, in which the larvae develop, should also be treated. A dust of DDT 1 part and pyrophyllite 10 parts kills the larvae but not the eggs. Benbrook (1959) recommends pyrethrum sprays or 1 gallon per 4000 sq.ft. of 5 per cent DDT for application to the environments. Turk (1959) recommends the application of malathion (4 per cent dust or 2·5 per cent spray) and burning of litter or debris. Strains of fleas resistant to DDT, methoxychlor, chlordane and BHC have appeared in various parts of the world and for these a 4 per cent dust or 0·5 per cent wash of malathion is recommended. Resistant strains of the dog and cat fleas to DDT may be treated with 1 per cent emulsions of diazinon, malathion, gamma BHC and chlordane.

   Echidnophaga gallinacea, the sticktight flea, presents a special problem, because the adult fleas are attached to the hosts. DDT at a concentration of 0·1 per cent in dip form is effective though this may be raised to 1 per cent without harmful effects. Dusts containing 5 per cent DDT kill the fleas but do not give prolonged protection as do the dips. A 5 per cent malathion dust has proved effective.

ORDER: DIPTERA

Species of this order have only a single pair of membranous wings. These are the mesothoracic pair, the metathoracic pair being modified to form the halteres (balancers). The mouth parts are adapted for sucking. Usually they form a proboscis, the labium having at its distal end a pair of fleshy lobes (*labella*). The mandibles are usually absent. The mesothorax, which bears the single pair of wings, is usually large and the prothorax and metathorax are small and fused with the mesothorax. The tarsi usually have five joints. The metamorphosis is complete, the larvae being apodous and often having a reduced head. The pupa may be coarctate and enclosed in the skin (puparium) of the last larval phase, or it may be obtect. The number of veins in the wings is reduced. Many species of this order cause diseases of farm animals. Examples of them are the mosquitoes and their relations, the house fly, the tsetse fly, the blow fly, the warble fly and the sheep-ked.

CLASSIFICATION OF THE ORDER DIPTERA

The Order Diptera is divided into the following three suborders:

SUBORDER: NEMATOCERA

The antennae of the adults are longer than the head and thorax. They have more than eight segments and the segments are, with the exception of the first two segments next to the head, all more or less alike. They have no arista. The larvae and pupae of Nematocera described in this book are aquatic. The larvae have a well-developed head and mandibles that bite horizontally. The pupae are obtectate.

The suborder contains several families of veterinary and medical importance, including: family Ceratopogonidae (biting midges); family Simuliidae (black-flies); family Psychodidae (sandflies); family Culicidae (mosquitoes).

Other families of no veterinary importance are Tipulidae (daddy-long-legs), Bibionidae, Chironomidae (non-biting midges).

SUBORDER: BRACHYCERA

The antennae are shorter than the thorax and consist of less than six segments, three only being often present, the last segment being annulated. An arista may be present on the antenna, but, when it is, it is terminal. The maxillary palps are held stiffly forwards (porrect). The abdomen usually has seven visible segments. The larvae have an incomplete and usually retractile head and the mandibles bite vertically. The pupa is obtectate. The only family of veterinary importance in this suborder is the Tabanidae.

SUBORDER: CYCLORRHAPHA

The antennae have only three segments and there is an arista, which is usually on the dorsal side of the antenna. The maxillary palps are usually small and consist of one joint only. The abdomen usually has fewer than seven visible segments. The larva has a vestigial head. The pupa is coarctate.

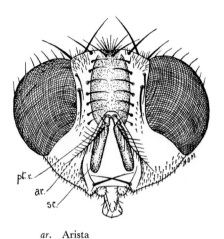

ar.   Arista
pt.r. Ptilinal ridge
sc.   Third antennal segment

FIG. 193. *Lucilia sericata*, Head, Anterior View (Original)

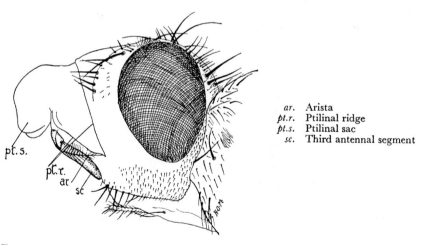

ar.   Arista
pt.r. Ptilinal ridge
pt.s. Ptilinal sac
sc.   Third antennal segment

FIG. 194. *Lucilia sericata*, Head of Fly just emerged from Puparium, showing inflated Ptilinal Sac; Lateral View (Original)

The head of the *Cyclorrhapha* has a horseshoe-shaped ridge, the *ptilinal suture* or frontal suture, which runs transversely above the antennae and downwards on either side of them. Along this suture the head capsule is invaginated in the form of a much convoluted membranous sac which functions only in the young fly. When the latter is ready to emerge from the puparium, it pushes out this *ptilinal sac* by inflating it, and thus breaks a circular piece off the anterior end of the pupal case. The sac is then gradually withdrawn and the ptilinal suture closes. Species of the Nematocera and Brachycera have no ptilinal sac and emerge from the pupal case through a T-shaped split on its dorsal surface.

The suborder Cyclorrhapha is divided into the following three sections:

Section: Aschiza

Frontal or ptilinal sature restricted, ptilinum absent. Generally of no veterinary importance except the Syrphidae (hover flies) which may occur in food material.

Section: Schizophora

Frontal or ptilinal sature distinct, ptilinum always present.

Superfamily Acalypterae. Squamae small, not concealing the halteres. Thorax without distinct transverse sature. Of no veterinary importance.

Superfamily Calypterae. Squamae well developed, concealing halteres. Thorax with a distinct transverse sature. Families of importance include: Anthomyidae (house flies, stable flies etc.); Tachinidae (blow flies) and Oestridae (bot flies).

Section: Pupipara

Head closely united with thorax, dorso-ventrally flattened, integument leathery or horny. Adapted for ectoparasitic life. Wings reduced or absent viviparous. Philinum present or absent. One family of veterinary importance; Hippoboscidae (louse flies).

SUBORDER: NEMATOCERA

Family: Ceratopogonidae

Species of this family are the minute insects that are called biting midges, punkies or in the U.S.A. 'no-see-ums'. In Australia they, and the Simuliidae as well, are often called 'sandflies'. Their mouth parts form a short proboscis adapted for sucking blood, the mandibles acting like scissors. The thorax is humped over the head. The long antennae of Ceratopogonidae are, like those of Culicidae (see later), plumose in the male and pilose in the female. The wings, however, unlike those of the Culicidae, have no scales, but they have hairs. The wings of some Ceratopogonidae are spotted and their anterior veins, which are stouter than the posterior ones, enclose two small areas called the first and second radial cells, and the other veins form two median forks, the branches of which end at the margin of the wing. The wings, are folded flat over the abdomen when they are at rest.

The eggs of Ceratopogonidae are laid in water and the wormlike larvae, like those of the non-biting midges, the Chironomidae, are aquatic or semi-aquatic, but, while the larvae of some Chironomidae are coloured red by haemoglobin and are called bloodworms, the larvae of Ceratopogonidae are whitish, with a small head and three thoracic and nine abdominal segments, the terminal segment bearing a few locomotory spines.

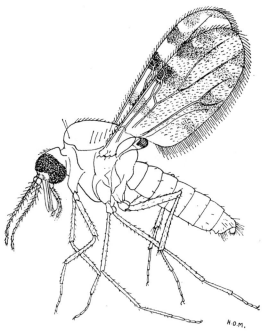

FIG. 195. *Culicoides* (Original)

At the posterior end there are three retractile anal gills, but the larvae also breathe through the skin. The brown, inactive, obtectate pupa is like the chrysalis of a butterfly. It has two long, respiratory trumpets on the sides of the mesothorax and nine abdominal segments, which end in two spines with which the pupa anchors itself in, or at the surface of, shallow water or in crevices in manure heaps or rotting vegetation. The whole pupa is covered with spines and tubercles.

Among the Ceratopogonidae the genus *Culicoides* has veterinary importance. Species of this genus are about 1–3 mm. long, and can pass through ordinary mosquito screens. The females of some species of this genus attack man and animals to suck blood, and can cause great annoyance if they occur in large numbers. Their bites cause itching and swellings, which may require treatment. Several species are vectors of Protozoa and filarioid nematodes. They are listed, together with the Protozoa and nematodes they transmit, and the literature about them, by Fallis & Bennett (1961). The following species are intermediate hosts of the filariid nematodes named: *C. grahami* and *C. austeni* of *Dipetalonema perstans* in Africa and *C. grahami* probably of *D. streptocara* in Africa; *C. nubeculosus* and possibly other species of *Onchocerca cervicalis* of horses in Britain; *C. pungens* and possibly three other species also of *O. gibsoni* in Malaya; *C. furens* of *Mansonella ozzardi* in South America. Species of *Culicoides* are also responsible for the transmission of virus diseases, especially that of blue-tongue of sheep in South Africa and also that of horse sickness in Africa. *C. robertsi* causes an allergic dermatitis of horses in Queensland described by Riek (1954), which is due to hypersensitivity to the bites of this insect and is associated with increase of histamine in the blood in the summer, rising to a peak in late afternoon and early morning when this species is most active.

Control of these species is difficult. Screens treated with repellents and insecticides prevent the entry of the insects. Their larvae may be attacked in their breeding grounds. Smith *et al.* (1959) found that the adults of *C. furens* can migrate for several miles over the salt marshes of eastern Florida. Ditching, dyking and pumping water from these marshes failed to control the insects breeding, but excellent control of the larvae was obtained by the application by aircraft of 5 per cent dieldrin granules and heptachlor was also effective. But in 1958 it was found that the larvae had become resistant to dieldrin, heptachlor, chlordane, lindane and endrin, but not to DDT. Parathion, malathion and Bayer L 21/199 were, however, highly effective against strains resistant to chlorinated hydrocarbons. Kettle *et al.* (1959) found that, in the boglands of Midlothian Scotland, spraying with dieldrin, chlordane and DDT controlled *C. impunctatus* and that 100 per cent control persisted for 3 years and seemed to improve with time. BHC was much less effective.

FAMILY: SIMULIIDAE

The small species of this family are often called black flies or buffalo gnats. The thorax is humped over the head and the piercing proboscis is short. The long antennae, which have eleven segments, differ from those of species of the families Ceratopogonidae and Culicidae, in not being plumose or pilose. The wings are broad and they are not spotted. They have no scales and they are not hairy, except for bristles on the thick anterior veins. The body is covered with short golden or silvery hairs.

The eggs are laid on stones or plants just below the surface of the water in running streams. The female inserts her ovipositor into the water to lay, and deposits several hundred eggs at a time. They hatch in 4–12 days, depending on the temperature. The larvae are cylindrical and attach themselves by means of a posterior sucker-like organ which is armed with small hooks, but they are able to move about. Anteriorly are the mouth parts and a pair of brush-like organs; the larvae are carnivorous. Near the anterior extremity the ventral surface bears an arm-

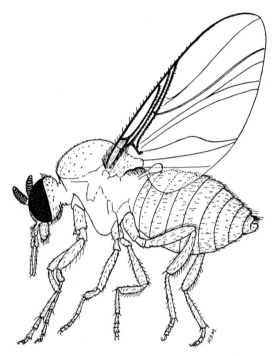

FIG. 196. *Simulium*

like appendage called the *proleg*, which has a circlet of hooks at its free end and the larva uses this when it moves about. The larvae moult six times; at the last moult the pupa appears. The mature larva spins a triangular cocoon on the surface to which it is attached, and in this the pupal stage is passed. The obtectate pupa has one dorsal and one ventral respiratory tube, the branches of which float out of the cocoon.

The simuliids occur in practically all parts of the world, but are troublesome especially in warm countries. They cause great annoyance and irritation. Swarms of these flies will keep cattle from grazing or cause them to stampede and hurt themselves. They bite on the legs and abdomen, or on the head and ears. The bites give rise to vesicles which burst, or wart-like papules, which may be very troublesome on the teats of cows and take weeks to heal. Poultry are often attacked and may even become anaemic from loss of blood. The flies are active in the morning and evening, resting during the hot part of the day on the under-side of leaves near the ground.

Simulium indicum, the potu fly, is active in the Himalayan mountains. Swarms of *S. columbaczense* on the shores of the River Danube in 1923 are reported to have killed 20,000 horses, cattle, sheep, goats and pigs, as

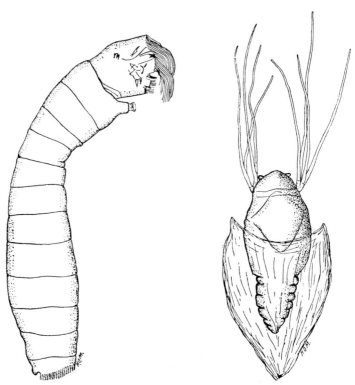

FIG. 197. *Simulium* Larva (Original)   FIG. 198. *Simulium* Pupa (Original)

well as deer, foxes, hares and other animals, and in 1934 even larger numbers of animals were killed by it. *S. pecuarum*, the southern buffalo gnat, has caused severe losses of cattle in the Mississippi Valley and may especially attack mules. Several species of *Simulium* are vectors of other kinds of parasites. Thus in North America *S. venustum* transmits the protozoon *Leucocytozoon anatis* of ducks, *L. smithi* of turkeys and *L. caulleryi* of the fowl. *S. rugglesi* may transmit *Haemoproteus nettionis* to ducks and geese (various species of *Anas*, *Melanitta perspicillata*, *Bucephala clangula americana*, *Clangula hyemalis*, *Aix sponsa* and *Mergus* sp.). In Canada *S. ornatum* is the intermediate host of the filariid nematode *Onchocerca gutturosa* of cattle. The intermediate hosts of *O. volvulus* of man are *S. damnosum* and *S. neavei* in Africa and, in Guatemala and Mexico, *S. metallicum*, *S. ochraceum* and *S. callidum*. It has been claimed that *S. decorum katmai* mechanically transmits tularaemia.

Control is difficult because the adults can fly 2–3 miles or more. Medicated screens may provide some protection against the adults. WHO points out that the adults prefer to get into clothing before they bite, so that repellents applied to clothing may help. Openings at the neck, wrists etc., should be closed and light-coloured clothes attract them less. For protecting poultry from these flies a dust bath of 0·5 per cent lindane (20 per cent lindane 1 part, inert dust 40 parts) is recommended but this may be toxic to young chickens and turkeys. Several workers have shown that 0·1–0·3 part per million of DDT will rid streams of the larvae for several miles. WHO states that *S. arcticum* was almost completely eradicated in Canada from 100 miles of stream by 0·13 ppm of DDT applied by aircraft and suggests as a guide the application of 0·1 ppm of DDT for 15 minutes at intervals of 1 mile, or 0·05 lb. of DDT per acre of water surface. These amounts will not kill fish, but may harm aquatic arthropods. *S. neavei* was eradicated from the whole of Kenya, excepting one small area, by the application of 0·05–1 ppm of DDT to the streams in nine cycles, each cycle lasting 10 days.

Family: Psychodidae

The Psychodidae, commonly known as 'sandflies' or 'owl midges', are small, moth-like flies, rarely over 5 mm. long. Their bodies and wings are hairy. The legs are long, rarely short. The wings are held roof-like over the abdomen during rest. The mouth parts are short or of medium length. The antennae are long, consisting of sixteen segments which often have a beaded appearance, and they are thickly covered with hairs. The palpi are recurved and hairy.

The eggs are laid in moist, dark places, e.g. in rock crevices and between stones. The female of *Phlebotomus papatasii* lays about forty to eighty eggs at a time. A temperature of over 15°C is required, else the embryo becomes dormant. Under favourable conditions the whole life-cycle can be completed in about 6 weeks. The larvae resemble small caterpillars and feed on faeces of lizards, bats and other animals and on dried leaves.

The flies are active at night only and hide during the day in dark corners. They are weak fliers and the females of some species are bloodsuckers. They can pass through ordinary nets, or will otherwise search for an opening to get through. Adler & Theodor (1957) summarise research in progress on the transmission of disease by phlebotomine sandflies and give a list of the various species of *Phlebotomus* involved. *P. papatasii*, *P. sergenti*, *P. major* and perhaps other species transmit the protozoon *Leishmania tropica*, the cause of cutaneous leishmaniasis, to man, dogs being reservoir hosts in some areas (e.g. Iran); and *L. tropica* is transmitted from gerbils and ground squirrels to man in Turkestan and Iran by *P. papatasii* and *P. caucasicus*. Various species of *Phlebotomus*

transmit *L. braziliensis*, the cause of South American cutaneous leishmaniasis (espundia), to man. *L. donovani*, the cause of kala-azar, is
transmitted by *P. argentipes* in India, by *P. chinensis* in China and probably
by several other species of *Phlebotomus* in the Middle East, Africa and the
Mediterranean region. Sandfly fever is transmitted in the Mediterranean
area by *P. papatasii* and in China possibly by *P. chinensis* and *P. mongolensis*.

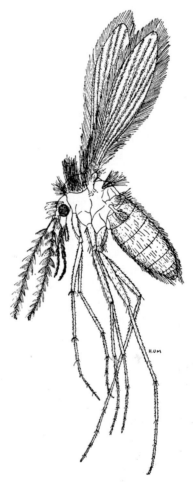

FIG. 199. *Phlebotomus* Sp. (Original)

Bartonella bacilliformis, the cause of Carrion's disease (Oroya fever), is
transmitted by *P. verrucarum* and in Colombia possibly by *P. columbianum*.

Control. Removal of dense vegetation discourages the breeding of these
flies. WHO states that single residual application of 100–300 mg. of DDT
per sq. ft. to the interiors of human and animal dwellings has given good
results and protection for 1–2 years, and that 22 mg. per sq. ft. of gamma

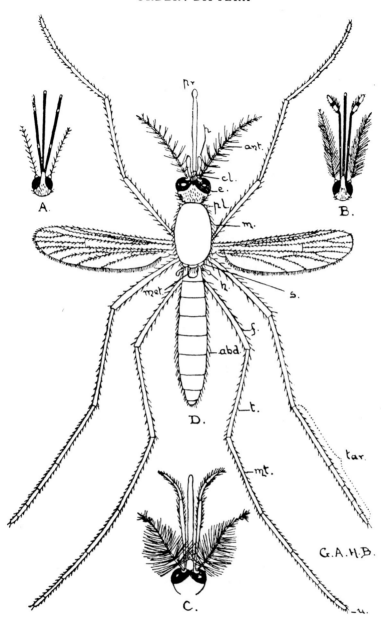

abd.	Abdomen	mt.	Metatarsus
ant.	Antenna	p.	Palp
cl.	Clypeus	pl.	Prothoracic lobe
e.	Eye	pr.	Proboscis
f.	Femur	s.	Scutellum
h.	Halter	t.	Tibia
m.	Mesothorax	tar.	Tarsus
met.	Metathorax or post-scutellum	u.	Ungues, or claws

Fig. 200. External Anatomy of Mosquitoes: A, Head of *Anopheles* sp., female; B, head of *Anopheles* sp., male; C, head of *Culex* sp., male, and D, *Culex* sp., female (After Bedford)

BHC also reduced the numbers of the flies for 3 months. Resistance of these flies to insecticides has not yet been reported.

Repellents, such as dimethyl phthalate, may be tried, and spraying rooms with DDT will kill the sandflies.

FAMILY: CULICIDAE

The mosquitoes are slender Nematocera with small, spherical heads and long legs. The antennae of fourteen to fifteen segments are conspicuous and are plumose in the males. The proboscis is long and slender.

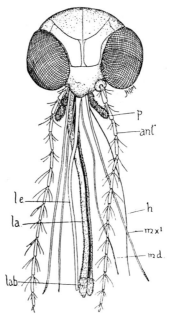

ant.	Antenna	*lab.*	Labellum
h.	Hypopharynx	*md.*	Mandible
la.	Labium	*mx.*[1]	First maxilla
l.e.	Labrum-epipharynx	*p.*	Palp

FIG. 201. Head and Mouth Parts of a *Culex* Female (Original)

The abdomen is elongate and the thorax is characteristically wedge-shaped, with the broad end dorsally. The wings are long, narrow and folded flat over the abdomen during rest. They bear elongate, leaf-like scales along the margins and on the veins.

The eggs are laid on water or on floating vegetable matter, and each species has its special requirements, which are usually very restricted. Some species lay their eggs only in fresh rain water, others in stagnant pools or in any vessel that contains water; others lay in quiet pools at the edges of streams, and some even lay in salt water. The temperature of the water, the nature of the microflora in it, the presence or absence of decayed matter and the acidity or alkalinity are all deciding factors. The eggs may be deposited in masses or 'egg-rafts' as in the case of *Culex*, or singly as in the case of *Anopheles* and *Aedes*. In the egg-rafts the eggs are arranged vertically with their anterior ends towards the water. The anopheline egg is boat-shaped and is provided with a float on either side and a frilled edge.

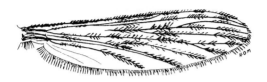

FIG. 202. Wing of a Mosquito (Original)

The larvae have a well-developed head and a distinct thorax and abdomen. The head bears eyes, antennae and several hairs. The mouth parts are masticatory, and are surrounded by brushes that produce currents in order to bring food particles to the mouth. The unsegmented

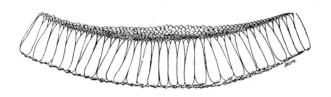

FIG. 203. *Culex* Egg-raft (Original)

thorax bears feathered hairs and the abdomen, which is segmented and also hairy, is provided in the anophelines with certain palmate hairs, by means of which the larva is able to cling to the surface of the water. The stigmata from which tracheae pass through the whole body are situated on the fused eighth and ninth abdominal segments. The tenth segment bears feathered hairs and tracheal gills, which are especially well developed in forms like *Aedes*, that feed at the bottom of the water. All mosquito larvae, except those of *Anopheles*, are provided with a siphon or tube which arises from the dorsal aspect of the eighth and ninth abdominal segments and surrounds the stigmata. It is closed at its apex by chitinous valves that open when the larva goes to the surface of the water to breathe. The larvae then hang down into the water at an angle, while anopheline larvae lie against the surface. The larvae moult four times, the last time at the moment of pupation.

The pupa has a rounded 'body', which consists of head and thorax, and an elongate abdomen, flattened dorso-ventrally and flexed underneath the body. Through the delicate cuticle of the latter the wings and appendages of the adult can be seen. From the dorsal aspect of the thorax,

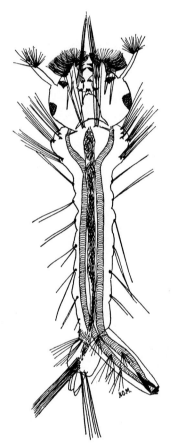

Fig. 204. Culicine Larva (Original)

and attached to the lateral stigmata, there arise a pair of tubes or respiratory trumpets, through which the pupa breathes at the surface of the water. The pupae are not quite as active as the larvae.

The time required for development differs according to the species and varies from about 7 to 16 days under favourable circumstances, which means especially a sufficiently high temperature. Cold weather may prolong the larval period to several months. The eggs of some species can also resist cold or drying for a considerable time. There are great variations in the seasonal prevalence of different species, mainly due to temperature requirements; most species breed in warm weather, but in warm climates some breed only in winter. Females which find it too late to lay may hide away and hibernate, or aestivate in hot climates, until the next season. The hiding-places are usually relatively dark surroundings with an even temperature, like cellars, barns and lofts under thatched roofs.

Apart from the presence of permanent water, rainfall has a marked influence on the number of mosquitoes for several reasons. If there is little or no rain, mosquitoes will be scarce because their numbers are

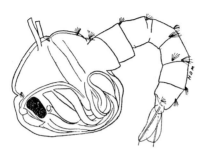

Fig. 205. Culicine Pupa (Original)

limited by their natural enemies in the permanent breeding-places. After a rain the numbers will increase, because the mosquitoes develop rapidly and are not restricted by enemies in the new breeding-places. Much rain, on the other hand, washes away the larvae and usually decreases the number of mosquitoes, unless pools remain afterwards. The young stages can be transferred to a new area by water which flows inter-mittently.

The adults may fly fair distances, especially anophelines, which, according to recent investigations, can travel several kilometres from their breeding-ground to feed and return in the morning. They may be carried much further by winds or cover long distances in successive stages. They can also be transported in all kinds of vehicles. Some species readily enter buildings, while others do not.

Mosquitoes can be fed on fruit juices and sugar water, and the males exist normally on such food, but the females are blood-suckers and require a meal of blood in order to lay eggs. The females seem to be attracted by the warmth radiating from the skin of their host. They are active at night and are attracted by light, while during the day they hide in dark corners.

The family Culicidae is divided into several Tribes, but veterinarians will be chiefly concerned with species belonging to the Tribes *Culicini* and *Anophelini*. The chief features distinguishing these two Tribes are given in the table on p. 404.

Although mosquitoes can be a great nuisance and cause painful bites, their chief importance lies in the fact that they are the intermediate hosts and vectors of several very important parasitic and virus diseases

DISTINGUISHING CHARACTERS OF ANOPHELINI AND CULICINI

	Anophelini	Culicini
Eggs	Laid singly, boat-shaped with paired lateral floats	Laid in rafts or singly (*Aedes*) No floats
Larva	No siphon tube	Well-developed siphon tube
	Rests parallel to water surface and feeds there	Hangs head down from water surface and feeds below it
	Palmate hairs on dorsal surface of abdomen	No palmate hairs
Pupa	Breathing trumpet short and broad in lateral view	Breathing trumpets long and narrow in lateral view
Adults	Rest with abdomen directed away from resting surface, i.e. proboscis and abdomen in a straight line	Rest with abdomen pointing towards resting surface. Proboscis and abdomen at an angle, imparting a humped-back appearance
	Female palps as long as proboscis	Female palps very short
	Male palps as long as proboscis, clubbed	Male palps as long as proboscis, not clubbed
	Scutellum evenly curved	Scutellum trilobed
Examples	*Anopheles maculipennis.* *Anopheles gambiae*	*Culex pipiens* *Aedes aegypti*

of man and domestic animals. Thus the definitive hosts of species of the protozoan genus *Plasmodium*, which cause human malaria, are various species of *Anopheles*, and those of the species of *Plasmodium* which cause bird malaria are species of *Culex*, *Theobaldia*.and *Aedes*. Various culicine and anopheline species are intermediate hosts of filariid nematodes. Thus those of *Wuchereria bancrofti* of man are numerous species of *Culex*, *Aedes* and *Mansonia*; those of *B. malayi* in Indonesia, Indo-China and Ceylon are species of *Mansonia* and *Anopheles*; and those of *Dirofilaria immitis* of the dog are species of *Anopheles*, *Culex*, *Mansonia* and *Myzorhynchus*. The spirochaete *Borrelia anserina* is transmitted to the fowl by species of *Aedes*. Rift Valley fever of man in South Africa is transmitted by species of *Mansonia*; yellow fever of man is transmitted chiefly by *Aedes aegypti* and perhaps by several other species of *Aedes*; eastern and western equine encephalitis and St. Louis and Japanese B encephalitis of man, and other forms of viral encephalitis in America and elsewhere, are transmitted by species of *Aedes* and *Culex*, as well as by *Dermanyssus gallinae*. Dengue fever is transmitted to man chiefly by *Aedes aegypti* and perhaps by other species of *Aedes*. It has been reported that *Aedes aegypti* may mechanically transmit tularaemia and that *A. aegypti* and species of *Culex* may mechanically transmit *Treponema pertenue*, the cause of yaws.

Control. In recent years campaigns against malaria and yellow fever have been remarkably successful in eradicating anopheline and culicine mosquitoes. Thus the WHO Chronicle (1960) briefly describes the eradication of *Aedes aegypti* from Brazil with DDT and this species has also been eradicated from Guyana, Mauritius and Venezuela with DDT, and *Anopheles darlingi* has been virtually eradicated from Venezuela and *A. funestus* from Mauritius. The larvae are attacked in their breeding places. Drainage will remove water from these and paraffin or other oils put on the water surface prevents the respiration of the larvae. Among insecticides which have been sprayed or otherwise applied to the breeding places are Paris green, pyrethrum, DDT, heptachlor, dieldrin, chlordane, lindane and BHC. The WHO Eighth Report of their Expert Committee on the control of Vectors (1958) and their Specifications for Pesticides (1961) give details of formulae used and of the use of hand- and fog-sprayers, fog generators and application by means of aircraft. For larvae of *Culex tarsalis* not resistant to chlorinated hydrocarbon insecticides 0·1 lb. of DDT, heptachlor, dieldrin or lindane are recommended and 84 g. of EPN or parathion or 450 g. of malathion per hectare have been successful; but in California strains of these larvae resistant of DDT and malathion have appeared, though the strain resistant to malathion is not resistant to parathion.

The adults are attacked by: (a) general measures such as the use of screens, mosquito nets, protective clothing etc., (b) repellents. Of the many compounds tested for their repellent action, indalone, dimethyl phthalate and Rutgers 612 seem to be the most effective. The WHO (1958) lists these and other repellents and warns that all of them must be used with care. Some of them damage clothing other than that made of cotton or wool and some repel Simuliidae and other insects as well. (c) The application of insecticides to places in which mosquitoes occur, such as the walls of buildings, aeroplanes etc., either by hand or other means or by aircraft to areas of land.

Control has been, in recent years, complicated by the appearance in some parts of the world of strains of mosquitoes resistant to chlorinated hydrocarbon insecticides, usually either to DDT or methoxychlor, on the one hand, or to dieldrin, aldrin and BHC on the other, but rarely to both, so that an insecticide suitable for each resistant strain can still be chosen.

The numerous species of mosquitoes proved to be resistant to various insecticides are listed by the WHO (1959, 1963) and the general problem of insecticide resistance is reviewed by Micks (1960) and WHO (1964).

Culicine species are attacked by much the same methods. The WHO Report (1958) recommends, for attacks on adults of *Culex quinquefasciatus* (*fatigans*), the application of 200 mg. of DDT per sq. ft., or of 0·25–0·5 g. of dieldrin per sq. m. or of 0·25–0·4 g. of BHC per sq. m. or of 1 g. of chlordane per sq. m. according to whether the strain attacked is resistant to the insecticide or not. The larvae can be attacked by the methods given above for the larvae of *C. tarsalis*. The species of *Mansonia* which transmit rural filariasis in Ceylon have been controlled by the application of methyl-chlorophenoxyacetic acid as a herbicide against the plant host, *Pistia stratiotes*, of this species.

SUBORDER: BRACHYCERA

The only family of this suborder that needs to be considered in this book is the family Tabanidae.

FAMILY: TABANIDAE

These insects, commonly known as 'horse-flies' or 'breeze flies', are large, robust flies with powerful wings and large eyes. The latter are almost contiguous (holoptic) in the males and separated by a narrow space in the females, and project posteriorly beyond the lateral margins of the thorax. The antennae have two short basal segments and a third which is large and usually ringed. The wing venation is very characteristic, especially the branching of the fourth longitudinal vein. The proboscis

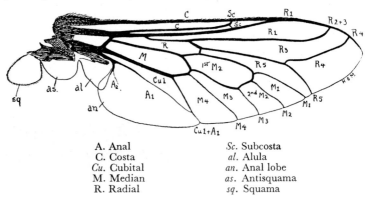

A. Anal	Sc. Subcosta
C. Costa	al. Alula
Cu. Cubital	an. Anal lobe
M. Median	as. Antisquama
R. Radial	sq. Squama

FIG. 206. *Tabanus,* Wing showing Veins and Cells. (Original)

is relatively short in *Tabanus* and *Haematopota,* longer in *Chrysops* and *very long* in *Pangonia.* These are the most important genera. In species of the genus *Pangonia* the proboscis is very long and projects forwards, and the third (terminal) segment of the antenna has six or seven annulations. The wings are held divergent when at rest. In species of the genera *Tabanus, Chrysops* and *Haematopota* the proboscis is soft and it hangs down. These three genera may be distinguished by their antennae. In species of the genus *Chrysops* the first and second segments of the antenna are long, the third (terminal) segment has four annulations, the wings have a dark band passing from the anterior to the posterior border of the wing, the wings are divergent when at rest, and the eyes are of a metallic colour. In species of the genus *Haematopota* the first segment of the antenna is large and the second segment narrower, while the terminal segment has three annulations and the wings have a characteristic mottling. In the species of the genus *Tabanus* the first two segments of the antenna are small and the third (terminal) segment has a tooth-like projection on its basal part and also four annulations (Fig. 208). Species of this genus have clear wings. They are frequently brown with longitudinal stripes on the abdomen, and hold their wings horizontal when at rest.

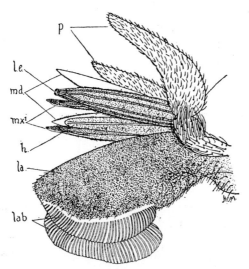

h. Hypopharynx	*l.e.* Labrum-epipharynx
la. Labium	*md.* Mandibles
lab. Labella with pseudo-tracheal	*mx¹.* First maxillae
membrane	*p.* Palps

FIG. 207.   Mouth Parts of *Tabanus* (Original)

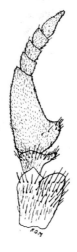

Fig. 208.   *Tabanus*, Antenna (Original)

Life-cycle. The eggs are laid in the vicinity of water, usually on the leaves of plants. The larger species lay 500–600 eggs, the smaller 300. The eggs are about 2 mm. long and light in colour, but turn dark after a while. The larvae hatch after 4–7 days and drop into the water, or on mud, into which they disappear. They are maggot-like and the body has eleven segments, besides the cephalic portion which is not conspicuous. Each segment has eight fleshy tubercles. The mouth parts are prehensile and masticatory; the larvae are carnivorous. There are three-jointed antennae and the large lateral tracheae open on the penultimate segment, which also bears a retractile siphon tube. The larvae feed on small crustacea or even on one another, and grow for 2–3 months,

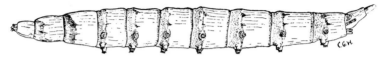

FIG. 209.   *Tabanus* Larva (× 5) (Original)

performing several ecdyses. Finally they pass through a quiescent stage and then pupate. The pupa is brown and subcylindrical; the abdominal segments are movable, and in the anterior part the appendages of the imago can be distinguished. This stage lasts about 10–14 days. The whole life-cycle takes 4–5 months under favourable conditions, but low temperatures prolong development and the larvae may hibernate. The eggs are parasitised by certain small Hymenoptera.

Biology of adults. The flies are seen in summer and are very fond of sunlight. They abound especially near their breeding-places and are most active on hot, sultry days. They attack chiefly large animals like horses and cattle. Some feed mainly on the under-side of the abdomen around the navel or on the legs; others also bite on the neck and withers. They bite a number of times in different places before they are replete, and from the wounds made by them small quantities of blood usually continue to escape and are sucked up by non-biting Muscidae. The flies feed about every 3 days. After feeding they rest on the under-side of leaves, or on stones or trees, for a few hours.

The bites of the Tabanidae are painful and irritating and may give rise to weals in soft-skinned animals. Horses and cattle are restless when troubled by these flies and may become unmanageable if they are in harness. The flies, as well as the Muscidae that come after them, may act as mechanical transmitters of bacterial diseases like anthrax and the virus of equine infectious anaemia. *Chrysops dimidiata*, the Mango fly, and *Chrysops silacea* are intermediate hosts of the filariid nematode, *Loa loa*. Various species are mechanical vectors of *Trypanosoma evansi*, the cause of surra of equines and dogs; *T. equinum*, the cause of Mal de Caderas of equines, *T. simiae* of pigs, *T. vivax* and *T. brucei*, which cause nagana of cattle, sheep, equines and other ungulates; and of *T. gambiense* and *T. rhodesiense*, which cause human African trypanosomiasis. *T. theileri* of cattle is transmitted cyclically by species of *Tabanus* and *Haematopota*.

Control is difficult. Where drainage is possible the breeding-places may be destroyed by this method. The flies have a habit of skimming over water and occasionally dipping their bodies into it; this led to the practice of pouring kerosene onto water, which kills the flies when they dip into it. Animals should be kept away from places where the flies abound during the hot part of the day. Nets which can be fixed to the harness of horses are obtainable in some countries. Aerial sprays of lindane, dieldrin and DDT have been tried in Canada, but neither these, nor pyrethrum, protect the stock for longer than 3 days or so. The methods given below for the control of *Stomoxys* and *Lyperosia* may be tried.

SUBORDER CYCLORRHAPHA
SECTION ASCHIZA

The insects in this group of Diptera are of no direct veterinary importance. However the Syrphidae or hover flies are frequently found in the summer on dung, rotting wood and decaying animal food. They are brightly coloured flies and superficially resemble wasps. A characteristic feature of the wing venation is a 'vena spuria'. One genus, *Eristalis*, has a larval stage with a long terminal flexible respiratory tube and hence it is referred to as a 'rat-tailed maggot'.

This may be found in decaying foodstuffs and may also occur accidentally in the digestive tract of animals (pigs especially) and man. The larvae cause no harm.

SUBORDER CYCLORRHAPHA
SECTION SCHIZOPHORA

SUPERFAMILY: CALYPTERAE

Squamae well developed, concealing halteres. Thorax with a distinct transverse sature. Families of importance Anthomyidae, Tachinidae, Oestridae.

FAMILY: ANTHOMYIDAE

Hypopleural bristles absent (see Tachinidae). Median (M) wing vein more or less parallel to radial $(R4+5)$ wing vein or curving towards it; no definite elbow bend in radial vein (see Tachinidae). Genera of importance *Musca*, *Stomoxys*, *Lyperosia*, *Glossina*, *Haematobia*, *Fannia*.

Genus: Musca Linné, 1758

M. domestica Linné, 1758, the common house fly, has a cosmopolitan distribution, and is important as a mechanical carrier of various infectious agents such as bacteria and worm eggs, and also as intermediate host of several parasitic worms. Some other species of this genus bear a close resemblance to *M. domestica*. Male 5·8–6·5 mm., female 6·5–7·5 mm.

long. The arista is bilaterally plumose up to the tip. In the wing the
M1+2 vein curves forward distally and the R5 (first posterior) cell is
closed or nearly so, while the second is widely open. The thorax is

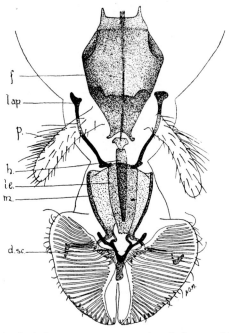

d.sc. Discal sclerite	*l.e.* Labrum-epipharynx
f. Fulcrum	*m.* Mentum
h. Hypopharynx	*p.* Palp
l.ap. Labral apodeme	

FIG. 210. *Musca domestica*, Mouth Parts, Dorsal View (Original)

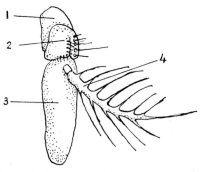

1, 2, 3, First, second and third segments of the antenna; 4, arista biplumose to its tip

FIG. 211. Antenna of *Musca domestica*

yellowish-grey to dark grey and has four longitudinal dark stripes which
are equally wide and extend to the posterior border of the scutum. The
abdomen has a yellowish ground colour and a median, black, longitudinal

stripe which becomes diffuse on the fourth segment. In addition to this stripe the abdomen of the female is marked on either side with a diffuse dark band.

The mouth parts are adapted for imbibing liquid food. The labium is expanded distally into two labella. These are capable of marked expansion when the fly is feeding. The median walls are covered by pseudotracheae which bear a system of channels serving to suck up food in fluid form. Twenty to thirty grooves occur. The labella are also hollow organs and their cavities are connected through that of the labium with the general body cavity or haemocoele. Pressure of the haemocoele fluid (blood) therefore causes the labella to expand and turn their medial surfaces forwards, so that they can be brought in contact with the food. Beginning at the periphery, these grooves converge towards the prestomum, the middle ones opening directly into it, while the dorsal and ventral grooves run first into larger collecting channels. Each groove is strengthened by a series of incomplete rings of chitin, standing closely side by side. The rings are bifid at one end and expanded at the other, and they are so arranged that the bifid and expanded ends alternate on either side of the groove. When the fly feeds the edges of the grooves are drawn together and the food is strained through the small openings which remain between the bifid and expanded ends of the rings. Under such conditions the house fly can swallow particles of only about 4 μ diameter, but it can swallow larger particles if the grooves are not so tightly shut, or particles of about 45 μ diameter if it separates the labella completely and sucks directly through the prestomum, although it is doubtful whether this is frequently done. Liquefiable solid food, such as sugar, may be made fluid before it is sucked up by ejection on to it of saliva and crop-fluid, these drops of fluid being called *vomit-drops*. These points are important in connection with the disease-transmitting powers of the fly.

Life-cycle. The house fly lays 100–150 eggs at a time and a total of about 600. Fresh horse manure is preferred above anything else, but the fly will also develop in the faeces of other animals and man, as well as in all sorts of decaying organic matter and refuse. The eggs are about 1 mm. long, rather elongate, creamy white in colour, and the dorsal surface has two curved, rib-like thickenings. The larva hatches in 12–24 hours, and grows into a maggot 10–12 mm. long in 3–7 days. The body of the larva is pointed anteriorly, and broad at the posterior end on which the stigmal plates are situated. The distance between the two plates is less than the width of a plate and each bears three winding slits. The second body segment also bears a pair of anterior spiracles which are fan-shaped, consisting of a stalk and five to eight papillae each. Anteriorly the body bears a pair of oral hooks which are connected to an internal cephalopharyngeal skeleton composed of darkly pigmented chitin. Three ecdyses occur during the larval life and the pupa remains in the last larval skin, which turns brown and becomes rigid to form the puparium. The full-grown larva leaves the material in which it has developed to pupate in the ground. The pupal stage lasts 3–26 days, depending on the temperature. Fertilisation and ovipostion take place a few days after emergence of the fly and the whole cycle may be completed in about 12 days, so

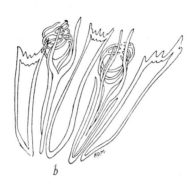

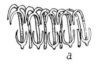

a, Chitinous supports of food channels; *b*, same at discal sclerite, with intervening tooth-like blades

FIG. 212. *Musca domestica*, Chitinous Structures of Pseudo-tracheal Membrane (Original)

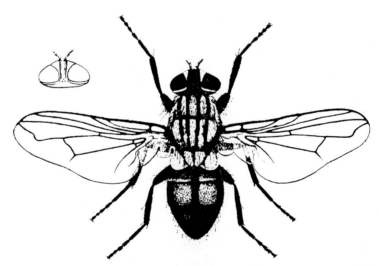

FIG. 213. *Musca domestica*, The House Fly, Female. Inset: Head of the Male (from the drawing in colour by C. G. Hewitt in Hewitt (1914), *The House-fly*, Cambridge University Press, by permission of the publishers)

that a number of generations develop in one summer. The adult flies live
a few weeks only in summer, but they live longer in cool weather. They
probably rarely hibernate. Development proceeds slowly even in winter,
but flies do not emerge in cold regions. The eggs, larvae and pupae can
resist a fair degree of cold when they lie protected, and they are responsible
for the new crop of flies in spring.

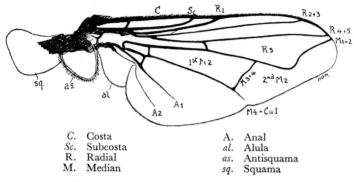

C.	Costa	A.	Anal
Sc.	Subcosta	al.	Alula
R.	Radial	as.	Antisquama
M.	Median	sq.	Squama

FIG. 214. *Musca domestica*, Wing (Original)

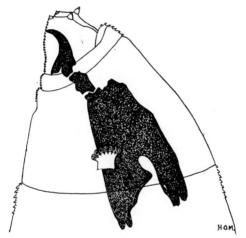

FIG. 215. *Musca domestica*, Anterior End of Third-Stage Larva, Lateral View, showing
Anterior Spiracle and Cephalopharyngeal Skeleton (Original)

Habits and importance. The breeding and feeding habits of *M. domestica*
and related species make them ready carriers of numerous pathogenic
bacteria and parasites. The larval stages developing in faeces become
infected with worm eggs which are present there. Pathogenic bacteria
in the faeces may also be swallowed and persist through the pupal to the
adult stage, but more frequently the adult fly infects itself by feeding on
material which contains these organisms. The hairy feet and legs of the
fly also act as suitable carriers of bacteria from material on which the
fly settles. The possibility of transferring disease germs is especially great
on account of the fact that flies feed on practically any edible matter,

even human faeces, and also on the food of man and animals. When the fly has fed it frequently regurgitates fluid from the crop, and it may deposit this to lick it up again later, or use it to moisten solid food like sugar. Although the house fly may frequently, though not habitually, feed on

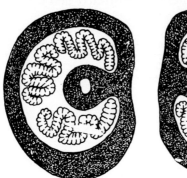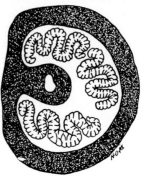

FIG. 216. *Musca domestica*, Posterior Spiracles and Stigmatic Plates of Third-Stage Larva (Original)

wounds, other related species are habitual blood-feeders and often follow a blood-sucking fly. When the latter has inserted its proboscis into an animal, these flies worry it until it leaves, and then they suck up the exuding blood.

The house fly and related species are known to act as carriers of several disease-producing organisms, including those of typhoid fever, cholera, tuberculosis, dysentery, anthrax and various viruses. *Musca domestica* is the intermediate host of several worm parasites of domestic animals, and it may act as a disseminator of the eggs of many others.

Control. The veterinarian is mainly concerned with control measures against the breeding of flies in connection with stables, stock-yards, abattoirs, drains, garbage etc.

Manure must be regularly and frequently removed from stables, sties etc. Its further treatment depends on prevailing conditions, and, as it is usually valuable as a fertiliser, it must be treated accordingly; but under certain conditions this consideration has to be disregarded. Chemical treatment is usually expensive and could therefore only be applied to small quantities of manure. It is not completely effective, because the eggs and larvae are not easily killed in this way. Moreover, such treatment reduces the fertilising value. Powdered borax well mixed with the manure at the rate of 1 kg. per cu. m. of manure (1 lb. per 16 cu. ft.) is stated to kill 90 per cent of the larvae and is harmless to the manure.

A simple method of manure disposal is direct transport to a field and broadcasting thinly. This is only effective in dry, hot weather and the ground should not be moist. In dull or moist weather, or when the manure is spread too thickly, flies will still breed in it.

If manure is stacked in large compact heaps it ferments and the heat thus produced kills the maggots, as well as the eggs and larvae of internal parasites, in the central portion of the material. The sides of the heap and the surrounding soil may be treated with insecticides.

Garbage should be collected in cans with tightly fitting lids, or the lid may overhang the top of the can and allow the entrance of flies, which are then caught in a trap placed over a hole in the lid (*Hodge's garbage can trap*). Garbage which is not used should be incinerated. If it is fed to pigs, not more should be given than can be eaten in a day.

For killing the adult flies pyrethrum gives a rapid knockdown, especially if synergists, such as piperonyl butoxide, are added. Fay & Kilpatrick (1958) discuss the use of these and also their combination with DDT, lindane, BHC and other chlorinated insecticides, which add a killing effect to the knockdown produced by pyrethrum. Cyclethrin, allethrin and similar compounds have also been used and aerosols containing Freon 11 and Freon 12. DDT, lindane, BHC and related compounds have also been recommended and have the advantage of a residual effect, though this varies according to various factors discussed by Fay & Kilpatrick (1958), such as the particle size of the compound used, the nature of the surface on which it is deposited, evaporation etc. A serious complication has been introduced by the appearance in many parts of the world of strains of house flies resistant to the chlorinated hydrocarbon insecticides. Against these some of the organophosphorus compounds (diazinon, malathion etc.) were at first successful, but strains resistant to these have also appeared. Thus Hansens (1960) reported resistance to diazinon and Dow ET-57 (Ronnel), as well as to DDT and lindane, and that malathion and dimethoate gave unsatisfactory control. La Brecque *et al.* (1959) tested the value of two carbamates (methyl carbamate and Pyrolan) against house flies resistant to malathion and DDT and suggest that both these compounds are better than DDT, though they may not remain so for long. La Brecque & Wilson (1960) reported that exposure of the flies to malathion only can cause rapid development of resistance to DDT, even if the flies have not been exposed to DDT.

Thus *Musca domestica* presents a very difficult problem of control. Fay & Kilpatrick (1958) record the use, in barns, dairies, halls and similar places, of cotton cords impregnated with parathion, diazinon or DDT, to which synergists may be added. A mixture of 10 per cent parathion and xylene used in this way gave season-long control and a mixture of Dilan, DDT and cottonseed oil, controlled resistant flies. Sugar (20 parts to 1 part of the insecticide) greatly increases the effect of diazinon, malathion, chlorthion, Dipterex and Cyanamid 4124, but the brief residual effect of these organophosphorus compounds is a disadvantage. Cotton cords impregnated with a mixture of 25 per cent Dow ET-57 (Ronnel) and xylene give good control for 8–16 weeks and are more effective than residual spraying, Dow ET-57 being of relatively low toxicity to mammals.

Poison baits. Fay & Kilpatrick (1958) discuss the use of these and refer to authors who suggest baits containing 0·15 per cent of lindane plus 0·06 per cent of molasses; or the surfaces on which the flies settle may be treated with a mixture of 1·5 g. of Dipterex, 4 oz. of water and 1 pint of Karo syrup, or baits containing malathion, diazinon or Dipterex may be tried. Deposits of lindane and diazinon have some fumigant action. For further literature see the periodical publications of the WHO (e.g. 1963, 1964).

M. autumnalis De Geer along with *M. bezzii* and *M. lusoria* are haematophagous species which, although they are unable to pierce the skin and suck blood, follow the blood-sucking flies. It seems they disturb the blood-suckers in the act of feeding and then feed on the blood and tissue fluids which ooze from the wound.

M. autumnalis is commonly found around the eyes and nostrils of cattle and horses; so much so that it is considered to be a pest of economic importance in parts of the U.S.A., where it is known as the 'face fly'. The flies gather chiefly around the eyes and nostrils, causing annoyance and irritation; horses huddle together in the shade, are nervous and interrupt their normal grazing behaviour. In cattle milk yield and growth may be interrupted.

Dorsey (1966) assessed various control measures on Quarter Horses in West Virginia. He found insecticide formulations smeared on the face to be uneffective, however, good to excellent control of face flies was achieved by the use of specially designed halters impregnated with Dichlorvos. These consisted of a halter to which a series of strands of plastic, 10 in. or more in length, were attached to the brow band at intervals of about 1 in. The free-swinging strands covered the face and the eyes. During a 3 year observation period none of the horses wearing the Dichlovos-treated halters showed any signs of toxic reactions.

Genus: Stomoxys Geoffroy, 1762

S. calcitrans Geoffroy, 1764 is the commonest species of this genus and is known as the 'stable fly'. It occurs all over the world. The flies are about as large as *Musca domestica*. The proboscis is prominent, directed horizontally forwards and has small labella. The M_{1+2} vein curves gently forwards and the R_5 cell is open, ending at or behind the apex of the wing. The thorax is grey and has four longitudinal dark stripes, of which the lateral pair are narrow and do not reach the end of the scutum. The abdomen is shorter and broader than that of the house fly, and has three dark spots on each of the second and third segments.

Life-cycle. *Stomoxys* sometimes lays its eggs in horse manure, but prefers decaying vegetable matter like straw and hay, especially when these are contaminated with urine. The material must be moist, otherwise it is unsuitable. A fly lays about twenty-five to fifty eggs at a time and may lay a total of 800. The eggs are dirty-white to yellow, about 1 mm. long, and bear a longitudinal groove on one side. They hatch in 1–4 days, or longer in cold weather. The larvae feed on the vegetable matter and in warm weather grow mature in 14–24 days. The full-grown larva resembles that of *Musca*, but its stigmal plates are far apart and each has three

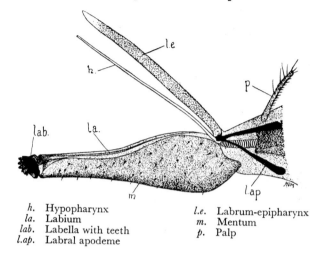

h.	Hypopharynx	*l.e.*	Labrum-epipharynx
la.	Labium	*m.*	Mentum
lab.	Labella with teeth	*p.*	Palp
l.ap.	Labral apodeme		

FIG. 217. *Stomoxys calcitrans*, Mouth Parts (Original)

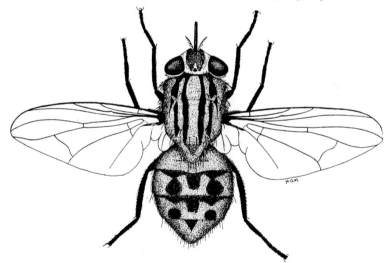

FIG. 218. *Stomoxys calcitrans*, Female (Original)

S-shaped slits. Pupation takes place in the drier parts of the breeding material and this stage lasts about 6–9 days, or much longer in cold weather. Oviposition begins about 9 days after emergence of the fly and after a few meals of blood have been taken. The complete life-cycle may cover about 30 days. *Trypanosoma evansi* (surra of equines and dogs in India) and *T. equinum* (Mal de Caderas of equines, cattle, sheep and goats in South America) are transmitted, mechanically only, by *Stomoxys*, which may also mechanically transmit *T. gambiense* and *T. rhodesiense*, the causes of human trypanosomiasis in Africa, and *T. brucei* and *T. vivax*, which cause nagana of cattle, sheep, goats and equines in Africa.

Habits and significance. The flies are most abundant in summer and autumn and live about a month under natural conditions. They prefer a fairly strong light, and are not seen in dark stables or houses. They enter

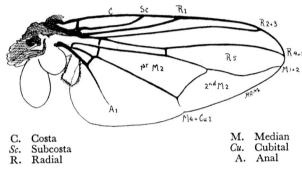

C.	Costa	M.	Median
Sc.	Subcosta	*Cu.*	Cubital
R.	Radial	A.	Anal

FIG. 219. *Stomoxys calcitrans*, Wing (Original)

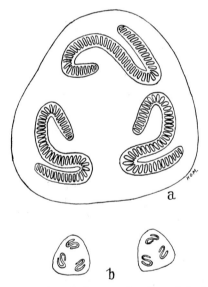

FIG. 220. *Stomoxys calcitrans:* a, stigmal plate, much enlarged; b, showing relative distance between stigmal plates (Original)

buildings only in autumn or during rainy weather. They are swift fliers, but are not inclined to travel long distances. Both males and females are blood-suckers, attacking man, horses, cattle and other mammals, and even birds and reptiles. About 3–4 minutes are required for a meal, and the fly often changes its position or flies to another animal to continue its feed.

Stomoxys is known to act as intermediate host of the nematode *Habronema microstoma*. It has been proved experimentally that this fly can act as a mechanical vector of equine infectious anaemia and anthrax. When the flies occur in large numbers they may become a source of great annoyance to domestic animals, resulting in decrease of milk yield and loss of weight. Sheep that have recently been shorn, as well as young lambs, are attacked along the back and suffer great annoyance.

Control. The fly is most troublesome in localities where suitable breeding-places are readily found. Control measures should therefore be directed toward destroying breeding-places by regular removal of moist bedding, hay and faeces from stables and yards, and food wastes from feeding troughs, and by preventing the accumulation of heaps of weeds, grass cuttings and vegetable refuse. The application of a suitable DDT preparation to animals will kill the flies attacking them. Dipping of cattle in a DDT-sodium arsenite dip for the control of tsetse flies (see below) free them from *Stomoxys* also. Insecticides applied to the habitations of the hosts may effect some control by killing the flies on their resting-places, but this control seems to last only for a few days. Methoxychlor and diazinon are effective for this, and chlordane is effective when sprayed on the breeding places.

Genus: Lyperosia Rondani, 1856 (syn. Siphona)

Several species of this genus may be encountered in various countries and are serious pest of cattle. The flies are some of the smallest of the blood-sucking anthomyids, measuring about 4 mm. in length. The face is silvery-grey, the thorax silvery-grey medially and dark laterally with two well-defined dark stripes. The wing venation is similar to that of *Stomoxys calcitrans*. The palps are yellowish, stout and of uniform thickness and as long as the proboscis. The aristae are haired on the dorsal surface only.

L. exigua (De Meijere, 1903) is the buffalo fly of India, Malasia, China and Australia, being distributed in the northern part of the latter country. The fly feeds on buffaloes and cattle chiefly and rarely leave the host except for a brief flight when disturbed, to transfer to another host or to lay eggs. Several thousand flies may occur on cattle, especially bulls. Weight gain and milk production are severely interferred with by heavy infections.

L. minuta Bezzi, 1892 occurs in Africa and has similar habits to the above.

L. irritans (Linné, 1758) is generally known as the horn fly, however in North America the horn fly is referred to as *Haematobia irritans* (see below). Smart (1939) states that *L. irritans* is the smallest of the British blood-sucking anthomyids, it is uncommon in that country being confined to the South.

Life-cycle. The eggs are laid in the fresh dung of cattle and buffaloes.

They are 1·3–1·5 mm. long and hatch in about 20 hours at a temperature of 24–26°C. Lower temperatures retard or arrest development and the eggs are rapidly killed by drying. The larvae burrow into the dung and feed on it, growing mature in about 4 days at a temperature of 27–29°C. Lower temperatures prolong development considerably. A fair amount of moisture is also required; Australian workers have found that 68 per cent of free water is optimal for *L. exigua* larvae and that development ceases if the moisture falls below 50 per cent. The pupae are found underneath drier dung heaps or in the surrounding soil. They require about the same temperature as the larvae and also suffer from too dry conditions. The pupal stage lasts 6–8 days.

Lyperosia is adapted to certain ranges of temperature and moisture and is able to exist only in a warm, moist climate. The distribution of *L. exigua* in Australia is markedly controlled by these factors. It becomes sluggish at temperatures below 70°F and comatose at 40°F and a wet-bulb temperature below 60°F is markedly unfavourable to it. It disappears in cold weather and is limited to areas with a high humidity, being prevalent along shaded watercourses. It is influenced also by the odour, warmth and sweat of the host. The flies are not inclined to fly about, but remain on their hosts for several days, feeding at intervals or darting down to lay eggs when the animal has defaecated. They are spread therefore chiefly by their hosts.

Control. This is similar to that for *Haematobia stimulans* (see below). Herzett & Goulding (1959) found that back-rubbers impregnated with 5 per cent rotenone dust protected dairy herds for an average of 6–7 weeks and that 5 per cent methoxychlor dust protected them for 3–5 weeks, while 4 per cent malathion and 25 per cent delphene dusts protected for only 1 week. Burns *et al.* (1959) found that back-rubbers impregnated with 0·25 per cent of Bayer L 21/199 (Co-Ral) or 1 per cent Dow ET-57 (Ronnel) gave results comparable to those obtained with toxaphene.

Genus: Haematobia Robineau-Desvoidy 1830

Smaller than *Stomoxys calcitrans* but larger than *Lyperosia*. Palps slightly shorter than the proboscis, clubbed. Aristae haired on both sides.

H. stimulans (Meigen, 1824). Smart (1939) states this fly to be generally distributed in the British Isles and its range does not seem to extend beyond Europe.

H. irritans (Linné, 1758). This is the 'horn fly' of North America. They may be found in thousands around the base of the horns and also on the back, shoulders and belly of cattle. They occasionally attack horses, sheep and dogs. The fly remains on the animal and leaves it only to pass to another host or to lay eggs when the animal defaecates. It is a marked blood-sucker and heavy burdens cause marked injury from loss of blood and irritation due to the constant piercing of the skin. The animal may develop sores and wounds and these attract the screw-worm fly.

Favourable climatic conditions for horn flies consist of hot, humid weather; hot, dry weather or cold weather is unfavourable. Studies by Morgan (1964) on the autecology of the horn fly indicate that the preferred macroclimate is a temperature of 73–80°F, a relative humidity of 65–90 per cent with scattered light showers and no wind. Within the mantle of the micro-environment of the skin of an animal the flies prefer an air temperature of 85°F, a skin temperature of about 97°F and a relative humidity of 65 per cent. Such a micro-environment was most commonly found by Morgan in the Holstein and there was a significant difference between the number of flies on animals of this breed than on Guernsey or Jersey heifers. The flies prefer the dark coloured areas of bicoloured cattle during the daylight hours, the black of the Holstein being preferred to the tan of the Guernsey. When the macrotemperature is about 85°F many flies are found on the white skin of the belly and udder areas.

Life-cycle. This is essentially the same as for *Lyperosia.*

Control. Since the flies remain for long periods on the animal, control of the adult is relatively easy. Regular spraying with DDT, BHC, the organophosphates and other insecticides gives good control. Where these are used for other control measures, e.g. tick control, the horn fly is often not a problem. However, within recent years insecticide resistance in horn flies has appeared and in these cases alternative insecticides must be used. With hand treatment (sprays etc.) the insecticide should be directed to the shoulders, sides, belly and the base of the horns. The introduction of 'back-rubbers' impregnated with a suitable insecticide has greatly simplified the control of horn flies, in that cattle may frequently acquire self-administered application of insecticides. Repeated application is necessary for continuous protection since protection from a single spray (e.g. of Ronnel, Co-Ral etc.) will last about 30 days. A single spraying, e.g., for the warble flies (*Hypoderma* spp.), does not give prolonged control of *H. irritans* (Khan & Lawson, 1965).

Genus: Glossina Wiedemann, 1830

The species of the genus *Glossina* or tsetse flies are undoubtedly the most important blood-sucking flies, since they transmit several species of trypanosomes which cause fatal diseases, for example, nagana of domestic animals and sleeping sickness of man. The tsetse flies occur only in the continent of Africa, except *G. tachinoides*, which is also found in southern Arabia. The flies are narrow-bodied, yellowish to dark brown and 6–13·5 mm. long. At rest the wings are held over the back, overlapping almost completely. The width of the forehead at the vertex is about half the width of an eye in the female and one-third to one-half in the male. The proboscis is long and held horizontally, ensheathed in the long palps, which are of an even thickness throughout. The antenna has a large, elongate third antennal segment which ends in a blunt, forwardly directed point, and an arista which bears seventeen to twenty-nine dorsal branching hairs. The thorax frequently has a dull greenish ground colour and is marked with insconspicuous stripes or spots. The abdomen is light to

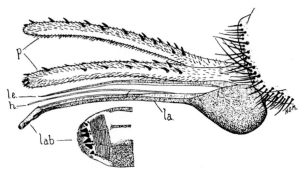

h. Hypopharynx	*lab.* Labellum (enlarged figure, medial
la. Labium strengthened by mentum	view, showing armature)
l.e. Labrum-epipharynx	*p.* Palps

FIG. 221. *Glossina pallidipes*, Mouth Parts (Original)

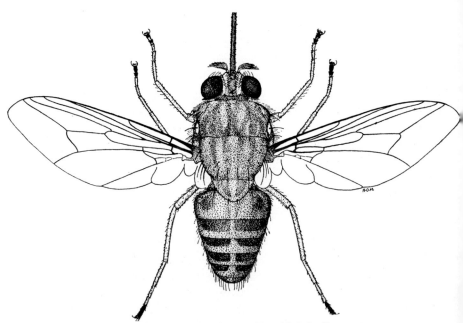

FIG. 222. *Glossina morsitans* (Original)

dark brown, and six segments are visible from the dorsal aspect. The venation of the wing is very characteristic, especially the course of the M_{1+2} vein. This runs obliquely backwards from its base, then bends forward to meet the very oblique anterior transverse vein, bends back sharply again towards the posterior transverse vein, and finally runs forward to reach the margin well in front of the apex. The R2 + 3 and R4 + 5 veins also turn forward at their extremities. The discal cell (first M2) has the shape of a butcher's cleaver.

A description of the different species of *Glossina* goes beyond the scope of this book. They are described by Smart (1956), Swynnerton (1936) and Buxton (1955).

Life-cycle. The female fly produces one larva at a time when the latter is full grown and ready to pupate. The larva grows in the uterus of the female, its mouth being attached to a 'teat' from which 'milk' is obtained for nourishment, and its posterior extremity, which bears the stigmal

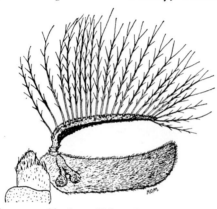

FIG. 223. *Glossina pallidipes*, Antenna (Original)

plates, lies near the vulva. The gestation period lasts about 10 days under suitable conditions, but is prolonged if food is scarce or in cold weather when the flies do not feed readily. The longevity of flies in nature is not well known, but it is estimated that a female can produce eight to ten, sometimes up to a total of twelve larvae. A female of *G. palpalis* has been kept alive under artificial conditions for 227 days, and a female of *G. morsitans* 233 days.

The larva is an oval, mobile maggot, about 7 mm. long. It wriggles into the soil to a depth of about 2 cm. and turns into a pupa after $1-1\frac{1}{2}$ hours. The larva has two large respiratory lobes at its posterior end, each perforated by about 500 spiracular openings. These lobes persist with the last larval skin, which forms the puparium covering the brown or black pupa, and they give the pupa the characteristic appearance shown in Fig. 225. They vary in different species and are used for the identification of the pupae of different species. The pupa is about 6–7 mm. long. The length of the pupal period varies according to the temperature and the species concerned. It usually lasts about 35 days, with limits from about 17–90 days. The pupal period of *G. pallidipes* varies from 31 days in the summer to 149 days, or more usually about 92 days, in the winter.

Habits. The bionomics of tsetse flies, especially of certain species, have been extensively studied and the knowledge obtained is recorded in a vast amount of literature. Reference should be made to Buxton (1955).

Tsetse flies are found mainly in the central part of Africa, extending from the southern boundaries of the Sahara to Bechuanaland, Rhodesia and Zululand. In these regions the flies are confined to definite areas known as 'fly-belts', the limits of which are controlled by various factors such as altitude, moisture, vegetation and the presence of hosts. The different species vary greatly in their adaptation to environment and consequently in their distribution. *G. palpalis* occurs mainly in the areas drained by the Senegal, Niger and Congo rivers; *G. morsitans* occurs from

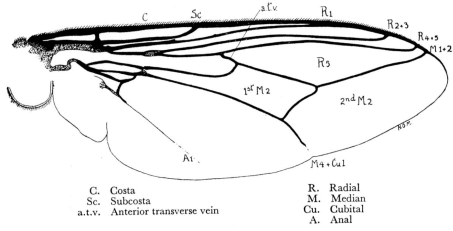

C.	Costa	R.	Radial
Sc.	Subcosta	M.	Median
a.t.v.	Anterior transverse vein	Cu.	Cubital
		A.	Anal

FIG. 224. *Glossina pallidipes*, Wing (Original)

Senegal to Ethiopia in the east and right down to Bechuanaland and Rhodesia. *G. pallidipes* is essentially an East African species and is found from Zululand to Uganda and Kenya. *G. tachinoides* can live at higher temperatures than most other species and is found in hot regions like Northern Nigeria.

The humidity of the atmosphere, the temperature and the presence of shade have an important bearing on the life of the fly. *G. palpalis* requires an almost saturated atmosphere and much shade, and is therefore found near water, especially along the banks of rivers or lakes surrounded by overhanging trees or bushes. It is killed within a short time by direct sunlight and by temperatures over 30°C, especially if the humidity is not high. Its natural range from water is about 30 m., but the fly will follow a host for 300 m. or sometimes more away from water. *G. morsitans* and *G. pallidipes* are much less restricted to moisture and shade conditions and are most active in a moderately dry and warm climate. They occur in open 'parkland' type of vegetation. *G. pallidipes* requires a moderate degree of humidity, and is less independent of cover than *G. morsitans*. Both these species require trees or scrub for shelter and the former especially does not venture far into open country.

The different species are each particularly associated with certain types of vegetation, an important factor which requires much further study. The vegetation as well as other controlling factors like the presence of water restrict the flies during bad seasons to certain areas known as 'primary fly centres' or permanent haunts, from which they migrate outwards along suitable courses to temporary haunts during favourable seasons. *G. palpalis* will, for instance, ascend to the upper limits of rivers in rainy seasons and again descend when dry conditions set in.

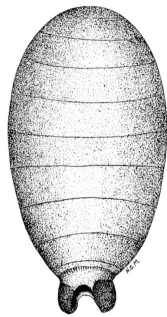

FIG. 225. *Glossina pallidipes*, Pupa (Original)

All the species of *Glossina* feed on the blood of vertebrates. *G. tachinoides* feeds on its dead mates in captivity and may therefore, perhaps, also feed on insects in nature. Some species of hosts are more suitable than others, and the prevalence of flies is dependent on the number and suitability of hosts. *G. palpalis* thrives best on the blood of warm-blooded animals and is stated to prefer human blood, but it can also feed on cold-blooded animals like crocodiles. It is generally agreed that this species is not dependent on big game for its existence. *G. morsitans* feeds on any large mammal or bird, but is not able to exist permanently where big game or cattle are absent. This fly disappeared from the Transvaal with the big game which was killed out by rinderpest. Occasionally *G. morsitans* has been found where big game was scarce, but since the pupal period is long, such flies may have emerged some time after the main stock of flies left the particular area. *G. pallidipes* is similarly dependent on big game or cattle for its existence, but warthogs are an important source of food for both species.

The flies fly low near the ground and hunt by sight. They are susceptible to the effects of light and shade and are attracted especially by moving objects. As a rule they prefer to bite on dark surfaces, probably being attracted by them just as they are attracted by a shadow. While it is being attracted by or following a host, the fly will leave its natural haunts and cover for variable distances, depending on the species of fly and the prevailing conditions. G. palpalis is attracted to boats moving on a river and G. morsitans may attack animals or human beings several hundred metres away from its bush cover. In this way the fly may reach new sites after leaving its host or after giving up the chase. When the host stops moving, the fly, especially G. palpalis, is apt to leave.

The flies feed about every 3 days, depending on the temperature and humidity. In a humid atmosphere longer starvation is possible, while a higher temperature shortens the interval. Most species are active in the forenoon and afternoon, disappearing during the hottest hours of the day. Some, like G. brevipalpis, are nocturnal in their habits, feeding especially on moonlight nights, but others may attack hosts around a camp fire at night. Rain or windy weather causes the flies to remain in shelter.

As the fly engorges, its abdomen becomes much distended. Finally the fly leaves its host and settles on the under-side of a leaf or a log or on the bark of a tree to rest. Soon a drop of dark fluid is voided through the anus, then several drops of clear fluid, and sometimes also a drop of fresh blood, which then fills the gut.

Towards the end of the gestation period the females do not feed but remain in shelter. Unsuitable food or starvation may cause the female to abort, and occasionally pupation occurs in the uterus and is invariably fatal to the fly.

The breeding-places of tsetse flies are carefully chosen and they are restricted by various factors. G. palpalis deposits its larvae usually not more than 25 m. from water and about a metre above water-level in dry, coarse sand or in humus around tree trunks, in forks of branches and cracks of bark up to 4 m. high above the ground. G. morsitans and G. pallidipes breed in loose, sandy soil rich in humus on sheltered and well-drained spots, usually near game paths where the flies abound. The pregnant female about to deposit a larva is attracted by objects which provide shelter, like fallen tree trunks or slanting rocks, and deposits the larva underneath them. Shade is essential to the pupae even though they lie covered in the soil. A few hours of sunshine per day rapidly kills them.

Natural enemies of the tsetse flies do not appear to play an important part in nature, although the pupae are frequently parasitised by small Hymenoptera and the flies themselves may be caught by predatory wasps and birds.

Control. The following methods have been used:

1. Catching and trapping. Catching with hand nets is not practicable except in small areas. It is a common method of determining the fly

density in a given locality. Numerous types of traps have been designed, mainly on the principle that the fly is attracted by a horizontal shadow and flies in underneath it. The traps cast such a shadow and catch the flies in a cage, into which they are drawn by light falling through from the top.

For many years the Harris trap has been used in Zululand. However, it has now been more or less abandoned as a means of direct control.

2. *Artificial breeding-places* may be valuable additional aids to reduce the flies, where the natural breeding-places are limited in number. Attractive sites are made under logs, rocks or planks, and the pupae are regularly removed or the covering object is placed in such a way that the pupae may be killed by the sunlight.

3. *Bush-clearing.* In the case of flies like *G. palpalis*, which require much shade, this measure is important and the clearing of bush around settlements, wells, landing-places and fords on rivers and on either side of roads has given excellent results in providing protection from the fly. Wholesale clearing of large areas, however, presents many difficulties, especially the expense incurred and the rapid regrowth of the bush. Only if clearing is followed by settlement can the advance be maintained.

G. pallidipes and *G. morsitans*, which prefer more open savannah country, present a different problem and bush clearing is less effective against them. Attempts have been made to erect barriers against such flies by planting broad strips of dense vegetation, in which they cannot live. *G. austeni*, on the other hand, prefers the coastal thickets of East Africa. Strip clearing is a method by which an area can be divided into sections for fly control and reinfection of cleared areas can be prevented by it. Selective clearing removes particular species of trees or other vegetation favoured by the different species of the flies.

4. *Burning of vegetation*, properly organised in areas to which it can be applied, destroys the shelter of the flies and may kill off pupae, either directly or by removing the moisture they require, or even by encouraging their ant enemies. Thus Glover *et al.* (1956), reporting on the control of *G. morsitans* in Northern Nigeria, found that reduction of vegetation and clearance of trees from shallow valleys at the headwaters of streams where the flies congregate reduced this species to such an extent that cattle could be kept free of the flies in the area thus treated.

5. *Destruction of big game* is designed to remove the food of the flies and also to break up their breeding areas. Removal of the big game (antelope) controlled *G. morsitans* in Rhodesia, a species which prefers to feed on antelope and other big game, but it failed to control *G. pallidipes* in Zululand, probably because this species feeds not only on big game, but also on bush pig, bush buck and other smaller hosts. *G. morsitans* also feeds on these, so that, as Du Toit (1954) says, these also should be removed, if game destruction is to succeed.

6. *Fly screens, repellents* and similar devices designed to prevent the flies

from gaining access to their hosts may be tried, but they can be, at most, only partially successful.

7. *Insecticides*. These have been applied, on the one hand, to the hosts and, on the other, to wide areas of country inhabited by the flies. DDT sprayed on to animals will kill tsetse flies and will discourage them from biting, but it does not adhere well to the hair of cattle and its effects therefore soon wear off. Davies (1960) reported control of *G. palpalis* with dieldrin.

The application of insecticides to large areas of country has been very successful and a large literature discusses it. Thus the British Colonial Insecticides, Fungicides and Herbicides Committee (1952) reported that spraying of 15 square miles of country in East Africa with DDT by means of aeroplanes reduced, a year after the spraying, *G. morsitans* by 99·1 per cent, *G. swynnertoni* by 95·6 per cent and *G. pallidipes* by 99·9 per cent, and that a gamma BHC smoke reduced *G. morsitans* and *G. swynnertoni* by 93 per cent. This method is more likely to be effective against species which inhabit open country. In Zululand, du Toit (1954) concentrated on the control of *G. pallidipes*. Several methods of control were used, these including the broadcasting of DDT or BHC from the exhausts of fixed wing aircraft, DDT smoke generators placed every 70 yards in dense bush, the dusting of bush mechanically and weekly dipping of cattle.

Genus: Fannia Robineau-Desvoidy, 1830

F. canicularis (Linné, 1761). This is a common species measuring 4–6 mm. in length, greyish to almost black in colour and possesses three dark longitudinal stripes on the dorsal aspect of the thorax. The aristae are bare. The larvae breed in all kinds of decaying vegetable matter and refuse and are readily recognised by the dorso-ventral flattening of the body and by the branched fleshy processes which project from the sides of the body.

F. scalaris (Fabricius). This is the latrine fly. It resembles *F. canicularis* and the larvae have fleshy processes which are more feathered than in *F. canicularis*. This fly breeds in human faeces.

Neither of the above flies actively parasitised animals, however their larvae may accidentally occur in the digestive tract.

FAMILY: TACHINIDAE

This is a large family of flies. They are usually bristly and are characterised by the presence of a row of bristles on the hypopleuron—the hypopleural bristles—which are placed like a screen on either side, in front of the metathoracic spiracles.

The family is divided into three subfamilies, Tachininae, Calliphorinae and Sarcophaginae. The Tachininae is the largest subdivision of the family, being the flower flies whose larvae are parasitic on other insects.

They are bristly flies generally with bare aristae. They are of no veterinary importance. The Calliphorina are the blowflies and are often metallic blue or green in colour. Several species are of veterinary importance. The Sarcophaginae includes the flesh flies which have a grey longitudinal striped thorax with a check-board marked abdomen.

SUBFAMILY: CALLIPHORINAE

Genus: Lucilia Robineau-Desvoidy, 1830 (syn. Phoenicia)

This genus contains the most important blowflies **L. cuprina** and **L. sericata.** The larvae of *L. cuprina* are the chief cause of blowfly strike of sheep in Australia and South Africa; those of *L. sericata* are its chief cause in Britain. Larvae of *L. sericata* have also been found in human wounds. These flies have bright metallic colours, being bright green, or a bronze colour in some kinds of lighting. They are called greenbottle or copper bottle flies. The eyes are brownish-red. The body is relatively slender, 8–10 mm. long. It is difficult to distinguish between these two species: the legs are black, but in *L. cuprina* the femora of the first pairs of legs are bright green.

Genus: Calliphora Robineau-Desvoidy, 1830

Species of this genus are often called bluebottle flies, the body having a metallic blue sheen.

C. erythrocephala Meigen (syn. *C. vicina*) is a large, stoutly-built fly about 12 mm. long, which buzzes loudly when it flies. The eyes are red and the genae are red with black hairs. **C. vomitoria** Linné is similar, but the genae are black with reddish hairs. Both species strike sheep in England. **C. stygia** Fabricus, **C. australis, C. nociva** Hardy, **C. augur** and **C. fallax** Hardy strike sheep in Australia.

Microcalliphora varipes and species of **Sarcophaga** are also sheep blowflies in Australia.

Genus: Phormia Robineau-Desvoidy, 1830

Species of this genus are sometimes called black blowflies. **P. regina** deposits its eggs in the wool of sheep in the United States. Its thorax is black, with a metallic blue-green sheen, the abdomen blue-green to black, the fly being 6–11 mm. long.

P. terrae-novae Robineau-Desvoidy strikes sheep in Britain and northern Canada, but in Canada *P. regina* is the most important cause of strike.

Genus: Chrysomyia Macquart, 1855

C. chloropyga Wiedemann and **C. albiceps** Wiedemann are sheep blowflies in South Africa; **C. rufifacies** Macquart, the hairy maggot fly, and **C. micropogon** Bigot, the steel-blue blowfly, are sheep blowflies in Australia; **C. bezziana** (Villeneuve), the Old World screw-worm fly, occurs in Africa and southern Asia. It is a medium-sized stout, bluish-green fly, with four black stripes on the prescutum; the face is orange-yellow. In India it may leg eggs on the skin of man and domesticated animals.

CALLIPHORINE MYIASIS OF SHEEP

This disease, commonly called 'strike', may be caused by the larvae of various species belonging to the genera *Lucilia*, *Calliphora*, *Phorma* and *Chrysomyia*. The condition should be distinguished from the form of myiasis caused by the larvae of the screw-worm flies belonging to the genera *Callitroga* and *Chrysomyia*. The latter is described in more detail on page 437.

Life-cycle of the species causing strike. The flies lay clusters of light yellow eggs in carcasses, wounds or soiled wool, being attracted by the odour of decomposing matter. While the fly is selecting a suitable spot to lay, it feeds on the moist matter present. A female blowfly lays about 1000–3000 eggs altogether and 50–150 in one batch. A meal of protein is required before the ovaries reach full maturity.

The larvae hatch from the eggs in 8 hours to 3 days, depending on the temperature, and begin to feed. They grow rapidly and pass two ecdyses, becoming full-grown maggots in about 2–19 days. The rate of growth depends on the amount and suitability of food, the temperature and the degree of competition with other larvae. The mature larvae roughly resemble those of *Musca*. They are about 10–14 mm. long, greyish-white or pale yellow in colour, sometimes with a pink tinge. The anterior extremity bears a pair of oral hooks and on the broad, flattened, posterior end the stigmatic plates are situated. The second segment bears a pair of anterior spiracles as in *Musca*.

Two groups of larvae can be recognised: 'smooth' larvae and 'hairy' ones. The 'hairy' larvae bear a number of thorn-like, fleshy projections with small spines at their tips on most of the body segments. The larvae of *Chrysomyia rufifacies*, *Chrysomyia albiceps* and *Microcalliphora varipes* are

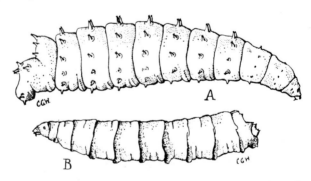

FIG. 226. A, Hairy Larva of *Chrysomyia albiceps*; B, Smooth Larva of *Lucilia sericata* (× 5)
(Original)

'hairy'; those of *Chrysomyia micropogon* and the other sheep blowflies mentioned above are smooth. The different species of larvae can be further differentiated by means of the structure of their spiracles and the cephalo-pharyngeal skeletons.

The mature larvae usually leave the host or the carcass to pupate in the ground, but some may pupate in dry parts of a carcass or even in the wool of the live animal. Before pupating the larvae may wander fair distances over or through the soil, and most species usually pupate below the surface. If conditions are not favourable, as in cold weather, pupation can be suspended for months and the larvae may hibernate. At pupation the larva loosens its skin, which turns brown and becomes rigid to form the puparium. The pupa therefore bears some resemblance to the last larval stage; the pupae of the 'hairy' maggots retain the projections on their covering. For the rest the pupae are slightly shorter than the mature larvae and their ends are more bluntly rounded.

The pupal stage lasts 3–7 days in summer to much longer in winter, hibernation also occurring in this stage. The fly emerges by pushing off the end of the puparium by means of the inflated ptilinal sac, which is further used for progression to the surface of the soil. The shortest time known for completion of the life-cycle is 7 days, so that several generations can develop in one year. Nine to ten generations may be completed in a year in certain parts of South Africa. The flies live a month or longer and can also hibernate.

Epizootiology. The factors which influence the occurrence of calliphorine myiasis in sheep can be classed into two groups: those controlling the prevalence of flies and those that determine the susceptibility of the sheep.

The *prevalance of flies* is seasonal, because the adults are adapted to definite ranges of temperature and to variations of humidity. They are most abundant in late spring and early summer, decreasing in numbers during the hottest part of the year and again increasing in the early autumn. The different species are, however, not all alike in this respect, some preferring lower temperatures than others, and consequently a number of overlapping 'waves' of different species succeed one another during the season.

The abundance and suitability of food for the adults as well as for the larvae is of great importance. The adult flies feed on liquefied protein and on the nectar of certain plants. Since protein food is required for the maturation of the ovaries, its relative abundance greatly influences the fertility of the females. The rate of growth of the larvae and the number that can develop also depend on the same factor. The larvae can obtain this food from either living sheep or dead carcasses of various animals (carrion) on which the adults lay eggs, and the flies can be classified into (a) *primary flies*, which initiate a strike by laying eggs on living sheep; (b) *secondary flies*, which do not usually do this, but lay their eggs on sheep already struck, the larvae extending the injury done by the larvae of the primary flies; (c) *tertiary flies*, which come last of all, the larvae of which do little further damage. This succession occurs on both living sheep and on carrion, the succession on carrion corresponding to the various stages of decomposition of the carcasses. Thus the larvae of the primary flies develop during autolytic and early bacterial decomposition, those of the secondary flies during the succeeding phase of liquefaction, while the tertiary flies follow when the carcass begins to dry out. In Australia, the primary flies occur in two principal waves, being most prevalent in the spring and autumn, and control and treatment are adapted to meet these waves. The waves vary in numbers in different years. The most important primary fly in Australia is *Lucilia cuprina*, other flies concerned being *Calliphora stygia*, *C. augur*, *C. australis*, *C. novica*, *C. fallax* and *Lucilia sericata*. In New Zealand *Lucilia laemica* causes strike over most of that country, but in Canterbury and Otago *L. sericata* is more important. In Britain the most important primary fly is *L. sericata*. In Australia the secondary flies include *Chrysomyia rufifacies*, *Chrysomyia micropogon*, *Microcalliphora varipes* and carrion flies of the Calliphorine genus *Sarcophaga*. The tertiary flies in Australia are *Musca domestica*, *Fannia australis* and *Peronia rostrata*. The succession of the secondary and tertiary flies is further influenced by competition between them for food. In the battle for this, the larvae of the secondary flies usually overcome those of the primary flies, so that, once the secondary flies have entered the competition, relatively few eggs of *Lucilia* and other primary flies give rise to adult flies. When the carnivorous larvae of *Chrysomyia* arrive, they feed on the larvae of the other species. The importance of this fact was realised in South Africa, where it was found that *Chrysomyia marginalis*, which never strikes live sheep but breeds in carcasses only, plays a very important role as a competitor in carcasses. This fly is active only during the warm summer months and then it completely prevents primary sheep blowflies from breeding in carcasses, since it has a strong repellent action on their larvae, as *C. rufifacies* has. During this period the primary sheep blowflies can therefore breed on live animals only, whereas in winter, when *C. marginalis* is inactive, they are able to breed in carcasses and they build up a large population of hibernating larvae and pupae in the soil, from which flies emerge in spring.

Lucilia cuprina, the most important primary fly in Australia and South Africa, prefers living sheep to carrion and it is possible that *L. sericata*, the most important primary fly in Britain, is also abandoning the habit of its relatives of feeding primarily on carrion. Species of this genus are therefore more likely to be derived from living sheep than from carrion.

The *susceptibility of the sheep* depends on inherent factors which can be influenced by selective breeding and temporary factors which can be otherwise controlled.

Sheep are struck most frequently in the breech (*breech strike, crutch strike*) and around the tail (*tail strike*), where the wool is soiled and the skin scalded by diarrhoeic faeces and by urine in the case of ewes. The major predisposing factors lie in the conformation of this region, especially narrowness of breech and wrinkling of the skin, which favour constant soiling by urine and faeces. Rams and wethers, in which the sheath has a narrow opening, soil the wool of this region with urine and become struck there (*pizzle strike*). Rams with deep head folds or with horns lying close to the head develop a 'sweaty' condition of the skin in these parts and attract blowflies, strike in this region being called *poll strike*.

Any other part of the body may become infected if an undressed wound is present, as the result of accidents, dog bites, contacts with barbed wire etc., or due to operations. The term *wound strike* is sometimes given to strikes which occur on wounded areas. They are seen especially on the scrotum after castration, on the tail after docking, and on the heads of rams that have been fighting. Myiasis in the dorsal region of the body (*body strike*) is usually due to prolonged wet weather, when the wool becomes soaked with rain and bacterial activity sets in. Areas over the withers are especially susceptible. Length and fineness of wool are important factors in this connection. Sheep with short or coarse wool, which dries rapidly, are less commonly affected in this way than those with longer or finer wool.

Pathogenesis. Unless a wound is present, attracting the flies and providing a suitable substrate for the larvae, bacterial activity appears to be important in preparing favourable conditions. In wool that is kept moist by prolonged wet conditions, the yolk, wool scales and skin scales become pasty and form a suitable medium for bacteria. These then produce decomposition, an odour that attracts the flies, and probably also an exudative reaction of the skin which provides food for the young larvae until they are able to pierce the skin. Where the skin becomes soiled by urine and faeces, it is directly affected and becomes inflamed, but even here bacteria probably assist to aggravate the condition and to attract flies. The larvae of the primary blowflies initiate the attack and create favourable conditions for those of the secondary flies. They secrete proteolytic enzymes which digest and liquefy the tissues of the host and then feed on this pre-digested material. Only when this stage has been reached are the secondary larvae able to develop in the lesion. It is believed that the secondary blowflies, whose larvae are predatory on primary larvae, originally deposited their brood in such lesions because the primary larvae were there to feed on, and that they themselves only later became parasites of the host animal.

Large wounds are usually produced and the larvae, especially those of the secondary flies, may form deep tunnels in the tissues and underneath the skin. The central portion of the lesion may heal with the formation of a thick scab, while the action of the larvae extends outwards. The smell emanating from the lesion attracts other flies to deposit eggs in it, and further batches of primary and secondary larvae may find suitable conditions for development. The maggot-infected wounds are strongly alkaline and only alkaline wounds are attractive to blowflies.

The lesion and the parasites are irritating, and the animal consequently does not feed properly, so that it becomes poor and weak. The immediate cause of death, however, is probably a toxaemia due to absorption of toxic substances from the lesion, or even septicaemia.

Clinical signs. The affected sheep usually stands with its head down, but does not feed, and presents a characteristic picture, so that it can be readily noticed. It may attempt to bite the affected part. When the lesion is situated around the tail or on the buttocks, the animal will stamp or jerk the hind-legs and wag the tail. Examination shows a patch of discoloured, greyish-brown, moist wool with an evil odour. The maggots may be found in the wool attacking the skin, and they crawl away into the surrounding wool when disturbed. In later stages there is an inflamed ragged wound from which a foul-smelling liquid exudes into the wool; the larvae are burrowing into the tissues and only their posterior extremities project. The temperature may be elevated. If the disease progresses, malnutrition and loss of milk occur and death may follow within a few days in bad cases.

Diagnosis is easily made from the clinical signs and by finding the larvae in the wound.

Treatment of strike lesions. This aims to kill larvae in the lesions, to promote healing and to prevent re-infestation with more larvae. The extent of the lesion is ascertained by clipping the wool and many larvae can be removed while this is being done. Larvae removed should be killed to prevent them from giving rise to adult flies. It may be difficult to remove larvae in deep pockets, but these also must be killed, especially when the fly concerned is a primary fly such as *L. cuprina* or, in Britain, *L. sericata*, which prefers to feed on living sheep. The dressing should be bland and not toxic to the sheep and should promote healing.

Several insecticides may be used, including 0·4 per cent dieldrin, 0·5 per cent BHC, 0·3 per cent aldrin and several of the organophosphorous insecticides, usually in the form of a 0·05 per cent wash. The latter may be applied as a spray from a portable knapsack sprayer. The organophosphates in use include chlorfenvinphos, dichlorfenthion, fenchloros, carbophenothion, pyrimithate etc.

In some countries, e.g. New Zealand, Australia, Britain, U.S.A. etc., the use of the chlorinated hydrocarbon insecticides (dieldrin, BHC etc.) is prohibited because of the persistence of the residues in the meat.

Prophylaxis. Prophylactic measures may be divided into those which attempt (1) to render the sheep less attractive to the flies; and (2) those which are directed against the flies themselves.

Treatment of the sheep to render them less attractive to the flies may be described under the following headings:

Selective breeding. It has been shown that narrowness of the breech and folds of skin in this region predispose sheep, especially ewes, to strike. Efforts have therefore been made to eliminate, or to lessen, the influence of these features by breeding sheep with plain, or plainer, breeches, and much progress has been made in this respect, although it has been necessarily slow.

Surgical removal of breech folds. Mules (1933, 1935) suggested the removal of the skin of the crutch which becomes stained and scalded with urine, and methods of doing this, called the Mules operation, have been evolved. It can be done on sheep of any age, but is conveniently done on lambs when they are being marked. It renders them non-susceptible to breech strike for the rest of their lives. Graham (1959) recommends the type of the operation which removes only two strips of skin down each buttock. A more radical procedure removes strips of skin on either side of the tail and down the postero-medial aspects of the legs to about 3 in. below the level of the vulva. Strips of $\frac{1}{2}$–$1\frac{1}{2}$ in. are removed, according to the degree of looseness of the skin. All lambs are thus treated, but about 10 per cent need further treatment a few months later.

Docking. Tests carried out mainly in Australia have shown that docking the tails of lambs behind the fourth instead of the usual second caudal vertebra reduces strike appreciably. The explanation seems to be that the tail, being pressed against the body of the animal, tends to flatten out small skin folds often present on either side of the vulva, which may become soiled when they are prominent. The longer tail is also held well away from the body when the ewe urinates. Thirdly, short docking tends to produce a stump surrounded by folds—the so-called 'rose tail'—which is often struck.

Crutching consists in clipping the wool from around the tail and in the breech. This is a very useful measure, tending to promote dryness in this region, and it is effective in preventing strike for 4–5 weeks under ordinary circumstances. Machine crutching is more effective than hand crutching, because the machine clips the wool shorter than the shears.

Treatment of sheep with insecticides. During the last two decades there has been extensive development and use of highly effective insecticides for the protection of sheep against blowfly strike. For many years the chlorinated hydrocarbon insecticides (DDT, BHC, dieldrin etc.) were used with marked success. With dieldrin especially a single dipping of sheep would give protection for several months and a single treatment only was necessary during a normal blowfly season. Where the challenge was heavy a second treatment may be necessary.

With the emergence of resistant strains of blowflies and, more significantly, the concern about insecticide residues in animal tissues, greater emphasis has been placed on the organophosphorous insecticides and in the major sheep rearing countries these insecticides are the ones that are now used for blowfly strike control. Several different organophosphate insecticides exist under a multitude of different proprietary names some of which have been mentioned above (treatment): all are highly effective and if properly applied will often give a whole season's protection. A second treatment may be necessary when the blowfly challenge is high.

Various methods are employed to apply the insecticides. The traditional one is dipping in which the sheep is completely immersed in a dipping tank. This allows good penetration of the insecticidal dip into the fleece. It is however laborious and slow and alternative techniques such as run-through-spray-races or spray-pens have been developed when large numbers of sheep are to be treated. Both rely on overhead booms and floor jets and the penetration of the insecticide is not as efficient as with plunge dipping, however for the purposes of blowfly control it is adequate. 'Tip spraying' may be used, in which a small volume of concentrated insecticide wash is applied as a light surface spray without any attempt being made to saturate the fleece.

Exhausting of the insecticide in the dip or spray solution may occur and this must be guarded against by frequent replenishments of the solution.

Control of the flies. To kill the flies in barns and similar places the methods used for the control of house flies may be tried. 200 mg. of DDT per sq. ft. applied to surfaces on which the flies rest gave control for 2 weeks and, when their night-time resting surfaces were treated, for 3 months. When strains resistant to chlorinated hydrocarbon compounds appear, organophosphorus insecticides may be tried.

Carcass disposal. The destruction of carcasses is only important during those seasons when they are the main breeding grounds of sheep blowflies and there is little or no competition from other species. During such periods—for instance, during the winter in South Africa—carcasses should be burnt or treated with insecticides and buried. The flies often deposit their eggs in the nostrils, ears and anus of an animal even before it is dead or, at any rate, soon after death, and ordinary burial would not stop development of the maggots nor emergence of the flies.

During the rest of the year, when the primary blowflies breed on live sheep and carcasses produce only harmless competitors such as *Chrysomyia marginalis*, carcasses may advantageously be buried without insecticide treatment in order to encourage the competitors.

Trapping as a measure to control blowflies has proved to be of little use and has generally been abandoned, mainly because the primary flies, which are the important ones, are attracted by relatively fresh meat bait only and it has not yet been possible to produce a more satisfactory artificial bait.

Destruction of maggots. The importance of the destruction of all maggots in strike wounds has already been stressed in the section on treatment, and it is obviously of far greater value than indiscriminate attempts at blowfly extermination, such as trapping. Combined with prophylactic insecticide application, curative larvicidal treatment of strike wounds may have far-reaching effects on the numbers of sheep blowflies.

Parasites and natural enemies of blowflies. Although much attention has been paid to biological control by means of hymenopterous parasites, which could be bred and released in large numbers, they do not appear to offer much promise of ever becoming significantly effective, even when artificially assisted.

Genus: Callitroga

This genus includes species the larvae of which cause myiasis of man and other animals and are called screw-worms (see below).

C. hominivorax (syn. *C. (Cochliomyia) americana*), the American screw-worm fly, occurs in North and South America.

C. (syn. *Cochliomyia*) **macellaria** is also an American species; its distribution extends from central Canada to Patagonia. The adults of these two species are 10–15 mm. long, the body being bluish-green, with three longitudinal stripes on the thorax and the face and the eyes are orange-brown; the palps of both species are short and thread-like and the antennae of both species are feathered to their tips. It is difficult to distinguish between the adults of these two species, but their larvae differ. Those of *Callitroga hominivorax* have pigmented tracheae and large posterior spiracles, while those of *Callitroga macellaria* have non-pigmented tracheae and small posterior spiracles.

SCREW-WORMS OF MAN, CATTLE AND OTHER ANIMALS

Screw-worm myiasis of man, cattle and other animals. The name screw-worm is given to the larvae of *Callitroga hominivorax* (syn. *Callitroga (Cochliomyia) americana*) and *Callitroga (Cochliomyia) macellaria*, both of which occur in North and South America and to those of *Chrysomyia bezziana*, the Old World screw-worm fly, which occurs in Africa and southern Asia.

Life-cycle of the screw-worm flies. The female flies deposit clusters of 150–500 eggs at the edge of a wound on the host. Both these species have become so closely adapted to parasitic life that they breed only in wounds and sores on their hosts and not in carcasses. The larvae hatch in 10–12 hours and grow mature in about 3–6 days, after which they leave to pupate in the ground. The mature larvae are about 15 mm. long and are well armed with bands of spines around the body segments. The pupal period lasts from 3 days (*C. hominivorax*) or 7 days (*C. bezziana*) to several weeks, according to the prevailing temperature. Hibernation occurs most commonly in the pupal stage.

Pathogenesis. Cattle, pigs and equines suffer most frequently, but other animals, including fowls, dogs and man, may also be affected. The flies deposit their eggs in wounds resulting from accidents, castration, dehorning, branding, scalding by dips, tick bites and so forth, as well as around the vulva of cows when there is a bloody discharge, or on the navel of young calves. Most cases occur during rainy weather. The maggots penetrate into the tissues, which they liquefy and thus extend the lesion considerably. The wound develops an evil odour and a foul-smelling liquid oozes out. Severe infections are common and death from screw-worm infection is frequent. At one time screw-worm infection was common in the U.S.A. and represented a serious pest to livestock in the Southern and South-western States. Now, for all practical purposes it has been eliminated by the use of irradiation-sterilised flies (see below).

Treatment and Prophylaxis. The wound is thoroughly cleaned and the maggots, especially those of *C. bezziana,* should be destroyed to prevent them from pupating. Dressings used for myiasis in sheep may be applied, and further infection guarded against. Prophylaxis requires proper dressing of all wounds and avoiding operations, such as branding, de-horning, earmarking etc., during the fly season. *C. hominivorax* is especially attracted to new-born animals, and it was recommended in the southern United States at one time that breeding should be so controlled as to have no young stock born between May 1 and November 15, while the fly was most active. Various dressings can be applied to wounds to prevent screw-worm infection. These include packing the wounds with BHC and washes containing organophosphorus insecticides. The compound Bayer L 21/199 used as a 0·25–0·5 per cent wash gives good protection and was previously widely used in the U.S.A.

The most dramatic campaign against these flies and their larvae was the one carried out for the eradication of *Callitroga hominivorax* from Florida by the release of male flies sterilised by irradiation. Knipling (1955) discusses the theoretical considerations relating to campaigns of this kind. The basis of it was the fact that this fly mates only once a year, so that mating with sterilised males prevents its breeding. The campaign itself is described by Baumhover *et al.* (1955, 1959), Bushland (1960) and Skerman (1958). For the eradication campaign 50 million irradiated flies a week were required and 40 tons of meat a week to feed their larvae, and Sherman describes the methods used to produce these large numbers and to distribute them by means of aeroplanes. The results of the campaign were that, after preliminary eradication of *C. hominivorax* from the island of Curaçao, it was eradicated from the whole of Florida and also from the Bahama Islands near to the coast of Florida. Surveys of the incidence of various flies in the Bahama Islands have shown, as Fenton (1960) records, that, although *Callitroga hominivorax* has apparently been eliminated there, *Callitroga macellaria, Callitroga aldrichi* and species of *Sarcophaga* are still present on the islands. The campaign has subsequently been applied to the whole of the Southern part of the U.S.A. with outstanding success. The majority of the cases of screw-worm infections which now occur are traceable to flies which have migrated across the U.S.A.–Mexican border, either on the wing or on animals.

Genus: Cordylobia Grünberg, 1903

C. anthropophaga Grünberg, 1903, the 'tumbu fly' or 'skin-maggot fly', is a stout, compactly built fly, about 9·5 mm. long. The general colour is light brown, with diffuse bluish-grey patches on the thorax, and a dark grey colour on the posterior part of the abdomen.

Life-cycle and habits.—The fly deposits some 500 eggs in the sleeping-places of man and various animals, on the ground or on straw, sacking

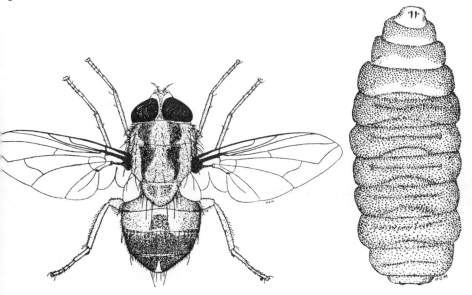

FIG. 227. *Cordylobia anthropophaga* (Original) FIG. 228. *Cordylobia anthropophaga*, Maggot (Original)

etc., sometimes apparently also on clothing that smells of perspiration. The larvae hatch after 2–4 days and penetrate into the skin, where they grow mature in 8–15 days. The mature larva is about 12 mm. long, and is covered with a large number of minute spines. It leaves the host and pupates in the ground for 3–4 weeks in summer before the fly emerges.

Clinical signs and diagnosis. The larva is situated in a swelling which is not very large—about 1 cm. in diameter—but is rather painful and has a small central opening. Of the domestic animals, especially dogs and rabbits are parasitised.

Treatment. The larvae can be easily pressed out and a disinfectant applied.

Prophylaxis. Cleanliness and regular disinfection of sleeping-places is important. In the case of valuable animals, like angora rabbits, which are frequently affected, protection can be afforded by keeping the flies out with gauze wire.

Genus: Booponus Aldrich, 1923

B. intonsus Aldrich, 1923 is the 'foot maggot' which attacks cattle, goats and carabao in Celebes and the Philippine Islands. The fly is about as large as a house fly, light yellow with light brown on the anterior dorsal part of the thorax. The eyes are relatively small. The head, abdomen and femora are evenly covered with short, black hairs. The veins of the wings are yellow. The flies are active mainly in the dry season.

The fly lays its eggs on the hairs along the coronet and the posterior part of the pastern. When the larvae hatch they penetrate the skin in these parts and produce wounds in which the hind ends of the larvae can be seen. After about 2–3 weeks they fall out and pupate in the ground for 10–12 days.

Affected animals are restless and show lameness, which may be serious in severe cases.

Treatment. The maggots should be destroyed and reinfection prevented by applications as in myiasis due to sheep blowflies. A grease containing dieldrin and Diazinon is effective.

Subfamily: Sarcophaginae

The 'flesh flies' are medium-sized to large and thick-set, of a light or dark grey colour. The arista is plumose to about its middle and bare in the distal portion. The thorax often has three longitudinal dark stripes and the dorsum of the abdomen has dark spots or is chequered dark and grey. Species of the family are larviparous and may lay their larvae in wounds or sores in which the larvae develop, although some species also lay their larvae in decomposing meat or other decaying matter.

Genus: Sarcophaga Meigen, 1826

Among the species of this genus which may lay their larvae in de-composing flesh, wounds, ulcers etc., are:

S. haemorrhoidalis Fallen, 1810, which occurs in Europe, America, Asia and Africa.

S. fusicauda Böttcher, 1913, which occurs in Australia, China, Japan and neighbouring countries.

S. carnaria (Linné, 1758), which, like the two species just mentioned, may lay its larvae in wounds etc., on the skin of man. This species can drop its larvae from a height of 26 in. through wire-gauze covers put over meat.

S. dux Thomson, 1868, the larvae of which have been found in skin lesions on a camel, cow and bullock in Madras.

Genus: Wohlfahrtia Brauer & Bergenstamm, 1889

Species of this genus are also larviparous and have habits similar to those of species of the genus *Sarcophaga*. Important species are:

W. magnifica (Schiner, 1862), the Old World Flesh Fly, which occurs in the Mediterranean area, Arabia, Turkey and Russia. It may deposit its larvae in the external ear of man, or in sores around the eyes or else-where on the bodies of man and other animals. It is an important pest of sheep in southern Russia.

W. vigil (Walker, 1919) which occurs in Canada and the northern United States.

W. meigeni, which occurs in the western United States.

These three species have similar habits and the severe disfigurements and suffering that they may cause in man, especially in children, are discussed in textbooks of medical entomology.

W. euvittata deposits its larvae in the egg packets of locusts or in the soft young bodies of these insects.

FAMILY: OESTRIDAE

The adults are hairy flies which have rudimentary mouth parts and do not feed. They usually lay their eggs on animals. The larvae are parasitic maggots and consist of twelve segments, of which the first two are fused together. Oral hooks are usually present, but there is no head. The posterior stigmata open through semicircular plates which may be retractile. The larvae moult twice during their parasitic life and leave the host when they are full grown to pupate in the ground. They feed on the body fluids of the host or on exudates which surround them.

Genus: Gastrophilus Leach, 1817

The larvae of several species of this genus are parasites of equines and are known as 'bots'. They are rarely found in dogs, pigs, birds and man. The adult flies are brown in colour and hairy, somewhat resembling bees, but have, of course, only one pair of wings. *G. intestinalis* (de Geer, 1776) (syn. *G. equi*) is the commonest species. The adults of this species are about 18 mm. long and a dark, irregular, transverse band runs across either wing. The third-stage larvae of the different species can be differentiated as follows:

1. Without spines . . . . *G. inermis* (Brauer, 1858)
   One row of spines on each segment . . *G. nasalis* (Clark, 1797)
   (syn. *G. veterinus* Linné, 1761)
   Two rows of spines on each segment 2
2. Dorsal surface with complete rows of spines only on segments two to five . . . . *G. pecorum* (Fabricius, 1794)
   Dorsal surface with complete rows of spines only on segments two to eight 3
3. Spines of first row larger than spines on second row
   G. intestinalis (de Geer, 1776)
   Spines of first row smaller than spines on second row
   G. haemorrhoidalis (Linné, 1761)

Biology. The adult flies occur during the latter half of the summer and

live only a few days, rarely up to 3 weeks. The female fly hovers about
the animal with its ovipositor extended, and repeatedly darts at it to glue
an egg to a hair. A large number of eggs may be laid in succession.
G. intestinalis deposits its eggs mainly around the fetlocks of the forelegs,
also higher up the legs and in the scapular region. *G. nasalis* lays on the
hairs of the intermandibular region, while *G. haemorrhoidalis* and *G. inermis*
deposit their eggs on the hairs around the mouth and on the cheeks. The
eggs of *G. pecorum* and *G. haemorrhoidalis* are dark in colour, those of the
other species pale yellow; they are elongate, pointed at the attached end
and operculate at the other.

The eggs are ready to hatch in 5–10 days or more. The eggs laid near
the mouth of the horse hatch spontaneously, while those of *G. intestinalis*
and *G. pecorum* require to be licked or rubbed by the animal. The larvae
are not swallowed directly into the stomach, but they penetrate into the
mucosa of the mouth, and gradually wander down in this way at least
as far as the pharynx. The larvae of *G. intestinalis* and *G. haemorrhoidalis*
are found chiefly in the mucosa of the tongue, those of *G. pecorum* and
G. inermis in the mucosa of the cheeks. The larvae of the latter species,
perhaps also those of *G. haemorrhoidalis*, even pierce the skin of the face
and wander in it to the mouth, leaving conspicuous tracks behind them
and this has been known to occur in man. *Gastrophilus*, however, though
it rarely infests man, may cause in him a cutaneous swelling at the point
at where the first larva penetrates the skin. More rarely the larvae reach

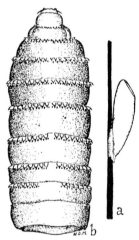

Fig. 229. *Gastrophilus intestinalis:* a, Egg on Hair; b, Larva, Dorsal View (Original)

the human stomach and cause irritation there. In other animals the
migratory larvae occasionally go astray and they have been found in
various thoracic and abdominal organs, the sinuses of the head and even
in the brain.

The larvae of *G. intestinalis*, after wandering in the tongue for 21–28 days,
become attached in the cardiac portion of the stomach, rarely in the fundus

or the pylorus; they have a reddish colour. Those of *G. nasalis* are pale yellow and attach themselves in the pylorus and the duodenum. The larvae of *G. pecorum* are blood-red in colour; the second and sometimes also the third stage is found in the pharynx and the upper part of the oesophagus, but the third stage is usually attached in the fundus of the stomach. The young stages of *G. haemorrhoidalis*, which are red, are occasionally found in the pharynx, but later they settle in the stomach.

The larvae remain in the host for 10–12 months and then pass out through the intestine. Those of *G. haemorrhoidalis* again attach themselves for a few days in the rectum. Some larvae may leave the host in the late autumn, but usually they pass out in the spring. They pupate in the ground for 3–5 weeks and then the flies emerge.

Pathogenesis. The flies which lay their eggs on or near the head of the host annoy the animals and may even cause them to become panicky and run away. The migrating larvae are found in the superficial layers of the buccal epithelium and produce no reaction. When later they attach themselves in the pharynx, stomach or duodenum, an inflammatory process produces a ring-like thickening around the larva. Very rarely perforations of the pharynx, oesophagus or stomach have been seen. Clusters of larvae around the pylorus interfere with the action of the sphincter and the passage of food. The larvae that pass through the intestine, and especially those that attach themselves anew in the rectum, cause an irritation by means of their spines.

However opinions vary about the importance of bots in horses. Many stock owners firmly believe that the parasites must be removed and institute regular treatments for this. There is little critical evidence that the bot is an important parasite, nevertheless it would seem unreasonable to assume that the, at times, extensive ulceration of the stomach by a large number of parasites is without a general effect. Debility due to bots has been ascribed to a hypersensitivity to the excretions of the larvae but there is no firm foundation for this belief.

Diagnosis. The eggs can be found by examining the sites in which they are deposited, and larvae in the pharynx can be seen at direct inspection, but there is no way of diagnosing the presence of the larval parasites in the stomach.

Treatment. Carbon bisulphide given as for *Habronema* or in a capsule is effective, as is carbon tetrachloride also, but these kill only larvae in the stomach. They should be given in the autumn after the flies have disappeared, and eggs on the hairs of the horses should also be then removed. A piperazine–carbon disulphide complex is effective against the second and third-stage larvae. It would appear, however, that this effect is due to the carbon disulphide released from this compound rather than to the piperazine, since piperazine by itself has no effect on the larvae. Drummond *et al.* (1959) reported that 37–40 mg. per kg. bodyweight of Bayer L 13/59 (Neguvon) given in the food controlled the larvae of *G. intestinalis* and *G. nasalis*, but that DOW ET 57 and Bayer 21/199 (CoRal) had no effect on the larvae.

Prophylaxis. Frequent grooming removes some eggs and the larvae of *G. intestinalis*, which hatch as a result of the friction. Singeing and clipping may be useful, but more advisable is the weekly application of a 2 per cent carbolic dip to those parts of the animal on which the eggs are deposited, in order to destroy them.

Genus: Oestrus Linné, 1761

O. ovis Linné, 1761, the 'sheep nasal fly', has a dark grey colour with small black spots which are especially prominent on the thorax, and it is covered with light brown hair. The flies hide in warm corners or crevices, and in the early morning they can be seen sitting against walls or other objects in the sun. They occur from spring to autumn, particularly in summer, but in warm climates they are active even in winter. The larvae occur in the nasal cavity and the adjoining sinuses in sheep and rarely in goats, and have also been found in the blesbock (*Damaliscus albifrons*) and, in Egypt, in the camel. *Oestrus* sometimes also deposits its larvae in the eyes, nostrils and on the lips of man, where they may develop causing serious trouble.

The flies deposit their young larvae around the nostrils of the host, whence they crawl upwards. Sometimes they enter into cavities which have small openings, like those of the turbinated bones or a branch of the frontal sinus, with the result that they are not able to get out when they have grown adult and so they die there. The rate of development of the first larval instar varies considerably, this instar remaining in the nasal passages for 2 weeks to 9 months during the cold months. The second instar passes into the frontal sinuses and may develop rapidly, leaving the sheep 25 days after infection or considerably longer. Finally the full-grown larvae crawl out and pupate in the ground for 3–6 weeks, or longer during the cold season, before the fly emerges.

The young larvae are white or slightly yellow; when they become mature, dark transverse bands develop on the dorsal aspects of the segments. The full-grown larva is about 3 cm. long, tapering anteriorly, and ending with a flat surface posteriorly. There are large, black, oral hooks, connected to an internal cephalo-pharyngeal skeleton. The ventral surface bears rows of small spines and the black stigmal plates are conspicuous on the posterior surface.

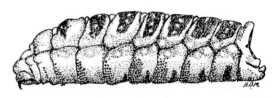

FIG. 230. *Oestrus ovis*, Larva, Lateral View ($\times 2\frac{1}{2}$) (Original)

PLATE XI

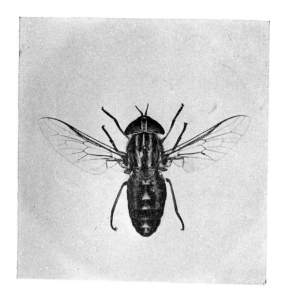

A. *Tabanus taeniola*, male

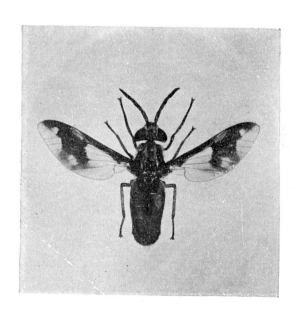

B. *Chrysops stigmaticalis*

PLATE XII

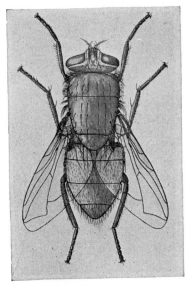

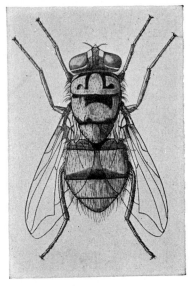

A. *Lucilia sericata*. (After Smit)   B. *Chrysomyia chloropyga*. (After Smit)

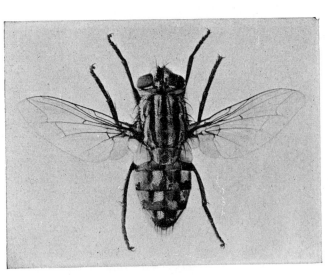

C. *Sarcophaga haemorrhoidalis*, female. (Original)

PLATE XIII

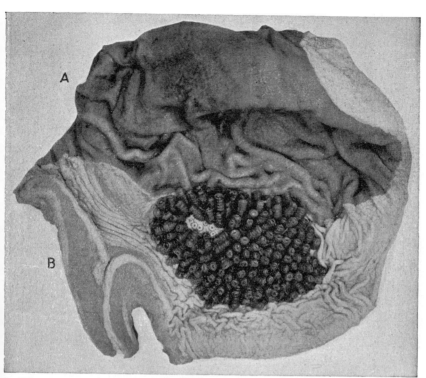

A. Muscous membrane of horse stomach affected with horse bots. (A) Pyloric end of stomach; (B) oesophageal (cardiac) end of stomach; the horseshoe shaped indentation at the bottom of the illustration is the oesophageal opening. Several bots have been removed to show the circular pits where the larvae have been attached (H. Thornton)

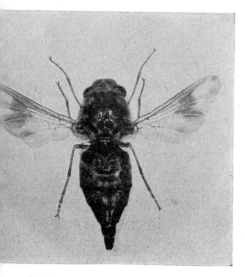

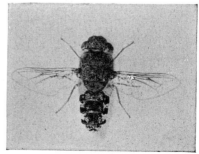

B. *Gastrophilus intestinalis*, female

C. *Oestrus ovis*, female (Original)

PLATE XIV

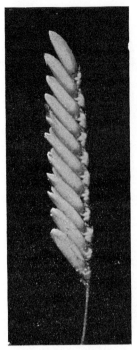

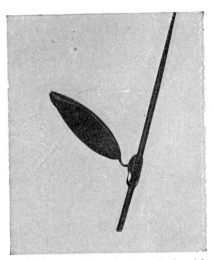

B. Single egg of *Hypoderma bovis* with two-lobed pedicle by which it is attached to an ox hair. × 32. (Crown copyright)

A. Eggs of *Hypoderma lineatum* on ox hair. × 15. (Crown copyright)

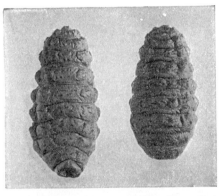

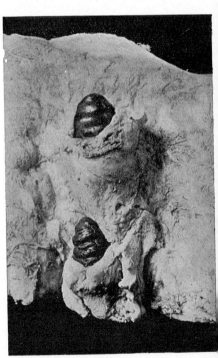

C. Full-grown larvae of *Hypoderma bovis* removed from skin of back. Left—dorsal view; right—ventral view. (Crown copyright)

D. *Hypoderma* larvae embedded in fat on under-surface of ox skin. (Crown copyright)

PLATE XV

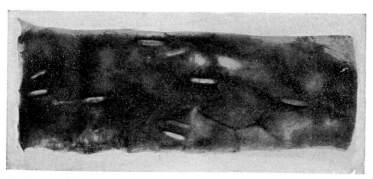

A. Larvae of *Hypoderma lineatum* in submucous tissue of bovine oesophagus. Some congested blood vessels can be seen, and are the result of the inflammatory condition produced. × ½. (H. Thornton)

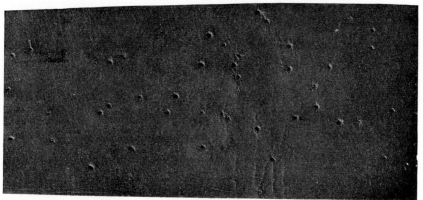

B. Portion of leather (butt) showing damage due to ox warbles. (Crown copyright)

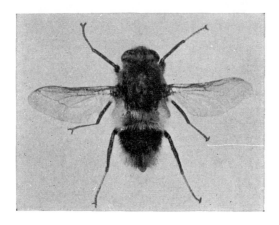

C. *Hypoderma bovis*, male. (Original)

PLATE XVI

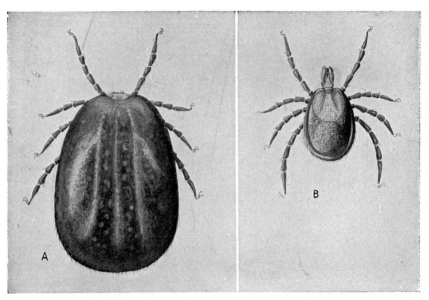

Ixodes ricinus. (A) Engorged adult female. (B) Unengorged adult female. The male tick is somewhat smaller and does not swell in engorging. × 5. (Burroughs Wellcome)

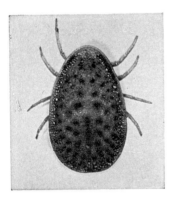

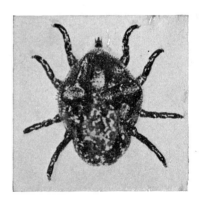

C. *Argas persigus*, dorsal view

D. *Otobius megnini*, nymph

PLATE XVII

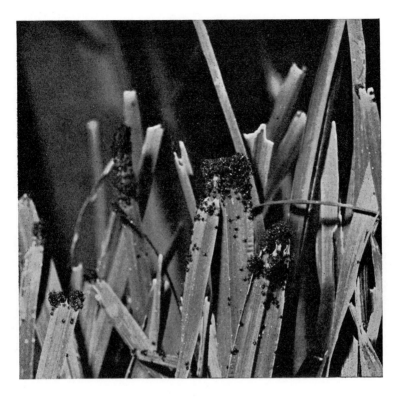

'Seed ticks' collecting on the tips of grass blades to await an opportunity to attach themselves to passing hosts.

(Reproduced by kind permission of the Liaison Officer, Agricultural Liaison Section, Commonwealth Scientific and Industrial Research Organisation, East Melbourne Australia)

PLATE XVIII

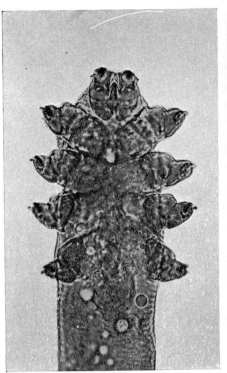

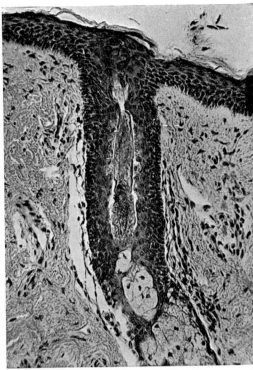

A. *Demodex folliculorum.* Adult female, stained with lignin pink. × 600

B. *Demodex folliculorum.* Vertical section of human skin, showing an adult male in the mouth of a hair follicle. × 140

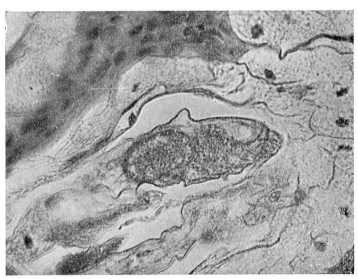

C. *Demodex folliculorum.* Vertical section of human skin, showing a ovigerous female in a sebaceous gland. × 275

(Photographs by Mr. Lunnan, Institute of Dermatology, University of London, from Spickett (1960), reproduced by kind permission of the author and of the Director of the Institute)

Pathogenesis. The flies cause great annoyance when they attack the sheep to deposit larvae, so that the animals stop feeding and become restless. They shake their heads or press their noses against the ground or in between other sheep. When the flies are plentiful, they may thus cause considerably interference with the feeding of the animals. The larvae irritate the mucosa with their oral hooks and spines, causing the secretion of a viscid mucous exudate, on which they apparently feed. Erosion of the bones of the skull may occur and even injury to the brain, and then such signs as high-stepping gait, incoordination, may suggest infection with *Coenurus cerebralis* (*q.v.*). For this reason the infection has been called 'false gid'. Infected sheep have a nasal discharge and sneeze frequently.

Diagnosis can only be made tentatively from the clinical signs, excluding other possible causes like lungworms and chronic bronchial or pulmonary diseases.

Treatment. This is difficult since the larvae are difficult to reach: frequently the openings into the sinuses are narrowed or occluded. At one time direct injections into the frontal sinus were made, using an emulsion of tetrachlorethylene, but this has now been largely discontinued. Instillation of BHC in oil (1–4 per cent) into the nostrils while the sheep is lying on its back have been practised in South Africa, with good results.

The use of systemic insecticides, such as the organophosphorus compounds, is a more rational approach. Sheep given 55–88 mg. per kg. of a mixture of 2 g. of Neguvon (Bayer L 13/59) and 0·2 g. of Asuntol (Bayer L 21/199) were cleared of the infection (Stampa, 1959).

Prophylaxis. This is difficult since the present fly repellents are short lasting. One method is to feed sheep in narrow troughs, the edges of which are smeared with tar. The animals automatically tar themselves and this acts as a repellent.

Genus: Hypoderma Latreille, 1818

The larval stages of *H. bovis* (de Geer, 1776) and *H. lineatum* (de Villiers, 1789) (syn. *H. lineata*), the 'ox warbles', are common parasites of cattle, rarely also of man and horses, in many countries in the northern hemisphere and cause great economic losses. Apart from infections in imported animals the genus is not established in the southern hemisphere. *H. bovis* is about 15 mm. long; *H. lineatum* measures 13 mm. Both flies are hairy and have no functioning mouth parts. The hairs on the head and the anterior part of the thorax are yellowish-white in *H. lineatum* and greenish-yellow in *H. bovis*. The abdomen is covered with light yellow hairs anteriorly, followed by a band of dark hairs, and the posterior portion bears orange-yellow hairs.

Life-cycle. The flies occur in summer, especially in June and July. They are most active on warm days, when they attack cattle to lay their eggs.

16

These are about 1 mm. long and are fixed to the hairs by means of small terminal clasps, especially on the legs, but more rarely on the body as well. *H. bovis* lays its eggs singly, while *H. lineatum* deposits a row of six or more on a hair. The flies are very persistent in approaching the animals, and one female may lay 100 or more eggs on one individual. The larvae hatch in about 4 days and crawl down the hair to the skin, through which they penetrate. They wander in the subcutaneous connective tissue up the leg and then towards the diaphragm, gradually increasing in size. The larvae of *H. lineatum* find their way into the oesophageal wall, where they come to lie in the submucous connective tissue for the rest of the summer and autumn, growing to about 12 mm. in length. Eventually during January and February they travel towards the dorsal aspect of the body and reach the subcutaneous tissue of the back. The larvae of *H. bovis* sometimes enter the spinal canal, but usually leave it again. When the parasites arrive under the skin of the back, swellings begin to form, measuring about 3 cm. in diameter. The skin over each swelling becomes perforated, and the larva then lies with its posterior stigmal plate directed towards the pore for the purpose of respiration. This stage lasts about 30 days. The younger larvae are almost white, changing to yellow and then to light brown as they grow older. Two ecdyses occur during the development of the larvae. The full-grown larva of *H. bovis* is 27–28 mm. long; that of *H. lineatum* 25 mm. Each segment

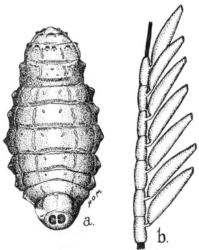

FIG. 231. a, Larva of *Hypoderma bovis*, Ventral View; b, Eggs of *H. lineatum* on Hair
(Original)

bears a number of flat tubercles and small spines are present on all segments but the last in *H. lineatum* and on all but the last two in *H. bovis*. In spring the mature larva wriggles out of its cyst and falls on the ground, into which it penetrates to pupate. The pupal case is black and the fly emerges from it, after 35–36 days, by pushing open an operculum at the anterior end. Among other hosts on which species of *Hypoderma* may lay eggs, especially when cattle are not available, are horses and man, though the larvae do not usually mature in these hosts, though in horses they may rarely enter the brain and cause death. Usually, however, they remain in the skin, causing sores there.

Pathogenesis. When the flies approach to lay eggs the cattle become scared and attempt to escape the attack by running away, and will even go into water. Since the flies are persistent the animals are constantly irritated and do not feed properly, which results in an appreciable loss of weight and decrease of milk yield. The animals may hurt themselves severely or at least become wounded and thus damage their skins.

The larvae irritate the tissues around them, the flesh becomes greenish-yellow and infiltrated, especially along the tracks where larvae have wandered, and thus depreciates in value.

Great damage is caused to the skin of the back by the perforation produced. The annual loss due to this factor alone is very high in some countries. It is uncertain whether the larvae have a toxic influence on the host, but animals which have been treated for the parasite show better growth and production.

Clinical signs. Except for poor growth in bad cases and decreased milk yield the animals show no appreciable signs until the larvae appear along the back, when the swellings can be felt and seen. The larva lies in a cyst which also contains a yellow purulent fluid.

Calves and young cattle are more frequently and more severely infected than older animals. It is possible that cattle develop a certain degree of resistance to the larvae. Older animals may have become sensitised during previous infections by the absorption of body fluids of larvae that die, so that they may show anaphylactic reactions when subsequently larvae die or are broken during extraction. Even abortions have been noted in such cases.

Diagnosis must be based on the presence of the larvae under the skin of the back. The eggs may also be found on the hairs of the animals in summer.

Mechanical removal of larvae. Mature larvae may be squeezed out of the warble swelling. This is less successful when the larvae are not mature. Rupture of the larvae during extraction may lead to a localised inflammation and abscess formation or even a generalised anaphylaxis in a few animals.

Insecticide treatment. Until the advent of the organophosphorus insecticides, derris, or its active principal rotenone, was widely used as a larvicide. Derris was usually used as a wash and applied to the back of infected cattle after the scabs covering the warble swellings had been removed by scrubbing with a soapy mixture. This treatment was highly effective but for adequate control repeated treatment of stock was necessary during the warble season. A disadvantage was that the warble fly larvae were killed only when they had migrated through the body and produced damage to flesh and hides. The introduction of the organophosphorus systemic insecticides allowed control of the larvae while they were in the early stages of migration and before they reached the backs of animals.

The systemic organophosphorus larvicides have now more or less replaced other methods of control. Those such as trichlorophon ('Dyvon') coumaphos ('Co-Ral'), Ruelene and several others are widely used. They are employed during the autumn and early winter with the aim of killing the younger larval stages. The compounds may be given orally, in drench or bolus form, but one of the more convenient methods is 'pour on' dressings in which a small volume of concentrated insecticide is poured along the animal's back. Enough insecticide is absorbed through the skin to kill warble fly larvae.

These compounds should be avoided in January and February since severe reactions may occur due to the death of larvae in the wall of the oesophagus (tympany) or spinal canal (paraplegia).

H. aeratum Austen, 1931 is a similar parasite of goats and sheep in Cyprus, Crete and Turkey, while **H. crossi** Patton, 1923 infects goats and sheep in India, especially in the dry, hilly regions of the North-West Provinces. The eggs are laid on the long hairs at the sides of the body and the larvae penetrate directly through the skin, remaining there to develop for about 7 months. **H. diana** Brauer, 1858 causes warbles of deer in Scotland, **H. actaeon** occurs in Central Europe and **H. silenus** Brauer, 1858 attacks equines and goats in the Balkans, Asia Minor and possibly in North Africa. **Oedemagena tarandi** (Linné, 1761 attacks reindeer and caribou in Northern Europe and America.

SUBFAMILY: CUTEREBRINAE

Genus: Dermatobia Brauer, 1860

D. hominis (Linné 1781) (syn. *D. ovaniventris*), also called the 'berne', 'nuche' or 'forcel', occurs in man in tropical America from Mexico to the Argentine. Cattle, dogs, cats, sheep, rabbits and other animals, including man, may become infected. The female is about 12 mm. long. The thorax is dark blue with a greyish bloom, the abdomen is short and broad and has a brilliant blue colour.

Life-cycle. The adult flies do not feed and nourishment is derived from food stores accumulated during the larval period. When the adult fly is ready to oviposit, she captures a mosquito, or other blood sucking fly, and glues a batch of eggs to the abdomen of the captive fly. When the transport fly alights on a warm-blooded host the larvae of *D. hominis* hatch from the eggs and penetrate the skin of the host, often using the skin puncture made by the blood-sucking fly. About 6 days are required for the egg to reach the stage of hatching, but this occurs only when the carrier fly settles on a suitable animal to feed. The most common vectors of *D.*

hominis larvae are members of the genus *Psorophora* though *Culex* and *Stomoxys* are also concerned and non-blood-sucking anthomyids have also been incriminated. Non-insect transmission may occur when *D. hominis* eggs are deposited on damp clothes or laundry. *D. hominis* breeds in forest country and domestic and wild mammals are commonly parasitised. Man is usually infected when he is associated with domestic animals. As the larva grows it produces a swelling which has a central opening through which it breathes. These swellings are usually very painful. Development in the host requires 5–10 weeks, after which the larva escapes and pupates in the ground for an equally long period before the fly emerges. The mature larva is about 25 mm. long and has a few rows of strong spines on most of the segments.

Diagnosis. The presence of a superficially situated swelling with a central opening, especially if more than one is present, would lead to the suspicion of myiasis. Specific diagnosis can be made only after extraction of the larva.

Treatment. In man the only satisfactory treatment is surgical removal of the parasite.

In cattle and other animals dips or washes containing BHC, DDT and toxaphene, applied regularly have given reasonable control and it is probable that the organophosphorus insecticides could be used to advantage.

Genus: Cuterebra Clark, 1815

Large flies (20 mm. or more in length), bodies bee-like, mouth parts vestigial. Larvae parasitic, large (25 mm. in length), stout and parasitic under the skin of rodents etc. North American forms.

The adult flies oviposit near the entrance of the burrows of rabbits (*C. buccata, C. americana, C. lepivora*), mice and chipmonks (*C. emasculator*). Larvae hatch at intervals and penetrate the skin of the above hosts producing cyst-like subcutaneous lesions in which the larvae mature. Mature larvae are produced in about 1 month, at which stage they are dark in colour and covered with bands of spines. Younger larvae are lighter in colour. Larvae leave the host to pupate in the soil.

Pathogenesis. A large subcutaneous cyst is produced with associated swelling. *C. emasculator* frequently parasitised the scrotum destroying the testes and causing parasitic castration.

Though these forms are usually found in wild rodents occasional infection of cats, dogs and humans may occur. In the cat larvae are frequently found in the neck or subandibular region and due to scratching the swelling may become secondarily infected. Infection of the cranial cavity of the cat has been reported as well as parasitic orchitis in the dog and cat. Human nasal and dermal infection may also occur.

Treatment. Surgical removal is the most satisfactory.

SUBORDER CYCLORRHAPHA
SECTION PUPIPARA

The Pupipara are a group of aberrant Diptera, related to the Antho-myidae. They are markedly adapted to a parasitic life. All the species, with one exception, live on the blood of mammals or birds. The body is broad and flattened dorso-ventrally; the abdomen is indistinctly seg-mented, and usually its wall is soft and leather-like. Wings are present in some species and absent in others. The antenna has one joint and lies in a pit on the forehead. The feet are provided with strong claws, by means of which the parasite clings to the hairs or feathers of its host. As the name Pupipara indicates, the females give birth to larvae which are ready to pupate.

FAMILY: HIPPOBOSCIDAE
Genus: Hippobosca Linné, 1761

Several species of this genus, especially **H. equina** Linné, 1758, **H. rufipes** Olfers, 1816, and **H. maculata** Leach, 1817, are common parasites of horses and cattle, particularly in warm countries. Other animals like dogs may also be attacked. The flies are about 1 cm. long to the tip of the abdomen and have a reddish-brown colour with pale yellow spots. There are two wings, the veins of which are crowded together towards the anterior border. The short, thick palpi ensheath the tip of the slender proboscis, of which the main portion is withdrawn into the head during rest.

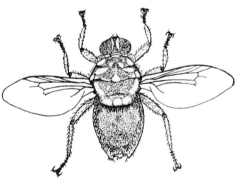

FIG. 232. *Hippobosca rufipes* (after Bedford)

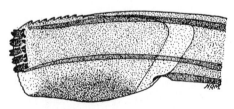

FIG. 233. *Hippobosca rufipes*, Distal End of Proboscis, Laterval View (Original)

Life-cycle and habits. The female fly deposits one larva at a time in sheltered spots where there is dry soil or humus. In Wales *H. equina* lays in humus at the roots of certain plants, mainly bracken (*Pteris aquilina*). The larvae pupate almost immediately, and gradually turn from yellow to black. The larva is sub-globular in shape; it measures about 5 by 4 mm. and possesses a dark spot at the posterior pole. The length of the pupal period is greatly influenced by the temperature. The flies are most frequent in summer and bite more particularly in sunny weather. They remain for long periods on their hosts and are not easily disturbed. They cluster in the perineal region and down between the hind-legs to the pubic region, but may also bite on other parts of the body. Distribution occurs almost exclusively with cattle and horses, since the flies are not inclined to travel more than a few metres, although they are strong fliers. These flies are a source of great irritation to animals which are not accustomed to them. They transmit the non-pathogenic *Trypanosoma theileri* to cattle and species of *Haemoproteus* to anatid and other birds.

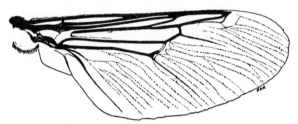

Fig. 234. *Hippobosca rufipes*, Wing (Original)

Control. The flies can be readily killed by applying DDT to those parts of animals where they congregate. Regular dipping or spraying for the control of ticks eliminates them.

H. capensis v. Olfers, 1816 (syn. *H. francilloni*) occurs in Africa and Asia and attacks chiefly dogs.

Genus: Melophagus Latreille, 1804

M. ovinus (Linné, 1758), the sheep ked, is found in most parts of the world. It is a wingless, hairy, leathery insect, 4–6 mm. long. The head is short, broad and not freely movable; the thorax is brown and the broad abdomen greyish-brown. The legs are strong and armed with stout claws.

Life-cycle and habits. The female attaches its larva to the wool of the sheep by means of a sticky substance. Parturition lasts a few minutes. The larva is immobile and soon turns into a chestnut-brown pupa. It is ovoid in shape with broad ends and 3–4 mm. long. The pupal stage lasts 19–23 days in summer to 36 days in winter, or even longer if the sheep are exposed to very cold conditions. The female ked lives 4–5 months on a sheep. Copulation occurs 3–4 days after emergence of the adult and each gestation lasts about 10–12 days. A female may produce ten to fifteen larvae. Engorged females can live up to 8 days off the host. Pupae removed from the sheep, for instance at shearing, can hatch if conditions are favourable, but the emerging adults die very soon if they do not find a sheep to feed on. They usually spread from sheep to sheep by contact and are most numerous in the autumn and winter. A summer decrease in numbers occurs on all sheep of any age or sex. Sheep with dense, long or clotted fleeces are more likely to spread the infestation, because the keds come to the surface of such fleeces.

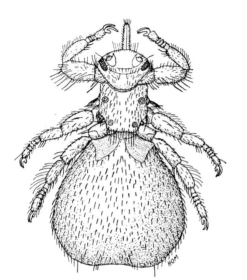

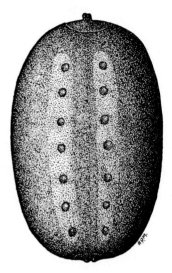

FIG. 235. *Melophagus ovinus*, Adult   FIG. 236. *Melophagus ovinus*,
(Original)   Pupa (Original)

Pathogenesis. The parasites live in the wool of the sheep and suck blood. Heavy infections can reduce the condition of the host considerably and even cause anaemia. They produce intense irritation, causing the sheep to bite, rub and scratch itself, thus damaging the wool. The faeces of the keds produce stains in the wool which do not wash out readily. The ked transmits *Trypanosoma melophagium* to sheep. Poorly fed animals or animals that are not protected against cold weather are most liable to suffer from keds, so that the parasites are particularly troublesome towards the end of winter.

Control. The ked population is markedly reduced by shearing. Where control measures are in operation for lice, blowflies, mange or ticks, these usually result in the control of *M. ovinus*. The insects are very susceptible to the chlorinated hydrocarbon (e.g. BHC) and organophosphorus insecticides and a single dipping will give several months protection. 'Tip spraying' is an effective control measure with short-fleeced sheep but with the long-woolled breeds a second treatment may be necessary.

Genus: Pseudolynchia Bequaert, 1925

P. canariensis (Macquart, 1840) (syn. *P. maura*) is a dark brown fly, 6 mm. long, which resembles the sheep ked, but has a pair of transparent, tapering wings with the venation reduced and concentrated along the anterior border. The claws are strong and spurred. The parasite is widely distributed in warm countries and lives on domestic pigeons and a few wild birds.

Life-cycle and habits. The flies move through the feathers, sucking blood and causing painful wounds, especially on young nestling pigeons 2-3 weeks old, when the feathers begin to grow and afford protection. When the bird is handled the parasites fly away and they are not easily caught. They may bite man. The female produces four to five young during her life of 43 days or so. Copulation takes place on the host and the larvae are laid in dark crevices of the pigeon-house in dry dust or in the nests. Benbrook (1959) states that they are laid on the host and roll off it. They are yellow with a dark posterior pole and measure about 3 by 2·5 mm.; they turn into black pupae in a few hours. The pupal stage lasts 23–31 days in warm weather. *P. canariensis* and species of related genera transmit *Haemoproteus columbae*, a blood protozoon of pigeons, and the related *H. lophortyx* of the quail.

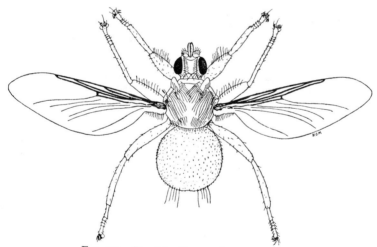

FIG. 237. *Pseudolynchia canariensis* (Original)

Control. Benbrook (1959) states that a spray composed of pyrethrum 1 part and kerosene 2 parts rids pigeon lofts of the flies, and he recommends rubbing derris powder or pyrethrum into the skin of the birds, or dipping them in 1½–2 oz. of derris in 1 gallon of water containing 2½ oz. of laundry soap; or dusting them with a dust containing 3 g. of 10 per cent DDT mixed with talc. The organophosphorus compounds may be of value in treatment and control.

CLASS: ARACHNIDA

This Class includes the king-crabs, scorpions, spiders, ticks and mites; and also other species which need not be considered in this book. The head, however, is absent from all species of this Class and they therefore have no antennae. The mouth of arachnids is small and they feed chiefly on the tissue-fluids of other animals which they suck up by means of a sucking pharnyx. They are thus carnivorous animals and many of them possess poison glands and poison-claws, with which they paralyse their prey before they suck the juices out of them. The first and second pairs of appendages are modified to help in feeding, the first pair being called the *chelicerae* and the second pair the *pedipalps*. Either of these two pairs of appendages may be pincers and poison-glands may be associated with them. The poison-glands of the scorpion are, on the other hand, situated on a terminal, postanal segment of the body. The basal joints of the pedipalps of arachnids, and also those of some of the walking legs behind them, may bear teeth which help in chewing the prey. Such basal joints are called *gnathobases*.

The segmentation of the body of arachnids differs from that of other arthropods and different terms are used to describe it. Less confusion arises if the terms thorax and abdomen are abandoned and the term *prosoma* is given to the first six segments of the body and the term *opisthosoma* to the remaining segments. The prosoma bears the chelicerae, pedipalps and the four pairs of walking legs. It may be divided into the *gnathosoma*, which bears the chelicerae and pedipalps, and the *podosoma*, which bears the four pairs of walking legs. The opisthosoma corresponds to the abdomen. The podosoma and the opisthosoma are sometimes together called the *idiosoma*. These subdivisions are not, however, evident on the bodies of ticks and mites, because the bodies of these species have lost external signs of segmentation. Most of them show a division into two parts only, (1) an anterior gnathosoma, which bears the chelicerae, and pedipalps, and also the median hypostome developed by these species only; the gnathosoma of ticks and mites is called the *capitulum*; (2) a posterior single piece, which represents the fused podosoma and opisthosoma and may therefore be called the idiosoma. The mouth parts of ticks and mites are modified for sucking the blood or tissue-fluids of their hosts, and for holding on to the host. They are further described below.

Arachnids breathe by means of the gill-books, lung-books and tracheae described above. *Gill-books* are present on segments nine to thirteen of the aquatic king-crabs. *Lung-books* and tracheae are present in the air-breathing species, which may breathe by means of either tracheae or lung-books or both. Some species, such as some aquatic and other mites have no special respiratory organs, but absorb oxygen through the cuticle. Various classifications of the Class have been proposed and the following division of it into three subclasses is convenient for the purposes of this book:

SUBCLASS I. PANTOPODA (PYCNOGONIDA)

These are small marine arachnids with a very small opisthosoma without appendages and four pairs of clawed legs on the rest of the body.

SUBCLASS II. MEROSTOMATA

These are aquatic arachnids one order of which, the *Eurypterida*, is extinct, while the other order, the *Xiphosura*, is represented by the marine king-crabs belonging to the genus *Limulus*.

SUBCLASS III. EUARACHNIDA

This subclass includes the scorpions, spiders, ticks and mites and a number of other related species. The Euarachnida breathe air and their bodies are divided into a prosoma and opisthosoma, except those of the ticks and mites whose bodies consist of one piece only, which is formed by fusion of the thorax and abdomen. This subclass may be divided into the following orders:

ORDER I. SCORPIONIDEA

These are relatively large, terrestrial arachnids which inhabit warm countries. The prosoma consists of a single piece covered by a single dorsal plate. Behind this, the opisthosoma is divided into a portion called the *mesosoma*, consisting of seven segments which are as broad as the segments of the prosoma, and a narrower portion behind this, consisting of five segments, called the *metasoma*, behind which is the terminal, post-anal *sting* containing the poison-gland. The chelicerae of Scorpionidea are small, but the pedipalps are large and bear pincers. There are four pairs of walking legs, and on the ventral sternal plates of segments ten to thirteen there are four pairs of stimata leading into the lung-books. The body ends in a post-anal segment called the sting, which contains a poison-gland and is provided with a sharp spine.

ORDER 2. PEDIPALPI

These are predatory species living in warm climates, which prey chiefly on insects. They have large pedipalps and the chelicerae bear claws, which may contain poison-glands. For this reason the bites of some species of this order may have severe effects.

ORDER 3. ARANEIDAE

These are the spiders, which breathe air. Their bodies are divided into a prosoma (cephalothorax) and an unsegmented soft abdomen, the first segment of which forms a stalk (pedicel) that joins these two parts together. The chelicerae have poison-glands and hooks for killing the prey and the pedipalps are relatively small. The bites of some spiders may have serious effects.

ORDER 4. PALPIGRADI

These are microscopic terrestrial species, which look rather like insects, because the prosoma is covered by three separate plates and the opisthosoma is a broader part of the body.

ORDER 5. SOLIFUGAE (SOLFUGAE)

These hairy, nocturnal, terrestrial species live in warm countries and breathe by means of tracheae. The first two, or according to some experts the first three segments, form a single piece that bears the very large and powerful pincer-like chelicerae, the leg-like pedipalps and the first pair of legs. This anterior part of the body is jointed to the rest of the body, so that it can be raised. The chelicerae can kill small mammals and birds, but Solifugae feed chiefly on insects.

ORDER 6. CHERNETIDEA (CHELIFERAE)

The small species of this order are often called chelifers or pseudo-scorpions. The prosoma is covered by a single plate and the opisthosoma is segmented. The chelicerae are small pincers, but the pedipalps, like those of scorpions, are large and end in pincers. Chelifers feed chiefly on insects and their larvae.

ORDER 7. PODOGONA

This order contains only two small species found in South America and West Africa. The prosoma is a single piece, the opisthosoma is segmented and both the chelicerae and pedipalps bear pincers.

ORDER 8. PHALANGIDEA

Species of this order breathe by means of tracheae and are sometimes called Harvestmen, but they should not be confused with the larvae of the mites belonging to the acarine genus *Trombicula*, which are often called harvesters. Phalangidea look rather like spiders, but the opisthosoma is segmented and it is joined to the podosoma across its whole width, so that there is no waist. The chelicerae bear pincers, but the long pedipalps do not. The very long walking legs are brittle.

ORDER 9. PENTASTOMIDA

This order includes the tongue-worm of the dog, which is further described below, and its relatives, all of which are parasitic in the upper respiratory passages of carnivorous vertebrates. Their bodies are elongated, soft, annulated and worm-like, the appendages having been greatly reduced. Their life histories are indirect, the intermediate hosts being usually herbivorous vertebrates, among which sheep and cattle are included. Man is an intermediate host of some species.

ORDER 10. ACARINA

The species of the order are the hard and soft ticks and their numerous small, or minute relatives, which are often, called mites. Apart from the ticks, most of the species of the order are minute. A few of the numerous species cause the various kinds of mange or inflict other kinds of injury on farm animals. The mouth parts consist of a pair of chelicerae, a pair of pedipalps and, between these, a median toothed structure called the *hypostome*. They are borne on the *gnathosoma*, which consists of a plate called the *capitulum* and the mouth parts just mentioned. The segmentation of the rest of the body is indistinct or absent.

The life history of Acarina begins with the *egg*, from which emerges a *larva*, which lacks the fourth pair of legs present in the later phases, so that the larva has only six legs. The larva moults to become the *nymph*, which usually resembles the adult, but has no sexual organs. One or more nymphal instars, sometimes called the protonymph, deutonymph and tritonymph, may precede the appearance of the adult phase. The other features of the species of Acarina described in this book are given below.

The order Acarina may be divided into six suborders. Of these the suborders Nostostigmata and Holothyroidea have no economic importance The remaining suborders, some species of which are further described below, are:

Suborder: Mesostigmata

This suborder includes species of the group Gamasides (gamasid mites), examples of which are the red mite of poultry (*Dermanyssus gallinae*), the tropical fowl mite *Bdellonyssus* (*Liponyssus*) *bursa* and their relatives.

Suborder: Ixodoidea (Ixodides)

This suborder includes the hard and soft ticks.

Suborder: Trombidiformes

This suborder includes species which are pests of various fruits and bulbs and also the species of the genus *Demodex*, which cause demodectic mange and those of the genus *Trombicula*, the larvae of which suck the tissue fluids of man and animals and may be important vectors of disease, such as scrub (mite) typhus.

Suborder: Sarcoptiformes

This suborder may be divided into (a) the *Oribatei* (oribatid mites), which are not parasitic, but some species of them are intermediate hosts of tapeworms belonging to the families Anopolocephalidae and Catenotaeniidae (of rats and mice). (b) The *Acaridae*, a group which includes the mites which cause sarcoptic and other forms of mange and also various species which injure grains, flour and other stored products.

ORDER: ACARINA

SUBORDER: MESOSTIGMATA

Species of this suborder are usually armoured with brown or dark-brown plates. The body, like that of the ticks, to which the species of this suborder seem to be related, is divided into two portions only, an anterior minute gnathosoma, which bears the mouth parts, and a posterior idiosoma. The name of the suborder refers to the fact that the single pair of stigmata are lateral and outside the coxae of the legs. Like the stigmata of ticks, they may be borne on peritremal plates. There are no genital suckers. Among the numerous species of the suborder Mesostigmata the only ones of veterinary importance belong to the group of the suborder called the Gamasides or gamasid mites. Some gamasid mites are not parasitic and live in soil, moss, decaying wood or vegetation or in litter. Others are parasitic on myriapods, beetles and other insects, snakes, birds, bats and other mammals. Among them is *Raillietia auris*, a small species about 1 mm. long, which has been found in the external ears of cattle in Europe (France, Austria and elsewhere), Madras and North America. The following species have veterinary importance:

FAMILY: DERMANYSSIDAE

Genus: Dermanyssys Dugès, 1834

D. gallinae (Degeer, 1778). This cosmopolitan species (Fig. 238) attacks the fowl, pigeon, canary and other cage birds and also many wild birds. It may also feed on man. It is often called the red mite of poultry, but is, like the other mites mentioned below, only red when it has recently fed on its host's blood; otherwise it is whitish, greyish or black. The engorged female adult is about 1 mm. long or larger, the other stages of the life history being smaller. The dorsal shield does not quite reach the posterior end of the body and its posterior margin is truncated. The setae on it are smaller than those on the skin around the dorsal plate. The anus is on the posterior half of the anal plate, whereas in *O. sylviarum* the anus is on the anterior half of this plate. The chelicerae are long and whiplike.

Life-cycle and habits. The eggs are laid, usually after a blood meal, in cracks and crevices in the walls of the poultry houses or in the nest of the birds, up to seven eggs being laid at a time. The eggs hatch, at outdoor summer temperatures, in 48–72 hours, liberating six-legged larvae which do not feed. These moult in 24–48 hours to become protonymphs, which feed on the host's blood and moult after 24–48 hours to become deutonymphs and these, after a blood meal, moult in 24–48 hours to become the adults. The whole life-cycle can be completed in 7 days under optimal conditions. The adults can, under experimental conditions, live for 4–5 months without a meal of blood.

The nymphs and adults periodically visit the hosts to suck blood and hide, during intervals between meals, in cracks and crevices in the quarters of the birds. Under favourable conditions the mites reproduce rapidly and may become a serious pest, causing much irritation and

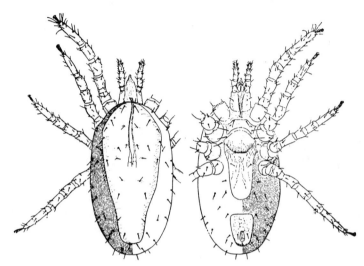

FIG. 238. *Dermanyssus gallinae*: left, dorsal view of female; right, ventral view of female
(Degeer)

anaemia due to loss of blood. The birds become listless and their egg production may be reduced and loss of blood may cause death. *D. gallinae* may be a frequent parasite of aviaries, especially when these are heated. *D. gallinae* is, in Australia, a vector of *Borrelia anserina*, the cause of *spiro-chaetosis* of the fowl. The parasite has been found naturally infected with the viruses of St. Louis encephalitis, Eastern encephalitis and Western encephalitis and consequently it may act as a vector for these infections. *D. gallinae* may occur as a temporary parasite on humans, causing skin lesions.

Diagnosis. The mites can be seen with the unaided eye, especially when they have fed recently on blood and are red. Other causes of anaemia, such as the soft tick, *Argas persicus* and Simuliidae and Cimicidae, should be eliminated.

Control. The nests of the birds should be removed and well-made houses free from crevices should be provided. Harrison (1960) reviews the considerable literature on acaricides used. He obtained good control with 0·25 per cent of Sevin (Carbaryl) applied to the houses and deep-litter houses and perches, repeated after 2–3 weeks. This did not taint the eggs nor affect egg production. Fiedler (1958) found dusts or sprays of malathion the easiest method of control and that BHC sprays are effective for treatment of the premises, but must not be used to treat the birds or their foods. For the treatment of the premises or litter good results have been obtained with 0·5 per cent lindane, 1 or 1·5 per cent DDT or 2 per cent chlordane or 2 per cent malathion dust spread over the litter at the rate of 1 lb. per 20 sq. ft. which has not been found toxic to the birds. Nicotine sulphate painted on the perches may have some fumigant action. Since cage birds are especially susceptible to the chlorinated hydrocarbon insecticides and some of the organophosphorous compounds, they should be avoided or used with great care. Alternatives are synergised pyrethrins or Sevin (Carbaryl) which may be used in the form of aerosol sprays. It should be remembered that the adult mites can live for 4–5 months without a meal of blood.

Genus: Ornithonyssus Sambon, 1928

(Bdellonyssus Fonseca, 1941, Liponyssus)

O. sylviarum (Canestrini & Fanzago, 1877). This species (Fig. 239), often called the northern mite of poultry, is found on the fowl and other birds in temperate climates generally and it has been found in England and in New Zealand. The elongate-oval adult mites are about 1 mm. long. *O. sylviarum* can be distinguished from the other species here described by

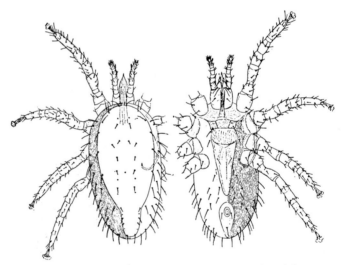

FIG. 239. *Ornithonyssus sylviarum*; left, dorsal view of female; right, ventral view of female (Canestrini & Fanzago)

the shape of its dorsal plate, which is wide for two-thirds of its length and then rather suddenly tapers to form a tongue-like continuation about half as wide for the remainder of its length. The setae on the dorsal plate, like those of *D. gallinae*, are smaller than the setae on the adjacent skin. The ventral plate, like that of *D. gallinae*, bears only two pairs of setae, a third pair being present on the skin immediately behind this plate or almost touching it. The anus, is on the anterior half of the anal plate.

Life-cycle and Habits. Under laboratory conditions, the sticky, whitish eggs are laid largely on the host, one to five eggs being laid after a blood meal. The eggs hatch after 1 day, or earlier, according to the temperature and humidity. They liberate six-legged larvae, which do not feed, but moult after 8–9 days to become the protonymphs, which feed on blood, needing, in the laboratory, two blood meals, and then moult to become, after 1–3 days, the deutonymphs, which do not feed, but moult, after 3–4 days, to become the adults. The whole life-cycle, from the female's blood meal before egg-laying to the adult stage, can occur in 5–7 days, but usually takes longer.

The mites are found on the birds or in their nests or houses and they feed intermittently on the birds, but seldom attack young chickens. They can bite through tender human skin and thus cause pruritus. Heavily infested birds may suffer irritation, loss of weight, reduction of egg production and even, when the loss of blood is great, death. This mite may transmit fowl pox and the viruses of St. Louis encephalitis and Western equine encephalomyelitis have been found in it

Control is difficult. Effective and safe control has been achieved with Sevin dust or emulsion and with dusts of Dow ET-57, Bayer L13/59 or Bayer 21/199 for periods up to 28 days. Harrison (1961) reported excellent control of this mite with a 5 per cent Sevin dust. Good results have been claimed for 4 per cent malathion dust applied to the vents and breasts of the birds or to their litter and nesting boxes and with dusts of 4 per cent nicotine, or 4 per cent malathion, or a mixture of these, which do not, it is claimed, affect the birds or the flavour of their eggs; success is claimed also for a 0·5 per cent emulsion of malathion. Chlordane, toxaphene and lindane have been found toxic to birds.

O. (*Bdellonyssus, Liponyssus*) **bursa** (Berlese, 1888). This species (Fig. 240), often called the tropical fowl mite, is found on the fowl, pigeon, sparrow and other birds in the warmer parts of the world, where some experts think it replaces *O. sylviarum*, with which it has been confused. It will attack man, causing pruritus, but this is temporary, because this species cannot survive for longer than 10 days away from a bird host. It has been found in South Africa, Mauritius, Zanzibar, India, China, Australia, Colombia, Panama and the United States. It can be distinguished from *O. sylviarum* by the shape of its dorsal plate, which gradually tapers to a blunt posterior end, although the setae on this plate are, like those on the dorsal plates of *O. sylviarum* and *D. gallinae*, smaller than those on the adjacent skin. The anus, like that of *O. sylviarum*, is on the anterior half of the anal plate; but in *O. bursa* the ventral plate bears all three pairs of setae, while in *O. sylviarum* and *D. gallinae* only two pairs of these setae are on the ventral plate, the third pair being on the skin behind the plate.

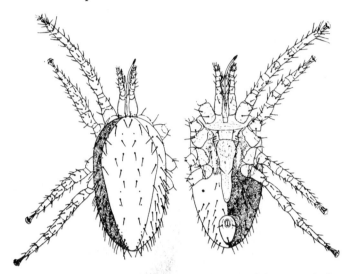

FIG. 240. *Ornithonyssus bursa*: left, dorsal view of female; right, ventral view of female
(Berlese)

Life-cycle and Habits. Baker *et al.* (1956) state that, in the laboratory, the eggs are usually laid in the litter, not on the host, but in birds in the field, large numbers of eggs may be found in the fluff of the feathers, as well as in the nests of the birds. On sparrows most of the life-cycle takes place in the nests and few mites are found on sparrows flying about. On poultry most of the mites are found on the fluff of the feathers, especially on those around the vent, and they tend to be present on few feathers, large numbers of them giving these feathers a dirty appearance. The distribution of the mites on the birds may be patchy, hundreds being found in small areas. The mites are not usually found on the roosts of the birds.

The eggs hatch in about 3 days, liberating six-legged larvae, which do not feed, but moult, after about 17 hours, to become protonymphs, which feed on the host's blood and, after about 1–2 days, moult to become deutonymphs, which also feed on the host's blood and become the adults. More details about the life-cycle are required.

Control. The methods suggested for the control of *O. sylviarum* may be tried.

O. (*Bdellonyssus, Liponyssus*) **bacoti** (Hirst, 1931). This species (Fig. 241), often called the tropical rat mite, is parasitic on rats and man all over the world. The adult female mite is from 650 μ to 1 mm. long. Its dorsal plate is narrower than that of the other species just described and it tapers gradually to a blunt point; on it are numerous setae, which are the same size as those on the adjacent skin. The chelicerae have no teeth and there is a spur on the distal segment of the pedipalp. The sternal plate bears three pairs of setae, the anterior pair being on the anterior margin of this plate, the posterior margin of which is concave. The anus is on the anterior half of the anal plate.

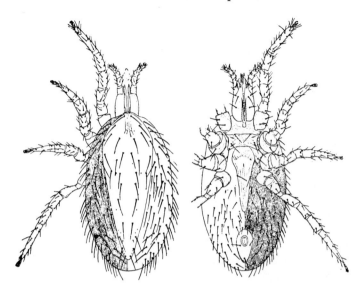

FIG. 241. *Ornithonyssus bacoti*: left, dorsal view of female; right, ventral view of female (Hirst, 1913)

Life-cycle and habits. The eggs are laid in the nests and burrows of the rats, not on the hosts. Baker *et al.* (1956) state that the female mite lays after a blood meal one to two eggs and may lay about ninety-eight eggs during her lifetime, temperature and humidity affecting the egg-laying. The eggs hatch in 1–2 days, liberating six-legged larvae, which do not feed, but moult after 24 hours to become protonymphs, which take a blood meal and moult to become the deutonymphs, which, like the larvae, do not feed, but moult, after 24–36 hours, to become the adults. Under laboratory conditions 75 per cent of the mites became adult in 11–16 days. Unfertilised eggs may develope parthenogenetically to provide males which can fertilise eggs.

It was formerly thought that this species can transmit *Rickettsia typhi*, the cause of endemic murine typhus, but Baker *et al.* (1956) quote literature which indicates that the part played by this species as a vector of this disease is negligible. The same authors state that this species cannot transmit *Pasteurella tularensis*, the cause of tularaemia, by its bites, although it can transmit this organism if mites infected with it are eaten. It has also been shown that *Pasteurella pestis*, the cause of plague, can be experimentally transmitted from rat to rat by the bites of the mites, by eating them or by the injection of infected mites. *O. bacoti* is the intermediate host of the filarial nematode, *Litomosoides carinii* of rodents.

Control. Measures should be taken to control the rats which are the hosts of this mite. Baker *et al.* (1956) report that a 10 per cent DDT dust applied to the runs or burrows of the rats reduces, but does not eliminate, the mites and that a dust containing 8 per cent DDT and 10 per cent sulphur is better. In laboratory animal houses a 10 per cent DDT dust can be applied to rats, but is toxic to mice, for which equal parts of talcum and derris root powder can be tried. The cages of the rats can be steam-sterilised. Malathion, DMC and Aramite have also been suggested. For human dwellings DDT, lindane or chlordane have been recommended.

Allodermanyssus sanguineus (Hirst, 1914). This relatively little-studied mite is called the 'house mouse mite' and occurs on the domestic rat, house mouse and spiny mouse (*Acomys*) in Egypt and the United States. It is generally believed that it may transmit *Rickettsia akari*, the cause of rickettsial pox of man. The mite may be differentiated from the other species just described by its two dorsal plates. The sternal plate bears all three pairs of setae. The life-cycle, which resembles that of the species just described, is completed, according to Baker *et al.* (1956), in 17–23 days.

Control should include control of the mice and the methods suggested for the other mites just described may be tried.

Other gamasid mites are the laelaptid mites among which are **Echinolaelaps echidninus** (Berlese, 1887), the spiny rat mite, which is the definitive host of the haemogregarine protozoon, *Hepatozoon*, of the rat and hamster; and other species parasitic on rodents described by Baker *et al.* (1956), who discuss their possible importance as vectors of diseases of man and other animals. Other interesting genera are *Halarchne* and *Orthohalarachne* parasitic in the respiratory passages of the seal and other Pinnipedia (cf. *Cytodites* below).

Genus: Pneumonyssus Banks, 1901

P. caninum Chandler & Ruhe, 1940. This species lives in the nasal passages and nasal sinuses of the dogs. It has been found in the United States, Hawaii, Australia and South Africa. Dogs of any age, breed or sex may be affected, but the effects are generally not serious and are usually confined to reddening of the mucosae, sneezing, shaking of the head and rubbing of the nose. The mites are oval and pale yellow, and measure 1–1·5 by 0·6–0·9 mm. Their smooth cuticle has scanty setae. The single dorsal plate is irregular in shape; the sternal plate is small and irregular and not well sclerotised; it bears two pairs of setae, the second pair not being on this plate. There are no genital plates and the genital opening is a transverse slit between the fourth coxae. The gnathosoma, visible from above, bears long, slender palps composed of five segments. The short chelicerae are chelate. The long, well-developed legs bear claws. Mature females often contain eggs and it has been said that they give birth to larvae, but little is known about the life history.

P. simicola is a related species parasitic in the bronchi of the rhesus monkey (*Macaca mulatta*). Apart from causing cough and sneezing, its effects seem to be mild, but it has been suggested that it may predispose the monkeys to other respiratory diseases. Its life history is little known and attemps to control it have so far failed.

SUBORDER: IXODOIDEA (IXODIDES)

This suborder contains the hard and soft ticks and is subdivided into two families, the Argasidae, which includes the fowl ticks and tampans, and the Ixodidae, or true ticks.

FAMILY: ARGASIDAE

The integument is leather-like, frequently mammillated, and there is no dorsal shield. In the nymph and imago the capitulum and mouth parts are situated anteriorly on the ventral surface and are not visible from the dorsal aspect. Eyes are absent, or there may be two pairs situated laterally in the supracoxal folds. There is one pair of spiracles situated postero-laterally to the third coxae. Sexual dimorphism not marked.

Genus: Argas Latreille, 1795

A. persicus (Oken, 1818), the 'fowl tick', is a common parasite in many warm and temperate climates, attacking fowls, turkeys, pigeons, ducks, geese, canaries, ostriches and certain wild birds, and it may also bite man. The imago measures 4–10 by 2·5–6 mm. and is oval in shape, narrower anteriorly than posteriorly. The edges of the body are sharp. The engorged tick has a slaty-blue colour, while the starved animal is yellowish-brown with the dark intestine showing through. As in other Argasidae there is little difference between the males and the females; the sexes can be distinguished only by the shape of the genital opening, which is situated anteriorly on the ventral surface and is larger in the female than in the male.

Life-cycle and habits. The eggs are laid in cracks and crevices of the fowl-house and under the bark of trees. They are small, spherical, brown in colour and are laid in batches of 20–100. The larvae hatch after 3 weeks or more; they have six relatively long legs and roughly circular bodies, which become spherical after engorging. The larvae attach themselves to the host, frequently under the wings, and engorge in about 5 days, rarely up to 10 days. They they drop off and hide away, to moult after about 7 days. There are two nymphal stages, each of which lasts about 2 weeks and engorges once during this time. The nymphs and the adults hide away in sheltered spots and attack their hosts at night, feeding for about 2 hours. The adults feed once a month, more or less, and the females lay a batch of eggs after each meal. The larvae can live without food for about 3 months. The nymphs and the adults survive starving for about 5 years.

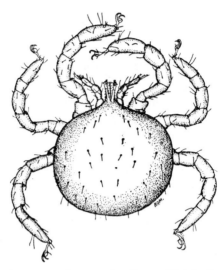

FIG. 242. *Argus persicus*, Larva (Original)

Pathogenesis. The fowl tick worries the birds at night so that they sleep restlessly, and in heavy infections anaemia results from the loss of blood. Egg laying decreases or may stop completely. *A. persicus* causes tick paralysis of ducks and transmits *Anaplasma marginale* in the United States and the poultry piroplasm *Aegyptianella pullorum* in Tunis and South Africa. It is also the vector of *Borrelia anserina*, the cause of fowl spiro-chaetosis; the spirochaete is passed through the egg to the offspring of an infected female tick, and so can be eradicated only with the ticks.

Diagnosis. The parasites will be found in cracks of the woodwork or the walls of the fowl-house.

Control. The classical procedure against fowl ticks in buildings is as follows: The birds must be removed from their run and houses and are placed in wooden crates. The larvae on the birds will drop off within 10 days and the fowls can then be returned to their quarters, which have meanwhile been cleaned. All birds subsequently introduced should be treated in the same way. The crates can be cleaned by scalding with boiling water or spraying with insecticide, or they can be burnt. It is best to burn unsatisfactory buildings, together with all rubbish, loose wood, the bark of trees etc. Metal buildings can be sterilised with a blow-lamp. Wooden structures may be thoroughly sprayed with in-secticide. Sprays of BHC (o·o5 per cent gamma isomer) are better than DDT for killing the larvae and adults. An emulsion containing 1·27 per cent gamma isomer of BHC, applied at the rate of 1·5 ml. per linear foot to roosts, does not taint the eggs or flesh of the birds. Organophosphorus insecticides are also valuable in control.

A. reflexus (Fabricius, 1794) occurs chiefly on pigeons and has been found in Europe, Russia and Algeria. It may transmit *Borrelia anserina* to poultry.

A. mianensis, Brumpt, 1921 the Persian miana bug, possibly transmits human relapsing fever there.

Genus: Otobius Banks, 1912

O. megnini (Dugès, 1883), the 'spinose ear tick', was introduced from America into Africa. Its larval and nymphal stages are most often parasites in the ears of dogs, sheep, horses, and cattle, but are sometimes also found in goats, pigs, cats, ostriches and man, and also on rabbits, deer and other wild animals. The engorged larvae are almost spherical. The nymphs are widest at the middle and their skin is mammillated and bears numerous spine-like processes; body colour is bluish-grey, while the legs, mouth parts and spines are pale yellow. Adults, which are not parasitic, have a constriction at the middle, giving the body a fiddle shape.

Life-cycle and habits. The eggs are laid in sheltered spots such as cracks of poles, under food-boxes or stones, or in crevices of walls. The infection is therefore mainly associated with sheds, yards and kraals, and is hardly ever seen in ranch animals that remain in the open pasture. The larvae hatch in 3–8 weeks and may live without food for 2–4 months. If they find a suitable host, they attach themselves in the ears below the hair-line and engorge in 5–10 days. The larvae suck lymph and, when they are engorged, they are $\frac{1}{8}$ in. long and are usually yellowish-white or pink. Their shape is almost spherical and the legs are relatively small. They moult in the ears, and the spined eight-legged nymphs feed there and remain in the ears for 1–7 months, unless they are accidentally dislodged. The fully-grown, engorged nymph measures $\frac{1}{3}$–$\frac{2}{5}$ in. long. They drop off the host and seek dry, protected places in crevices of buildings, fences and trees, where they moult after a few days to become adults, the skins of which are not spiny. The adults do not feed, but the females lay 500–600 eggs. Oviposition may last for as long as 6 months. When it ends the females die, but unmated females may live longer than a year. The eggs may hatch 10 days after they are laid and the larvae that hatch from them are then ready to feed on a host.

Pathogenesis. Masses of these ticks may be present on the host. They suck blood and cause marked irritation, which results in inflammation. Secondary bacterial infection may extend inwards with serious results. The infected animals appear dull and worried; they do not feed well, lose condition, and dogs especially shake the head and scratch the ears. A waxy or oily exudate from the ear is usually present. The ticks, when they are numerous, can remove much blood.

Diagnosis. Heavy infestations with the ear-canals packed with ticks are readily diagnosed. In other cases the waxy exudate is removed and the ear probed by means of a suitable piece of wire with a small loop at the end, which will assist in dislodging and extracting a few parasites if they cannot be seen by direct inspection.

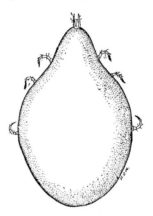

FIG. 243. *Otobius megnini*, Engorged Larva (after Mönnig)

Treatment and prophylaxis. The United States Department of Agriculture (1947) recommends, among other remedies, 1 part of BHC (15 per cent of the gamma isomer), 2 parts of xylol and 17 parts of pine oil, all by weight, which penetrates the ear wax, kills the larvae and protects for 3–4 weeks; or 40 per cent chlordane emulsion 1 part and pine oil 15 parts may be instilled into the ear.

Infected sheds or kraals are most satisfactorily treated by the use of insecticide sprays.

O. lagophilus is similar to the above being found on rabbits in the Western United States.

Genus: Ornithodoros Koch, 1844 (emend Ornithodorus, Agassiz, 1845)

O. moubata Murray, 1877, the eyeless tampan, lives in native huts and in the sand under trees where animals and human beings frequently seek shelter. The female lays batches of about 100 eggs in the sand. The larvae do not hatch, but moult in the egg so that the nymphs hatch out. Several nymphal instars are passed through and the nymphs, like the adults, attack their hosts for short periods only to feed. This tampan sucks blood on man and various domestic and wild animals, including birds and even tortoises. In certain localities, for instance in South-west Africa, this parasite causes much trouble by feeding on sheep at their resting-places in the pasture and it is very difficult to combat it under such conditions. It is the only vector, under natural conditions, of *Borrelia* (*Spirochaeta*) *duttoni*, the cause of African relapsing fever of man. It is also cited as a vector of Q fever and may transmit *Borrelia anserina* and *Aegyptianella pullorum* of the fowl.

O. savignyi Audouin, 1827 is a tampan which possesses eyes. Its habits are similar to those of *O. moubata*, but its larvae hatch from the eggs, though they do not feed. It occurs in Africa, India and the Near East on the camel, fowl and other domesticated animals, but may bite man.

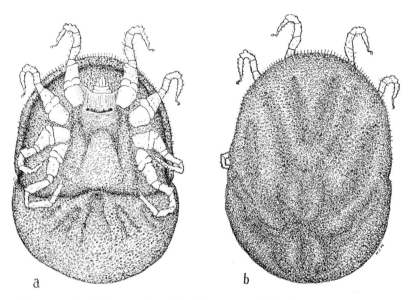

FIG. 244. *Ornithodoros moubata*, Female: *a*, ventral; *b*, dorsal view (Original)

O. turicata (Duges, 1876) occurs in the U.S.A. especially the South-western and Western States. It is referred to as the relapsing fever tick since it is responsible for transmission of that disease to man in the South-west. Neitz (1956) cites this as a vector, together with *O. hermsi*, *O. parkeri*, *O. erraticus* and *O. gurneyi*, of *Coxiella burnetii*, the cause of Q fever. He also cites *O. lahorensis* as a vector to goats of *Theileria ovis* and *Anaplasma ovis* and as a cause of tick paralysis of sheep in Central Asia.

O. talaje (Guérin-Méneville, 1845) is found in the South-western States of the U.S.A. and in Florida.

FAMILY: IXODIDAE

Ticks of this family possess a hard, chitinous shield or scutum which extends over the whole dorsal surface of the male and covers only a small portion behind the head in the larva, nymph and female. The mouth parts are anterior and well visible from the dorsal aspect. Eyes when present consist of one pair situated on the lateral margin of the scutum. The imago has one pair of spiracles situated postero-laterally to the fourth coxae.

The basis capituli or capitulum, which is inserted into the body anteriorly and carries the mouth parts and palps, shows two dorsal porose areas in the female. The scutum has bilateral cervical and lateral grooves, varying in depth and length in different species. The body of the female may have a pair of lateral 'marginal grooves' behind the scutum, while

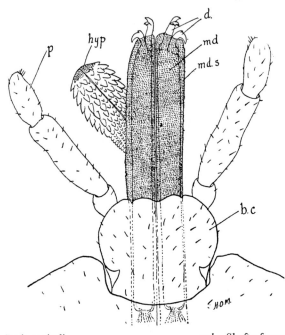

b.c. Basis capituli	*md.* Shaft of mandible
d. Digits of mandible	*md.s.* Mandibular sheath
hyp. Hypostome, twisted to show it sventral surface	*p.* Palp.

FIG. 245. *Amblyomma hebraeum*, Anterior End, Dorsal View (Original)

postero-lateral and median grooves are usually present on the dorsum in both sexes. The posterior border of the body is frequently notched, forming the 'festoons', which are generally eleven in number. The genital opening is a ventral transverse slit in front of the middle, the anus being posterior. The male may have ventral plates. *Ornate ticks* have coloured, enamel-like areas on the body, *inornate ticks* have not.

Bionomics. The *Ixodidae* lay their eggs in sheltered spots: under stones and clods of soil or in crevices of walls and cracks of wood near the ground. The eggs are small, spherical, yellowish-brown to dark brown in colour and are laid in large masses. The female lays all her eggs in one batch, numbering up to 18,000 in some species, and then dies. The whole process of development to the adult stage is greatly influenced by the prevailing temperature, cold weather causing marked prolongation of the different stages, especially hatching of the eggs and the pre-oviposition period of the engorged female.

The newly hatched larvae or 'seed ticks' (Plate XVII) climb on to grass and shrubs and wait there till a suitable host passes, to which they attach themselves with their claws. Lees & Milne (1951) described this and the other habits of *Ixodes ricinus* in detail. After having engorged, the larva moults and becomes a nymph. The integument of the latter requires a few days to harden, and then the nymph engorges and moults, to become an imago. After hardening of the integument, and often also after copulation, which may take place on the ground or, more usually, on the host, the female engorges, drops off and seeks a sheltered spot to lay. The males remain much longer on the host than the females, in some cases 4 months or even longer, and consequently they accumulate on the host. Although it is not definitely known whether the males of all species feed on the host, many of them certainly do so for a few days and then go in search of females. If no males are present on the host, the females may remain attached for much longer periods than under normal conditions.

According to the number of hosts they require during their life-cycle, ticks can be classed in three groups:

1. *One-host ticks*. All three instars engorge on the same animal, the two ecdyses also taking place on the host—e.g. *Boophilus decoloratus, B. annulatus*.

2. *Two-host ticks*. The larva engorges and moults on the host and the nymph drops off after also having engorged; it moults on the ground and the imago seeks a new host—e.g. *Rhipicephalus evertsi, R. bursa*.

3. *Three-host ticks*. These require a different host for every instar; they drop off each time after having engorged and moult on the ground. Examples are *Ixodes ricinus, Rhipicephalus appendiculatus* and most other ticks.

Each species of tick is adapted to certain ranges of temperature and moisture, some occurring only in warm regions with a fair degree of humidity, while others are winter ticks most active in a dry climate. They suck blood and sometimes lymph and are in general not very specific with regard to hosts, although some species, or certain instars of a species, show a particular preference for certain host species, or there may be a definite adaptation to certain hosts. When a tick attaches itself to feed, it buries its mouth parts deeply into the tissues of the host and remains attached until it is engorged. If it should be detached before engorgement is complete, it will rarely feed again in the same instar.

The following key to the genera of *Ixodidae* is adapted from Bedford (1932):

1. Anal grooves surrounding the anus anteriorly (Prostriata). *Ixodes.*
   Anal grooves surrounding the anus posteriorly (Metastriata) (in *Boophilus* and *Margaropus* the anal groove is faint or obsolete) 2
2. Hypostome and palpi short 3
   Hypostome and palpi long 8
3. Eyes absent . . . . *Haemaphysalis*
   Eyes present 4

4. Festoons present 5
   Festoons absent 7
5. Males with coxae IV much larger than coxae I to III; no plates or
   shields on ventral surface of male 6
   Males with coxae IV not larger than coxae I to III, a pair of adanal
   shields and usually a pair of accessory adanal shields on ventral surface of the male. Species usually inornate; basis capituli generally
   hexagonal dorsally . . . . *Rhipicephalus*
6. Species ornate; basis capituli rectangular dorsally . . *Dermacentor*
   Species inornate; basis capituli hexagonal dorsally with prominent
   later angles. Coxae IV of male with two long spines . . . . .
   Rhipicentor
7. Inornate; coxae I with a small spine. Male with median plate projecting backwards on either side of the anus and with a caudal protrusion when engorged. Fourth pair of legs of male dilated . .
   Margaropus
   Inornate; coxae I bifid. Male with a pair of adanal and accessory
   shields and a caudal protrusion. Fourth pair of legs normal
   Boophilus
8. Eyes present 9
   Eyes absent or rudimentary. Species occurring almost exclusively on
   reptilia . . . . *Aponomma*
9. Festoons absent or present. Males with a pair of adanal shields and
   two posterior abdominal protrusions. Accessory adanal shields absent
   or present . . . . *Hyalomma*
   Species usually ornate; festoons present. Male without adanal shields,
   but small plaques may be present on the venter near the festoons .
   Amblyomma

Various species of Ixodidae are vectors and reservoirs of important
viral, rickettsial and protozoan parasites of man and other animals.
The protozoal diseases are discussed in the section on Protozoology. A
general consideration of ticks and disease is given by Arthur (1962).

Genus: Ixodes Latreille, 1795

The anal groove surrounds the anus anteriorly. Palpi long. Inornate. Eyes and festoons absent. Ventral surface of male armed with
pregenital, median, anal, epimeral, and adanal shields, the latter two
being paired. Stigmatic plates oval in male, circular in female.

I. ricinus (Linné, 1746), the 'castor-bean tick', is common in Europe,
and occurs also in some other countries. It is frequently found on dogs,
but also occurs on other domestic and wild mammals, while nymphs
and larvae have been recorded from lizards and birds. The tarsi taper
away to their ends and are not humped. The postero-internal angle of
coxa I bears a spine which is long enough to overlap coxa II. The

following data on the life-cycle of the parasite are compiled from various authors:

Pre-oviposition period	7–22 days
Oviposition lasts	About 30 days
Eggs hatch (depending on temperature) . .	2–36 weeks
Larvae engorge	2–6 days
Larvae moult (depending on temperature) . .	4–51 weeks
Nymphs engorge	3–7 days
Nymphs moult (depending on temperature) .	8–28 weeks
Females engorge	5–14 days
Unfed larvae survive	13–19 months
Unfed nymphs survive	24 months
Unfed adults survive	21–27 months, extreme 31 months

Campbell (1953), Lees & Milne (1951) and others have shown that in Britain the life history of *I. ricinus* extends over 3 years, the larval stage lasting through the first year, the nymphal stage through the second year, and the adult stage through the third year. In Northumberland and Southern Scotland each of these phases feeds only in the spring (March–June) and these ticks are called spring-feeders. In Cumberland, Wales, Ireland and Western England and Scotland there are, however, not only spring-feeders but others that feed chiefly in the autumn (August–November). Spring-feeders can be turned in the laboratory into autumn-feeders by raising the temperature to quicken the development, but they then remain autumn-feeders. Wood *et al.* (1960) state that, in Britain, *Ixodes ricinus* is usually found attached to the face, ears, axillae and to the inguinal region where the hair is short or the skin bare, that is to say, to parts of the body constantly brushed by vegetation on which the ticks are waiting.

I. ricinus transmits redwater of cattle caused by *Babesia divergens* and *Babesia bovis*, which pass through the egg of the tick, *Anaplasma marginale*, and the viruses of louping ill and Rickettsial 'tick-borne fever' of sheep. In Britain this species is associated with the spread of pyaemia caused by *Staphylococcus aureus*, which especially affects lambs 2–6 weeks old. Neitz (1956) cites the tick as a cause of tick paralysis in Crete, of Czechoslovakian encephalitis and Russian spring–summer encephalitis and of *Coxiella burnetii* in Germany. It also transmits Bukhovinian haemorrhagic fever.

I. persulcatus (Schulze, 1930) is a Eurasian form and transmits several species of *Babesia*.

I. hexagonus Leach, 1815, sometimes called the hedgehog tick, is found on the hedgehog, dog, otter, ferret and weasel in Britain. The tarsi are humped and the postero-internal angle of coxa I bears a sping that is not long enough to overlap coxa II.

I. canisuga Johnston, 1849, often called the British dog tick, has been iound on the dog, sheep, horse and mole. It may be very numerous in dog-kennels and possibly is a parasite of the fox. Its tarsi are humped, but there is no spine on coxa I.

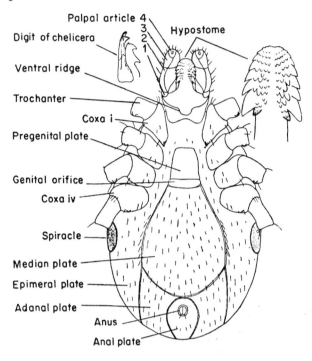

FIG. 246. *Ixodes pilosus*, Ventral Surface of Male (after Bedford)

I. pilosus (Koch, 1844), the russet or sourveld or bush tick, occurs, according to Theiler (1950), at most seasons in most areas of South Africa. It is not, as is often stated, a winter tick and, although it has been accused of causing tick paralysis and has therefore been called the paralysis tick, it does not cause paralysis and statements that it does are probably due to wrong identification. Its hosts are cattle, sheep, goats, horses, dogs, cats and wild ungulates.

The life-cycle may be summarised as follows:

Pre-oviposition and incubation period (summer) . 43–93 days
Pre-oviposition and incubation period (winter) . . 222–309 days
Larvae engorge . . . . 2¾ days or longer
Larvae moult (summer) . . . . 27 days
Nymphs engorge . . . . 4 days
Nymphs moult (autumn) . . . . 52 days
Females engorge (males present) . . . . . . 5–6 days

I. rubicundus Neumann, 1904 is the paralysis tick of South Africa. Theiler (1950) described its distribution there. It is confined to the moister areas of the Karrooveld which are hilly or mountainous. It is active in that country from April–May till July and only exceptionally in the summer. Stampa & du Toit (1958) discussed its biology and life history. The chief hosts of the adults are domesticated sheep, goats and cattle. Other hosts are wild Artiodactyla, Carnivora and Lagomorpha. The immature stages feed on the red hare, elephant shrew, bush hare and wild Canidae (e.g. the red jackal and dog), but it is never found on the cat or horse or on birds.

Life-history. This requires 2 years. The engorged females lay eggs for 6 weeks from the end of August to early September. The eggs are susceptible to dry heat and do not hatch at humidities below 70 per cent; all of them hatch at humidities between 80 and 100 per cent. The larvae are active from March to mid-August, with a peak of activity in April–May, when the peak incidence of the tick paralysis also occurs. After 73–149 days the larvae moult, after feeding, to become nymphs, which are active from July to November, with a peak of activity in September–October. They moult 6 months after engorgement. The adults feed for 4–7 days, attaching on the radial aspects of the legs from the knee or fetlock downwards and on the ventral parts of the host's body. On sheep they prefer woolled to bare areas. The adults are active from February to mid-November of the second year of the cycle, with a peak of activity in April–May, when the tick paralysis also occurs. At high altitudes the ticks are more active in August.

Treatment and Control. Stampa & du Toit (1958) found that, because these ticks attach to the legs and undersides of the bodies of their hosts, shallow dips, through which the hosts were made to walk, gave good control, but they should be repeated every 4–6 weeks. Any small numbers left probably maintain themselves on the hare. The dip should be some 26 in. deep and may contain an insecticide standing 18 in. deep. Removal of the ticks is, in some instances, though not in all, followed by recovery from tick paralysis caused by them.

I. holocyclus Neumann, 1899 is the paralysis tick of Australia. It is a coastal species confined to bush and scrub country. It occurs along the northern and east coast of New South Wales and Queensland and in Victoria and Tasmania. It occurs on man, dogs, cats, other domestic animals and the long-nosed bandicoot, the opossum and spiny anteater. Its brown legs and long, prominent mouth parts distinguish it from *Boophilus*. Seddon (1951) describes its life history. It is very susceptible to variations in temperature and humidity. The female lays 2000–3000 eggs and each instar engorges normally in 4–7 days.

This species transmits *Coxiella burnetii* in Australia. Seddon (1951) describes the paralysis caused by the adult females, of which one may suffice, or, rarely, by large numbers of nymphs. The paralysis is mainly of importance in dogs. It usually begins towards the end of the fourth or the beginning of the fifth day after attachment of the ticks. If there are many ticks on a small pup, signs may appear at the beginning of the fourth day. There is a rapidly progressing motor paralysis affecting first the hind-quarters and then the forelegs, the muscles of the head and neck and the respiratory muscles. Vomition may be marked. Initially there may be a fever, but soon the temperature drops to subnormal. Death appears to be due to respiratory paralysis.

Recovered animals are temporarily immune and dogs can be hyperimmunised by frequently allowing ticks to engorge on them. The serum of such dogs has a highly curative value and is the only effective remedy. Preventive measures consist of weekly applications of derris dust or washes, a bath or spray containing BHC and DDT given weekly and frequent examination of dogs and the removal of ticks.

I. scapularis Say, 1821 is the 'shoulder tick' or 'black legged tick' occurring on cattle, sheep, horses and dogs and cats in North America. It occurs in the South Atlantic, South Central, Southern North Central and North Atlantic States. It may be responsible for the transmission of anaplasmosis in some areas.

I. cookei Packard, 1867 occurs on cattle in California and Oregon, horses in Massachusetts, and on dogs and cats in the South Eastern and North Eastern States of the U.S.A. and in South Eastern Canada.

I. pacificus Cooley & Kohls, 1945, the 'California black legged tick', occurs on cattle, sheep, horses and dogs and cats in California, Oregon, Utah and British Columbia.

Several other species of the genus *Ixodes* occur in North America and these include:

I. angustus (Oregon, Washington; dogs), **I. kingi**, (the 'rotund tick', Idaho, Montana, Dakotas, Wyoming, Utah and Ontario; dogs), **I. muris** (the 'mouse tick', Maine; dog), **I. rugosus** (California, Oregon, Washington; dog), **I. sculptus** (Oregon, Wisconsin; dog) and **I. texanus** (Iowa, British Columbia; dog).

Genus: Boophilus Curtice, 1891

Anal groove obsolete in female, faint in male and surrounding the anus posteriorly. Inornate. Eyes present. Festoons absent. Palps and hypostome short; palps with prominent transverse ridges. Coxa I bifid. Spiracles circular or oval. Males small, provided with adanal or accessory shields and a caudal process; fourth pair of legs of ordinary size.

B. annulatus (Say, 1821), the 'North American cattle tick', is native to North America. It occurs usually on domestic and wild ungulates, but has also been found on other animals and man.

Various authors give the following data on the life-cycle:

Pre-oviposition period . . . . 3–25 days
Oviposition lasts . . . . 14–59 days
Larvae hatch . . . . 23–159 days
Parasitic period on host . . . . 15–55 days
Unfed larvae survive up to 8 months

This species, like other members of the genus, is therefore a one-host tick. At one time *B. annulatus* was extensively distributed in the Southern part of the U.S.A. being of considerable importance since it was responsible for the spread of *Babesia bigemina* infection, or Texas cattle fever. A campaign started in 1906 has resulted in the eradication of the tick from the U.S.A.

B. decoloratus (Koch, 1844), the 'blue tick', is a one-host species which occurs throughout the Ethiopian region, especially in humid areas. It is parasitic chiefly on cattle and equines, but is also found on sheep and goats, wild ungulates and dogs. The engorged females have a slaty-blue colour and pale yellow legs.

The female lays up to 2500 eggs, which hatch in 3–6 weeks under favourable conditions. This is a one-host tick, requiring 22 days (summer) to 38 days (winter) for its development on the host. Unfed larvae survive up to 7 months.

This species transmits *B. bigemina* and possibly *B. bovis* also, *Anaplasma marginale* of cattle, spirochaetosis (*Borrelia theileri*) of cattle, horses, goats and sheep, and *Babesia trautmanni* of pigs in East Africa. In all instances the infection passes through the eggs of the tick.

Control can be effected by dipping at intervals of 14–21 days, and regular dipping of all animals for about 9 months should exterminate the tick.

B. microplus (Canestrini, 1887) (syn. *B. australis* Fuller, 1899) the Tropical cattle tick, occurs in Australia, West Indies, Mexico, Central America, South America, Asia and South Africa. According to Neitz (1956) it transmits *Babesia bigemina* in Australia, Panama and South America, *B. argentina* in Australia and the Argentine, *Anaplasma marginale* in Australia and South America, *Coxiella burnetii* in Australia and *Borrelia theileri* in Brazil.

B. calcaratus (Birula, 1895) transmits, according to Neitz (1956), *Babesia bigemina* and *B. berbera* in North Africa and *Anaplasma marginale* in the northern Caucasus.

Genus: Margaropus Karsch, 1879

This genus, of which *Boophilus* is regarded as a synonym by some authors, differs from the latter genus in that the males are large, their fourth pair of legs is markedly thickened, and they have a median ventral plate which is prolonged into two spines projecting on either side of the anus; coxa I has a small posterior spine.

M. winthemi Karsch, 1879, the 'Argentine tick', is a native of South America which has also been introduced into South Africa. It is a parasite of horses and sometimes occurs also on cattle. The engorged female resembles that of *B. decoloratus*, but has dark bands at the joints of the legs.

This is a one-host tick which is especially prevalent in winter. It is not known to transmit any disease.

Genus: Hyalomma Koch, 1844

Inornate, sometimes ornate. Eyes present. Festoons present or absent. Hypostome and palps long. Male with a pair of adanal shields and sometimes accessory adanal shields; frequently a pair of chitinous protrusions behind the adanal shields. Spiracles comma-shaped in male, triangular in female. The pathogenic agents transmitted by various stages of the species of *Hyalomma* are: *Babesia caballi*, *B. equi*, *Theileria parva*, *T. annulata*, *T. dispar*, *Coxiella burnetii*, *Rickettsia bovis*, *R. conori* and the causes of haemorrhagic fevers in Russia. Neitz (1956) listed the parasites transmitted by the various species.

There is much confusion in the literature regarding the species of the genus *Hyalomma* and further information about it may be obtained from Feldman-Musham (1954) and Hoogstraal (1956). Rousselot (1953) and Kaiser & Hoogstraal (1964) have divided the genus into three subgenera viz.: *Hyalomma*, *Hyalommina* and *Hyalommosta*. Keys are given for these in both publications and full descriptions of species are given by Kaiser & Hoogstraal (1964).

Arthur (1966) has renamed or synonymised various species of the genus as follows:

H. plumbeum plumbeum (= *H. marginatum*) in Southern Europe, the Southern U.S.S.R. and also in the Nile Delta; **H. excavatum** (= *H. anatolicum*) in Egypt, Israel, Greece, Asia Minor and extending east through Southern U.S.S.R. to India; **H. detritum scupense** (= *H. volgense*, *H. uralense*) in Transcaucasia. Other species are **H. dromedarii** in North Africa, **H. impressum** near **planum** in East Africa and **H. detritum mauretanicum** in North Africa.

Hyalomma spp. are usually two host ticks, though three hosts may be used in some species. A general life-cycle is detailed below:

Pre-oviposition period	4–12 days
Oviposition lasts	37–59 days
Larvae hatch	34–66 days
Larvae engorge	5–7 days
Larvae moult	2–15 days
Nymphae engorge	7–10 days
Nymphae moult	14–95 days
Larvae and nymphae on host	13–45 days
Females engorge	5–6 days
Unfed larvae survive	12 months
Unfed nymphae survive	3 months
Unfed adults survive	14 months or longer

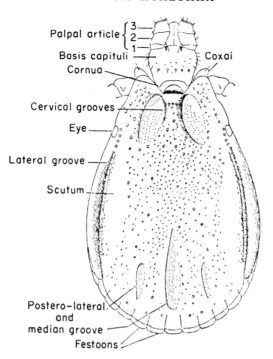

Palpal article { 3 2 1

Basis capituli

Cornua

Coxai

Cervical grooves

Eye

Lateral groove

Scutum

Postero-lateral and median groove

Festoons

FIG. 247. *Rhipicephalus appendiculatus*, Dorsal View of Male (after Bedford)

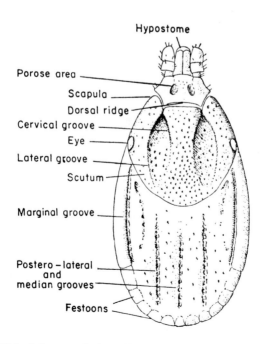

Hypostome

Porose area

Scapula

Dorsal ridge

Cervical groove

Eye

Lateral groove

Scutum

Marginal groove

Postero-lateral and median grooves

Festoons

FIG. 248. *Rhipicephalus appendiculatus*, Dorsal View of Female (after Bedford)

Genus: Rhipicephalus Koch, 1844

Usually inornate. Eyes and festoons present. Hypostome and palpi short. Basis capituli hexagonal dorsally. Coxae I with two strong spurs. Males with adanal and usually also accessory adanal shields; frequently with a caudal prolongation when engorged. Spiracles comma-shaped, short in the female and long in the male. This genus contains a large number of species which are difficult to differentiate and are important vectors of infectious diseases.

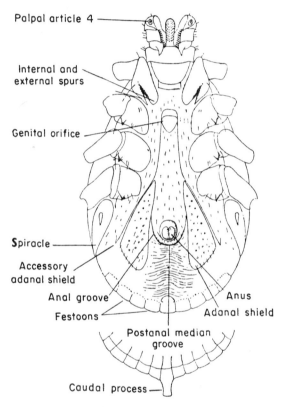

FIG. 249. *Rhipicephalus appendiculatus*, Ventral View of Male (after Bedford)

R. appendiculatus Neumann, 1901, the 'brown ear tick', is widely distributed in Africa south of the equator. It is absent from West Africa. It is parasitic on cattle, equines, sheep, goats, wild antelopes, and has also been found on the dog and wild rodents.

This is a three-host tick. The female lays about 3000–5000 eggs.

Pre-oviposition period . . . . 5–40 days
Eggs hatch (summer) . . . . 28 days
Eggs hatch (winter) . . . . 3 months
Larvae engorge . . . . 3–7 days
Larvae moult . . . . 10–49 days

Nymphs engorge	3–7 days
Nymphs moult	10–61 days
Females engorge	4–10 days
Unfed larvae survive	7 months
Unfed nymphs survive	6½ months
Unfed adults survive	14 months, sometimes longer and exceptionally over 2 years

This species occurs in a relatively warm climate only. It attaches most frequently under the tail and in the ears, but may also be found on other parts of the body. This tick is the chief vector of East Coast fever (*Theileria parva*) of cattle. It also transmits *Hepatozoon canis* and exanthematic fever of dogs, *Theileria mutans* and *Babesia bigemina* of cattle, and *Rickettsia conori* and the viruses of Nairobi sheep disease and louping-ill. In none of these cases, except *B. bigemina*, does the infection pass through the egg of the tick.

R. capensis and **R. simus**, both three-host ticks, transmit East Coast fever (*T. parva*), and the last-mentioned also transmits *Anaplasma marginale*.

R. neavei, R. jeanelli and **R. ayrei** transmit *T. parva* in Africa.

R. sanguineus (Latreille, 1806), the 'brown dog tick', which was probably a native tick of Africa originally, has a more or less cosmopolitan distribution. It is mainly parasitic on dogs and is frequently associated with kennels, but has also been found on various other animals.

This is a three-host tick. The female lays 2000–3900 eggs.

Eggs hatch	17–30 days or longer
Larvae engorge	2–4 (–6) days
Larvae moult	5–23 days
Nymphs engorge	4–9 days
Nymphs moult	11–73 days
Females engorge	6–21 days
Unfed larvae survive	Up to 8½ months
Unfed nymphs survive	Up to 6 months
Unfed adults survive	Up to 19 months

This tick transmits canine piroplasmosis or biliary fever, the infection passing through the egg of the tick. There is some confusion in the literature as to the protozoa, rickettsiae, bacteria and viruses that this species can transmit. It seems clear, however, that it transmits *Babesia canis* of dogs, *B. vogeli, B. equi* and *B. caballii* of equines, *Anaplasma marginale* in North America, *Hepatozoon canis* of dogs, *Coxiella burnetii, Rickettsia conori, R. canis, R. rickettsii, Pasteurella tularensis, Borrelia hispanica* and the viruses that cause Nairobi sheep disease and other viral diseases of sheep in Africa. For further information see Neitz (1956), Zumpt (1958) and Arthur (1962). It also causes tick paralysis of the dog. It has been incriminated as a vector of *B. bigemina, B. equi* and *Theileria annulata*.

R. evertsi Neumann, 1897, the 'red-legged tick', is common in

Africa south of the equator and occurs on many species of domestic and wild mammals. This tick was found in 1960 in game farms in Florida and New York. It was eradicated from the U.S.A. in 1962. This species can be distinguished from other members of the genus by its red legs; the shield is black and densely pitted and in the male it leaves a red margin of the body uncovered. This is a two-host tick; the larval and nymphal stages engorge on the same host.

Pre-oviposition period	6–24 days
Eggs hatch	4–10 weeks
Larvae and nymphs on host	10–15 days
Nymphs moult	42–56 days
Females engorge	6–10 days
Unfed larvae survive	7 months
Unfed adults survive	14 months

The larvae and nymphs are usually found in the ears or the inguinal region, the adults mainly under the tail.

This species transmits East Coast fever (*T. parva*), redwater (*B. bigemina*) and *T. mutans* of cattle, *Borrelia theileri* to various animals, and biliary fever (*Babesia equi*) of horses and *R. conori*. In the case of redwater and spirochaetosis, the infections pass through the egg of the tick.

R. bursa Canestrini & Fanzago, 1878 is widely distributed in Southern Europe, Africa and elsewhere, and transmits *Babesia ovis*, *B. equi*, *B. caballi*, *B. berbera*, *Theileria ovis*, *Anaplasma marginale*, *Rickettsia ovina*, *Coxiella burnetii* and the virus of Nairobi sheep disease.

Genus: Haemaphysalis Koch, 1844

Inornate. Eyes absent. Festoons present. Palps usually short and conical, the second articles having conspicuous lateral projections. The trochanter of the first pair of legs bears a dorsal process. Spiracles in female ovoid or comma-shaped; in males ovoid. Ventral surface of male without chitinous plates. Species usually of small size. A large number of species occur in this genus and further information may be obtained from Hoogstraal (1956).

H. leachi leachi (Audouin, 1826), the 'dog tick', occurs in Africa, Asia and Australia. It is mainly parasitic on domestic and wild carnivora, frequently also on small rodents and rarely on cattle. This is a three-host tick. The female lays about 5000 eggs.

Pre-oviposition period	3–7 days
Eggs hatch (20°C)	26–37 days
Larvae engorge	2–7 days
Larvae moult	about 30 days
Nymphs engorge	2–7 days
Nymphs moult	10–16 days
Females engorge	8–16 days
Unfed larvae survive	6 months or longer

Unfed nymphs survive . . . . 2 months or longer
Unfed adults survive . . . . 7 months or longer

The tick lives on the head and body of its host and transmits canine piroplasmosis (*B. canis*), the infection being passed transovarianly, and tick-bite fever (*Rickettsia conori*) and *Coxiella burnetii*.

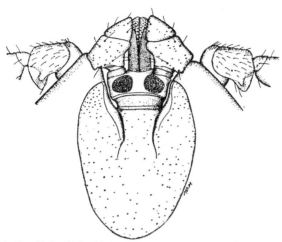

FIG. 250. *Haemaphysalis leachi leachi*, Anterior End of Female, Dorsal View (Original)

H. cinnabarina punctata Canestrini & Fanzago, 1878 occurs in Europe, Japan and North Africa.

While the adults parasitise cattle and other mammals, the larvae and nymphs are also found on reptiles (lizards and snakes). In Europe this species has been found on sheep, goats, deer, cattle, horses, rabbits, hedgehogs, the bat *Plecotus auritus* and on the partridge, missel-thrush and curlew. In Asia it has been found on the wolf and bear.

The female lays 3000–5000 eggs
Pre-oviposition period . . . . 10 days to 7 months
Oviposition lasts . . . . 24–29 days
Larvae hatch (14°C) . . . . 38–82 days
Larvae engorge . . . . 4–19 days
Larvae moult . . . . 14–238 days (winter)
Nymphs engorge . . . . 4–33 days
Nymphs moult . . . . 7–295 days (winter)
Females engorge . . . . 6–30 days
Unfed larvae survive . . . . 10 months
Unfed nymphs survive . . . . $8\frac{1}{2}$ months
Unfed adults survive . . . . $8\frac{1}{4}$ months

This species transmits *Babesia bigemina*, *B. motasi* and *Anaplasma marginale* and *A. centrale* and causes paralysis of sheep and cattle.

H. leporis-palustris Packard, 1867, the 'rabbit tick', is widely distributed in the United States, from Massachusetts to California and it also occurs in South America. It transmits Q fever (*Coxiella burnetii*),

Rocky Mountain spotted fever and tularemia (*Pasteurella tularensis*) to man. The infection passes through the egg of the tick.

H. cinnabarina Koch, 1844 (syn. *H. chordeilis* Packard) the 'bird tick' occurs in North and South America and is stated to attack poultry occasionally. It transmits tularemia. Deaths in turkeys and wild game birds have been ascribed to heavy infestations with this tick.

H. humerosa Warburton & Nuttall, 1909 transmits Q fever (*Coxiella burnetii*).

H. bispinosa Neumann, 1897 is the New Zealand cattle tick or bush tick. It has a wide distribution throughout the East occurring in India, Burma, Malaysia, China, Japan, Australia, New Zealand and is also present in East Africa. In Australia it occurs in south-east Queensland and Northern Coastal areas of New South Wales.

It occurs on man, cattle, sheep, horse and dog, wild mammals and birds.

Pre-oviposition	10–60 days
Oviposition	20–30 days
Incubation	37–90 days
Larval engorgement	3–9 days
Larval moult	19–22 days
Nymphal engorgement	5–7 days
Nymphal moult	23–97 days
Female engorgement	7 days

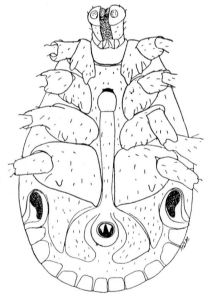

FIG. 251. *Dermacentor rhinocerotis*, Male Ventral View (Original)

It is a three-host tick, but males are scarce and parthenogenesis has been observed in this species. Unfed larvae may survive up to 217 days, unfed nymphs 263 days and unfed females 249 days.

Heavy infestation may be seen in cattle and at times dogs, horses and sheep may be severely parasitised. *H. bispinosa* is a vector of *Babesia gibsoni* of dogs in India and of *Coxiella burnetii* (Q fever).

Other species of *Haemaphysalis* include: **H. bancrofti** ('Wallaby tick'; Queensland; marsupials, cattle), **H. inermis** (Central Europe); and **H. parmata** (antelope, various carnivors; Africa).

Genus: Dermacentor Koch, 1844

Usually ornate. Eyes and festoons present. Hypostome and palps short. Coxa I bifid and coxa IV of male much larger than coxae I to III. No plates on ventral surface of male.

D. reticulatus (Fabricius, 1794) (syn. *D. marginatus*) occurs mainly in Asia and Southern Europe. It is parasitic on many domestic and wild mammals.

Larvae hatch	2–3 weeks
Larvae engorge	2 days or more
Larvae moult	about 2 weeks
Nymphs engorge	several days
Nymphs moult	2–3 weeks

This is a three-host tick which transmits *Babesia caballi, B. equi* and *B. canis*, the infection passing through the egg of the tick.

D. venustus Banks, 1908 (syn. *D. andersoni*, Stiles, 1905, the Rocky Mountain wood tick, is the vector of Rocky Mountain spotted fever and occurs in the United States between the Cascade and the Rocky Mountains. The larvae and nymphs occur on practically all available small mammals, especially rodents, while the adults suck blood mainly on horses and cattle, also on other large mammals and man. It is a three-host tick.

The females lay about 4000 eggs	
Pre-oviposition period	7–41 days
Oviposition lasts	about 30 days
Eggs hatch	15–51 days
Larvae engorge	3–8 days
Larvae moult	6–21 days
Nymphs engorge	3–9 days
Nymphs moult	over 3 weeks
Females engorge	8–14 days
Unfed larvae survive	21–117 days
Unfed nymphs survive	300 days or longer
Unfed adults survive	413 days

This tick transmits Rocky Mountain spotted fever and tularemia (*Pasteurella tularensis*) to man, as well as equine encephalomyelitis (western type). In all cases the infection passes through the egg of the tick. It also transmits *Anaplasma marginale, Babesia canis, Coxiella burnetii* and *Leptospira pomona* and causes paralysis in man, cattle, sheep and the dog. In such cases of paralysis the ticks are usually found attached along the back of the neck near the vertebral column. The clinical signs develop in the course of about a week after attachment of the tick; there is a progressive paresis of the limbs and usually incontinence of urine at the height of the disease.

D. variabilis (Say, 1821), the 'American dog tick', which is common on dogs in the United States, transmits Rocky Mountain spotted fever and St. Louis encephalitis. This species also transmits *Anaplasma marginale* of the cattle and tularemia to man and causes tick paralysis of dogs in North America. The larvae and nymphae feed on wild rodents, especially the 'short-tailed meadow mouse', *Microtus* spp. This is a three-host tick.

The females lay 4000–6000 eggs

Pre-oviposition period	3–58 days
Oviposition lasts	14–32 days
Eggs hatch	20–57 days
Larvae engorge	2–13 days
Larvae moult	6–247 days
Nymphs engorge	3–12 days
Nymphs moult	16–291 days
Females engorge	5–27 days
Unfed larvae survive	14–540 days
Unfed nymphs survive	29–584 days
Unfed adults survive	up to 1053 days

The seasonal incidence of the adults varies in different parts of the United States, but in general they are most numerous in the spring and early summer; in the south they are found throughout the year and breed slowly through the winter. In colder areas all stages may survive through the winter, except the eggs, which usually hatch before winter comes. The larvae and nymphs are found on mice and other small mammals throughout the winter.

Control. Climatic factors, especially dryness, are probably the most important means of natural control, but *D. variabilis* is very resistant to cold. Many are destroyed by poultry, wild birds and mice. The effects of *Hunterellus hookeri*, a parasite of *D. variabilis*, need investigation. Otherwise control is difficult. Correlated with the fact that the larvae and nymphs feed on field mice and small rodents is the fact that this tick tends to congregate alongside roads, tracks etc. For this reason strips of land 20–30 ft. wide on each side of the road and tracks are sprayed with a mixture of 0·05 per cent DDT, 2·5 per cent pine oil and 97 per cent water. The mice should be controlled, undergrowth and grass should be kept cut and human beings should wear protective clothing when they traverse infected areas.

D. nitens Neumann, 1897 is the 'tropical horse tick' of Mexico, Central and South America, the Caribbean and also occurs in Florida in the U.S.A. Equines are the preferred hosts though the tick may also occur on sheep, cattle and deer. The preferred site of attachment is the ear though in heavy infections any part of the body may be infested. *D. nitens* is a one-host tick.

The females lay 2000–5000 eggs

Pre-oviposition period	3–15 days
Oviposition lasts	15–37 days
Eggs hatch	19–39 days
Larvae engorge and moult	8–16 days
Nymphs engorge and moult	7–29 days
Females engorge	9–23 days
Unfed larvae survive	71–117 days

D. nitens is a vector of equine piroplasmosis. Suppuration of the ears may occur in heavy infections.

D. albipictus (Packard, 1869) is the 'winter tick' or 'moose tick' occurring in the Northern part of the U.S.A. from Maine to Oregon and through the Western states to Texas. It is common in Canada. The preferred host is the moose but it also occurs on elk, horse, cattle, antelope, bear, deer, beaver, bighorn sheep, coyote, mountain goat and mountain sheep. It is most numerous in upland and mountain country. It is a one-host tick.

The females lay 1500–4400 eggs

Pre-oviposition period	7–180 days
Oviposition lasts	19–42 days
Eggs hatch	33–71 days
Larvae engorge and moult	9–20 days
Nymphs engorge and moult	10–76 days
Females engorge	8–30 days
Unfed larvae survive	50–346 days

Heavy infestation may occur in the long winter coat of animals during autumn and winter, causing debility, anaemia and at times death of horses and moose especially when there are food shortages. *D. albipictus* is a vector of *Klebsiella paralytica*, the cause of paralysis in moose, of anaplasmosis and possibly also of Rocky Mountain spotted fever.

D. occidentalis (Marx, 1897), the 'Pacific Coast tick'. It is found in the area between the Sierra Nevada Mountains and the Pacific Ocean from Oregon to Southern California. Adult ticks occur on deer and also cattle, horse, donkey, rabbit, sheep and man while the immature forms occur on a variety of rodents. *D. occidentalis* is a three-host tick. It is a vector of anaplasmosis, Colorado tick fever, possibly Q fever and tularaemia.

D. nigrolineatus (Packard, 1869), the 'brown winter tick' is closely related to *D. albipictus* and some authors consider it to be a variety of the latter species. It is widely distributed in the Eastern U.S.A. The preferred host is the white-tailed deer but it also occurs on horses and cattle. It is a one-host tick.

Other species of the genus include: **D. marginatus** (Asia, Central Europe); **D. nuttalli** (Asia; transmits Siberian tick typhus); **D. silvarum**

(Soviet Union; transmits Siberian tick typhus), and **D. halli** (North America).

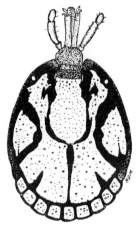

Fig. 252. *Amblyomma hebraeum*, Male, Dorsal View, not showing the Legs (Original).

Genus: Rhipicentor Nuttall & Warburton, 1908

This genus closely resembles *Dermacentor*, but differs from it especially in the following points: it is inornate, the basis capituli is hexagonal dorsally and has prominent lateral angles, and coxa IV in the male bears two long spurs. There are several species, none of which are known to transmit any disease.

Genus: Amblyomma Koch, 1844

Usually ornate. Eyes and festoons present. Hypostome and palpi long. Male without ventral plates, but small chitinous plaques may be present close to the festoons. The species are usually large and broad.

A. hebraeum Koch, 1844, the 'bont tick', occurs frequently in the warmer parts of South and Central Africa and is parasitic on all domestic and many wild mammals; the young stages also attack birds. This is a three-host tick.

The female lays up to 20,000 eggs

Pre-ovipositon period	6–26 days
Larvae hatch	4–13 weeks
Larvae engorge	4–7 (–20) days
Larvae moult	25–66 days
Nymphs engorge	4–20 days
Nymphs moult	21 days to 3 months
Adults engorge	10–20 days
Unfed larve survive	7 months
Unfed nymphs survive	6 months
Unfed adults survive	7–20 months

The tick attaches usually in the perineal and genital regions of its host and may produce bad wounds. Zumpt (1958) says that the larvae and nymphs feed on birds, which may carry them over long distances. The species transmits *Rickettsia ruminantium*, the cause of heartwater of cattle, sheep and goats, which is also transmitted by **A. pomposum** in South Africa and in Kenya by **A. gemma**. *A. hebraeum* also transmits *Rickettsia canori* of tick-bite fever. It is very resistant to dipping, especially the adult stage.

A. variegatum (Fabricius, 1794), the 'variegated tick', is an African species. It feeds on many species of mammals and rarely on birds, and transmits heartwater, Nairobi sheep disease and *Coxiella burnetii*.

A. americanum (Linnaeus, 1758). This is the 'lone star tick' occurring in the U.S.A. from Texas and Missouri eastwards to the Atlantic Coast. It is given the name because of a single large white spot on the scutum of the female. It has a wide range of hosts and although larvae and nymphs occur on the same hosts as the adults, larger populations of the larval stages are found on foxes and smaller mammals. The ear is the favoured site of attachment but in heavy infestations the head, belly and flanks are also parasitised. It is a three-host tick.

The female lays 1000–8000 eggs

Pre-oviposition period	5–13 days
Larvae hatch	23–117 days
Larvae engorge	3–9 days
Larvae moult	8–26 days
Nymphs engorge	3–8 days
Nymphs moult	13–46 days
Adults engorge	9–24 days
Unfed larvae survive	48–279 days
Unfed nymphs survive	3–476 days
Unfed adults survive	393–430 days

Apart from the painful bites caused by this tick it transmits Q fever, Rocky Mountain spotted fever and tularaemia. It is associated with tick paralysis in the Eastern and Southern U.S.A.

A. cajennense (Fabricius, 1787), the 'cayenne tick' occurs in Southern Texas in the U.S.A. but is widespread in Mexico, South and Central America and the Caribbean. The horse is chiefly parasitised but other hosts are a wide range of wild animals. It is a three-host tick with a developmental cycle similar to that of *A. americanum*.

This species transmits spotted fever in South America and *Leptospira pomona*.

A. maculatum (Koch, 1844). This is the 'Gulf Coast tick' occurring in areas of high temperature and humidity on the Atlantic and Gulf of Mexico seaboards of North America. Larvae and nymphs occur mainly on ground-inhabiting birds (e.g. larks) and also occur on rodents. Adults are found on cattle and also horse, sheep, dog and man. It is a three-host tick.

The female lays 4500–18,000 eggs

Pre-oviposition period	3–9 days
Larvae hatch	21–142 days
Larvae engorge	25–100 days
Larvae moult	7–121 days
Nymphs engorge	4–11 days
Nymphs moult	17–71 days
Adults engorge	5–18 days
Unfed larvae survive	up to 179 days
Unfed adults survive	up to 411 days

This species is not known to transmit disease but it causes severe bites and painful swellings and is also associated with tick paralysis.

Genus: Aponomma Neumann, 1899

Eyes vestigial or absent, otherwise resembles *Amblyomma*. The species of this genus occur almost exclusively on reptiles.

TICKS AS PARASITES

Ticks may harm their hosts by: (a) injuries done by their bites, which may predispose the hosts to attacks by blowflies, screw-worm flies and biting flies generally; (b) sucking blood; (c) transmitting the viruses, rickettsiae, bacteria and protozoa mentioned above.

The harm done by their bites and blood-sucking has been reduced by control measures taken to control the diseases transmitted by ticks, but these two forms of harm are themselves important, especially in warm climates. The various stages of the ticks may be very numerous on some hosts. Estimates of the amount of blood removed vary according to the species under consideration. It has been estimated that a single adult female will remove 0·5–2·0 ml. of blood and thus where an animal carries several thousand ticks a substantial blood loss may occur. Such theoretical figures may not apply under natural conditions, for example 20,000 adult *Boophilus* failed to kill a steer whereas 500 did kill a calf (Barnett, 1961). Heavy infections of *Dermacentor albipictus* may kill moose and horses especially during winter when food supplies are low.

Though the very heavy infestations mentioned above do occur in nature the more usual is for animals to carry a few hundred ticks. These produce a less tangible effect generally known as 'tick worry'. This is probably a combination of several entities including irritation from the tick bites, local skin infection, blood loss, and secondary attack by flies. Systematic control of ticks almost always results in improved weight gains and yields from animals as well as making them look sleeker.

The secondary effects of tick attack are infection of the local area, producing suppurative lesions (e.g. of the ears, legs etc.) and in lambs the local infection may become pyaemic (e.g. tick pyaemia in lambs in Great Britain). Attacks by blowflies and screw-worm flies are much encouraged by ticks.

A further effect is the damage produced to hides.

Tick paralysis. This condition is caused by the injection of a 'toxin' by certain developmental stages of ticks, chiefly the adult female, but sometimes by the nymphs. Ticks of the genus *Ixodes* are particularly associated with the condition but other genera, especially *Dermacentor* (*D. venustus = andersoni*) are concerned and it has also been ascribed to infestations with *Ornithodorus lahorensis* (Mihailov, 1957) and *Argus persicus*.

Tick paralysis is a motor paralysis which begins at the extremities, especially the hind legs, and gradually ascends affecting ultimately the whole body, but respiration is not affected until just before death, which may occur 1–4 days after the onset of the clinical signs. In general the degree of paralysis is proportional to the length of time the tick has been feeding and frequently also on the number of ticks attached. Removal of the ticks is usually followed by recovery provided the heart and respiratory centres have not been affected.

In some instances paralysis seems to be produced only by ticks when they are attached near the head or along the spinal column (e.g. *D. venustus = andersoni*), however this situation is the preferred feeding site for this tick and with other species (e.g. *I. ricinus, I. rubicundus, I. holocyclus*) the preferred feeding sites are the axillae, udder and along the belly. Consequently local injury to underlying nervous tissue does not explain tick paralysis.

Tick paralysis is mostly caused by engorging females but the nature of the 'toxin' produced is obscure. It appears to be elaborated in the tick concomitantly with egg production and it has been suggested that the toxin accumulates in the ovaries and passes to the salivary glands in the late stages of engorgement. Toxin, apparently identical with that injected by the engorging tick, has been obtained from the eggs of ticks which induce tick paralysis, however a similar substance can also be obtained from the eggs of ticks which are not usually associated with tick paralysis (e.g. *Rhipicephalus evertsi, Boophilus decoloratus, Haemaphysalis leachi* etc.) and consequently there is some doubt that the effective toxin is produced in the ovaries. It would seem rather that the toxin is produced in the salivary glands and some support for this comes from observations that engorging larvae of *I. holocyclus* can induce paralysis (Arthur, 1962). Furthermore, unmated females of *D. venustus* (*= andersoni*) readily produce paralysis (Gregson, 1958). Gregson (1959) also found that 4–6 days of engorgement were required to produce paralysis with *D. venustus*, but when ticks were transferred from paralysed animals to normal animals signs of paralysis appeared in 12–18 hours. Martin (personal communication) has observed that three different types of glandular acini occur in the salivary glands of female ticks, one of which has the same morphological structure as the poison glands of snakes: it is possible that the toxin is produced in these. Such acini are present in ticks which have fed for several days.

The 'toxin' apparently causes a neuromuscular block. Conduction is normal in the motor nerves and muscles respond normally to direct stimulation (Rose & Gregson, 1956; Murnaghan, 1958). However degenerative changes have been observed in the spinal cord and the medulla of paralysed animals. In some cases capillary haemorrhages are present around nerve cells and in the adventitia sheath, such being accompanied by infiltrations of mononuclear cells (Arthur, 1962).

Animals that recover from tick paralysis develop an immunity to the 'toxin' and in the absence of further infestation, may remain refractory to tick paralysis for 8 weeks to 8 months, the longer period being seen with *I. holocyclus*. Such immunity however, should not be confused with that directed against the engorgement of the tick in which a marked local cellular reaction at the site of attachment interferes with engorgement and prevents full repletion. Serum from animals exposed to ticks may be used for curative purposes (see *I. holocyclus*).

Eleven ixodid ticks and one argasid tick have been associated with tick paralysis in mammals, while in poultry *Argas persicus* has been recognised as a cause of the condition. A large number of hosts are affected including cattle, sheep, goats, pigs, dogs, various wild ruminants and man. Experimentally the groundhog (*Marmota flaviventris avara*), the hamster and, to a lesser extent, the guinea-pig are susceptible to paralysis. The species which are particularly associated with paralysis are *I. holocyctus*, especially in dogs in Australia, *I. rubicundus*, the cause of Karoo paralysis in South Africa and *D. venustus* (= *andersoni*) which causes paralysis in cattle, deer and man in the north-western United States and western Canada. In the eastern and southern United States, *D. variabilis*, *A. maculatum* and *A. americanum* are implicated (Wilkinson, 1965). In Western and Central Europe *Haemaphysalis inernis*, *H. punctata* and *I. crenalatus* are responsible.

Another disease caused by tick 'toxins' is sweating sickness of South, Central and East Africa. It also has been reported from India and Ceylon. This affects cattle, sheep, goats and pigs and is at its highest incidence during the summer months. The tick chiefly concerned is *Hyalomma transiens* (= *truncatum*) though other species (e.g. *H. rufipes rufipes* and *H. rufipes glabrum*) have been incriminated. The adult stage of the tick is responsible for donating the 'toxin' to the animals. Neitz (1959) has stated that ticks reared for many generations on unsusceptible animals still retain the ability to transmit the toxin.

Treatment and control of tick infection. Although ticks are in themselves important parasites, and should be combated for this reason, control measures are, as a rule, directed against the diseases of which the ticks are the vectors, and are therefore based on the epizootiology of these diseases as well as on the habits of the ticks. Barnett (1961) summarised the conclusions of an international Committee appointed by the Food and Agricultural Organisation and the Organisation Internationale des Epizootiques to consider the harm done by ticks and their control.

Because ticks attach to various parts of the bodies of animals, treatment has to be applied to the whole body and is usually carried out by dipping the animals in a suitable tank containing the dip in an aqueous solution, suspension or emulsion; however spray races, showers etc. are replacing conventional plunge dips since they are labour-saving and economical. These modern forms of apparatus drain the dipping fluid and filter it after it has been sprayed on the animals and return it for use again. The various dipping baths and sprays which are available for various animals are discussed in detail by Barnett (1961), who should also be consulted for the other considerations on tick control.

The various stages of ticks may stay on their hosts for only a few days during each year and are often on the hosts only at certain times of the year. Dipping for control of ticks is therefore planned with knowledge of the biology of each species of tick, the duration of each of its stages and of its feeding times and the duration of the whole life history. An important consideration is whether the tick is a one-host tick, all the stages of which feed on the same individual host, a two-host species, which uses one individual host for the larvae and nymphs and another for the adult, or a three-host tick, each stage of which requires a separate individual host. The one-host tick is obviously much easier to control than the others. Acaricides act differently on the different stages of the life history. Thus Hitchcock (1953), combating the one-host tick *Boophilus microplus* in Australia, found that the adults of a strain of this were resistant to BHC, but that the larvae were not and were killed by 500 p.p.m. of BHC; and in South Africa it was found that adults of a strain of *Boophilus decoloratus* were resistant to toxaphene, while the larvae were killed by dipping every 7 days with 0·25 per cent of toxaphene and that this gave excellent control of this strain.

Barnett (1961) gives an extensive account of the acaricides which may be used for tick control. A few years ago control was achieved by the use of the chlorinated hydrocarbon insecticides (e.g. DDT, BHC, toxaphene etc.), toxaphene having been used extensively against all species of ticks. It has a very good residual effect. With the increased interest in insecticide residues in meat and the development of resistance of *Boophilus* spp. to the chlorinated hydrocarbon insecticides a greater emphasis was placed on the organophosphorus and carbamate insecticides. Several of these are available and are discussed by Barnett (1961). Where *Boophilus* spp. have become resistant to all three groups of insecticides it may be necessary to resort to arsenic dips, in some cases, however, the resistance is limited to the adult stage of the tick and an increased frequency of dipping, even with the insecticide to which the adults are resistant, may still result in control.

The acaricides of choice are detailed by Barnett (1961) as follows.

Acaricide	Short interval treatment (5–7 days)	Long interval treatment (2–5 weeks)	Single treatment
Arsenic	0·16	0·175–0·2	—
Asuntol (Co-Ral, Bayer 21/199, Coumafos)	0·03	0·06	0·75
BHC (gamma isomer)	0·025–0·035	0·035–0·05	0·05
DDT	0·25	0·5	—
Delnav (Dioxathion)	0·05	0·1	0·15
Diazinon	0·05	0·1	0·15
Dieldren	0·05	0·1	—
Toxaphene	0·25	0·5	0·5

All figures given as percentage concentrations.

Apart from the control measures just described, there are other measures which have a more limited value; they are useful more especially against two- and three-host ticks, which spend relatively long periods of their lives off the host and on the pastures. These methods are:

Burning of pastures. This may kill large numbers of the larvae and other stages, especially if it is correlated with the times of the year when these stages may be expected to be off the hosts.

Cultivation of land. This undoubtedly tends to reduce tick life by controlling the movements of domestic and wild animals, as well as by creating conditions unsuitable for ticks, as, for instance, exposure of eggs to sunlight, or burying them deeply by ploughing. Good drainage helps to reduce the humidity on which the ticks depend. Another practice found effective in Australia, to which the term 'pasture-spelling' has been given, works on the principle of removing cattle from pastures infected with ticks for long enough to ensure that most, if not all, of the larval ticks on the pastures are killed off by starvation or climatic effects. Rotational grazing systems are devised to apply this method of control and considerable control has been obtained by it, only one dipping with DDT being then found necessary, instead of dippings every 7 weeks.

Starvation. In general this method is not practicable, because ticks live for long periods without food and wild animals may serve as hosts.

Repellents may be useful in certain circumstances, the most effective ones being indalone, dimethyl phthalate and Rutgers 612.

Natural enemies. Certain small hymenopterous parasites of ticks, for instance species of *Ixodiphagus* and *Hunterellus*, are known and have been studied. They parasitise especially the nymphs, in which they lay their eggs, and which are literally 'eaten out' by the larvae of the parasite. Certain ants as well as birds (*Bubulcus ibis*, *Buphagus erythrorhynchus*, *B. africanus*) destroy a large number of ticks. Specific diseases of the parasites are also known. It is, however, questionable whether biological control by means of parasites and other agents would be able to diminish the number of ticks to a point below which they are no longer important as disease transmitters. It is, for instance, frequently difficult to find a *Rhipicephalus* on cattle which have for some months been regularly dipped in an East Coast fever area, and yet the few remaining ticks may still be sufficient to cause cases of the disease.

Infected buildings, such as stables, kennels and homes or railway trucks and ships, may be cleaned of ticks by thorough fumigation with cyanide. Where such treatment is not possible, all litter should be removed and the buildings should be sprayed with a suitable preparation of DDT, BHC or pyrethrins, or one of the organophosphorus compounds.

SUBORDER: TROMBIDIFORMES

FAMILY: TROMBICULIDAE

This family contains the mites, whose parasitic larvae are called 'harvest mites', 'chigger mites', and various other names. The term 'chigger' is, however, also given to the flea, *Tunga penetrans*. Trombiculidae usually have a scarlet, red, orange or yellow colour and the adults may be very large. The nymphs and adults are free-living and feed either on invertebrates or plants. Their bodies are covered with dense hairs which give them a velvety appearance. Their bodies are divided into a gnathosoma, a propodosoma bearing the first two pairs of legs, and a hysterosoma which bears the third and fourth pairs of legs. The last segment of the large pedipalps opposes a claw on the last segment but one, much as a finger and thumb do. Much the same features define the family Trombidiidae, in which family some authorities include the Trombiculidae. The larvae are parasitic on various animals and man, causing marked irritation, and in some cases they transmit important diseases. The larval mites occur most frequently in autumn and attack grazing animals and human beings working in low-lying fields. The natural hosts of the larvae are in most cases small rodents, such as field-mice. The larval mites attach themselves to the host and their salivary secretion hydrolyses the cuticle of the host, forming a tube called the *stylostome*, through which the larva sucks up the host's tissue fluids. When they are ready to moult they drop off and moult to become the non-parasitic nymphal stage.

Trombicula (*Neotrombicula*) **autumnalis** (Shaw, 1790). The larvae of this and other species of this genus attack man and practically all species of domestic animals, including poultry. The latter may be killed by heavy infections. The larger animals are usually attacked on the head and sometimes the neck. The larvae of this species may cause generalised pruritus and lesions in the interdigital spaces of the dog, and they may be the cause of 'heel-bug' of racehorses. The adults live in the soil and in Britain the parasitic larvae are most numerous in the late summer and autumn. They are commonest on chalky soils and on grassland, corn-fields, heathland and scrubby wood-land; they are less common on clay soils. The unfed larvae are about 0·21 mm. long and have a deep red colour; when they are full-fed, they are 0·4 mm. long and have a pale pink or yellow colour.

T. akamushi (Brumpt, 1910) found in Japan and New Guinea, T. delhiensis Walch, 1922 which extends from India to China and Australia, and possibly other species of this genus and also possibly species of Euschöngastia, may be vectors of Rickettsia tsutsugamushi, the cause of scrub or mite typhus (tsutsugamushi disease, Japanese river fever) of man. For further information about these and other related species which transmit Korean fever and other diseases, see Baker et al. (1956).

Control. For area control of the species which transmit scrub-typhus, the WHO (1958) recommend the application to the infested ground of 2 lb. per acre of toxaphene or chlordane or ½ lb. per acre of lindane as a spray or dust. DDT is relatively ineffective.

As a repellent benzyl benzoate may be applied to the clothes, especially to openings in them, either by hand or as a spray, or the repellent may be dissolved in a dry cleaning fluid, or in acetone or a soapy solution, or the clothes may be impregnated with one of these; it remains in the clothes after one or two washes.

T. sarcina is the cause of blacksoil itch (leg itch) of sheep in Queens-land.

This species occurs in areas in Australia which have the true black earths (not 'black soils'), the normal hosts being the kangaroo and wallaroo. The golden-yellow larvae feed on dogs, especially between the toes, and also attack man and sheep and sometimes the horse.

Pathogenesis. The irritation due to the larvae causes stamping and the skin of the coronet, heels and pasterns becomes reddened and abraded. Secondary infection may lead to swelling, thickening of the skin and scab formation and in severe infections similar lesions on the legs may swell to twice their normal thickness. The lesions have a repulsive odour.

Treatment. Dressings of kerosene in oil have been used but a foot-bath of 0·1 per cent BHC is more satisfactory.

Lime-sulphur solutions kill, but do not eradicate, the larvae and DDT has not been successful. Possibly some of the organophosphorus com-pounds would be effective. Dibutyl phthalate may be tried as a repellent. Baker et al. (1956) describe T. minor, the scrub-itch mite of Queens-land, which attacks man and rats; and other related species, among which is Acomatacarus australensis, which attacks man and dogs in Queensland and New South Wales, for the control of which BHC and dibutyl phthalate are suggested.

T. alfreddugési is the common red bug of the United States, though it ranges from Canada to South America and the West Indies and has different local names in different countries. Its larvae are commonest on the borders of forests and in swamps. It attacks many mammals, birds, reptiles and Amphibia and also man. On man the larvae attach themselves on parts of the body constricted by clothing and the lesions produced may be like those due to *Sarcoptes scabiei*. Baker *et al.* (1956) describe this and related species, among which are **T. spendens** and **T. batatas,** which attack man and other hosts in North and South America and Australia.

Neoschöngastia americana (Hirst) attacks fowls in the southern United States, Mexico, Guatemala and Jamaica and a related variety occurs in Japan and the islands of the Pacific. These attack chickens, quail and turkeys and may cause skin lesions which affect the market value of the birds. For further information about these and related mites, see Baker *et al.* (1956).

Diagnosis. This is done by finding the reddish to yellowish larvae in scrapings taken from the lesions.

FAMILY: PEDICULOIDIDAE

Pediculoides ventricosus (Newport, 1850), the 'grain itch mite', is frequently found as a parasite on insects or their young stages that live in grain or straw. From such infected grain the mites may pass on to human beings or domestic animals, which they attack, causing a dermatitis known as 'grain itch'.

Treatment and Prophylaxis. The mites on animals can be killed by an application of a suitable dip or disinfectant. Symptomatic treatment to relieve itching may be necessary; for this purpose benzyl benzoate ointment is recommended. When grain and straw are examined before use to determine their suitability, the possible presence of these mites should be remembered. Infected material is best destroyed by burning.

FAMILY: DEMODICIDAE

Genus: Demodex Owen, 1843

This is a very specialised group of parasitic mites which live in the hair follicles and sebaceous glands of various mammals, causing demodectic or follicular mange. The parasites which occur on different species of hosts are usually regarded as distinct species, although it is difficult to distinguish between them morphologically, since the main difference is that of size. Most of the species are called after their hosts; for instance, *D. canis*, *D. ovis*, *D. caprae*, *D. bovis*, *D. muscardini* of the dormouse, *D. criceti* of the hamster etc., while *D. folliculorum* occurs on man and *D. phylloides* on the pig.

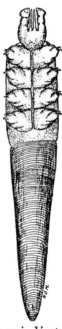

FIG. 253. *Demodex canis*, Ventral View (Original)

The parasites are elongate, usually about 0·25 mm. long, and they have a head, a thorax which bears four pairs of stumpy legs, and an elongate abdomen which is transversely striated on the dorsal and ventral surfaces. The mouth parts consist of paired palps and chelicerae and an unpaired hypostome. The penis protrudes on the dorsal side of the male thorax and the vulva is ventral in the female. The eggs are spindle-shaped.

Life-cycle. This is not well known. The mites develop in the skin of the host where they live. The larva has three pairs of legs and there are apparently three nymphal stages.

The parasites are fairly resistant, being able to survive for several days off the host in moist surroundings. Under experimental conditions the mites lived up to 21 days in pieces of skin that were kept moist and cool.

Infection is transmitted by direct contact or by mechanical means. Artificial infection is rarely successful, probably because the condition of the host is a strong factor in determining susceptibility. In the case of dogs predisposing factors are youth, short hair, poor condition, debilitating diseases—particularly distemper—and possibly too frequent washing of animals with a tender skin, especially if an alkaline soap is used. The parasites can be recovered from the healthy skin, especially that of older dogs, and some authors think that *Demodex* is a very prevalent parasite and occurs in practically all dogs, but produces mange only when the general health and condition are markedly affected.

Pathogenesis. The mites enter the hair follicles and sebaceous glands, producing a chronic inflammation with proliferation and thickening of the epidermis and loss of hair. A secondary bacterial invasion, usually by *Staphylococci*, frequently takes place and leads to the formation of pustules or abscesses. The infection may be spread by wandering of the parasites, contact of different parts of the body or wrong treatment. Death is due to toxaemia or emaciation.

Clinical signs. Two forms of the disease are usually recognised. In the *squamous* or scaly form there is loss of hair, thickening and wrinkling of the skin, which becomes scaly and is usually reddened, later becoming bluish-green or acquiring a coppery-red colour. The *pustular* form is due to bacterial infection and is usually preceded by the scaly form; pustules a few millimetres in diameter develop, or large abscesses may form, and necrotic foci are sometimes seen. Itching is less severe.

In the dog both forms are seen; pustules frequently form on the abdomen, the insides of the legs, the face, the elbows and the feet.

In the pig large abscesses usually develop. In cattle the rump, neck and shoulders are mainly affected with hard, crusty thickenings of the skin, and abscesses may sometimes be seen. In goats the pustular form is the most common. In sheep the disease is rare and usually the scaly form develops. In horses both forms occur. Cats, like dogs, usually develop lesions on the head, but they are rarely affected.

Diagnosis. The mites can be found in deep scrapings and in the contents of pustules and abscesses.

Treatment. This is often difficult and requires much care and patience. Turk (1959) regards rotenone as the remedy of choice. This is applied in oil (e.g. olive oil), at about a 2 per cent concentration, which is applied by massage of the affected parts every 4–5 days for several weeks. This represents one of the legion of remedies for demodectic mange, which can be extremely intractable. The most satisfactory treatment at present appears to be repeated systemic and topical applications of the systemic organophosphorus compounds such as fenchlorphos ('Ectoral') and trichlorphon. Another treatment, recommended by Koutz (1955), consists of an emulsion containing 20 per cent benzyl benzoate and 0·25 per cent BHC. Fiedler & du Toit (1955) claimed that the *delta* isomer of BHC will cure even severe infestations, but this finding needs further investigation.

FAMILY: CHEYLETIDAE

Genus: Psorergates Tyrrell, 1883

The genus is classified by Baker *et al.* (1956) in this family, but Till (1960) places it in a family called the Psorergatidae.

P. ovis Womersley, 1941. This species is a parasite of the skin of sheep and has been found in Australia, Tasmania, New Zealand, and in the

U.S.A. in Ohio, California and New Mexico. The mites are very small, the female measuring only 189 by 162 μ and the male only 167 by 116 μ. The body is almost spherical, with sides slightly indented between the legs, which are radially arranged and have paired claws. The femur of

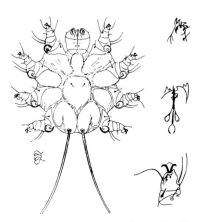

FIG. 254. Left: *Psorergates simplex*, (Tyrell) female; right: *Psorergates ovis* (Womersley, 1941), palps, chelicera and tarsus 1. (Courtesy of Baker *et al.* (1956) and the National Pest Association, New York).

each leg bears relatively long setae and, on the ventral side, a large, curved spine directed inwards. The chelicerae are very small stylets and the pedipalps are short and conical. There is a single dorsal plate. The female has, on the ventral side, near the posterior end, two pairs of long setae which arise from two lobes. The male has only one pair of ventral setae near the posterior end, which arise from a median lobe. The penis is on the anterior half of the dorsal surface of the body. The spherical eggs are 48 μ in diameter.

Life-cycle and habits. Womersley (1941) described the larva, proto-nymph, deutonymph and adults, but little more is known of the life-cycle. The mites live in the surface layers of the skin and have so far been found in fine-wooled Merino sheep and also in Polwarths, Corriedales, Come-backs and Border Leicesters. They cause a mild, but chronic, irritation which leads to occasional biting and scratching, so that the wool is disturbed in affected areas, showing a pale tip or even tufts which have been pulled out. The wool growing on affected areas becomes thready, forming pointed tufts. It contains dry scabs and breaks easily. The general appearance is that of a louse-infested sheep. The skin is hardly altered except that it is covered with dry scales. Microscopically there is a hyperkeratosis and marked desquamation; the deeper layers show round-cell infiltration and sometimes eosinophilia in the immediate vicinity of a parasite. The mites apparently do not penetrate into the skin. The in-fection spreads very slowly over the body, requiring some 3–4 years to become generalised.

Diagnosis. Scrapings are taken after moistening the skin with a light mineral oil and directly examined in the oil.

Treatment. The mite is not controlled by the conventional preparations of BHC (which rely on the gamma isomer) and South African workers have suggested that its increase in that country may be due to wide use of DDT and BHC instead of the sulphur dips.

Lime–sulphur dips are the most satisfactory, using a concentration of 1 per cent of polysulphide sulphur. The addition of a wetting agent is required to insure good penetration of the fleece. Fiedler & du Toit (1955) assessed various preparations from the treatment of the mite and found the delta and epsilon isomers of BHC, Bayer L 13/199 and malathion gave promising results. A single dipping with 0·1 per cent delta isomer BHC or 0·2 per cent malathion cured infestations (see Skerman *et al.*, 1960).

P. simplex Tyrrell. This closely-related species has been found in pustules on the skin of *Mus musculus* in Canada. It has also been found in the multimammate rat (*Rattus natalensis*) used in laboratories in South Africa.

P. oettlei was found by Till (1960) on *Rattus natalensis*.

P. bos Johnston, 1964 is a recently discovered itch mite of cattle in New Mexico and Texas, U.S.A. Roberts & Meleney (1965) believe the mite to be a widely distributed parasite of cattle in the U.S.A. but because of its small size and lack of any marked pathogenic effect it has, hitherto, been undetected. Mites may occur on apparently normal skin and itching or scratching are not features of the infection. In one animal alopecia and desquamation occurred along the sides of the neck, but there appears to be no constant recognisable lesion associated with the infection.

Genus: Syringophilus Heller, 1880

S. bipectinatus (Heller, 1880) may be found inside the quills of the feathers of the fowl, **S. columbae** (Hirst, 1920) inside the quills of the feathers of the pigeon, and **S. (Cheyletoides) uncinata** (Heller, 1880) inside the quills of the feathers of the peacock. These mites have elongated bodies adapted to their life inside the quills of the feathers. Hughes (1959) states that species of this genus found inside the quills of the flight feathers of geese and 'similar birds' may prey on the mite *Syringobia*, although they probably also feed on the material inside the quills.

Genus: Cheyletiella Canestrini, 1886

C. parasitivorax (Mégnin, 1878), the rabbit fur mite, has been found on the fur of rabbits and cats, and Hart & Malone (1958) found it on four dogs in England. Since then it has been found on several occasions on dogs, being associated with a dry scaly dermatitis. The infection may also occur on humans in contact with infected dogs, the lesions consisting of a mild dermatitis to a more extensive papular eruption.

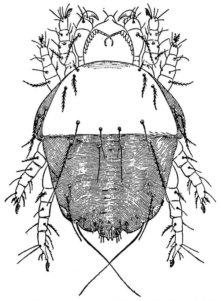

FIG. 255. *Cheyletiella parasitovorax* (Mégnin); Dorsal View of Female

The mites measure 386 by 266 μ and are readily recognised under the microscope by the numerous feathered bristles and the 'combs' on the tarsi.

Satisfactory control is achieved with derris washes or dusts, DDT, BHC or the organophosphorus compounds.

FAMILY: MYOBIIDAE

The small- or medium-sized mites of this family are related to the Cheyletidae and *Psorergates ovis* has been classified with them. They have a striated, unarmoured skin. Baker *et al.* (1956) describe species found on rats and state that these can cause a mild dermatitis.

Genus: Myobia v. Heyden, 1826

M. musculi may be found on laboratory and other mice being associated with loss of hair and dermatitis. It can be controlled with sulphur rubbed into the skin of the mice, though this may cause dermatitis; or by frequent application of a 1 per cent lindane dust, though this does not kill the eggs of the mites. Chlordane may be tried.

Genus: Sarcopterinus Railliet, 1893

S. (*Harpirhynchus*) **nidulans** lives in the feather follicles of various birds. Hughes (1959) states that *S. pilirostris* may be found in the skin on the head of the sparrow.

SUBORDER: SARCOPTIFORMES

This group includes a large number of species which are mostly free living and small in size. A few species are important parasites or vectors of disease. The legs are frequently grouped in two pairs on either side in the nymph and adult and they end in suckers, claws or hairs. Some species, in unfavourable environment, produce nymphs adapted to resist adverse conditions. They are called *hypopial nymphs* or *hypopi* and are often provided with groups of suckers and hooks on their legs which they can use to adhere to transport hosts which carry them to more favourable situations. The most important species of the suborder are those that cause mange. These species belong to the families *Sarcoptidae* and *Psoroptidae*, whose distinguishing features are summarised as follows:

FAMILY: SARCOPTIDAE

1. *Genera:* (a) *Sarcoptes*, species of which cause scabies of man and sarcoptic mange of sheep, goats, cattle, pigs, equines, dogs, foxes, rabbits and other animals. (b) *Notoedres*, species of which cause notoedric mange of cats, rabbits and rats. (c) *Cnemidocoptes*, species of which cause scaly leg (*C. mutans*) and depluming itch (*C. gallinae*) of poultry.

2. Species of this family burrow more or less deeply into the substance of the skin, causing marked thickening of the skin, rather than the formation of scabs.

3. The body of the mite is globose.

4. The striae of the skin are often interrupted by scaly or spinose areas. Species of the genera *Sarcoptes* and *Notoedres* have dorsal dentate spines with sharp points, which are larger in *Sarcoptes* than in *Notoedres*. They are absent from species of the genus *Cnemidocoptes*, which are further distinguished by the presence of two long bristles on the posterior margin of the abdomen.

5. Species of the genera *Sarcoptes* and *Notoedres* have two vertical setae on the dorsum of the propodosoma. Species of the genus *Cnemidocoptes* have, on the dorsal side, two longitudinal chitinised bars running from the bases of the pedipalps to the level of legs, where they are united by a transverse bar. The dorsal surface has ridges, grooves and scales.

6. The legs are short.

7. There are bell-shaped suckers (caruncles) on stalks (pedicels) on the tarsi of some or all of the legs.

8. The pedicels of the tarsal suckers of all species are *not* segmented. In *Sarcoptes* and *Notoedres* the pedicels are long; in *Cnemidocoptes* they are shorter and the females have no suckers on any of the legs.

9. Legs 3 and 4 *of the females only* end in bristles instead of suckers (caruncles).

10. The anus is terminal (except in *Notoedres*, in which it is dorsal).

11. The male has no adanal suckers (copulatory discs).

12. The posterior margin of the abdomen of the male not bi-lobed.

FAMILY: PSOROPTIDAE

1. *Genera:* (a) *Psoroptes*, species of which cause psoroptic mange of the sheep (sheep-scab), goats, cattle and equines. (b) *Otodectes*, species of which cause otodectic mange of dogs, foxes, cats and ferrets. (c) *Chorioptes*, species of which cause chorioptic mange of equines and of cattle.

2. Species of this family do not burrow into the skin, but are parasitic in its surface layers, causing the formation of thick, heavy scabs rather than thickening of the skin.

3. The body of the mite is oval.

4. There are no dorsal spines.

5. There are no vertical setae on the dorsum of the propodosoma.

6. The legs are longer and project beyond the margin of the body.

7. There are bell-shaped suckers (caruncles) on stalks (pedicels) on the tarsi of some or all of the legs.

8. The pedicels of the tarsal suckers are long and composed of three segments (in *Psoroptes*), or are short and not segmented (*Otodectes* and *Chorioptes*).

9. Legs 3 *of the females only* end in bristles instead of suckers (caruncles). Legs 4 *of the females only* of *Otodectes* are feebly developed and legs 4 *of the males* of all three genera are shorter than legs 3.

10. The anus is terminal.

11. The male has adanal suckers (copulatory discs).

12. The posterior margin of the abdomen *of the male* is produced into two lobes, which are prominent in species of the genera *Psoroptes* and *Chorioptes*, but are not prominent in species of the genus *Otodectes* or in other species of this family.

LEG SUCKERS IN SARCOPTIDAE AND PSOROPTIDAE

Genus	Male				Female			
	I	2	3	4	I	2	3	4
Sarcoptes ..	S	S	—	S	S	S	—	—
Notoedres	S	S	—	S	S	S	—	—
Cnemidocoptes	S	S	S	S	—	—	—	—
Psoroptes ..	S	S	S	—	S	S	—	S
Chorioptes ..	S	S	S	S	S	S	—	S
Otodectes ..	S	S	S	S	S	S	—	—

FAMILY: SARCOPTIDAE

Genus: Sarcoptes Latreille, 1806

The mites belonging to this genus are parasitic on a number of different domestic and wild mammals, causing a disease known as mange. They are regarded by some authors as belonging to different species and by others as biological or physiological races of the species *S. scabiei*, which are specific to their hosts. It has, however, been found possible to transmit the mites from various species of hosts to others, so that they might be considered as host varieties in process of evolution, but still able to pass from one species to another.

Sarcoptes scabiei is a minute parasite, roughly circular in outline. The female measures 330–600 μ by 250–400 μ and the male 200–240 μ by 150–200 μ. All the legs of both sexes are short and the third and fourth pairs do not project beyond the margin of the body. The positions of the caruncles on the legs are given in the table above, but some or all of these may no longer be present on the legs of specimens found in scrapings from the skin. The dorsal surface is covered with fine folds and grooves mainly transverse in arrangement, and bears a number of small triangular scales. The female bears on either side of the mid-line anteriorly three short spines and posteriorly six longer spines with bifid tips, in addition to a few hairs.

Life-cycle. The life-cycle of *S. scabiei* var. *humani* is described by Mellanby (1952). Probably the life-cycle of the varieties found on other animals is similar. The female burrows into the skin and lays forty to fifty eggs in the tunnel it forms. The eggs are laid one or two at a time about three to five being deposited daily. These hatch in 3–5 days to produce a six-legged larva. The larvae escape from the breeding tunnels and wander on the skin, but some remain in the parent tunnel or side pockets of it and continue their development there as far as the nymphal stages. Of those that reach the surface many perish; others burrow into the stratum corneum to construct almost invisible moulting pockets, in which they also feed. There are two nymphal stages which may stay in the larval pockets or wander and make new pockets. The nymphs have four pairs of legs, but no genital apertures. Finally, males and females are produced, the development from the time the eggs are laid lasting about 17 days. The adult female remains in the moulting pocket until fertilised by a male. She then extends the pocket into a tunnel or makes a new one, and, after 4–5 days, begins to lay eggs, three to five a day. The female probably does not live longer than 3–4 weeks. Infection is spread mainly by contact by the wandering larvae, nymphs and fertilised young females.

The mites are very susceptible to dryness and cannot live more than a few days off their host. Under optimal laboratory conditions the mites have been kept alive for 3 weeks.

Pathogenesis. The parasites pierce the skin to suck lymph and may also feed on young epidermal cells. Their activities produce a marked irritation which causes intense itching and scratching, which aggravates the condition. The resulting inflammation of the skin is accompanied by an exudate which coagulates and forms crusts on the surface, and is

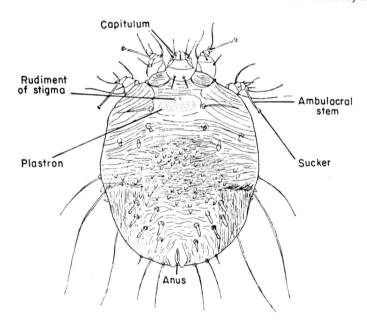

FIG. 256. *Sarcoptes scabiei*, Dorsal View of Female (After Bedford, Modified)

further characterised by excessive keratinisation and proliferation of connective tissue, with the result that the skin becomes much thickened and wrinkled. There is a concomitant loss of hair which may be very widespread.

Clinical signs. *Sarcoptes* prefers those parts of the body that are not covered by much hair, such as the face and ears of goats, sheep and rabbits, the hock, elbow, muzzle and root of the tail in dogs and foxes, the head and neck in equines, the sacral region and the neck in cattle, and the back of pigs. When the disease is allowed to spread, all parts of the body may eventually become affected. The disease is rare in woolled sheep. The local signs are obvious from the pathogenesis; the skin is more or less bare, thick and wrinkled and covered with dry crusts. In young lesions there are red papules or vesicles and fresh exudate. The lesion is exceedingly irritating and causes much biting and scratch-

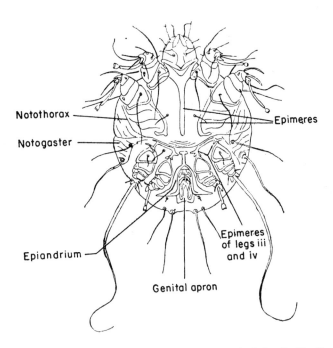

FIG. 257. *Sarcoptes scabiei*, Ventral View of Male (after Bedford)

ing. Small foci of mange have little or no effect on the general health of the host, but larger lesions produce progressive emaciation and even death. In pigs excessive thickening of the skin may occur: this may then crack open leaving deep wounds which frequently become secondarily infected. It is important to note that mange is a disease of poor-conditioned animals, and is therefore most frequently seen towards the end of winter and in early spring.

Diagnosis. The lesion is scraped by means of a knife until the moist layers of the skin are exposed and the material is examined for the presence of the parasites. It may be difficult to find specimens that can be identified with certainty and clinical signs should also be considered.

Differential diagnosis. In dandruff the skin is soft and pliable and no parasites are found. Ringworm does not cause thickening of the skin either, while the fungus spores can be found in the shafts of the hairs. Lice may produce crusts and matting of the hair, but they are readily detected and as a rule the skin is not thickened. Psoroptic, notoedric and chorioptic mange usually occur on other parts of the body and can be recognised by the different appearance of the parasites. Demodectic mange may be of the pustular or squamous kinds described above and *Demodex* is easily recognised. Harvest mites (Trombiculidae) cause scaly lesions from which the hairs fall out and are found mainly on the heads of animals that run on pasture; the skin remains soft and the mites, which are larval forms, have a scarlet-red colour.

Treatment. The gamma isomer of BHC is an effective remedy for sarcoptic mange on farm animals and dogs. It may be applied as a wash, dip or spray at a concentration of 0·016–0·03 per cent and should be repeated on two or three occasions at an interval of 10–14 days. Repeat treatment is necessary to kill larvae hatching from eggs. Various organo-phosphorus compounds may also be used either orally or by topical application. These include fenchlorphos ('Ectoral'), trichlorphon and diazinon.

Other remedies that have been recommended are:

Lime-sulphur dip containing 1·5 per cent polysulphide sulphur is applied as a spray or by means of a brush. Treatment is repeated three to six times, as required, at weekly intervals. For man sulphur ointment may be tried.

Benzyl benzoate is used as an emulsion or mixed with equal parts of soft soap and isopropyl alcohol or methylated spirits. It is painted on and allowed to dry.

Tetraethylthiuram monosulphide (Tetmosol) is used as a freshly-prepared watery solution, usually 5 per cent. It may be rubbed into the skin by hand after a bath and left on for 24 hours. For prophylaxis a 20 per cent Tetmosol soap may be used.

Good feeding and exercise are valuable additional measures. Spontaneous recovery is not uncommon in animals that are well fed and cared for.

Prophylaxis. All infected premises should be cleaned out and disinfected by spraying with BHC solution or lime-sulphur dip, and they are best left unused for 14–17 days. Utensils such as curry-combs, brushes and harness should also be disinfected or locked up for 3 weeks, when the mites on them will have died.

Genus: Cnemidocoptes Fürstenberg, 1870

C. gallinae (Railliet, 1887) is a small mite, resembling *Sarcoptes*, which cause 'depluming itch' in fowls. The mites burrow into the skin alongside the shafts of the feathers and cause an itching, inflammatory condition. The feathers break off readily and they are pulled out by the birds. The lesions are mostly seen on the back and wings, more rarely on the head and neck. The feather mite, *Megninia cubitalis*, may apparently cause a similar disease (see p. 517).

Diagnosis can be made by pulling out a few feathers at the edge of the lesion and searching for the mites on them.

Treatment. The birds are dipped in a mixture of sodium fluoride, sulphur, soap and water. Lindane or pyrethrum may be used.

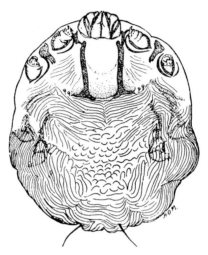

FIG. 258. *Cnemidocoptes mutans*, Dorsal View of Female (Original)

C. mutans (Robin, 1860) causes the condition known as 'scaly leg' in fowls and turkeys. The mites apparently get on to the feet of the birds from the ground, since the lesion usually develops from the toes upwards. The parasites pierce the skin underneath the scales, causing an inflammation with exudate that hardens on the surface and displaces the scales. This process, accompanied by marked keratinisation, is responsible for the thickened scaly nature of the skin. The disease may lead to lameness and malformation of the feet. In rare cases the comb and neck may be affected.

Treatment. Birds may be satisfactorily treated by dipping the legs in a bath containing 0·1 per cent gamma isomer of BHC. Other treatments consist of dipping the affected legs in kerosene to moisten the scales and then applying a 10 per cent sulphur ointment. This should be repeated several times at 10 day intervals. A further treatment consists of dipping the legs in a 0·5 per cent solution of sodium fluoride. This should be repeated weekly.

Further measures include cleaning poultry houses and spraying perches etc. with creosote, kerosene or BHC.

C. pilae. This species was described by Lavoipierre & Griffiths (1951) as the cause of scaly leg in a budgerigar or parakeet (*Melopsittacus undulatus*) in Britain. It affected the shanks and pads of the feet. Oldham & Beresford-Jones (1954) found that *C. pilae* affected the junction of the beak and feathers of budgerigars 6–12 months old and they also found it on an Alexandrian parakeet. *C. jamaicensis* is described as the cause of scaly leg of the golden thrush (*Turdus aurantiacus*) in Jamaica, which is related to *C. fossor*, found on the Maja finch (*Munia maja*).

Genus: Notoedres Railliet, 1893

N. cati (Hering, 1838) is a minute mite which attacks mainly cats and rabbits. Possibly there are different varieties of the parasite on the two hosts. It occurs chiefly on the ears and back of the neck, but may extend to the face, foot, hind paws and, in young cats, to the whole body. These mites burrow into the skin, causing mange-like lesions. Their life history is similar to that of *Sarcoptes*.

Since cats are especially susceptible to the toxic effects of the chlorinated hydrocarbon insecticides and also to several of the organophosphorus compounds, special care is necessary in the treatment of *N. cati*. An effective, though somewhat old-fashioned, treatment is to apply sulphur in oil (12 per cent) on several occasions. English (1960) has recommended malathion, cats being submerged for 1–2 seconds in a 0·25–1·25 suspension of the drug. It is stated that the taste of malathion is objectionable, this preventing the cats from acquiring a toxic dose by licking. Preparations containing piperonyl butoxide may be of value.

FAMILY: PSOROPTIDAE

Genus: Psoroptes Gervais, 1841

This genus contains a number of parasites which, unlike the species of the Sarcoptidae, are specific to their hosts, although morphologically they may be difficult to distinguish. They are oval in shape and the tarsal suckers have jointed pedicles. As a rule these parasites live on the skin of parts of the body well covered with hair or wool or in the ears of their hosts.

Sweatman (1958b) studied the validity of the so-called species of *Psoroptes* and recognised as valid only the following:

P. ovis (Hering, 1838) Gervais, 1941, the cosmopolitan body mite of domesticated sheep and cattle and of the horse and possibly also of the donkey and mule.

P. equi (Hering, 1838) Gervais, 1941, the body mite of the horse and possibly also of the donkey and mule, which occurs only in England.

P. natalensis Hunt, 1919, the body mite of domesticated cattle, the zebu and Indian water buffalo in South Africa, South America, New Zealand and probably France.

P. cervinus (cervinae) Ward, 1915, found on American hosts.

P. cuniculi (Delafond, 1859) Canestrini & Kramer, 1899, a cosmopolitan species which occurs in the ears of the rabbit, goat, sheep, horse, donkey, mule and possibly gazelle.

These names will be adopted in this book.

18

P. ovis is the cause of sheep-scab, an important disease which has been eradicated from Australia and from Britain but still occurs in certain states of the U.S.A. and elsewhere. The parasite cannot be transmitted to other species of animals. The mites are oval and have a white body with brownish legs. The larvae have three pairs of legs and the other stages four pairs. All bear suckers with jointed pedicles on the first and second pairs of legs; the larvae have two long bristles on the third pair; the nymphae, pubescent females and ovigerous females have bristles on the third pair and suckers on the fourth; the third pair of the male is long and suckered, while the fourth pair is very short and bears only hairs. The pubescent female is provided with a pair of posterior copulatory tubercles which are absent in the ovigerous female, while the latter has a wide genital aperture on the anterior aspect of the ventral surface. The male has posteriorly, on the ventral surface, a pair of brown copulatory suckers and terminally a pair of large tubercles which each bear several hairs. The dorsal surface of the body is devoid of scales and spines, but the cuticle shows very fine striations.

Life-cycle. The eggs are laid on the skin at the edges of the lesion and hatch normally in 1–3 days. Eggs separated from the skin by crusts may hatch in 4–5 days. Eggs removed with wool from the body or drawn away from the skin to the extent of several centimetres may hatch up to 10 days after having been laid, or otherwise die.

The larvae feed and, 2–3 days after hatching, moult to the nymphal stage, passing the last 12 hours in a state of lethargy. The nymphal stage lasts 3–4 days, including a lethargic period of 36 hours before the moult occurs. The smaller nymphs usually become males. As a rule the pubescent females appear before the males, sometimes as soon as $5\frac{1}{2}$ days after hatching, while the males do not appear before the sixth day. Copulation begins soon after ecdysis and lasts 1 day; if there are many more females than males, the period may be shorter. As a rule the proportion of males to females is 1–2 : 4. The pubescent female moults 2 days after the commencement of copulation and the ovigerous female begins to lay 1 day later or 9 days after hatching from the egg. The shortest period observed is 8 days. Even in winter, on sheep that are well clothed, the cycle is not much longer.

The female lives 30–40 days and lays about five eggs daily and a total of 90 or more.

Pathogenesis. The mites puncture the epidermis to suck lymph and stimulate a local reaction in the form of a small inflammatory swelling richly infiltrated with serum. The latter exudes on to the surface and coagulates, thus forming a crust. The altered conditions cause the wool to become loose and to fall out, or it is pulled out by the sheep in biting and scratching the lesion, which itches severely. The bare crusty patches are unsuitable for the mites, which therefore migrate to the margins of the lesion and thus extend the process outwards.

Clinical signs. Scab lesions may occur on all parts of the body that are covered with wool or hair, but occur most frequently around the shoulders and along the sides of the body in woolled sheep, and along the back, the sternum and the dorsal aspect of the tail in hairy sheep.

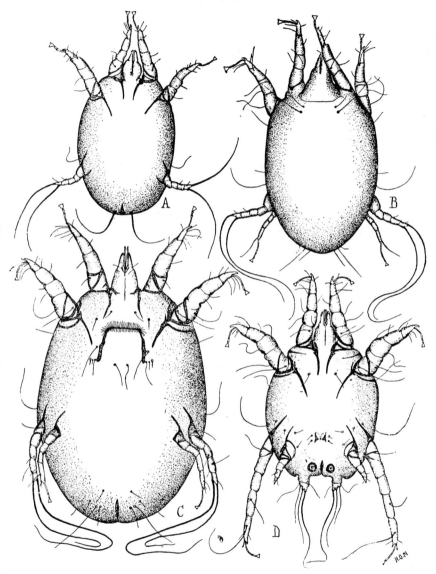

FIG. 259. *Psoroptes communis ovis :* A, larva, ventral; B, nymph, dorsal; C, ovigerous female, ventral; D, male, ventral view (Original)

In early lesions the wool is disturbed over the lesion by the biting and scratching of the sheep and usually has a lighter colour than the sur-rounding wool. A lesion of 2–4 days old appears as a small papule, about 5 mm. in diameter, with a yellowish colour and a moist surface; the mite will as a rule be found on the affected spot. From about the fifth day onwards the exudate begins to coagulate, forming pale yellow crusts, and the lesion extends outwards as the number of parasites increases. Older lesions are easy to detect on account of the loss of wool and presence of scab, while the mites are producing fresh foci in the surrounding covered parts. In some cases large portions of the body may be affected around an old lesion without showing on the surface. If the wool is opened, it is found to be matted together above the skin by scabs, underneath which numerous parasites are located.

In hairy sheep the scab lesion is, as a rule, drier than in woolled sheep. So-called 'latent' cases, in which a small lesion may exist for months, are seen in the form of small, dry lesions on the scrotum, in the perineum, along the sheath, on the sternum, in the ears and infra-orbital fossae and at the bases of the horns. Sheep scab is most active in autumn and winter, while latency tends to occur in summer, on account of less active feeding and decreased oviposition by the mites.

Diagnosis. It is relatively simple to diagnose the active disease in a scabby flock, but the latent lesions described above make it more difficult to declare a large flock free of scab.

In the latter case particular attention should be paid to the infra-orbital fossa, the base of the horns and, in rams, the scrotum. Scraping of suspect lesions should be taken for microscopic examination.

Treatment consists in dipping the sheep in a suitable dip and hand-dressing bad lesions, as well as the hiding-places of the mites. Particular care should be taken to treat the sites of the latent form of the disease described above. Though this disease was formerly a serious problem, it can now be controlled with BHC.

A single treatment with 0·02 per cent gamma BHC is frequently sufficient for cure. All the sheep of a flock should be treated and treatment may be repeated after about 2 months, especially in mountainous regions etc. where a total 'gather' of sheep may be difficult at any one time. A dip containing 0·03 per cent dieldrin is similarly effective. In countries where the chlorinated hydrocarbons are prohibited because of insecticide residues in the meat the organophosphorus compounds may be used. The latter may also be necessary where *P. ovis* has become resistant to BHC. An old, but effective treatment consisted of dipping twice, with an interval of 14 days, with a lime-sulphur dip, containing 1·5 per cent of poly-sulphide sulphur.

Genus: Chorioptes Gervais, 1859

The different species of this genus live on the skin of several species of domestic mammals, causing chorioptic mange. The parasites resemble *Psoroptes*, but the tarsal suckers have unjointed pedicles.

The so-called species of this genus have been named after the hosts on which they occur. Thus the form found on the fetlocks of horses has been called *C. equi* (Gerlach, 1857); the form found on the pasterns of sheep, *C. ovis*; the one found on goats, *C. caprae*; and the form found in the ears of rabbits *C. cuniculi*. The life history is completed in 3 weeks; it resembles that of *Psoroptes*. Sweatman (1957) concluded that the species called *C. bovis*, *C. equi* and *C. ovis* all belong to the species *C. bovis* (Hering, 1845); Gervais & van Beneden, 1859 and that the only other valid species is *C. texanus* Hirst, 1924, found on a domestic goat in Texas, and on Canadian reindeer.

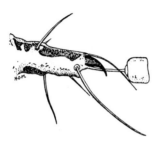

FIG. 260. *Chorioptes*, Extremity of Leg with Sucker (Original)

C. bovis. In horses this species causes the disease called 'foot mange' or 'itchy leg', characterised by itching, scab-like lesions on the fetlocks, especially on those of horses with long hair (feather) in this region, which make the horses rub, stamp, scratch and bite the legs and kick frequently, especially at night. It occurs especially on the pasterns, particularly those of the hind limbs, causing the formation of papules and, later, scabs. In cattle the root of the tail is frequently affected and if untreated the condition may spread to the sacral region and other parts of the body. It is most numerous in the winter.

Diagnosis of all the 'species' of this genus is made by finding them in skin scrapings.

Treatment. BHC washes are effective for chorioptic mange as are the organophosphorus insecticides such as fenchlorphos, trichlorphon or diazinon. An older, but effective, remedy is a lime–sulphur wash applied several times at intervals of 10 days.

Genus: Otodectes Canestrini, 1894

O. cynotis (Hering, 1838) occurs in the ears of the dog, cat, fox, red fox, ferret and other carnivores, causing ear or otodectic mange. The parasites resemble *Chorioptes*; they have tarsal suckers with unjointed pedicles on the first and second pairs of legs in the female and on all four pairs in the male. The fourth pair of legs in the female is small. In the male the copulatory tubercles are not prominent.

Life-cycle and pathogenesis. The eggs are laid singly, and the life history, which resembles that of *Psoroptes* takes 3 weeks. Sweatman (1958a) concluded that there is only one valid species, namely, *Otodectes cynotis* (Hering, 1888); Canestrini, 1894. The mites spend all their lives in the ears of the host, less often on its body, and Sweatman concluded that, like *Chorioptes*, they feed on epidermal debris which they chew and that they do not, as has been stated, pierce the skin to obtain body fluids. The clinical signs are seen in dogs at an earlier stage than in cats and foxes, which usually do not appear to be affected until the disease has reached an advanced stage. The animal shakes its head and scratches the ears in ordinary cases, while in more advanced stages the ears droop and there is a discharge. There may be torticollis or the animals turn about in a circle, and even more marked nervous signs like epileptiform fits may be seen. If the disease is allowed to take its course, a purulent inflammation of the external ear frequently sets in and perforation of the tympanic membrane may occur as the result of ulceration, leading to serious affections of the middle and inner ear and the brain.

Diagnosis. After removal of the crusts, the mites are readily found in material scraped from the skin of the external ear passage. They must be differentiated from *Sarcoptes scabiei* and *Notoedres cati.*

Treatment. The ear should be well cleaned of wax and detritus and an insecticide ointment or cream smeared in the meatus. A concentration of 0·1 per cent BHC is satisfactory and should be repeated after about 2 weeks to kill mites which have hatched from eggs. Benzyl benzoate emulsion (20 per cent) is also effective.

In advanced infections, especially when secondary bacterial infection has occurred antibiotics or sulpha drugs are indicated. Surgical intervention may be necessary to insure drainage.

FAMILY: ACARIDAE (SYN. TYROGLYPHIDAE)

Mites of this family feed on organic material, some are found in flour, grain, cheese, copra and similar products and may become accidental parasites on or in man and animals which handle or feed on such infested materials. At times enormous numbers may be present in old food material such as animal feed, flour etc. They are distinguished from the parasitic mites by the absence of well-marked suckers, the absence of a distinct 'thumb-print' pattern on the body surface; they usually have many more bristles than the parasitic forms and their nymphs may develop hooks and suckers which enable them to cling to other hosts to be transported to a more suitable environment (*Hypopi*; hypopial nymphs).

Acarus siro (syn. *Tyroglyphus siro*) (Linnaeus, 1758) is the cheese mite but is also found on other stored foods. It measures 500–550 μ in length and the body is covered with hairs. It is frequently found in food stores and upon accidental ingestion in large numbers may cause gastric or intestinal catarrh with diarrhoea. In food handlers, continued exposure may result in papular eruptions.

Acarus farinae (De Geer, 1778) (syn. *Tyroglyphus farinae*). This is similar to the former, being 330–600 μ in length, there is a distinct line or suture across the body and it is covered with numerous hairs. The mite lives in a variety of stored food products, especially cheeses and grains. In man it may cause digestive upsets if eaten in large numbers and may also cause skin lesions.

Tyrophagus longior (Gervais, 1844) the 'corpra mite' is found in grains, seeds and copra and is responsible for 'copra itch'.

Glyciphagus domesticus (de Geer, 1808). This is a very common species, being found in many stored food products. It is the cause of 'grocer's itch' of humans.

FAMILY: CYTODITIDAE (SYN. CYTOLEICHIDAE)

Genus: Cytodites Mégnin, 1879 (syn. Cytoleichus)

C. nudus (Vizioli, 1870), the 'air-sac mite', is a small, oval, creamy-coloured mite with suckered legs and practically no hairs, which lives in the respiratory passages and air-sacs and has also been found in other organs of fowls, turkeys and pheasants. The life-cycle is unknown, but the parasites are probably spread by mucus from the respiratory passages which is coughed up or passed with the faeces.

As a rule the parasites are not pathogenic. In South Africa this mite is very common, but it has not been recorded as a cause of disease. It has been stated that heavy infections may predispose to pulmonary disorders.

FAMILY: LAMINOSIOPTIDAE

Genus: Laminosioptes Mégnin 1880

L. cysticola (Vizioli, 1870), the 'subcutaneous mite' of the fowl, is a small oval parasite; the anterior two pairs of legs each end in a claw, and the posterior two pairs each in a claw and suckerless pedicle.

Life-cycle—unknown.

Significance. The live parasites are rarely seen, but they may be found in the subcutaneous tissues. Usually the presence of the parasites is only indicated by the occurrence of small, flat, oval nodules, which resemble bits of fat in the subcutis. These nodules have a caseous or calcified content and are formed around the dead mites, of which the remains may still be present. The parasites are not pathogenic, but large numbers of these nodules may reduce the value of birds intended for human consumption.

Treatment and *Prophylaxis*—unknown.

FAMILY: EPIDERMOPTIDAE

The very small species of this family are not more than 0·4 mm. long.

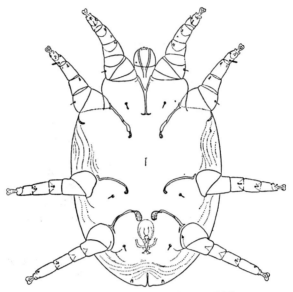

FIG. 261. *Cytodites nudus*, Ventral View

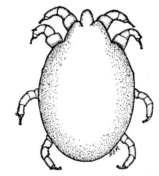

FIG. 262. *Cytodites nudus*, Dorsal View (Original)

They have circular, soft bodies; the males have adanal and copulatory suckers; all the legs bear suckers. *Epidermoptes bilobatus* and *E. (Rivoltasia) bifurcata* may be found in the skin of the fowl and may, if the mites are numerous, cause ill health.

FAMILY: LISTROPHORIDAE

Species of this family may be found on the hair of small laboratory mammals and on the ferret. Their bodies may be laterally compressed and the pedipalps, legs and sternal region may be modified for clasping the hairs of the host. **L. gibbus** may occur on the rabbit, **Chirodiscoides caviae** on the guinea-pig. **Myocoptes musculinus** may occur on laboratory mice and guinea-pigs and may be associated with a mange-like condition. Animals may be treated with a 0·1 per cent BHC wash or an organophosphorus insecticide.

Other species of the order Sarcoptiformes, the 'feather mites', are parasitic on the feathers of birds, although some of them may enter the quills of the feathers. They belong to the following families of their order:

FAMILY: ANALGESIDAE

Species of this family live chiefly between the barbules of the feathers and only rarely enter the quills. The bodies of the adults have an undivided posterior margin and the legs of the males are exceptionally well developed, but cannot be used for walking. Among species of this family are *Analges passerinus* found on the feathers of passerine birds, *Mégninia cubitalis* found on the feathers of the fowl, *M. velata* on those of the duck, *M. phasiani* on those of the pheasant and peacock, and *M. columbae* on those of the pigeon. *Mégninia ginglymura* occurs on the fowl in Madras. Lavoipierre (1958) found that *M. cubitalis* was the only detectable cause of a form of depluming itch in a hen, *Cnemidocoptes gallinae* being absent.

FAMILY: DERMOGLYPHIDAE

Both sexes of species of this family have a propodosomal shield and there may be other dorsal plates. Remarkable modifications of the legs, chelicerae and pedipalps may occur among the males. *Dermoglyphus elongatus* and *D. minor* may enter the feathers, the latter species having an elongated body adapted to this habitat resembling that of the trombidiform species *Syringophilus* mentioned above. *Pterolichus obtusus* lives on the feathers of the fowl, *P. bicaudatus* on those of the South African ostrich, *Freyana chanayi* on those of the turkey, *Pteronyssus striatus* on those of the sparrow, linnet and chaffinch, and *Falculifer rostratus* and *F. cornutus* on those of the pigeon. The nymph of the last-named species may enter the subcutaneous tissues or even the peritracheal tissues of the internal organs, and formerly, when they were found in these situations, they were given the names *Hypodectes*, *Cellularia* and *Hypodera*. The nymphs that enter the tissues are *hypopial nymphs*. Control of Dermoglyphidae (chiefly *Pterolichus*) of parakeets and cockatoos may be obtained by scattering malathion powder on the bare floor of the cage and leaving birds to make contact with it (Cross *et al.*, 1956).

FAMILY: PROCTOPHYLLOIDEA

Species of this family have several shields on the body and the posterior end of the female is bilobed and bears leaf-like appendages. Their habits are like those of the species of the two families just mentioned. An example of the family is *Pterophagus strictus*, which lives on the feathers of the pigeon.

CLASS: PENTASTOMIDA

This is a group of Arthropoda allied to the mites. They occur as internal parasites in the respiratory organs of vertebrates.

The parasites are elongate, often tongue-shaped. The cuticula is transversely striated or sometimes deeply ringed, so that the body may have a beaded appearance in its posterior part. The anterior end is thick, and its flattened ventral surface is armed with two pairs of strong, hooked claws, situated on either side of the elongate oral aperture. The small buccal cavity leads into a pharynx which has a suctorial function, and is followed by an oesophagus, an intestine and a rectum. The anus opens posteriorly. The females are usually larger than the males. As a rule the latter have two elongate testes, and a cirrus sac with a cirrus or penis is present. The male genital opening is situated near the anus. The female has one elongate ovary, but a double oviduct which leads into a uterus. The vulva is anteriorly or posteriorly situated. The eggs contain a fully-developed embryo when they are laid.

Life-cycle. The egg contains a larva with two or three pairs of rudimentary clawed legs and hatches in the intestine of the intermediate host. The larva bores into the intestinal wall and passes with the blood to the mesenteric glands, liver and lungs, whence it finds its way into a suitable organ, where it becomes encysted. After several ecdyses, during which the legs are lost, a nymphal stage which is infestive for the final host appears. The final host acquires the infection by eating the intermediate host containing the young parasites.

FAMILY: POROCEPHALIDAE

The female genital aperture opens posteriorly. The larva has two pairs of legs.

Genus: Linguatula Fröhlich, 1789

L. serrata Fröhlich, 1779, the 'tongue-worm', is a cosmopolitan parasite and occurs in the nasal and respiratory passages of the dog, fox and wolf, more rarely in man, the horse, goat and sheep. The parasite is tongue-shaped, slightly convex dorsally and flattened ventrally. The cuticle is transversely striated. Male 1·8–2 cm., female 8–13 cm. long. The eggs measure about 90 by 70 μ.

Life-cycle. The eggs are expelled from the respiratory passages of the host and, when swallowed by a suitable herbivorous animal such as a horse, sheep, goat, bovine, or rabbit, they hatch in the alimentary canal and the larva reaches the mesenteric lymph glands, in which it develops to the infective nymphal stage. The latter resembles the adult; it is 5–6 mm. long and has a white colour. It usually lies in a small cyst surrounded by a viscid, turbid fluid. Dogs become infected by eating infected rabbits or glands of larger animals.

Pathogenesis. The parasites attach themselves high up in the nasal passage and produce a severe irritation which causes the animals to sneeze and cough at intervals. Fits of difficult breathing, uneasiness and restlessness are observed. The animal often rubs its nose with the forefeet and snores in its sleep. A mucous discharge, often blood-stained, may exude from the nostrils. The parasites live about 15 months, after which the animal usually recovers.

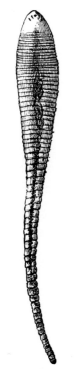 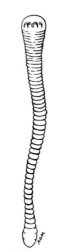

Fig. 263. *Linguatula serrata*, Female, Ventral View (after Neumann)

Fig. 264. *Porocephalus subclavatus*, Ventral View (× 1½) (Original)

Diagnosis is made from the clinical signs and by finding the eggs in the faeces or the nasal discharge.

Treatment is difficult. Injections and inhalations are not very effective. Trephining the nasal passages and removal of the parasites, followed by irrigation if necessary, is the most satisfactory method.

Prophylaxis. The infection can be avoided by preventing dogs and foxes from eating any possibly infected material.

Species of **Porocephalus** occur in the respiratory passages of large snakes. The body is deeply ringed and may have a beaded appearance posteriorly. The young stages are found in the mesenteric lymph glands.

and other organs of various wild and domestic animals, including Herbivora, Carnivora, and man.

Injurious Non-parasitic Arthropoda

Although the poisonous nature of some arthropods is sometimes much exaggerated, a number of species can be poisonous to man and animals in various ways.

1. *Piercing or biting species* inject poisonous or irritating substances into a wound made by their mouth parts or poison claws—e.g. spiders, mosquitoes, centipedes.

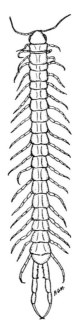

FIG. 265. A Chilopod, Dorsal View (Original)

2. *Stinging species* inject a poison by means of a sting situated at the end of the abdomen, e.g. scorpions. Such a sting is frequently a modified ovipositor—e.g. bees.

3. *Nettling species* have hairs or scales which possess irritating properties —e.g. certain caterpillars.

4. *Cryptotoxic species* contain irritant or poisonous body fluids—e.g. the blister beetles.

Myriapoda. The millipedes (*Diplopoda*) are circular in transverse section and have two pairs of legs on each of most of the segments. They are not poisonous, but it is stated that some of the large tropical species eject, when they are irritated, poisonous or pungent fluids from cutaneous glands. The centipedes (*Chilopoda*) are flattened dorso-ventrally and have a single pair of legs per segment. They have the first pair of legs modified as claws which contain poison glands. These are carnivorous animals and they use the poison claws to stun their prey. The smaller forms can at most cause a painful local reaction in larger animals or man, but the large forms, e.g. the tropical *Scolopendra gigantea*, can cause death.

Insecta: (1) *Piercing or biting species.* These and their effects have been described above.

(2) *Stinging species.* The stinging insects are *Hymenoptera*, the sting being a modified ovipositor found only in the females. In the bee there is a poison reservoir and the poison glands are of two types, one producing an alkaline and the other an acid secretion. When the bee stings, the tip of the abdomen with the whole poison apparatus breaks off and remains in the wound. The muscles of the organ remain active for a considerable time and force poison out of the reservoir into the tissues, so that it is necessary to remove the sting as soon as possible.

The sting produces a local necrosis with infiltration of lymphocytes, hyperaemia and more or less extensive oedema. Some individuals are much more sensitive to bee stings than others and some human beings have a high susceptibility. The stings of a large number of bees may cause death following collapse, shock or suffocation, the latter being due to oedema of the head and neck.

Some species, like bumble-bees, hornets and wasps, sting several times and the sting does not break off so easily. Most ants also possess poison glands and stings, but seldom use them. Some species have no stings, but make a wound by biting and then inject the poison into it.

(3) *Nettling species.* Many hairy caterpillars produce intense irritation by means of their hairs, which are hollow and bear a poison gland at the base. The hairs break off and remain in the skin of the affected animal or person. The scales of the 'brown-tail moth' (*Porthesia chrysor-rhoea*) and of some other moths may cause dermatitis and bronchitis, and the caterpillars of *Porthesia* are also stated to cast off hairs which are very irritating.

Poisonous caterpillars are known to cause stomatitis and even enteritis in animals if they are numerous on a pasture. In cases of dermatitis the application of ammonia, followed by 10 per cent ichthyol ointment, is recommended.

(4) *Cryptotoxic species.* The well-known Spanish fly or blister beetles (*Meloidae*) possess very irritating body fluids, containing cantharidin as the active principle. Powdered beetles or extracts have long been used for blistering and formerly also as aphrodisiacs. The action in the latter case is due to irritation and the kidneys suffer severely. Cases of poisoning of cattle from ingesting these beetles with their food are known, and the flesh of such animals is believed to be poisonous for human beings.

Of other cryptotoxic insects the most important are the caterpillars of the cabbage butterfly (*Pieris brassicae*), which cause stomatitis, colic, and paralysis of the hind-legs in animals.

Arachnida. In *scorpions* a post-abdominal segment forms the sting, which contains a pair of well-developed poison glands and ends in a hollow spine. The smaller species may cause painful stings, but these are not fatal. The larger tropical and subtropical species are frequently very poisonous. The poison causes elevation of blood pressure and increased glandular activity, especially lacrimation, salivation and a nasal discharge. There are also muscular spasms, and death is due to asphyxia.

Treatment consists in the application of a ligature proximal to the wound —not to be maintained for longer than half an hour—and the injection of a 1 per cent permanganate solution, as in the case of a snake bite. The stings of slightly poisonous forms can be treated by the local injection of procaine and adrenaline, which alleviates pain. For very poisonous forms antivenoms are prepared by hyperimmunisation of animals, and such a serum, prepared from one species, protects against closely related forms, but not against others. The scorpions themselves appear to contain antitoxins, so that they can resist the stings of other scorpions. The WHO (1958) recommends, for control, the application of 50 mg. per sq. ft. of gamma BHC to walls, attics etc., and to other places in which scorpions hide and the removal of wood stacks, loose bricks and any shelters of these arachnids.

The Araneidae, or spiders, have poison glands which lie in the cephalothorax and open through pores on the tips of the chelicerae. The poison is used to kill small animals, especially insects, for food, and most spiders are not able to bite through the skin of larger animals and man, nor are they sufficiently poisonous to do much harm. There are, however, a few other species that are well known to be very dangerous.

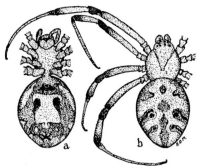

FIG. 266. *Latrodectus*, a South African Species, showing Characteristic Shape and Ornamentation: *a*, ventral; *b*, dorsal view (× about 1½ natural size) (Original)

The name 'tarantula' is derived from a spider of the family Lycosidae, *Lycosa tarantula*, which was believed to be the cause of an hysterical condition, and it was greatly feared in the Middle Ages. This spider is not poisonous to man or domestic animals. The name 'tarantula' is now usually applied to many large spiders of the Aviculariidae, which may inflict severe bites, but are not fatally poisonous. The wounds they make may become infected with bacteria from their mouth parts.

The most poisonous spiders are species of the genus *Latrodectus*, which occur in many tropical and sub-tropical countries, and are called 'hour-glass spiders', on account of a red hour-glass-shaped spot which is frequently present on the ventral side of the abdomen. *L. mactans*, the 'black widow', is one of the best-known species. The female measures up to 3 cm. in length, including the legs. The body is glossy black; on the dorsal side of the abdomen the males and young females have several lighter, spotted stripes which are transversely arranged and run down the sides. On the ventral surface there are brick-red spots which may form the shape of an hour-glass or of a cross. The legs are long and tapering. In the lighter-coloured species the joints of the legs are usually dark. The spiders live in buildings or in shrubs and spin a coarse web, and their eggs are laid in spherical masses with an irregular surface. These spiders are very poisonous and frequently also aggressive.

The symptoms are general rather than local, although severe local pain may occur. A general convulsive trembling of medullary origin is stated to be characteristic in guinea-pigs. In man shooting pains in the hips and marked abdominal pains are common, and are followed by numbness and paresis of the lower limbs. Dizziness and a general feeling of oppression occur. The blood pressure is elevated, there is marked salivation and cold perspiration, later followed by thirst and sometimes retention of urine. The respiratory system is affected, resulting in dyspnoea and cyanosis. Sometimes vomiting and constipation are seen. The course may be from a few hours to about 3 days. In cases that die soon, pulmonary oedema is the prominent lesion; in later cases necrotic foci are seen in the liver, kidneys, spleen and adrenals. Recovery is not infrequent.

Treatment in general as for snake-bite. Potassium permanganate is stated to destroy the poison rapidly. Warm baths give relief. Antivenoms are made and used with success, but must be injected very soon after the bite has occurred.

Chiracanthrium nutrix is a European spider which may cause symptoms of poisoning, and some of the Epeiridae, or orb-weavers, contain poisonous substances in their body fluids and eggs which may give rise to clinical signs in animals that swallow them accidentally.

REFERENCES

INSECTA—GENERAL

IMMS, A. D. (1948). *A General Textbook of Entomology.* London: Methuen
WIGGLESWORTH, V. B. (1950). *The Principles of Insect Physiology.* 4th edn. London: Methuen

PHTHIRAPTERA

HARRISON, I. R. (1961). Further observations on 1-naphthyl-N-methyl carbonate as a veterinary insecticide. *Vet. Rec.*, **73**, 290–293

HOFFMAN, R. A. (1960). The control of poultry lice and mites with several organic insecticides. *J. econ. Ent.*, **53**, 161–162

KRAEMER, J. P. (1959). Relative efficacy of several materials for control of poultry ectoparasites. *J. econ. Ent.*, **52**, 1195–1199

ROBERTS, F. H. S., O'SULLIVAN, P. J., RUMBALL, P. & McLAUCHLAN, A. W. (1947). Observations on the value of DDT for the control of the poultry stick-fast flea, *Echidnophaga gallinacea* Westwood. *Aust. vet. J.*, **23**, 148–152

SCOTT, M. T. (1950). Observations on the bionomics of *Linognathus pedalis*. *Aust. J. agric. Res.*, **1**, 465–470

SKERMAN, K. D. (1959). The efficiency of new insecticides for control of the body louse of sheep (*Damalinia ovis*) by dipping. *Aust. vet. J.*, **35**, 75–79

APHANIPTERA

BENBROOK, E. A. (1959). External parasites of poultry. *Diseases of Poultry* (Ed. by H. E. Biester & L. H. Schwart). Iowa State University Press

FIEDLER, O. G. H. (1958). Die Bekämpfung der Rinderzecken in Südafrika. *Vet.-Med. Nachr.*, **3**, 133–146

MEAD-BRIGGS, A. R. & RUDGE, A. J. B. (1960). Breeding of the rabbit-flea *Spilopsyllus cuniculi* (Dale); requirement of a 'factor' from a pregnant rabbit for ovarian maturation. *Nature, Lond.*, **187**, 1136–1137

ROTHSCHILD, M. (1965). The rabbit-flea and hormones. *Endeavor*, **24**, 162–168

TURK, R. D. (1959). Canine dermatoses. *Canine Medicine* (Ed. by M. A. Fincher, W. J. Gibbons, K. Mayer, & S. E. Park) 2nd Edn. Santa Barbara, California: American Veterinary Publications

YOUNG, J. D., BENFAMINI, E., FEINGOLD, B. F. & NOLLER, H. (1963). Allergy to flea bites. V. Preliminary results of fractionation, characterization and assay for allergenic activity of material derived from the oral secretion of the cat flea *Ctenocephalides felis felis*. *Exp. Parasit.* **13**, 155–166

DIPTERA—NEMATOCERA

ADLER, S. & THEODOR, O. (1957). Transmission of disease agents by phlebotomine sand flies. *Ann. Rev. Ent.*, **2**, 203–206

FALLIS, A. M. & BENNETT, G. F. (1961). Ceratopagonidae as intermediate hosts for *Haemoproteus* and other parasites. *Mosquito News*, **21**, 21–28

KETTLE, D. S., PARISH, R. H. & PARISH, J. (1959). Further observations on the persistence of larvicides against *Culicoides* and a discussion on the interpretation of population changes in the untreated plots. *Bull. ent. Res.*, **50**, 63–80

MICKS, D. W. (1960). Insecticide resistance. A review of developments in 1958 and 1959. *Bull. Wld Hlth Org.*, **22**, 519–529

RIEK, R. G. (1954). Studies on allergic dermatitis (Queensland itch) of the horse: The aetiology of the disease. *Aust. J. agric. Res.*, **5**, 109–129

SMITH, C. M., DAVIS, A. N., WEIDHAAS, D. E. & SEABROOK, E. L. (1959). Insecticide resistance in the salt marsh sandfly *Culicoides furens*. *J. econ. Ento.*, **52**, 352–353

WORLD HEALTH ORGANIZATION (1958). Insect resistance and vector control. *Tech. Rept. Series No.* **157**. Geneva

WORLD HEALTH ORGANIZATION (1959). *Tech. Rept. Series No.* **162**. Geneva

WORLD HEALTH ORGANIZATION (1961). *Tech. Rept. Series No.* **214**. Geneva

WORLD HEALTH ORGANIZATION (1963). Insecticide resistance and vector control. 13th Rept. of the W.H.O. Expert Committee on Insecticides. *Tech. Rept. Series No.* **265**. Geneva

WORLD HEALTH ORGANIZATION (1964). Genetics of vectors and insecticide resistance. Report of a W.H.O. Scientific Group. *Tech. Rept. Series No.* **268**. Geneva

DIPTERA—CYCLORRHAPHA

BAUMHOVER, A. H., GRAHAM, A. J., BITTER, B. A., HOPKINS, D. E., NEW, W. D., DUDLEY, F. H. & BUSHLAND, R. C. (1955). Screw-worm control through release of sterilized flies *J. econ. Ent.* **48**, 462–466

BAUMHOVER, A. H., HUSMAN, C. N., SKIPPER, C. C. & NEW, W. D. (1959). Field observations on the effects of releasing sterile screw-worms in Florida. *J. econ. Ento.*, **52**, 1202–1206

BENBROOK, E. A. (1959). External parasites of poultry. *Diseases of Poultry* (Ed. by H. E. Biester & L. H. Schwart). Iowa State University Press

BUSHLAND, R. C. (1960). New research results with systemic insecticides. *Proc. 62nd Ann. Mtg. U.S. Livestock Sanitary Assn.*, pp. 192–197

BURNS, E. C., McCRAINE, S. E. & MOODY, D. W. (1959). Korlan and co-ral for horn fly control on cable type back rubbers. *J. econ. Ento.*. **52**, 648–650

BUXTON, P. A. (1955). *The Natural History of Tsetse Flies: An Account of the Biology of the Genus Glossina (Diptera)*. Memoir No. 10 London School Hygiene and Tropical Medicine. London: H. K. Lewis

Davies, J. B. (1960). Attachment of immature Simuliidae to other arthropods. *Nature, Lond.*, **187**, 84

Dorsey, C. K. (1966). Face-fly control experiments on quarter horses—1962–64. *J. econ. Ent.*, **59**, 86–89

Drummond, R. O., Jackson, J. B., Gless, E. E. & Moore, B. (1959). Systemic insecticides for the control of Gasterophilus bots in horses. *Agric. Chem.*, **14**, 41–42

DuToit, R. (1954). Trypanosomiasis in Zululand and the control of tsetse flies by chemical means. *Onderstepoort J. vet. Sci.*, **26**, 317–387

Fay, R. W. & Kilpatrick, J. W. (1958). Insecticides for control of adult Diptera. *Ann. Rev. Ent.*, **3**, 401–420

Fenton, B. K. (1960). The screw-worm in the Bahamas. *Vet. Rec.*, **73**, 75–77

Glover, P. E., Jackson, C. H. N., Robertson, A. G. & Thomson, W. E. E. (1956). The extermination of the tsetse fly *Flossina morsitans* Westw., at Abercorn, Northern Rhodesia. *Bull. entolocl. Res.*, **46**, 57–67

Graham, N. P. H. (1959). The control of fly strike. *Wool. Techn. Sheep Breeding*, **6**, 111–115

Hansens, E. J. (1960). Field studies of house fly resistance to organophosphorus insecticides. *J. econ. Ent.*, **53**, 313–317

Herzett, L. Y. T. & Goulding, R. L. (1959). Rotenone and methoxychlor dust in backrubbers for horn fly control in dairy herds. *J. econ. Ento.*, **52**, 762–763

Kahn, M. A. & Lawson, J. E. (1965). Summer treatments for cattle grub control and their effects on horn flies and cattle weight gains. *Can. J. Anim. Sci.*, **45**, 43–50

Knipling, E. F. (1955). Possibilities of insect control or eradication through the use of sexually sterile males. *J. econ. Ent.*, **48**, 459–462

LaBrecque, G. C., Wilson, H. C. & Carrvel, N. (1959). Effectiveness of two carbonate against DDT and malathion-resistant house flies. *J. econ. Ent.*, **52**, 178–179

LaBrecque, G. C. & Wilson, H. E. (1960). Effect of DDT resistance on the development of malathion resistance in house flies. *J. econ. Ent.*, **53**, 320–321

Morgan, N. O. (1964). Autecology of the adult horn fly *Haematobia irritans* (L.) (Diptera: Muscidae). *Ecology*, **45**, 728–736

Mules, J. H. W. (1933). Surgical treatment for blowfly menace. *Pastoral Rev.*, **43**, 678

Mules, J. H. W. (1935). Crutch strike by blowflies in sheep. A preventive operation. *Queensld. Agric. J.*, **44**, 237–241

Skerman, K. D. (1958). The efficiency of new insecticides for control of the body louse of sheep (*Damlaina ovis*) by dipping. *Aust. vet. J.*, **35**, 75–79

Smart, J. (1939). Cychorrhapha. *British Blood Sucking Flies* (Ed. by F. W. Edwards, H. Oldroyd & J. Smart). London: British Museum

Smart, J. (1956). *A Handbook for the Identification of Insects of Medical Importance*. London: British Museum

Swynnerton, C. F. M. (1936). The testse flies of East Africa. *Trans. R. Soc. Lond.* **84**

Stampa, S. (1959). The control of internal parasites of sheep with Neguvon and Asuntol. A preliminary report. *Jl. S. Afr. vet. med Assoc.*, **30**, 19–26

World Health Organization (1963). Insecticide resistance and vector control. 13th Rept. of Expert Committee on Insecticides. *Tech. Rept. Series No.* **265**. Geneva

World Health Organization (1964). Genetics of vectors and insecticide resistance. Rept. of WHO Scientific Group. *Tech. Rept. Series No.* **268**. Geneva

MESOSTIGMATA

Baker, E. W., Evans, T. M., Gould, D. J., Hull, W. B. & Keegan, H. C. (1956). *A Manual of the Mites of Medical or Economic Importance*. New York: National Pest Control Association

Fiedler, O. G. H. (1958). Die Bekämpfung der Rinderzecken in Südafrika. *Vet.-Med. Nachr.*, **3**, 133–146

Harrison, I. R. (1960). The control of poultry red mite with 1-naphthyl-N-methyl carbonate. *Vet. Rec.*, **72**, 298–300

Harrison, I. R. (1961). Further observations on 1-naphthyl-N-methyl carbamate as a veterinary insecticide. *Vet. Rec.*, **73**, 290–293

U.S. Department of Agriculture (1947). *Farm Bulletin No. 980*

IXODIDES

Arthur, D. R. (1962). *Ticks and Disease*. Oxford: Pergamon Press

Arthur, D. R. (1966). The Ecology of ticks with reference to the transmission of Protozoa. *The Biology of Parasites* (Ed. by E. J. L. Soulsby). New York: Academic Press

Barnett, S. V. (1961). The Control of Ticks on Livestock. *FAO Agricultural Series No. 54*. Food and Agriculture Organization of the United Nations, Rome

Bedford, G. A. H. (1932). A synoptic check-list and host-list of the ectoparasites found on South African Mammalia, Aves, and Reptilia. *18th Rept. Dir. Vet. Ser. Anim. Ind. S. Africa*. pp. 223–523

Campbell, J. A. (1953). Studies on the control of the sheep tick, *Ixodes ricinus* L., *Proc. 15th Internat. Vet. Cong.* (Stockholm, Aug. 9–15), **1**, 450–455

FELDMAN-MUHSAM, B. (1954). The identity of *Rhipicephalus sanguineus* in the U.S.A. *J. Parasit.* **39**, 670

GREGSON, J. D. (1958). Host susceptibility to paralysis by the tick *Dermacentor andersoari* Stiles. *Can. Entomol.* **90**, 421–424

GREGSON, J. D. (1959). Tick paralysis in groundhogs, guinea-pigs and hamsters. *Can. J. comp. Med.*, **23**, 266–268

HITCHCOCK, L. F. (1953). Resistance of the cattle tick *B. microplus* (Canestrini) to benzene hexachloride. *Aust. J. agric. Res.*, **4**, 360–364

HOOGSTRAAL, H. (1956). *African Ixodoidea*, Vol. I, *Ticks of the Sudan*. Research Report Naval Medical 005.050.29.07. U.S. Navy

KAISER, M. N. & HOOGSTRAAL, H. (1964). The Hyalomma ticks (Ixodoidea, Ixodidae) of Pakistan, India, and Ceylon, with keys to subgenera and species. *Acarologia*, **6**, 257–286

LEES, A. D. & MILNE, A. (1951). The seasonal and diurnal activities of individual sheep ticks (*Ixodes ricinus* L.). *Parasitology*, **41**, 189–208

MIHAILOV, M. (1957). Incidence of *Ornithodorus lahorensis* and tick paralysis in sheep in Bitola, Yugoslavia. *Vet. Glasn.* **11**, 814–818

MURNAGHAN, M. F. (1958). Tick paralysis; a neurophysiological study. *Proc. 10th Int. Congr. Entomol.* (Montreal, 1956), **3**, 841–847

NEITZ, W. O. (1959). Sweating sickness: The present state of our knowledge. *Onderstepoort J. vet. Res.*, **28**, 3–38

NEITZ, W. O. (1956). A consolidation of our knowledge of the transmission of tick-borne disease. *Onderstepoort J. vet. Res.*, **27**, 115–163

ROSE, I. R. & GREGSON, J. D. (1956). Evidence of a neuromuscular block in tick paralysis. *Nature, Lond.*, **178**, 95–96

ROUSSELOT, R. (1953). *Notes de Parasitologie Tropicale*, Vol. II, Ixodes. Paris: Vigot Freres

STAMPA, S. & DU TOIT, A. (1958). Paralysis of stock due to the karoo paralysis tick *I. rubicundus*. *S. Afr. J. Sci.* **54**, 241–246

SEDDON, H. R. (1951). *Diseases of Animals in Australia*, Part 3, *Tick and Mite Infestations*. Publication No. 7 Commonwealth of Australia Department Health Service Publications

THEILER, G. (1950). Zoological survey of the Union of South Africa: tick survey. VI. *Onderstepoort J. vet. Sci.*, **24**, 34–52

WILKINSON, P. R. (1965). A first record of paralysis of a deer by *Dermacentor andersoni* (Stiles) and notes on the 'host potential' of deer in British Columbia. *Proc. ent. Soc. Brit. Columbia*, **62**, 28–30

WOOD, J. C., SPARROW, W. B., PAGE, K. W. & BROWN, P. P. M. (1960). The use of Dieldrin, Aldrin and Delnav for the control of the sheep tick *Ixodes ricinus*. *Vet. Rec.*, **72**, 98–101

ZUMPT, F. (1958). A preliminary survey of the distribution and host specificity of ticks (Ixodoidea) in the Bechuanaland Protectorate. *Bull. Ent. Res.*, **49**, 201–223

TROMBIDIFORMES

BAKER, W. E., EVANS, T. M., GOULD, D. J., HALL, W. B. & KEEGAN, H. C. (1956). *A Manual of the Mites of Medical or Economic Importance*. New York: National Pest Control Association

FIEDLER, D. G. H. & DU TOIT, R. (1955). Some observations on the control of the itch mite of sheep (*Psoregates ovis* Womersley). *Jl. S. Afr. vet. med. Ass.*, **2**, 231–235

HART, C. B. & MALONE, J. C. (1958). The occurrence of the rabbit fur mite *Cheyletiella parasitivora* (Megnin 1878) on the dog. *Vet. Rec.*, **70**, 991–993

HUGHES, T. E. (1959). *Mites or the Acari*. University of London, The Athlone Press

KOUTZ, F. R. (1955). *Demodex folliculorum* studies. IV. Treatment methods. *North Am. Vet.*, **36**, 129–131, 136

ROBERTS I. H., & MELENEY, W. P. (1965). Psorerogatic acariasis of cattle. *J. Am. vet. med. Ass.*, **146**, 17–23

SKERMAN, K. D., GRAHAM, N. P. H., SINCLAIR, A. N. & MURRAY, M. D. (1960). *Psorergates ovis*—the itch mite of sheep. *Aust. vet. J.*, **36**, 317–321

TILL, W. M. (1960). *Psorergates oettlei* n. sp., a new mange-causing mite from the multimammate rat (Acarina, Psorergatidae). *Acarologia*, **2**, 75–79

TURK, R. D. (1959). Parasitic dermatoses. *Canine Medicine* (Ed. by M. A. Fincher, W. J. Gibbons K. Mayer & S. E. Parks,) 2nd edn. Amer. Vet. Publ., Santa Barbara, California: American Veterinary Publications

WOMERSLEY, H. (1941). Notes on the Cheyletidae (Acarina, Trombidoidea) of Australia and New Zealand, with descriptions of new species. *Rec. South Aus. Mus.* **7**, 51–64

WORLD HEALTH ORGANIZATION (1958). Insect resistance and vector control. *Tech. Rept Series No.* **153**. Geneva

SARCOPTIFORMES

CROSS, R. F. & FOLGER, G. C. (1956). The use of malathion on cats and birds. *J. Am. vet. med. Ass.*, **129**, 65–66

ENGLISH, P. B. (1960). Notoedric mange in cats with observations on treatment with Malathion. *Aust. Vet. J.*, **36**, (3) 85–88

LAVOIPIERRE, M. M. J. (1958). Some mites responsible for skin disease in birds. *Trans. R. Soc. trop. Med. Hyg.*, **52**, 300

LAVOIPIERRE, M. M. J. & GRIFFITHS, R. B. (1951). A preliminary note on a new species of *Cnemidocoptes* (Ascarina) causing scaly leg in a budgerigar (*Melopsittacus undulatus*) in Great Britain. *Ann. trop. Med. Parasitol.*, **42**, 253–254

MELLANBY, K. (1952). *Scabies.* Oxford University Press

OLDHAM, J. N. & BERESFORD-JONES, W. P. (1954). Observations on the occurrence of *Cnemidooptes pilae.* (Lavoipierre and Griffiths, 1951) in Budgerigars and a Parakeet. *Br. vet. J.*, **110**, 29–30

SWEATMAN, K. (1957). Life history, non-specificity, and revision of the genus *Choreoptes* a parasitic mite of herbivores. *Can. J. Zool.*, **35**, 641–689

SWEATMAN, G. K. (1958). Biology of *Otodectes cynotis*, the ear canker mite of carnivores. *Can. J. Zool.*, **36**, 849–862

SWEATMAN, G. K. (1958b). On the life history and validity of the species in *Psoroptes*, a genus of mange mites. *Can. J. Zool.*, **36**, 905–929

PROTOZOA

Protozoa

THE protozoa are unicellular animals in which the various activities of metabolism, locomotion, etc., are carried out by organelles of the cell. Comparable forms in the plant kingdom are the protophyta (unicellular plants), and, in general, protozoa are differentiated from these by the absence of chlorophyll-containing chromatophores and their mode of nutrition (holozoic). The protophyta are frequently bounded by a fairly rigid cell wall made of cellulose, and the nuclear material is often dispersed in the cell. The protozoa, on the other hand, have a well defined nucleus and do not have a rigid cell wall, allowing, at times, a marked variation in size and shape. Nevertheless, these distinctions cannot be rigidly applied to all forms, and there is an assemblage of organisms which share the characters of both plants and animals. The term *protista* was introduced for such forms, but this has not been generally adopted.

Since the discovery of protozoa by Antoni van Leeuwenhoek, some 30,000 species have been described. The majority of these are free living and are found in almost every habitat on land and in water. Though the parasitic protozoa are smaller in numbers, they nevertheless assume an important role as producers of global disease which, apart from producing death or deformity, sap the energy and initiative and decay the moral fibre of mankind in many parts of the world. Of no less importance is the untold loss of livestock and livestock products which is frequently a burden in those communities and areas of the world that can least support it.

Structure of Protozoa

Nucleus

Usually only one nucleus is present, though in some forms more than one nucleus may be present in some or all stages of development. The *vesicular* type of nucleus consists of a nuclear membrane which bounds the nucleoplasm in which, lying more or less central, is an intranuclear body, the endosome (or karyosome) or the nucleolus. An endosome is devoid of deoxyribonucleic acid, whereas a nucleolus does possess DNA. Chromatin material (Feulgen positive for DNA) frequently occurs on the inner surface of the nuclear membrane and may also be seen as strands radiating from the karyosome to the nuclear membrane.

The vesicular type of nucleus is seen most commonly in the Mastigophora and the Rhizopoda.

The *compact* type of nucleus contains a large amount of chromatin and a small amount of nucleoplasm. This type is found in the ciliates as a macronucleus, it divides amitotically and regulates the cytoplasmic functions of the organism.

Cytoplasm

This is the extranuclear part of the protozoan cell. It may be differentiated into an outer ectoplasm and an inner endoplasm, the former often being homogeneous and hyaline in appearance and the latter frequently containing granules, vacuoles and sometimes pigment. In some forms (e.g. Rhizopoda) there is no definite limiting membrane, but usually a pellicle serves as such in the majority of species.

Locomotion

Protozoa may move by gliding, or by means of pseudopodia, flagella or cilia.

Gliding is seen in Toxoplasma, Sarcocystis and other forms, this being achieved without the aid of cilia or flagella.

Pseudopodia are used by the amoeba-like organisms, the structures being temporary locomotor organelles which are formed when required and retracted when not needed.

Flagella are whiplike filamentous structures which arise from a basal granule or kinetoplast in the cytoplasm of the organism. They are composed of a central axial filament, the axoneme, which is surrounded by a contractile cytoplasmic sheath. Ultrastructure studies indicate the axoneme to be composed of two central filaments surrounded by nine peripheral filaments. In some forms the flagellum may be attached to the body of the protozoan by an undulating membrane. Flagella are most commonly seen in the Mastigophora.

Cilia are fine, short, flagella-like structures originating from a kinetosome embedded in the pellicle or ectoplasm. They are the organs of locomotion in the ciliates, but they may also aid in the ingestion of food or serve as tactile structures. Their ultrastructure is similar to that of the flagella, and they usually occur in large numbers, being arranged in rows over the body of the protozoan.

Organelles for Nutrition

In the amoeba-like forms particulate food material is acquired by means of pseudopodia. An advance on this is a specialised opening called the cytostome through which food particles are engulfed and passed to food vacuoles. In the ciliates the cytostome may be lined with cilia which further assist in the ingestion of food.

Food vacuoles occur in the cytoplasm and contain particulate material in various stages of digestion. Non-digestible material may be extruded from the cell either via a temporary opening or through a permanent cytopyge.

Excretion of waste products may occur directly through the body wall or by means of contractile vacuoles which periodically discharge waste material through the body wall or, in a few instances, through an anal pore.

Nutrition of Protozoa

Nutrition may be holophytic, holozoic or saprozoic.

The *holophytic* protozoa are forms which possess some characteristics of plants, carbohydrates being synthesised by chlorophyll which is carried in chromatophores or in the bodies of algae or other protophyta which inhabit the cytoplasm of the protozoan. None of these forms are of medical or veterinary importance.

The *holozoic* protozoa utilise preformed food material derived from living animals or plants. Food material is ingested by pseudopodia or through a cytostome and passes to a food vacuole for digestion. Some forms (e.g. *Entamoeba, Balantidium*) ingest the tissue cells of the hosts.

The *saprozoic* protozoa absorb nutrients through the body wall, these being utilised directly by the organisms.

Stored food material may be visible as glycogen granules or chromatoid material.

Reproduction of Protozoa

Binary fission is the commonest form of asexual reproduction. In this two daughter cells result from a 'parent' cell, division being along the longitudinal axis, though in ciliates it is along the transverse axis. The nucleus divides first and cytoplasmic division follows.

In *multiple fission* or *schizogony* the nucleus divides several times before the cytoplasm does. In some of the sporozoans the nucleus of the parent cell divides mitotically into a large number of nuclear bodies, each of which becomes associated with a portion of cytoplasm and little or nothing of the parent cell remains except the greatly expanded limiting membrane. The dividing form is known as a schizont, and the daughter forms are merozoites. Schizogony is an asexual form of reproduction.

Budding is an asexual reproductive process in which two or many daughter forms are produced by the 'parent' cell. There is usually an unequal fragmentation of the nucleus and cytoplasm, but the budded forms are separated off and then grow to full size.

Conjugation is a form of sexual reproduction which occurs in the ciliates. In this two organisms pair and exchange nuclear material (from the micronucleus). The individuals separate and nuclear reorganisation takes place.

Syngamy is sexual reproduction in which two gametes fuse to form a zygote. The male gamete is a microgamete and the female a macro-gamete which are produced from microgametocytes and macrogameto-cytes, respectively. The process of gamete formation is gametogony, and the gametes may be similar in size (isogamy) or may markedly differ (anisogamy).

Sporogony normally follows syngamy, and a number of, or very many, sporozoites are formed within the walls of a cyst. This is an asexual pro-cess of multiple fission.

Classification of Protozoa

CLASS: MASTIGOPHORA
One or more flagella.

SUBCLASS: PHYTOMASTIGINA
With chromatophores. Nutrition holophytic. (Of no veterinary or medical importance.)

SUBCLASS: ZOOMASTIGINA
Without chromatophores. Nutrition holozoic.

ORDER: PROTOMONADIDA
One or two flagella.

FAMILY: TRYPANOSOMATIDAE
ORDER: POLYMASTIGIDA
Three to eight flagella.

FAMILY: TRICHOMONADIDAE
ORDER: RHIZOMASTIGIDA
One to three flagella and pseudopodia.

FAMILY: MASTIGAMOEBIDAE
ORDER: HYPERMASTIGIDA
Many flagella. (Of no veterinary or medical importance.)

CLASS: SARCODINA
Have pseudopodia, rarely flagella.

SUBCLASS: RHIZOPODA
FAMILY: ENDAMOEBIDAE
Parasitic amoebae.

CLASS: SPOROZOA

No organs of locomotion (except in gamete stages). Produce cysts. Reproduction asexual and sexual. Parasitic.

SUBCLASS: CNIDOSPORIDIA
Spores with polar filament. (Of no veterinary or medical importance.)

SUBCLASS: ACNIDOSPORIDIA
Spores without polar filament. One sporozoite produced. (Of no veterinary or medical importance.)

SUBCLASS: TELOSPORIDIA
Spores without polar filament. One or many sporozoites produced.

ORDER: COCCIDIA
Trophozoites intracellular, zygote non-motile. Sporozoites enclosed.

FAMILY: EIMERIIDAE
Gametocytes develop independently.

FAMILY: HAEMOGREGARINIDAE
Gametocytes develop attached to each other.

ORDER: HAEMOSPORIDIA
Schizogony in vertebrate host, sporogony in invertebrate host. Zygote motile.

FAMILY: PLASMODIIDAE
With the characters of the order. Pigment formed from host cell haemoglobin.

FAMILY: HAEMOPROTEIDAE
Schizogony in the endothelial cell of inner organs. Pigment produced.

FAMILY: BABESIIDAE
Small, nonpigment-producing forms of erythrocytes.

FAMILY: THEILERIIDAE
Small, pleomorphic forms of erythrocytes. Schizogony in lymphocytes or histiocytes.

CLASS: CILIATA
Possess cilia. Two types of nucleus, micronucleus and macronucleus.
FAMILY: BALANTIDIIDAE

ORGANISMS OF UNCERTAIN CLASSIFICATION

ENCEPHALITOZOON BESNOITIA
TOXOPLASMA SARCOCYSTIS

CLASS: MASTIGOPHORA Diesing, 1866

The *Mastigophora* are flagellate protozoa possessing one or more thread-like flagella. In some forms a flagellum may pass along the body, being attached to it by an undulating membrane (e.g. *Trypanosoma, Trichomonas*). The nucleus is usually vesicular and reproduction is generally by longitudinal binary fission. In a few parasitic forms encystation may occur, and this is a common phenomenon in the large number of the free-living forms, which make up the major part of the group.

The neuromotor apparatus consists of a granular blepharoplast or basal granule from which arises the axoneme. Electron micrographs indicate that the axoneme forms the axial structure of the flagellum and consists (in trypanosomes) of two central and nine peripheral fibrils. These are surrounded by a flagellar sheath which extends to the distal end of the axoneme. Closely posterior to the blepharoplast there is often a deeply staining granule, the kinetoplast. Under the electron microscope this structure is seen to consist of lamellae or a spiral and is considered by some to be mitochondrial in function. In the case of *Trypanosoma mega*, Steinert (1963) considers it responsible for the synthesis of DNA and the provision of genetic information for the synthesis of mitachondrial enzymes.

The Mastigophora are divided into two major groups, the *Phytomastigina* and the *Zoomastigina*. The Phytomastigina possess chromatophores, which contain chlorophyll, responsible for the synthesis of organic compounds from inorganic materials. Their nutrition is said to be *holophytic*, and the Phytomastigina are of no veterinary or medical importance. The Zoomastigina lack chromatophores and they feed in a *holozoic* manner; thus they use organic materials from plants or animals as food.

The Zoomastigina are classified into four orders:

Protomonadida, one or two flagella (e.g. *Trypanosoma*)

Polymastigida, three to eight flagella; one or two nuclei (e.g. *Trichomonas foetus*)

Rhizomastigida, one to three flagella and pseudopodia (e.g. *Histomonas meleagridis*)

Hypermastigida, many flagella. Parasites of termites and cockroaches. Of no veterinary importance.

ORDER: PROTOMONADIDA BLOCHMAN, 1895

FAMILY: TRYPANOSOMATIDAE DOLFEIN, 1901

Members of this family, the trypanosomes, are all parasitic and were originally parasites of the alimentary canal of insects. Now, many are found in the blood and/or tissues of mammals and birds. They are characteristically leaf-like in shape; they have a single flagellum and this is attached to the body of the organism by an undulating membrane.

During their life-cycle at least one further developmental stage is undergone (with the exception of a few mammalian forms), the various stages being morphologically distinct. Some confusion may arise, however, in that the descriptive names for the developmental stages are also used as the genetic names for other members of the family.

Developmental stages

Trypanosome stage, a blade-like form with a kinetoplast posterior to the nucleus and usually near the posterior extremity. An undulating membrane is well developed and a free flagellum is often present. This stage is usually found in the vertebrate host but it is also found in arthropods as the infective stage for the vertebrate host.

Crithidial stage. The kinetoplast and axoneme lie anterior to the nucleus and the undulating membrane is short. In a few species this stage is found in the vertebrate as part of the vertebrate developmental cycle but it is principally a stage in arthropods.

Leptomonad stage. The kinetoplast and axoneme are at the anterior tip of the body. There is no undulating membrane. It is found in arthropods or plants.

Leishmania stage. The body is rounded; a flagellum is absent or is represented by a short fibril; the kinetoplast is present. The body is found in vertebrates and arthropods.

The family includes the following genera:

Trypanosoma, occurs in vertebrates and arthropods; development may include the trypanosome, crithidial, leptomonad and leishmania stages. In many species, only the trypanosome stage occurs in the vertebrate host, but in a few more primitive forms, leishmanial and crithidial stages occur in the vertebrate.

Herpetomonas, found in invertebrates. Development may include the trypanosome, crithidial, leptomonad and leishmania stages.

Crithidia, found in arthropods and other invertebrates. Developmental stages include crithidia and leptomonads.

Leptomonas, found in invertebrates. Developmental stages include leptomonads and leishmania.

Phytomonas, found in plants and arthropods. Developmental stages include leptomonads and leishmania.

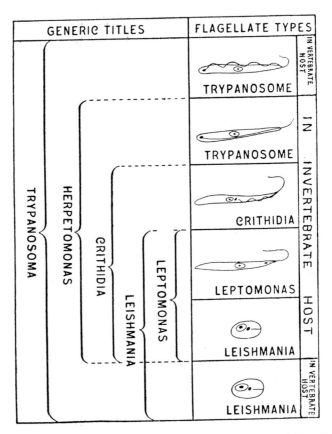

Fig. 267. Diagram of Classification of the Trypanosomes and Allied Flagellates. (From Wenyon, 1926)

Leishmania, found in vertebrates and arthropods. Developmental stages include leishmania and leptomonads, the latter in the invertebrate.

Most of the members of the Trypanosomatidae undergo cyclical development. In those genera of veterinary importance (e.g. *Trypanosoma, Leishmania*), the life-cycle alternates between the vertebrate and the invertebrate host. When the invertebrate host is infected from the vertebrate host, a cycle of development and multiplication takes place in the invertebrate host, usually involving a developmental stage different from that in the vertebrate host. Thus in the genus *Trypanosoma*, the trypanosome form occurs in the vertebrate but it is the crithidial form which predominates in the arthropod host.

Since the developmental stages of several genera may occur in invertebrates, it is not possible, with certainty, to identify any individual developmental stages as belonging to any specific genus. The stage may be a true parasite of the invertebrate or a developmental stage of a mammalian pathogen in the invertebrate.

Genus: Trypanosoma Gruby, 1843

Members of this genus occur in vertebrates, principally in the blood and tissue fluids, although a few may invade tissue cells. They are transmitted by blood-sucking arthropods in which the developmental stages mentioned above occur. A few species are transmitted mechanically; that is, there is no cyclical development in an arthropod.

Cyclical development may be 'anterior station' or 'posterior station' in type. In the former, developmental stages (e.g. crithidia) multiply in the gut of the arthropod, and infective stages, metacyclic trypanosomes (which are smaller than the vertebrate forms), accumulate in the mouth parts or salivary glands so that infection is transmitted when the arthropod takes a blood meal. This is the inoculative method of transmission. In the 'posterior station' forms, the metacyclic trypanosomes accumulate in the hindgut and are passed in the faeces of the arthropod. Infection of the vertebrate occurs by contamination of the skin or skin wounds.

Any trypanosome can be transmitted mechanically without cyclical changes taking place. Experimentally, this can be done by 'syringe passage' and in nature it is accomplished by blood-sucking insects (and possibly also vampire bats) which feed several times on different animals before repletion. There are a few species, however, where the ability to undergo cyclical development in arthropods has been lost and mechanical transmission is the only means available.

Hoare (1964) has divided the genus into two sections as follows:

Stercoraria (Posterior Station Group; Lewisi Group; Group A)

Morphology. Kinetoplast large and not terminal, posterior extremity tapering, free flagellum present, undulating membrane not well developed.

Biology. Multiplication in vertebrate host discontinuous: may occur in trypanosome, crithidial or leishmanial forms. Metacyclic trypanosomes in 'posterior station' in arthropod host and transmitted by contamination through faeces. Often nonpathogenic. Blood forms with a high respiratory quotient and low sugar consumption. Cyanide inhibits oxygen consumption.

Four subgenera are recognised by Hoare, namely *Megatrypanum*,

Herpetosoma, Schizotrypanum, and *Endotrypanum.* Only the first three contain forms of veterinary or medical importance, these being indicated in Table 6.

TABLE 6. STERCORARIA

Subgenus	Species	Vertebrate hosts	Arthropod hosts	Stage in which multiplication occurs in vertebrate hosts
Megatrypanum	*Trypanosoma theileri*	Cattle	Tabanid flies	Crithidia (binary fission)
	Trypanosoma melophagium	Sheep	Ked (*Melophagus ovinus*)	Uncertain
Herpetosoma	*Trypanosoma lewisi*	Rats	Fleas	Crithidia (multiple fission)
	Trypanosoma duttoni	Mice	Fleas	Crithidia (multiple fission)
	Trypanosoma nabiasi	Rabbits	Fleas	Leishmania (multiple fission)
Schizotrypanum	*Trypanosoma cruzi*	Man, dog, cat, armadillo, opossum etc.	Bugs	Leishmania (binary fission)
	Trypanosoma rangeli	Dogs, opossum etc.	Bugs	Trypanosome (binary fission)
	*Trypanosoma avium**	Rooks, jackdaws etc.	Hippoboscid flies	? May not multiply, only get larger

* This species and others from birds do not readily lend themselves to classification. See text later.

Salivaria (Anterior Station Group; Group B)

Morphology. Kinetoplast smaller, terminal or subterminal. Posterior extremity blunt, there may be no free flagellum, undulating membrane varying in development.

Biology. Multiplication in vertebrate host continuous in the trypanosome stage. Metacyclic trypanosomes in the 'anterior station' of the arthropod host, and transmission is by inoculation. Frequently highly pathogenic. Some species are atypical and are transmitted *non*cyclically by arthropods or by coitus. Four subgenera are recognised by Hoare, namely *Duttonella, Nannomonas, Pycnomonas* and *Trypanozoon.* All four contain species of veterinary and medical importance, which are detailed below:

Subgenus: Duttonella

Kinetoplast terminal. Posterior end of body rounded, poorly developed undulating membrane, free flagellum present, shows great motility, monomorphic. Development occurs in the proboscis of *Glossina* spp. only. Blood forms have a low respiratory quotient and high sugar utilisation.

The species include:
Trypanosoma vivax (long forms) in cattle, sheep, goat, antelope.
Tyrpanosoma uniforme (short forms) in cattle, sheep, goat, antelope.

Subgenus: Nannomonas

Kinetoplast marginal. Small size, no free flagellum, undulating membrane moderately developed, monomorphic and polymorphic. Development in midgut and then in proboscis of *Glossina* spp. Blood forms have high respiratory quotient and low sugar utilisation. Cyanide inhibits oxygen consumption.
The species include:

Trypanosoma congolense, monomorphic (short forms), in cattle, sheep, horses, pigs.
Trypanosoma dimorphon, monomorphic (long forms), in cattle, sheep, horses, pigs.
Trypanosoma simiae, polymorphic in pigs, cattle, horses.

Subgenus: Pycnomonas

Monomorphic, stout and short species: kinetoplast small, subterminal, free flagellum short. Development in midgut and salivary glands of *Glossina* spp. One species of importance: *Trypanosoma suis*, in pigs.

Subgenus: Trypanozoon

Monomorphic or polymorphic. In latter, long, intermediate and stumpy forms occur with long free flagellum, short free flagellum and no flagellum respectively. Undulating membrane well-developed, kinetoplast small and subterminal. Blood forms have low respiratory quotient, low sugar utilisation. Cyanide does not inhibit oxygen consumption.
For the purpose of this book the subgenus can be divided into two subgroups depending on the biology:

A. Cyclical development in midgut and salivary glands of *Glossina* spp.
Species include:

Trypanosoma brucei (polymorphic), in domestic animals and antelopes.
Trypanosoma rhodesiense (polymorphic), in man and antelopes.
Trypanosoma gambiense (polymorphic), in man.

B. No cyclical development in arthropod, transmission mechanical.
Species include:
Trypanosoma evansi (polymorphism inconstant), in cattle, camels, equines, dogs etc.
Trypanosoma equinum (polymorphism inconstant), in equines.
Trypanosoma equiperdum (polymorphism inconstant), in equines.

The Biology of Trypanosomes

In the Definitive Host. No sexual process has been observed in the life-cycle of trypanosomes and all multiplication is by binary or multiple fission. Division commences at the kinetoplast followed by the nucleus and then the cytoplasm. In the Salivaria, division is chiefly in the trypanosome stage in the blood or in the lymph glands. In a few instances other developmental stages have been detected; for example, leishmanial forms have been found in the heart of monkeys infected with *T. brucei* (Noble, 1955). With the Stercoraria, however, reproduction in the crithidial or leishmanial form is usual. *Trypanosoma lewisi* undergoes multiple fission in the crithidial stage producing rosettes of organisms. With *T. cruzi*, multiplication is intracellular, cells of the reticuloendothelial system and the striated muscle, especially of the heart, being filled with leishmanial forms.

As well as the different developmental stages in the several species, polymorphism also occurs and a variation in shape and size is seen. In *T. brucei* the three types (long, intermediate and stumpy forms) have been ascribed an essential role in the biology of the organism. Thus Fairbairn & Culwick (1946) have suggested that in cyclically transmitted strains only the slender forms are capable of division and Wijers & Willett (1960) consider that only the stumpy forms are capable of infecting *Glossina* spp. It is likely, however, that such statements are an oversimplification.

Some species and strains of trypanosomes can be adapted to abnormal hosts by serial subpassage (Desowitz, 1963). This may be a short or prolonged process but is associated with an increasing virulence for the new host. Rat strains of *T. vivax* have been established by supplementing rats with sheep serum and ultimately the dependence on sheep serum has been lost (after 37 subpassages). Such strains produce lethal infections in the rat (Desowitz & Watson, 1953). Studies with *T. lewisi* in mice by Lincicome (1957) have shown that as little as 0·01 ml. of rat serum would support *T. lewisi* in the normally refractive mouse. In such cases, the infection has been passaged by mechanical means and it is not known whether the same can be accomplished with forms which are passaged through the arthropod vector. In fact, a loss of ability to infect the arthropod host, and to undergo cyclical development in it, are features of cyclically transmitted forms which are transmitted continuously by mechanical means. The loss of ability to undergo cyclical transmission is unexplained though the associated loss of polymorphism, especially the loss of the stumpy forms (of *T. brucei*), may deplete the system of forms capable of infecting insects. A loss of virulence for the normal host when organisms are passaged in a new host is not an invariable event with all species or strains, though it is a common phenomenon especially when the passage is by mechanical means. Cyclical maintenance in an abnormal host may preserve normal host infectivity for long periods and *T. rhodesiense* has been passaged cyclically in sheep for 18·5 years without losing its infectivity for man (Ashcroft, 1959). Similar reports exist of its maintenance in antelope and monkeys for several years.

Physiological alterations include an increased oxygen uptake and a similar, but not so marked, increase in glucose utilisation. These differences are quantitative rather than qualitative, the oxidative metabolism apparently being similar in long-adapted strains and newly isolated cyclical strains (Grant & Fulton, 1957). Since fulminating infection occurs with adapted strains it is not surprising that metabolism is at a higher level.

Alterations in drug sensitivity may be marked and may lead to difficulty in drug testing and development. An increase in sensitivity to drugs may be spectacular and this is illustrated with *T. rhodesiense* which develops an increased sensitivity to arsenical compounds on mechanical passage in abnormal hosts. Desowitz (1956) found that the rat-adapted *T. vivax* was 15 times more sensitive to antrycide than the normal sheep strain.

The immunological changes consequent to mechanical passage in the laboratory host have provided a fertile field for study. The principal feature of artificially maintained strains is the apparent unlimited ability of them to produce relapse strains with different antigenic characteristics. This is a feature of both natural and artificial passaged strains and were it to continue unmitigated the essential species characteristic would be lost. However, under natural conditions a limitation is imposed on this, and the antigenic variation is reversible and is stabilised by cyclical transmission through the *Glossina* fly (Broom & Brown, 1940; Gray, 1963; Willett, 1961). Antigenic variation is related to antibody production in an infected animal and during the course of infection a series of antibody peaks coincide with development of a new variant organism. However each antibody peak is specific for the preceding strain of organism and not the strain which co-exists with the antibody. Using newer techniques, especially the preservation of strains in liquid nitrogen, more than twenty such strains have been demonstrated in the *Trypanozoon* subgenus (*Brucei* group). The production of such variants from a clone indicates that antigenic mutation is a principal mechanism for this. Work by Weitz (1963) has demonstrated that the antigens of the *Brucei* group of organisms are variable, some being species- or strain-specific while others are common to the species and strains of the group as a whole. Work with the agglutination test (Cunningham & Vickerman, 1961) and the precipitating reaction (Weitz, 1960; Gray, 1960) has greatly advanced knowledge on trypanosome antigens. Using these tests, two major antigenic components have been identified, a soluble 'exoantigen' which is present in the plasma of infected animals and 'bound' antigens which are liberated when the organisms are disintegrated. The exoantigen is not solely a surface substance but is liberated continuously into the surrounding fluid medium. The exoantigen stimulates agglutinating antibodies for homologous trypanosomes and it precipitates only with homologous antiserum; furthermore, when mice or rats are immunised with it they are protected against infection with the homologous organisms but not with heterologous species or strains (Weitz, 1962).

The bound antigens, though they contain exoantigens, are distinct from them. While the exoantigen appears to be species-specific the bound antigens may give cross reactions with other species, e.g. *T. brucei* with *T. vivax* (Weitz, 1963). When mice are immunised with bound antigen of one species a degree of protection is induced for another species.

The chemical nature of the antigens of trypanosomes has received attention from Brown (1963). Electrophoretic studies of trypanosome homogenates on starch gel revealed up to 11 components consisting of a nuclear protein-nucleic acid material, four slowly moving components and six more components. These could be divided into two main groups according to their resistance to heat, protease and periodate oxidation. An S-4 component (m.w. $4\text{-}8 \times 10^4$) and an S-1 component (m.w. $1\text{-}2 \times 10^4$) were identified, but these were essentially similar in two un-related strains and their antigenic variants (Brown & Williamson, 1962; Williamson & Brown, 1963; Weitz, 1963). The latter author comments that the changes in antigenicity are perhaps still too subtle for chemical determination by existing methods.

Though a detailed antigenic analysis of the pathogenic trypanosomes has only recently caught the imagination, studies on the antibody response to *T. lewisi* in the rat have been carried on for many years. In the rat, parasitaemia increases rapidly to about the 10th day after the infection when a crisis occurs, reducing the number of organisms in the circulation. The remainder survive for a longer time but are finally removed by a second crisis. The two periods of reduction of parasitaemia are due to circulating lytic antibody. However, Taliaferro (1923, 1932) has recog-nised a further substance, in addition to the lytic antibody, which speci-fically inhibits the reproduction of the parasites. It has no effect on the viability or infectivity of the organisms (Taliaferro, 1948) and has been given the name of 'ablastin.' Transfer of *T. lewisi* organisms along with ablastin to a new host prevents division of the organism in the new host. Ablastin is transferable from mother to offspring through the milk. A remarkable character of it is that it is not absorbable *in vitro* from immune serum with dividing forms of the organism. Ablastin is a 7S type of globulin similar to the first lysin whereas the terminal lysin is 19S in character. Ablastin greatly reduces nucleic acid synthesis (Pizzi & Taliaferro, 1960) and by about the 10th day of infection this is completely inhibited. Protein synthesis though reduced by the 10th day continues to decrease for some time. Taliaferro suggests that ablastin is a very weakly avid antibody and its continued presence in large amounts is necessary to maintain an adequate anti-reproductive effect.

Recently, however, Ormerod (1963) has advanced a counter-hypothesis suggesting that two antigens are concerned in the immune mechanism to *T. lewisi*, the developmental forms and the adult trypanosomes possessing separate and unrelated antigens. He suggests that dividing forms stimulate antibody which eventually eliminates them from the blood leaving the adult forms to survive until they, too, are removed by the second antibody crisis. The debate on the nature of ablastin has still to be resolved and further details of this should be sought in Ormerod (1963) and Taliaferro (1963). Other discussions on the immunology and biology of trypanosomes will be found in Weitz (1963).

In Insect Vector. With the exception of a few species, the majority of trypanosomes undergo cyclical development in an arthropod vector. When non-cyclical transmission (mechanical) occurs it is usually by the agency of biting-flies such as *Stomaxys* and *Tabanus*. The biting-fly is immediately infective after feeding but it remains so for a short time only and must feed on another animal very soon if the trypanosomes are to be transmitted. *Trypanosoma evansi* and *T. equinum* are solely transmitted in this way while *T. equiperdum* is transmitted mechanically by coitus. It should be stressed that even the cyclical forms may be transmitted mechanically and even by the arthropod in which they also develop cyclically.

In cyclical development, mammalian blood containing the trypanosomes is taken into the intestine of the arthropod and subsequent development depends on whether 'anterior' or 'posterior' station development occurs.

Anterior Station Development. This is exemplified by trypanosomes of the *Trypanozoon* (*brucei*) group. Ingested forms localise in the posterior part of the midgut of *Glossina* where they multiply in the trypanosome stage for the first 10 days. It has already been noted that the stumpy forms of a polymorphic population are possibly those which are destined for cyclical development. Initially, the dividing forms in the midgut are broad with a kinetoplast midway between the nucleus and the posterior end. By the 10th–11th day, however, long slender forms are produced and these migrate backwards and enter the space around the peritrophic membrane and then penetrate into the proventriculus, being found here 12–20 days after infection. They subsequently migrate anteriorly to the oesophagus and pharynx and then to the hypopharynx and salivary glands. In this latter situation, crithidial forms are produced and further multiplication takes place. In another 2–5 days the metacyclic or infective forms are produced. Metacyclic trypanosomes are small stumpy forms which somewhat resemble the stumpy forms in the blood. These are injected into the host along with saliva when the fly bites, several thousand being injected with each bite.

The developmental cycle of *T. brucei* in *Glossina morsitans* takes 25 days or more and flies are not infective until the metacyclic forms have been produced. A detailed account of factors which modify this infection rate and the species of flies which are concerned will be found in Buxton (1955).

If a trypanosome is transmitted by one species of *Glossina* then it is probably transmissible by all species (Hornby, 1952). Thus all species of *Glossina* which have been investigated appear capable of transmitting *T. vivax*, *T. congolense* and *T. brucei*. The differences in transmission by various species in nature are largely due to factors which determine the prevalance of the species of *Glossina*; e.g. host, feeding, climate, etc. (see Buxton, 1955).

Posterior Station Development. This is exemplified by *Trypanosoma lewisi* of the rat. Ingested trypanosomes enter cells which line the stomach of the rat flea, *Ceratophyllus fasciatus*. Within the cells the trypanosomes round up to pear-shaped organisms which increase in size while the nuclei and kinetoplasts divide, ultimately giving a large number of trypanosome forms. The cells rupture and the liberated trypanosome stages pass from the stomach to the rectal region. During this migration they change to crithidial forms, the kinetoplast being displaced anterior to the nucleus. The crithidial stages attach themselves to the lining cells of the posterior gut, multiply as crithidia and then produce metacyclic trypanosomes. The total cycle takes about 5 days in the rat flea. Metacyclic trypanosomes are passed in the faeces and infection of another rat is by contamination of a flea bite wound with faeces. Alternatively the infected flea may be ingested and then the metacyclic trypanosomes penetrate the mucous membrane of the digestive tract.

The Pathogenic Trypanosomes of Domestic Animals

Section: Salivaria (Anterior Station Forms)

Subgenus: Duttonella (Vivax Group)

Trypanosoma vivax Zieman, 1905 (syn. *T. cazalboui*; *T. caprae*; *T. angolense*, etc.). This is a monomorphic species, 20 μ–27 μ (average 22·5 μ) by 3 μ. The posterior part is distinctly broader and bulbous, the kinetoplast is large and terminal and the free flagellum is short, being 3–6 μ in length. The organism is very motile in fresh blood, moving rapidly across the field pushing red cells aside as it goes.

Its hosts include cattle, sheep, goats, camels, horses; but dogs and pigs are refractory to infection. In Africa antelopes serve as reservoir hosts and in South America deer act as such. Laboratory rodents are not readily infected, though white rats can be infected if the infection is supplemented with sheep blood (Desowitz, 1963).

Geographically it occurs throughout Africa being transmitted by tsetse flies (especially *Glossina morsitans* and *Glossina tachinoides*), development taking place in the anterior station and in the proboscis only. It is also established in Central and South America, the West Indies and Mauritius where it is transmitted mechanically by biting-flies. Despite the wide geographical locations, the African and South American strains are very similar.

Cattle are the principal hosts affected. The parasite generally causes a mild disease in cattle in East Africa but in West Africa more pathogenic entities are seen (Fairbairn, 1953). Virulence differs with strain and the strain characteristics tend to remain constant. In sheep, *T. vivax* has a moderate virulence and central nervous system complications sometimes occur. In goats virulence usually is low. In horses a chronic disease with spontaneous recovery is produced. This consists of a mild to moderate anaemia, progressive weakness and emaciation with oedema of the sub-cutaneous tissues. Pathogenicity is low in the camel.

Diagnosis of infection is best done by lymph node smears. Though early infections are characterised by a high parasitaemia, organisms are difficult to find in the more chronic infections. Sheep may be inoculated with blood and in these the prepatent period for the appearance of organisms is 7 to 10 days.

Trypanosoma uniforme Bruce *et al.*, 1911. This is similar to *T. vivax* with an average length of 16 μ (12–20 μ) by 1·5 μ–2·5 μ. The free flagellum is shorter than that of *T. vivax*. It infects cattle, sheep, goats, and antelope but is not transmissible to laboratory rodents. It occurs in Uganda and the Congo, being transmitted cyclically by tsetse flies. The disease process is similar to that produced by *T. vivax*, but it is more or less nonpathogenic for goats.

Subgenus: Nannomonas (Congolese Group)

Trypanosoma congolense Broden, 1904 (syn. *T. pecorum*; *T. nanum*; *T. montgomeryi*). This is a small monomorphic form, 9 μ–18 μ in length and it is the smallest of the African trypanosomes. The posterior extremity is blunt and the kinetoplast is typically marginal being some distance from the posterior end. Characteristically there is no free flagellum though the tapering anterior extremity may, inadvertently, give the appearance of one. Though the undulating membrane is inconspicuous the organism is active and it exhibits marked but non-progressive movements in fresh blood.

Its hosts include all domestic animals, and wild game animals such as antelope, zebra, warthog, and even the elephant, may act as reservoir hosts. The organism is readily transmitted to laboratory rodents. However, its chief association is with cattle and it is the principal cause of the disease 'nagana', this name being derived from a Zulu word meaning 'to be in low or depressed spirits'. It was used by the Zulus to describe trypanosomiasis in cattle, and Bruce, in 1898, brought the word into common usage. The parasite is renowned for the great number of strains which occur; these differ both in virulence and antigenicity.

Geographically *T. congolense* is widely distributed in tropical Africa and is transmitted cyclically by several *Glossina* spp. Different species of *Glossina* are of importance in different areas. Thus *G. morsitans* is more effective than *G. tachinoides* and *G. palpalis* in transmission in northern Nigeria, *G. longipalpis* more than *G. palpalis* and *G. submorsitans* in Guinea and *G. austeni* more than *G. morsitans* in East Africa. Of course, development may occur in any species of *Glossina* if it is present. Development occurs in the anterior station in the midgut and the proboscis. Mechanical transmission by biting-flies is common.

In cattle the parasite may cause acute, subacute or chronic disease. In the acute form death may occur in 10 weeks and in the chronic recovery may occur after about one year (Hornby, 1952). In the acute disease lymph nodes are swollen and oedematous, the liver is congested, haemorrhages occur in the cardiac muscle and kidneys, and the bone marrow is depleted. The whole disease process is associated with anaemia and emaciation. The organisms are regularly found in the circulation and generally do not leave it. The more chronic disease is associated with enlargement of the lymph nodes and the liver, chronic degeneration of the kidney and disturbances of the bone marrow. In unsuccessfully treated cases heart lesions may occur due to the plugging of capillaries by degenerate and abnormal forms, which Fiennes (1952) has designated as 'cryptic' forms. A similar disease occurs in sheep, goats and horses but pigs are more resistant.

Diagnosis is usually by the demonstration of the organisms in the blood. In some chronic infections it may be necessary to resort to animal inoculation (guinea pigs) for diagnosis.

Trypanosoma dimorphon Laveran and Mesnil, 1904. This is now recognised as a valid species (Hoare, 1959), previously it having been a synonym of *T. congolense*. It measures 11 μ–24 μ (mean 16·2 μ), is monomorphic, slender, has no free flagellum and the kinetoplast is marginal and subterminal.

It occurs in domestic animals and is distributed similarly to *T. congolense*.

Trypanosoma simiae Bruce *et al.*, 1911 (syn. *T. porci*; *T. ignotum*; *T. rodhaini*). This is a polymorphic form resembling *T. congolense*. The majority are 16 μ–24 μ, being long and stout with a distinct undulating membrane. About 7 per cent of a population are long and slender with an inconspicuous undulating membrane and a few are short with a poorly developed undulating membrane.

Its natural host is the warthog (*Phacophoerus*). It is highly pathogenic for pigs and camels and fulminating infections lead, in a few days, to death. Only mild infections occur in sheep and goats, while in horses, cattle and dogs, though infection occurs, there is no pathogenic effect.

It is distributed in tropical East and Central Africa. Transmission in nature is chiefly by *Glossina morsitans* and *G. brevipalpalis*, development occurring as in *T. congolense*. The *Glossina* flies probably introduce the parasite to domestic pigs but thereafter transmission is mechanical by *Stomoxys* and *Tabanus*. Severe outbreaks of disease may occur in the absence of *Glossina* but with an abundance of biting-flies.

Since the infections are peracute in pigs there is usually little difficulty in demonstrating the organism in the peripheral blood.

Subgenus: Pycnomonas

Trypanosoma suis Ochmann, 1905. This parasite was once thought to be *T. simiae*, but this is now recognised as a distinct species (Peel & Chardome, 1954). It is monomorphic, $14\,\mu$–$19\,\mu$ in length, stout and with a short free flagellum.

It occurs in the Congo being transmitted by *G. brevipalpis* and cyclical development occurs in the midgut and the salivary glands. *T. suis* is pathogenic for pigs. It causes an acute disease with death in 2 months or less in young swine and a more chronic disease in older animals. Attempts by Peel & Chardome (1954) to transmit it to various other domestic and laboratory animals have failed.

Subgenus: Trypanozoon (Brucei group)

Cyclically Transmitted Forms

Trypanosoma brucei Plimmer and Bradford, 1899 (syn. *T. pecaudi*). This is a polymorphic trypanosome, slender, intermediate and stumpy forms occurring. The undulating membrane is conspicuous in all forms; the kinetoplast is subterminal and the tail pointed. In laboratory animal infections, a fourth type may occur, the 'posterior nuclear' form, in which the nucleus is posterior in position.

The slender forms are $25\,\mu$–$35\,\mu$ (mean $29\,\mu$) in length, have a long free flagellum and a pointed posterior end. The intermediate forms average $23\,\mu$, the posterior end is more blunt and a free flagellum is present. The stumpy forms average $15\,\mu$, the posterior end is broad, the kinetoplast more terminal and the flagellum is lacking. Movement is snake-like or wriggling, the organism seldom moving out of the field.

All forms may occur in the blood at the same time but usually one form predominates, the peaks in length being significantly different. When the species is transmitted to laboratory animals polymorphism disappears, as does the ability to undergo cyclical development.

Trypanosoma brucei is widely distributed in tropical Africa between the latitudes of $15°$ north and $25°$ south. Transmission is principally by *Glossina morsitans*, *G. tachinoides* and *G. palpalis* but any of the *Glossina* species may be responsible if they are present. Development occurs in the anterior station, in the midgut and the salivary glands of the fly. Transmission may also be mechanical by biting-flies.

The parasitism is seen in its most severe form in equines. Horses may rapidly succumb to the infection in riverine areas, and numerous trypanosomes are found in the blood 4–8 days after infection. The animal shows an irregular rising temperature, is dull and lethargic, anaemia develops rapidly and a marked loss of condition occurs. There may be muscular stiffness and atrophy, an unsteady gait, corneal opacity and oedema of the legs and abdomen. Death, which is inevitable in untreated cases, may occur from 20 days to 4 months after infection.

Trypanosoma brucei infection may also be acute in dogs. Infections usually result from bites of *G. palpalis* and *G. tachinoides*; the disease is rapid in onset and there is a marked intermittent rise in temperature, dullness and prostration. The parasites are found in the blood 7–10 days after infection. Anaemia and loss of condition are marked and conjunctivitis and keratitis with blindness are common sequelae. Oedema may develop on the head and the limbs, and the lymph nodes are swollen. In the final stages the central nervous system involvement produces nervous signs and paralysis.

Acute infections may occur in sheep and goats, the condition being similar to that seen in equines.

In cattle the infection is seldom severe and most infections are mild and transient, many being symptomless. Pigs are relatively resistant to *T. brucei* and, at the most, only a mild chronic disease occurs. Of the laboratory animals, the mouse is highly susceptible, a fatal fulminating infection developing within a few days. In rabbits and guinea pigs a more chronic infection is produced but this may also terminate fatally.

Diagnosis of acute cases is by the demonstration of organisms in the peripheral blood. In chronic infections organisms are scanty and thick blood smears are necessary. Preferably these should be taken over several consecutive days. Lymph node smears may also be of value. Mouse inoculations may be resorted to in chronic infections, the mouse infections becoming patent in 3–4 days.

Trypanosoma gambiense Dutton, 1902 (syn. *T. ugandense*; *T. hominis*; *T. nigeriense*). This is the cause of Gambian sleeping sickness, or trypanosomiasis, of humans. It is morphologically indistinguishable from *T. brucei* of animals, occurring in a polymorphic condition of slender, intermediate, and stumpy forms.

T. gambiense occurs on the west coast of Africa between the latitudes of 15° north and 18° south with Lake Victoria as an eastern limit. The principal tsetse flies concerned in transmission are the riverine types *Glossina palpalis* and *G. tachinoides*. Development occurs in the anterior station, similar to *T. brucei*, and mechanical transmission due to biting-flies may also occur.

In the early part of the century much information accumulated on the mammalian reservoirs of *T. gambiense* (Wenyon, 1926). This must be accepted with reservations since much of the identification of trypanosomes in animal hosts at that time is now open to question. It is currently believed that under normal circumstances tsetse flies acquire their infection only from humans and that man is the only mammalian host for the parasite. It is possible to create artificial infections in antelopes, pigs, and other domestic animals but though the infection may persist for some time, the ability to undergo cyclical transmission is lost, even though the infection was cyclically induced (van Hoof, 1947). Consequently, even if such animals were infected in nature (which has never been demonstrated) they would not provide suitable hosts for the maintenance of the parasite.

Gambian sleeping sickness is a chronic disease. Initially there is invasion of the blood stream, then the lymph nodes and finally the central nervous system with the production of leptomeningitis and perivascular infiltrations around blood vessels. Diagnosis is based on symptoms, habitat and demonstration of the parasites in the blood, lymph nodes and the cerebrospinal fluid.

Trypanosoma rhodesiense Stephens and Fantham, 1910. This is the cause of Rhodesian trypanosomiasis or East African sleeping sickness of humans. The parasite is morphologically indistinguishable from *T. brucei* and *T. gambiense* and some authors prefer to refer to the three as the *Brucei* subgroup. The organism is polymorphic, showing the three forms, similar to the other species. Geographically it is more restricted than *T. gambiense*, being found in Zambia, S. Rhodesia, Nyasaland, Tanzania, Bechuanaland, in the southern Sudan and around the shores of Lake Victoria. The principal transmitting flies are the savannah tsetses, chiefly *G. morsitans* and, in some areas, *G. swynnertoni* and *G. pallidipes*. Development occurs in the anterior station, similar to *T. brucei*.

T. rhodesiense is pathogenic for the rat and other laboratory animals.

The source of human infection with *T. rhodesiense* is, of course, man but there is strong circumstantial evidence that game animals play an important part as reservoir hosts. The organism has been isolated from game (Bushbuck, *Tragelaphus scriptus*), and this produced disease in man (Heisch, McMahon & Manson-Bahr, 1948).

However, *T. rhodesiense*, from an untreated human, has been cyclically passaged by *G. morsitans*, through sheep, and later antelope and gazelle, for 16 years (Buxton, 1955; Willett, 1950; Fairbairn & Burtt, 1946). At intervals the strain was cyclically transmitted to human volunteers, and though the infectivity for man varied, after 16 years seven out of ten volunteers became infected. However, due to the limited number of experiments involving human volunteers the true incidence of *T. rhodesiense* infection in domestic cattle and game is not known. The only positive method of accurate identification of *T. rhodesiense* is to use human volunteers. The morphologically identical *T. brucei* does not develop in man.

Circumstantial evidence that *T. rhodesiense* is a zoonosis is based on the fact that the principal vectors of the organism are the game tsetses *G. morsitans*, *G. swynnertoni* and *G. pallidipes*. Contact between tsetse flies and man is diffuse in the area for Rhodesian trypanosomiasis, which would suggest that infections frequently do not go directly from man to man but rather through some reservoir host.

The clinical disease produced by *T. rhodesiense* is more acute than the Gambian form of the disease. The early stages are similar to the West African form but the climax is reached before any marked involvement of the central nervous system occurs. The marked sleeping sickness stage is not a strong feature of the infection. A fatal termination is common in untreated cases, which may be a matter of months only.

Mechanically transmitted forms

Trypanosoma evansi (Steel, 1885) Balbiani, 1888 (syn. *T. annamense*; *T. berberum*; *T. cameli*; *T. hippicum*; *T. soudanense*; *T. venezuelense*).

This was the first trypanosome shown to be pathogenic for mammals and was identified by Griffiths Evans, a British veterinarian.

In the majority of infections this parasite is monomorphic in character but polymorphism occurs sporadically. The typical form is indistinguishable from the slender form of *T. brucei*, being 15μ–34μ in length (mean 24μ), the kinetoplast is subterminal, the undulating membrane is well developed and there is a substantial free flagellum. Stumpy forms may appear sporadically. Forms which lack a kinetoplast may arise spontaneously, especially after drug treatment (Hoare, 1954).

Geographically *T. evansi* occurs typically in the Indian subcontinent. However, it is now widespread throughout the Far East; it also occurs in the Near East, in North Africa north of latitude $15°$ north, and in the Phillipines, and Central and South America. Transmission is by biting-flies such as *Tabanus*, *Stomoxys* and *Lyperosia*. No cyclical development occurs in these. An essential factor in mechanical transmission is interrupted feeding on the part of flies which go quickly from one host to the other in order to become replete. Trypanosomes do not survive for more than 10–15 minutes in the proboscis of a fly. In Central and South America the vampire bat may also act as a vector, though the bat may die of infection about a month after an infected blood meal.

Trypanosoma evansi affects a wide range of hosts including horse, dog, camel, buffalo, elephant, pig, cat, tapir, capybara and (in Mauritius) deer. Laboratory rodents such as mice, rabbits, rats and guinea pigs are readily infected.

The classical disease entity in the Indian subcontinent occurs in horses and is known as surra (a Hindi word meaning rotten). Surra is nearly always fatal to horses if treatment is not applied, death occurring in a few days to a few months depending on the virulence of the strain of organism. Emaciation and oedema are the most common clinical signs, the oedema varying from urticarial plaques on the neck and the flanks to oedema of the legs and lower parts of the body. The plaques may necrose in the centre and haemorrhages occur at the junction of the skin and mucous membranes, especially at the nostrils, eyes, and anus. An intermittent fever may be present but in some cases the condition is so acute that this is not obvious. On post mortem there is a marked anaemia, emaciation, enlargement of lymph nodes and splenomegaly. Petechiae occur on the serous surfaces and in the parenchyma of the liver and kidneys.

Diagnosis of surra in horses is usually relatively easy since the organisms are readily demonstrated in fresh stained blood smears.

An acute and fatal type of disease is usual in dogs in the East, death possibly occurring in 2–4 weeks. Oedema is marked, corneal opacity is common, and due to oedema of the larynx, voice changes similar to those which occur in rabies may be noticed. Diagnosis is similar to that in horses.

In camels in the East the disease is chronic. The animals become progressively weaker and emaciated and the infection runs a course of about 3 years.

Cattle and water buffalo are considered to be the main reservoirs of the infection for equines. In these the infection is subclinical in nature; nevertheless, occasional outbreaks of acute disease occur with quick death. This is often associated with the introduction of the parasite or a new strain of it into a new area or to additional stress on animals, such as foot and mouth disease vaccination.

In the elephant, surra follows a course similar to that seen in camels; animals become emaciated and show marked muscular weakness.

The diagnosis of *T. evansi* in the camel or other chronically infected animals may present difficulty because parasitaemia is usually low. Various indirect tests have been used including the complement fixation test which, though giving a group reaction, is of value when no other trypanosomes occur in the area. Other indirect diagnostic tests depend on disease-induced alteration of serum proteins. A mercuric chloride test consists of adding one drop of serum to one ml. of a 1 in 30,000 solution of mercuric chloride in distilled water, the tube being shaken gently. A white opalescence which appears in a few seconds indicates infection of one month or more standing. The stilbamide test (in India) consists of adding one drop of serum to a 0·3 per cent solution of stilbamide in distilled water. A positive reaction consists of an opalescence of precipitate after 1–2 minutes. Such tests are to a great extent nonspecific and undoubtedly animal inoculation, using rats or guinea pigs, is more satisfactory.

In the Sudan *T. evansi* is almost entirely restricted to the camel, the infection being known as 'Gufar'. Because of the differences between this form and that in Asia causing surra, the parasite was formerly referred to as *T. soudanense*. Generally, the course of the disease is chronic, death occurring only after several months. However, in a few cases it may be acute, producing death in 2–3 weeks. The incubation period is about 2 weeks, fever being followed by progressive weakness and emaciation; oedema of the dependent parts occurs and paralysis may develop. Occasionally horses in the Sudan show a chronic disease which may end fatally, but donkeys show a mild fever which terminates in a spontaneous cure.

The South American form of *T. evansi* infection produces similar disease entities as described above. In horses the infection is referred to as murrina (Panama) or derrengadera (Venezuela). A chronic disease associated with high mortality occurs in dogs, untreated animals dying 1–2 months after infection (Gomez Rodriguez, 1956). The capybara, though normally a reservoir host for the horse, may suffer an acute fatal infection similar to that in the horse.

Trypanosoma equinum Voges, 1901. This is a large monomorphic form, 22 μ–24 μ in length, differing from *T. evansi* only in lacking a kinetoplast. The axoneme of the flagellum arises from a small blepharoplast. It occurs in Central and South America, the enzootic areas being Argentina, Bolivia and Paraguay. Transmission is mechanical by biting-flies.

Trypanosoma equinum is chiefly an infection of equines, the horse being most seriously affected, and the clinical condition is referred to as 'mal de caderas'. Mules and donkeys are less susceptible while dogs, cattle, sheep and goats, in that order, can be infected with a mild disease. The capybara (*Hydrochoerus capybara*) is susceptible to infection and may serve as a reservoir host for the equine infection. The parasite is responsible for high mortality of horses in wet areas, particularly swamps, where the incidence of blood-sucking flies is high.

The disease in horses is rarely acute but in such cases death occurs in a few weeks after the onset of clinical signs. More usually it runs a chronic course with death occurring 2–6 months after infection. The incubation period is 4–10 days, after which pyrexia and parasitaemia appear. Emaciation commences early in the disease and a marked weakness of the hindquarters (mal de caderas) results in a staggering gait. This is progressive and the animal finally becomes recumbent. Associated lesions are conjunctivitis, keratitis and oedema of the eyelids. Transient cutaneous plaques occur over the neck and the flanks, these lose their hair and later scab over. On post mortem there is splenomegaly, enlargement of lymph nodes and anaemia. The kidneys show petechial haemorrhages, ascites may be present and there is often an oedematous infiltration in the spinal canal.

Diagnosis in the acute stage of the disease is based on the demonstration of organisms in the peripheral blood. In more advanced infections organisms are difficult to find and inoculation of blood into laboratory rodents (e.g. mice) is the most satisfactory means of diagnosis.

Trypanosoma equiperdum Dolfein, 1901. This species is morphologically identical to *T. evansi*. It causes a venereal disease of horses, 'dourine' (Arabic for unclean), that, at present, occurs in Asia, North and South Africa and southeastern Europe. The infection was once widespread in the United States but this country has now been free from the infection for several years. *Trypanosoma equiperdum* is ordinarily transmitted mechanically by coitus; rarely is it transmitted by biting-flies and by infective discharges contaminating mucous membranes.

The disease is naturally found in horses and asses. The jackass may be a symptomless carrier and is therefore especially dangerous. Of the other species, dogs may be infected with some strains of the parasite; cattle are generally resistant to infection, but laboratory mice, rats and rabbits are susceptible, though a second passage may be necessary to establish satisfactory infections. The organism varies in its virulence; some infections may never become clinical whereas others run a more definite clinical course, albeit chronic in character.

The clinical entity of dourine usually progresses through three distinct phases following an incubation period of 2–12 weeks or several months. In some latent cases the disease entity may only be precipitated by other severe disorders. The first phase, the stage of oedema, is initiated by a mucoid vaginal or urethral discharge, a degree of nymphomania and a mild fever with oedema of the genitalia. In the stallion the prepuce and scrotum are swollen and the oedema may extend under the belly as far forward as the chest. In the mare the vaginal mucosa is hyperaemic and ulcers may be present. There is deep pigmentation of circumscribed areas of the vulva and the penis. This phase lasts 4–6 weeks and in mild cases may go unnoticed, but in severe forms frequent micturition and even abortion in pregnant mares may be evident.

The second phase, the urticarial phase, is characterised by the appearance of oedematous plaques under the skin, especially of the flanks but any part of the body may be affected. The plaques are circular, sharply circumscribed and are 1 to 4 inches in diameter. They are classically referred to as 'dollar spots' since they appear as if a silver dollar had been inserted under the skin. They may persist for a few hours or 3–4 days, then disappear, but may reappear again. Though they are not an invariable consequence of *T. equiperdum* infection, their presence is almost pathognomonic for the disease and the affected areas may be left depigmented when the swelling has resolved, giving good evidence of their previous presence.

The third phase of infection is that of paralysis. The muscles of the face and nostrils are usually affected first but later paralysis of the muscles is associated with complete paralysis and recumbency, which is followed by death. Mortality varies from 50–70 per cent.

At post mortem the carcase is emaciated with marked muscular atrophy, there is oedematous infiltration of the perineal tissues and the abdominal wall and ulcers may occur on the body where the horse has lain. Serous infiltration is present along the large nerve trunks supplying the hind-limbs, and histological examination shows cell infiltrations, oedema and degeneration of these and also the posterior spinal cord.

The clinical disease is typical enough to allow diagnosis in an endemic area. Trypanosomes are not readily detected in the blood but they may be found in the vaginal or preputial discharges or in the serous fluid squeezed from the urticarial plaques. Material may also be inoculated into mice, rats, rabbits, etc. but a second passage may be necessary in order to demonstrate the parasites. The complement fixation test (Watson, 1915) is useful in both clinical and latent cases and has been used with marked success in the United States' eradication programme. Serum antibodies develop 3–4 weeks after infection and though a few nonspecific reactions may occur, the number of false negatives is small.

Section: Stercoraria (Posterior Station Forms)
Subgenus: Megatrypanum

Trypanosoma theileri Laveran, 1902 (syn. *T. americanum*). This is a relatively large species, 60 μ–70 μ in length, but forms up to 120 μ in length may be found, especially in chronic infections. Such forms have been reported as *Trypanosoma ingens* in the African antelope by Hoare (1949). The posterior end is long and pointed and the kinetoplast lies some distance from the posterior end. The undulating membrane is well developed and the free flagellum is well defined.

T. theileri is transmitted cyclically in the posterior station by tabanid flies such as *Tabanus* and *Haematopota*, infection of the bovine being by contamination. In the bovine both trypanosome and crithidial forms occur but multiplication occurs in the crithidial stage, chiefly in the lymph nodes and inner organs. *T. theileri* is readily cultured in a variety of culture media. In those incubated at 27°C only crithidial forms occur but in cultures incubated at 37°C both crithidial and trypanosome stages develop (Splitter & Soulsby, 1967).

Under ordinary circumstances *T. theileri* is a nonpathogenic form and probably occurs in cattle throughout the world. Occasionally, however, it may appear in a parasitaemic form following splenectomy or when stress conditions arise. For example, it has been incriminated as a cause of death in cattle following Rinderpest vaccination. In some animals the infection was peracute in nature producing an anthrax-like disease. It has also been associated with 'turning sickness' in Uganda (Carmichael, 1939), depressed milk production in three cows (Ristic & Trager, 1958) and abortion in cattle (Levine, Watrach, Kantor & Hardenbrood, 1956; Dikmans, Manthei & Frank, 1957).

Trypanosoma melophagium (Flu, 1908). This is a nonpathogenic form of sheep. It is 50 μ–60 μ in length and generally resembles *T. theileri*. It is transmitted cyclically in the posterior station by the sheep ked, *Melophagus ovinus*. Infection is by contamination of the skin and, also,

PLATE XIX

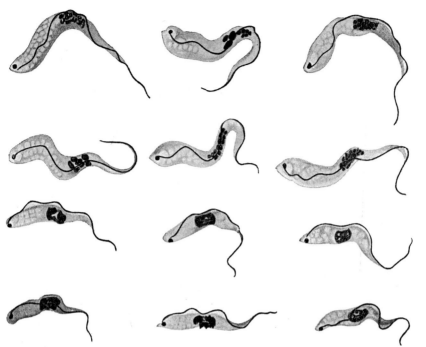

A. Trypanosomes of the subgenus *Duttonella*. Upper 2 rows *T. vivax*, lower 2 rows, *T. uniforme* (× 2000). (From Wenyon, 1926)

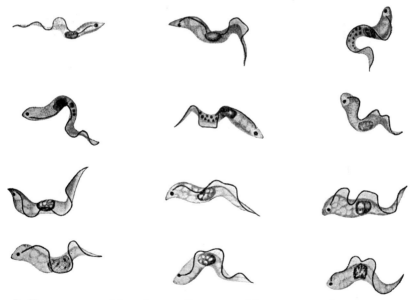

B. Trypanosomes of the subgenus *Nannomonas*. *Trypanosoma congolense* (× 2000). (From Wenyon, 1926)

PLATE XX

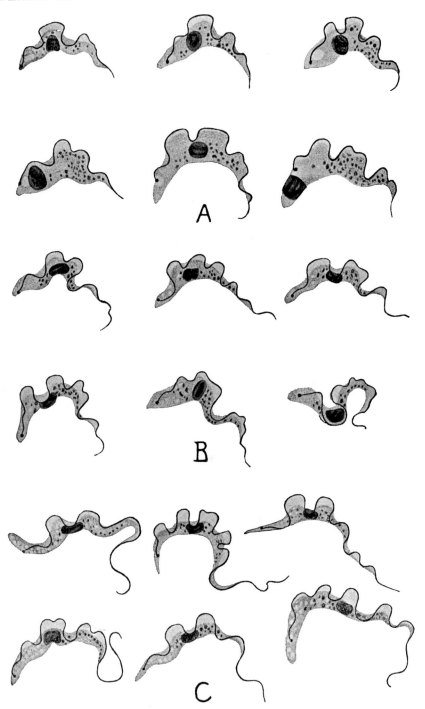

Trypanosoma brucei (× 2000). (From Wenyon, 1926). A. Broad stumpy form; two posterior nuclear forms are shown, one with kinetoplast behind the nucleus, and one with it in front. B. Intermediate form with short flagellum. C. Long slender form with flagella.

PLATE XXI

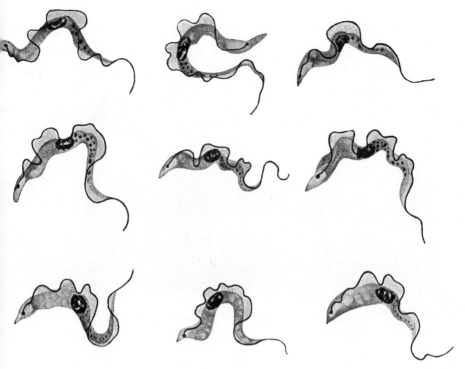

Trypanosoma evansi from blood of various animals (× 2000). (From Wenyon, 1926)

PLATE XXII

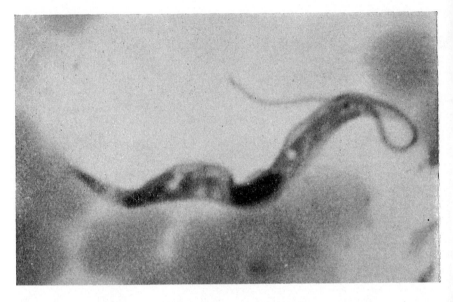

A. *Trypanosoma theileri* of cattle. Stained Geimsa. (× 2000)

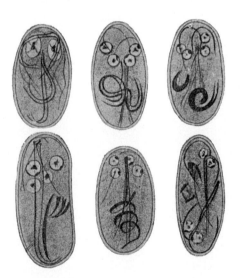

B. *Giardia lamblia:* Encysted forms from th
human intestine. (× 3000). (From Wenyor
1926). 1, Form with two nuclei; 2–5, Form
with four terminal nuclei; 6, Form in whic
two of the nuclei have migrated to the oppo
site pole and the flagellate is dividing wit
the cyst

if a ked is eaten the metacyclic trypanosomes may penetrate the buccal mucosa.

The organism is widespread. Usually it is demonstrable only by culture techniques but occasionally it may be demonstrated microscopically in the peripheral blood.

Trypanosoma theodori Hoare, 1931. This is similar to *T. melophagium*. It is nonpathogenic and occurs in goats in Palestine. It is transmitted by the hippoboscid fly *Lipoptena caprina*.

Subgenus: Herpetosoma

. Members of this subgenus are of little medical or veterinary importance. Some of the species have provided good models for research, especially on the immunological aspect of host–parasite relationships.

Trypanosome lewisi (Kent, 1880) Laveran and Mesnil, 1901. This occurs in rats and is transmitted by the rat flea *Ceratophyllus fasciatus*. It is 26 μ–34 μ in length, has a pointed tail and the kinetoplast is some distance from the posterior end. Normally this trypanosome is nonpathogenic to rats but it may cause death in nursling rats.

Trypanosoma nabiasi Railliet, 1895. This occurs in rabbits in Europe and is transmitted by the rabbit flea, *Spilopsylla cuniculi*. It is nonpathogenic.

Trypanosoma rangeli Tejera, 1920 (syn. *T. ariarii*; *T. guatemalense*). This species was first described from the crithidial stages in the reduviid *Rhodnius prolixus*. Later it was shown to occur in the blood of man, dog, cat, opossum and monkey. The blood forms, which are the only known stages in mammals, measure 26 μ–36 μ; the nucleus is anterior to the middle of the body and the kinetoplast is small and subterminal. The undulating membrane is relatively broad and rippled and the free flagellum is short. Reproduction is by longitudinal binary fission.

Development occurs in triatomid bugs, *R. prolixus* being the main vector. Others such as *Panstrongylus geniculatus*, *Triatoma dimidiata* and *T. nitida* have been incriminated. Development occurs in the fore- and hind-gut, a giant crithidial stage being produced. Metacyclic trypanosomes may migrate to the salivary glands and infection is either by inoculation or by contamination.

The organism does not appear to be pathogenic for the mammalian host and its principal importance is the differentiation of it from *T. cruzi*.

Subgenus: Schizotrypanum

Trypanosoma cruzi Chagas, 1909 (syn. *Schizotrypanum cruzi*; *T. escomeli*). This is the main pathogenic species of the Stercoraria. It is the cause of American human trypanosomiasis or Chagas disease in South America. In the blood it is monomorphic, 16 μ–20 μ in length, and crescent-shaped with a pointed posterior end. The kinetoplast is large and subterminal and fills the body of the trypanosome at that point. The nucleus is midway along the body and there is a moderately well developed undulating membrane and free flagellum. No division takes place in the trypanosome stage and division occurs in the leishmanial form. The dividing forms appear as bodies $1.5\,\mu$–$4\,\mu$ in diameter in muscle and other cells, especially the heart muscle cells.

The geographic distribution of human infection with *T. cruzi* is chiefly South America extending from Argentina northwards, and it also occurs in Central America. A wide variety of animals may be infected and serve as reservoir hosts. Thus dogs, cats, pigs, foxes, ferrets, squirrels, opossums and monkeys may, amongst others, be hosts and the dog is a frequent host in South America, up to 35 per cent more being infected (Neghme, 1940). Animal infection has been detected in the southeastern United States and various reports indicate a substantial prevalence (Olsen, Shoemaker, Turner & Hays, 1964).

Trypanosoma cruzi is of greatest importance in man, chiefly affecting young children and infants. The principal reservoir hosts in South America are the armadillo and the opossum; in Central America the opossum acts as such and in the U.S.A. woodrats and racoons may be important in this respect. The close association of man and dog makes the latter a likely source also of human infection. The knowledge that *T. cruzi* is much more widespread in the animal population of the United States than hitherto thought has posed the question of the importance of this zoonosis to human health in that country. Two autochthonous human cases have been diagnosed in the U.S.A., one in a child in Corpus Christi, Texas (Woody & Woody, 1955), and one in a child in Bryan, Texas (Goble, 1958).

Under natural conditions *T. cruzi* is transmitted by blood-sucking bugs of the family Reduviidae, development occurring in the posterior station. Metacyclic trypanosomes are passed in the faeces of the infected bug 8–10 or more days after initial infection. The human, or mammalian host, is infected when the metacyclic trypanosomes are rubbed into the wound made by the insect, into other skin abrasions or through the mucous membranes. Reduviids (kissing bugs) usually defaecate after feeding and they commonly feed on the thin skin near the eyes and lips. The infected material is therefore easily rubbed into the mucous membranes and the wounds. Animals may be infected by licking the faeces of the bugs or by ingesting infective bugs.

A large number of species of reduviid bugs have been found naturally infected and several more have been infected experimentally. The most important vectors in South America are *Panstrongylus megistus*, *Eutriatoma sordida*, *Panstrongylus geniculatus*, *Triatoma infestans* and *Rhodnius prolixus*. In the United States at least fifteen species have been shown to be infected, the two principal species being *T. protracta* and *T. sanguisuga* (Faust, 1949).

Following infection of a wound with metacyclic trypanosomes the organisms enter histiocytes and proliferate in the leishmanial form at the local site. There is a local inflammatory response and later encapsulation by fibrous tissue, the whole blocking the local lymphatics and producing oedema of the local area. This is the primary lesion or 'chagoma'. Leishmaniae pass from the primary site to local lymph nodes and then by the lymphatic system to the whole body. The liver, lungs, spleen, bone marrow, the cardiac muscle and the brain cortex are affected. Here the organisms multiply as leishmaniae. Large-scale rupture of host cells releases trypanosomes into the blood and this is associated with fever.

The disease in man may be acute or chronic in character, the former usually occurring in infants and young children. Death may occur in 2–4 weeks after the onset of symptoms in acute cases or they may resolve to the chronic form of the infection. The chronic disease is the usual form found in adults. The clinical manifestations depend on the location of the organisms but the cardiac form is common. The pathological changes consist of massive destruction of the reticulo-endothelial and muscle cells so that almost every organ of the body may be affected. The leishmanial forms are found in cyst-like nests in host cells which ultimately rupture, other cells are then infected and the process continues.

In dogs debility, anaemia and splenomegaly occur, young animals being especially susceptible. Myocardial involvement also occurs in dogs but it is not as extensive as in man. In cats, convulsions and posterior paralysis may be seen. The disease may also be produced in mice and guinea pigs but the reservoir hosts for the parasite appear to suffer little from the infection.

Diagnosis of the acute stage is based on the demonstration of the trypanosome stage in thick blood films. However, as the disease progresses the organisms become infrequent in the blood and are present in detectable numbers only during bouts of fever. In such cases blood may be injected into puppies, kittens or guinea pigs, or spleen or lymph gland biopsies made and the leishmanial bodies sought for. Xenodiagnosis, that is, the feeding of triatomid bugs on the suspect or allowing bugs to feed on the patient's blood through a membrane may be a valuable technique. Laboratory-reared and *T. cruzi* free triatomes are used and if the suspected material is positive, metacyclic trypanosomes are found 7 to 10 days later in the droppings of the bug (Pifano, 1954).

A complement fixation test using an alcoholic extract of cultured forms has been widely used in diagnosis. Cross reactions may occur with *Leishmania* infection. A purified antigen has been prepared by Knierin (1959) which is stated to give a 90 per cent diagnostic accuracy.

Trypanosomes of Birds

Several species of trypanosomes occur in avian hosts but, as far as is known, they are all nonpathogenic. *Trypanosoma avium*, Danilewsky, 1885, occurs in a wide range of birds in Europe and in Canada Geese in North America. *Trypanosoma calmetti*, Mathis & Leger, 1909, occurs in ducklings in South East Asia and *Trypanosoma gallinarum*, Bruce *et al.*, 1911, was reported from fowls in Uganda.

Treatment of trypanosomiasis

Reviews of the chemotherapy of trypanosomiasis are given by Goodwin & Rollo (1955), Goodwin (1964) and Whiteside (1962) and of the structure and activity of trypanocidal drugs by Barber & Berg (1962). It is intended to give a brief account only of the major compounds which are in use at the present time.

Essentially, the trypanocidal drugs available are curative or prophylactic. The latter, in some cases, may give protection against infection for 4–6 months.

Prior to 1938 and the discovery of the phenanthridinium compounds the only satisfactory drug available was tartar emetic. This is useful in the treatment of *T. congolense* and *T. vivax* in cattle and *T. evansi* in the camel but it is of little value for *T. brucei* in horses. It is given intravenously in 1 g. doses dissolved in 20–35 ml. of saline or water and is repeated 6 to 8 times at weekly intervals. Necrosis may occur if the drug leaks from the vein and it must be used freshly prepared to avoid toxicity. Other compounds of this vintage are Antimosan (40–50 ml. of 6·3 per cent solution weekly for 5 weeks in cattle). Fuadin (Stibophen) and Surfen C (Congasin). The latter causes marked reactions following intramuscular injection.

Suramin (syn. Antrypol; Bayer 205; Naganol; etc.) This has been used for many years as the drug of choice for *T. brucei* and it is similarly useful for *T. evansi*, *T. equinum* and *T. equiperdum*. In the horse a single dose of 4 g. per 100 lb. body weight is given intravenously, or it can be divided into three parts given over a period of 3 weeks. For dogs 0·3 g. intravenously is repeated for 6 days. Suramin is the drug of choice for *T. evansi* in camels in which it is well tolerated. It is given intravenously at the rate of 1–2 g. per 100 kg. body weight.

Phenanthridinium Series. The first of the series, phenidium chloride, though active against *T. vivax* and *T. congolense* suffered from the disadvantage of causing muscle necrosis. It was superseded by dimidium bromide. This, given intramuscularly as a 1 per cent solution at the rate of 1 ml. per kg. (Wilde, 1949), produced a high percentage of cures of *T. congolense* and *T. vivax* infections in cattle. High concentrations of the drug may lead to liver malfunction and photosensitisation, especially in cattle in East and West Africa. Such reactions are less obvious in Central and South Africa. In 1952 dimidium bromide was replaced by ethidium bromide (Wilde & Robson, 1953) which is a much less toxic compound. It has been in extensive use as a curative drug for *T. vivax* and *T. congolense* in cattle but its protective action lasts only about 5 weeks (Whiteside, 1962).

It is also of value for *T. congolense* infection in horses and dogs. It is given at the rate of 1 ml. per kg. body weight. When used continuously in an area, resistance of trypanosomes to the drug frequently develops and then other compounds, for example berenil, are indicated (see Drug Resistance in trypanosomes).

More recent additions to the phenanthridinium series include prothidium and metamidium, both of which offer good protection against trypanosomiasis. Prothidium has been widely used in East Africa and is given as a 4 per cent solution at the rate of 2–4 ml. (2 mg.) per kg. subcutaneously. This dose is active against *T. congolense* and also *T. vivax* and *T. brucei* and under conditions of relatively low tsetse fly density will give protection for 70–300 days against trypanosomiasis (Leach & El Karib, 1960, Robson, 1961). Where the prevalence of flies is high the period of protection is much shorter (Whiteside, 1962), however even in such circumstances, more frequent treatments enable animals to withstand severe challenge. The major disadvantage of the continued use of prothidium is the apparent ease with which trypanosomes become resistant to it. Furthermore, strains of organisms resistant to prothidium also have an increased resistance to the other phenanthridinium compounds. The toxicity of prothidium is generally low, but hard swellings may appear at the site of the subcutaneous injections.

Metamidium (the *p*-amidino-phenyldiazo-amino derivative of ethidium chloride) is used both curatively and prophylactically for *T. vivax* and *T. congolense* in cattle. At a dose of 5 mg. per kg. intramuscularly up to 204 days prophylaxis may result (Stephen, 1960). In combination with suramin, metamidium forms a depôt of drug which can give 111 days protection at 10 mg. per kg. Other uses of metamidium include the treatment of *T. simiae* in pigs (3–6 mg. per kg.) and in general the drug is particularly useful since, at therapeutic dose, it is able to eliminate infections resistant to quinapyramine (Antrycide) (Whiteside, 1960). Toxicity is seen with doses of 10 mg. per kg. and over.

Berenil (4,4-diamidinodiazoaminobenzene aceturate). This is a curative drug for *T. congolense* and *T. vivax*, being given at a dose of 2 mg. per kg. It has little action against the *brucei* group and a dose of 3·5 mg. per kg. is ineffective against *T. evansi* in camels (Leach, 1961). Berenil has no prophylactic effect, being rapidly excreted from the body, but it is particularly useful as a 'sanative drug' in that it cures infections which are resistant to other drugs (Whiteside, 1962). As far as is known resistance to berenil has not developed in the field. Toxicity is low at the therapeutic levels of the drug.

Antrycide [4-amino-6-(2-amino-1,6 dimethylpyrimidinyl-4-amino)-1,2 dimethyl-quinoline] (quinapyramine). Three forms of this compound are in use at present, namely antrycide methyl sulphate, antrycide chloride and antrycide pro-salt (a mixture of the methyl sulphate and chloride). Antrycide methyl sulphate is very soluble in water, forming a stable solution which, on injection, reaches a therapeutic level quickly. It is, however, also rapidly excreted and it is used essentially as a curative drug. It is highly active against *T. congolense*, *T. evansi*, *T. equinum* and *T. equiperdum*. Good action is obtained against *T. brucei* and it has been used for *T. simiae* in East Africa but it has failed to cure this infection in West Africa. *Trypanosoma vivax* is slightly less affected by the drug and Davey (1950) originally recommended 5 mg. per kg. for this species. The present recommendations for antrycide methyl sulphate are 4·4 mg. per kg. for *T. vivax*, *T. brucei* and *T. simiae*, 3 mg. per kg. for *T. evansi*, *T. equiperdum* and *T. equinum* and 2·2 mg. per kg. for *T. congolense*. It is given as a 10 per cent solution subcutaneously. The compound has been used to treat *T. brucei* in horses but these animals are more susceptible to toxicity than cattle, and a marked local reaction may occur. For dogs 1 mg. per kg. is satisfactory for *T. congolense* infection but 5 mg. per kg. is necessary for *T. brucei* infections. The drug has no effect against *Trypanosoma cruzi*. In the field, 5 mg. per kg. is generally adopted as the maximum tolerated dose. Signs of acute toxicity consist of increased salivation, muscular tremors of the head muscle, distressed breathing and collapse. Chronic toxicity may produce a marked enteritis, severe enough to cause death. Young animals are more susceptible to toxicity than the old.

Antrycide chloride is almost insoluble in water, remaining at the site of injection and being poorly absorbed. It is used for prophylaxis and is usually combined with the methyl sulphate under the common name of antrycide pro-salt. The proportions are 1·5 g. of the methyl sulphate to 1 g. of the chloride. The benefit of the pro-salt is that sufficient methyl sulphate is given to serve as a curative dose while depôts of the chloride are formed in subcutaneous tissues from which the drug is slowly absorbed. Davey (1950) recommends a dose of 12 mg./kg. given every 8 weeks. However the level of protection obtained varies with the density of infected flies. Thus Whiteside (1962) found in one group of animals given treatment every 2 months that cattle showed no infection over a 7-month period. In another area, however, where the density of flies was 10 times as great, protection began to fail before 2 months and at the end of 6 months, 20 per cent of animals were infected. In other words, the higher the incidence of trypanosomiasis, the shorter the period of prophylaxis achieved. As with the other trypanocidal drugs, resistance is a recurrent problem in the field (see below).

Drug Resistance in Trypanosomes. This has been a continuing problem in the treatment of trypanosomiasis and it is particularly common with *T. congolense*. Bishop (1959, 1962) has discussed the biological aspects of drug resistance while Whiteside (1960, 1962) has considered it from the field aspect. The latter author states that cattle trypanosomes readily become resistant to all existing drugs, except berenil, which is rapidly excreted from the body. Drug resistance develops in the treated host and naturally occurring drug-resistant trypanosomes have not yet been observed. Resistant strains of trypanosomes can be transmitted by tsetse flies but these disappear after 6 to 12 months provided that the cattle source of the resistant organisms is removed.

Resistance can be developed with relative ease by subcurative doses of drugs, which allow a relapse. Usually three to six such treatments are required for this (Whiteside, 1962) and thereafter the organisms are 40 to 80 times more resistant to the normal curative doses. Such strains can develop in an individual animal and resistance is retained for at least 1 year when the infection syringe is passaged to other cattle. Though the essential factor in the development of drug resistance is underdosing, this can inadvertently arise in several ways, especially with the prophylactic drugs. Thus where the incidence of infected flies is high, subcurative levels of a drug may exist towards the end of the protection period; animals may be exposed to infection for too long after a single prophylactic treatment and a further aspect is that a seasonal increase in prevalence of trypanosomiasis may produce a shortening of the protection period which in turn leads to a subcurative level of the drug.

Cross Resistance to Drugs. With the development of resistance to one compound, trypanosomes may show resistance to compounds of the same series and also to those of other series. Thus in the phenanhridinium series, resistance to prothidium leads to resistance to metamidium and ethidium. There is also cross-resistance between quinapyramine and the phenanthridinium series. In some cases the resistance developed is not great, and large, but tolerated, doses of other drugs will cure the infection (e.g. metamidium). The stage may be reached, however, where the level of resistance exceeds the maximum tolerated dose of other drugs (Whiteside, 1962). The degree of cross-resistance depends on the degree of direct resistance developed. A strain of *T. congolense*, resistant to 4 times the minimal curative dose of quinapyramine, was susceptible to the normal doses of ethidium chloride and berenil; two further exposures to normal doses of quinapyramine resulted in resistance to ethidium but not to berenil; another two exposures to quinapyramine resulted in resistance to berenil (Whiteside, 1962). Direct resistance to berenil appears to be rare in the field but berenil-resistant strains have been produced experimentally (Whiteside, 1962). Cross resistance to berenil may be induced in the field by antrycide (quinapyramine) and also prothidium (Whiteside, 1960; Smith & Scott, 1961); however Whiteside (1962) now considers the latter report to be doubtful.

No significant differences in metabolism have been found between normal and resistant strains of trypanosomes and Bishop (1962) has suggested that drug resistance develops by mutation. She quotes work in which DNA from resistant strains will transfer resistance to normal trypanosomes. A relationship between drug resistance and antibody resistance has been observed by Soltys (1959). A strain of 'antibody-resistant' *T. brucei* was less sensitive to suramin and antrycide than one which had not been exposed to antibody.

The control of drug resistance in the field is discussed by Whiteside (1962). In a curative programme ethidium chloride and berenil are used alternatively, since neither produces cross-resistance to the other. Ethidium is used over a wide area until evidence of resistance appears; it is then completely withdrawn and berenil is used instead for at least one year. This drug cures infections whether or not they are resistant to ethidium and it also cures animals reinfected with ethidium-resistant forms. After one year the ethidium treatment is recommenced.

With prophylactic drugs the situation is more difficult. The two commonly used drugs, quinapyramine and prothidium, induce reciprocal cross-resistance. Development of resistance is indicated by a reduction in the length of protection and when this occurs berenil or metamidium is introduced and is continued until such time as the resistant strain dies out. Prolonged treatment may be necessary when the resistant strains are introduced into *Glossina*.

Control of Trypanosomiasis

Under field conditions the control of trypanosomiasis is chiefly dependent on chemotherapy. However, many factors mitigate against complete control by chemotherapy, the development of drug-resistant strains being a major one. The control of *Glossina* offers a much more long-term control measure and this is discussed on p. 426.

The destruction of game, which serves two purposes, that of depriving *Glossina* of its food and of reducing the reservoir of trypanosomes, is a control measure which has aroused much controversy and antagonism. On the one hand, people may rightly fear the demise of a majestic and priceless inheritance while others fear that in the absence of the large game animals, tsetse flies will feed more on cattle. This subject has been masterfully and thoroughly discussed by Buxton (1955). In southern Rhodesia game destruction has resulted in the disappearance of *G. morsitans*, but other species of tsetse, which feed on a variety of small and large game, are little affected by game destruction. In some areas, such as West Africa, game destruction would be pointless since these animals form an unimportant source of the tsetse food supply. Controlled elimination of game by trained hunters may be of value in certain areas to create zones between game areas and those for agricultural development.

The breeding of trypanosome resistant strains of cattle has been considered on many occasions (Chandler, 1958; Mulligan, 1951). In West Africa, the N'Dama and Maturu breeds (or crosses with a large proportion of N'Dama blood) are little affected, carrying nonpathogenic burdens of trypanosomes. This is an acquired resistance since animals reared in non-tsetse areas are susceptible to infection (Desowitz, 1959), and may show a short bout of infection when moved to a new area (Stewart,

1951). A major disadvantage of such crosses is that the animals are economically inferior to the improved breeds.

Control of *T. evansi* and *T. equinum* is dependent on therapy and the elimination of blood-sucking flies (see p. 409). Since the capaybara may act as a reservoir host for *T. equinum*, the destruction of this animal will help control measures.

The control of *T. equiperdum* is achieved by quarantine regulations. The complement fixation test is used to detect infected animals, and reacting animals are destroyed. For Chagas disease, control is more difficult since poor economical conditions play an integral part in the epidemiology of the infection. The elimination of triatomic bugs from dwellings is a practical proposition and the destruction of wild animal reservoirs is also important.

Genus: Leishmania Ross, 1903

Developmental stages of this genus occur in the leishmanial form in vertebrates and in the leptomonad form in the insect vector and in culture. All the species of the genus are morphologically similar and their differentiation is based on the pathological entity they produce and on their geographical distribution.

Morphology. The leishmanial stages in vertebrates are found in the endothelial and macrophage cells of the body. They are circular or oval in outline and 2 μ–4 μ in diameter. When stained with Romanowsky stains the cytoplasm is blue, the oval nucleus is red and lies to one side and at right angles to it is a red- to purple-staining kinetoplast. The parasites multiply in the cytoplasm of cells forming clusters of organisms; dividing forms may be seen in smears. A more detailed account of the morphology is given by Adler (1964).

The Cycle in the Insect. A variety of *Phlebotomus* spp. (*Psychodidae*: *Nematocera*) have been shown to serve as vectors. During a blood meal the *Phlebotomus* (sandflies) ingests leucocytes and large mononuclear cells containing leishmanial bodies. These develop in the mid-gut of the sandfly and enormous numbers of leptomonads are produced. These pass to the oesophagus and pharynx of the fly and their number may be so great as to block the food canal. When a fly attempts to feed, a plug of organisms may be dislodged and injected into the mammalian hosts. Infection may also occur when infected sandflies are crushed on the skin.

Speciation of Leishmania

Though the leishmaniae are separated into species on pathological, immunological and geographical features there is considerable diversity and overlap between the various 'species'.

The speciation of the genus has been considered by Hoare (1949), Biagi (1953) and Adler (1964).

Leishmania donovani (Laveran & Mesnil, 1903) Ross, 1903 (syn. *Piroplasma donovani; Leishmania infantum; L. chagasi*). This organism is morphologically identical with the other species. It is the cause of kala azar, dumdum fever or visceral leishmaniasis in humans and dogs. In some areas dogs may serve as important reservoir hosts for the infection. Biagi (1953) has classified the different types of kala azar as follows:

Indian Kala Azar: Dundum fever, the classical form of *L. donovani*. It occurs in India affecting young adults, 60 per cent of infection being in the age group 10 to 20 years. There is no known reservoir in dogs, though they can be infected experimentally. Transmitted by *Phlebotomus argentipes.*

Chinese Kala Azar: Chiefly in northern China, mainly a condition of children with dog as a reservoir. Transmitted by *Phlebotomus chinensis* and *P. sergenti.*

Mediterranean (Infantile) Kala Azar: Chiefly in the Mediterranean area, southern Europe and parts of tropical Africa. Eighty per cent of cases occur in children under 5 years of age and 94 per cent in those under 10 years. Dogs serve as a reservoir host and in these infection rates may be as high as, or higher than, in the human population. Transmitted by *P. perniciosus* and *P. major*. (Some authors prefer to refer to this form as *L. infantum.*)

African Kala Azar: Occurs in Kenya and the Sudan. It resembles Indian kala azar in that 66 per cent of cases occur in young adults.

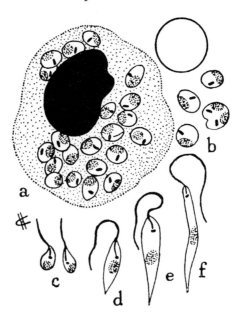

FIG. 268. *Leishmania donovani* and *L. tropica* (×2000). (After Hoare, 1950.) a. Macrophage containing rounded parasites ("Leishman-Donovan bodies"); b. Parasites outside host cell (one dividing); c–f. Flagellate (leptomonad) forms as seen in sandfly and in cultures. Erythrocyte drawn to scale.

Naturally infected dogs have not been found in endemic foci; however, natural infections have been found in a *Cercopithecus* monkey, a gerbil (*Tatera vicina*) and a ground squirrel (*Xerus rutilus*). Characterised by the early skin lesion which appears before the signs associated with the visceral infection. Transmitted by *P. orientalis* and *P. martini*.

Russian Kala Azar: This is an infection with a zoonotic reservoir in dogs and jackals in the Caucasus, Turkistan and other republics of the U.S.S.R. The transmitting fly is *P. arkaplensis*.

American Kala Azar: This occurs from Mexico to southern Argentina, though two cases of visceral leishmaniasis have been reported in dogs in the U.S.A. (Thorson, Bailey, Hoerlein & Siebold, 1955), both being imported cases. It occurs in humans of all ages but is more common in children. The dog and the fox (*Lycalopex vetulus*) serve as reservoir hosts. Transmitted by *P. intermedius* and *P. longipalus*.

In summary, therefore, the Indian and the African forms of visceral leishmaniasis are not dependent on canine infection (the latter may be a zoonosis since rodents may serve as reservoirs); with the Chinese, Mediterranean and American forms there is a definite zoonotic infection in dogs.

Pathogenesis of Visceral Leishmaniasis

Kala azar, especially the Indian form, is frequently a fatal disease in man. Following inoculation, leptomonads proliferate at the local site in macrophages and, after a period of weeks or months, they then invade the inner organs to multiply in the spleen, liver, bone marrow and elsewhere, destroying the macrophages in the process. In advanced cases involvement of the digestive tract results in diarrhoea, there is marked emaciation, a distended abdomen and mortality may reach 70–90 per cent in untreated cases, death occurring from a few weeks to a few years after infection.

On post-mortem there is emaciation, anaemia, a markedly enlarged spleen which is congested with prominent Malpighian corpuscles, and an enlarged liver shows fatty infiltration. Endothelial and macrophage cells contain masses of leishmaniae. The lymph nodes are usually enlarged and the cells parasitised. In the dog the same general pathology is seen as in humans, thus anaemia, emaciation and ultimately death occur, diarrhoea being a terminal clinical sign. On post mortem there is enlargement of the spleen, liver and lymph glands. Cutaneous lesions may occur, with ulcerations developing on the lips and eyelids. In chronic cases a chronic eczema may be seen and skin ulceration may be evident.

Immunity in Visceral Leishmaniasis. Recent reviews of this subject have been given by Adler (1963), Manson-Bahr (1963) and Stauber (1963). Adler (1963) comments that spontaneous cure is seldom seen in visceral leishmaniasis but he suggests that the massive lymphocyte-macrophage hyperplasia may have the effect of prolonging life. Treated human cases of kala azar, however, are immune and second infections do not occur in cured patients in endemic areas. Some of the cured cases show a post kala azar dermal 'leishmanoid', which contains numerous parasites, but such cases do not show generalised infection. In the dog, however, only temporary clinical improvement may occur after treatment, the infection persisting in the animal. Adler (1964) suggests that it is doubtful whether an effective immunity occurs to the Mediterranean form in the dog.

The relationship of protective immunity to circulating antibody is by no means proved (Stauber, 1963). Complement-fixing antibodies, using leishmanial antigens, have been demonstrated and these accompany marked changes in the *gamma* globulin fraction of the serum. There is, however, no quantitative relationship between the complement-fixing antibodies and *gamma* globulin and it would appear that the infection induces proliferation of clones of cells which produce *gamma* globulin without antibody specificity. The complement fixation technique has been used for surveys of canine leishmaniasis (Nussenzweig, 1959). Cross reactions occur with other protozoal infections, such as Chagas disease.

Nonspecific 'serological' tests such as the formal gel test of Napier (1927) and the urea stilbamine test of Chopra *et al.* (1927) have been used in India and China. These depend on the marked alterations in the albumin: globulin ratios which occur.

Diagnosis of Visceral Leishmaniasis. The only certain method of diagnosis is the demonstration of organisms in spleen pulp, lymph nodes, bone marrow, liver or fixed smears of peripheral blood. The first three may be taken by a biopsy and sternal puncture is increasingly used in diagnosis. In the dog, scrapings should be made from the periphery of skin ulcers or eczematous areas. Cultivation of biopsy or post-mortem material on NNN or a similar medium will demonstrate the leptomonads; however, growth may take one to several weeks to become evident.

Animal inoculation, using the golden hamster, is not usually resorted to for diagnosis, since infection takes some time to develop.

Treatment of Visceral Leishmaniasis. This has been reviewed by Goodwin & Rollo (1955). An early drug was tartar emetic but many doses had to be given for a cure. It has been replaced by the pentavalent organic antimony compounds such as Neostibosan, Solustibosan (sodium antimony gluconate) and the diamidine compounds such as hydroxystilbamine isethionate. In all cases several treatments are required.

Treatment of canine infection is less effective than that of the human forms, and the Mediterranean type responds poorly to Neostibosan, however, Solustibosan is reported to be effective.

Control of Visceral Leishmaniasis. A major control measure is the routine control of sandflies. The various chlorinated hydrocarbon, or organo-phosphorus, insecticides are useful, but measures against the breeding places of flies are also necessary. The latter include the removal of decaying vegetation and the clearing of dense vegetation around the houses. Where kala azar is a zoonosis involving dogs, these should be treated or destroyed. Control of stray dogs should be instituted.

Leishmania tropica (Wright, 1903) Lühe, 1906 (syn. *Helcosoma tropica, Herpetomonas tropica* etc.). The organism is morphologically identical with the other species. It is the cause of Old World cutaneous leishmaniasis, Oriental sore, Aleppo button, Delhi boil etc. The usual host is man. Dogs may suffer from dermal lesions, while in some areas the gerbil and other rodents are important reservoir hosts.

The organism is found in macrophages, endothelial cells of capillaries and the adjacent lymph nodes of the skin; it seldom invades the inner organs.

Types of Cutaneous Leishmaniasis

There are differences of opinion about the specific identities of the various cutaneous leishmaniases, but the situation is somewhat clarified if the view of Pessôa (1961) is adopted. He considers that each form of South American cutaneous or mucocutaneous leishmaniasis is caused by one of five distinct varieties of *Leishmania braziliensis*. This view will be adopted here. Consequently, cutaneous leishmaniasis of the Old World can be regarded as being due to *Leishmania tropica*.

Old World Cutaneous Leishmaniasis

The classical Oriental sore is found in Middle Eastern and Eastern countries with a hot, dry climate. It occurs in countries bordering the Mediterranean and the Black Sea, in the Sudan, Egypt, Equatorial Africa and West Africa, in the Middle East from the Lebanon to Turkey and thence eastwards to India, Pakistan and Ceylon. In these areas dogs are commonly infected and serve as zoonotic hosts. Sandflies are the natural vectors of the infection, the most common being *Phlebotomus papatasii* and *P. sergenti*. The former is chiefly concerned in the East and Africa and the latter in the Mediterranean littoral.

Russian authors distinguish an urban and a rural form of leishmaniasis in Turkestan, the former being caused by *Leishmania tropica* var. *minor* and the latter (the rural form) by *L. tropica* var. *major*. The latter organism produces a moist or wet lesion as compared with the dry lesion of *L. tropica* var. *minor*, this being similar to the classical Oriental sore infection and is possibly synonymous with it. *L. tropica* var. *major* is found in a variety of rodents of which the gerbil (*Rhombomys opimus*) is the most important. The sandflies *P. caucasicus* and *P. papatasii* live in the gerbil burrows and maintain the infection in these animals. *Phlebotomus papatasi* probably plays the more important role in the transmission of the gerbil infection to man since it more readily feeds on humans than *P. caucasicus*.

Pathogenesis of Old World Cutaneous Leishmaniasis. Following introduction of the leptomonads into the skin they are taken up by macrophages in which they multiply, they then rupture the cell and infect other cells. The first detectable lesion occurs 3 days to 6 weeks after the *Phlebotomus* bite, appearing as a reddish papule which gradually develops a crust, forming a shallow ulcer. The ulcer gradually enlarges and may reach several centimetres in diameter: ulcers may coalesce to form larger areas. In an uncomplicated infection the ulcers heal in 2–12 months leaving a deeply pigmented, depressed scar. The infection is very seldom fatal.

Skin leishmaniasis in the dog is similar to that in the human, ulcers being found on the skin.

In the dry type of infection in Turkestan (*L. t. minor*) there is a long incubation period, a prolonged clinical phase with papules persisting for several months and these contain large numbers of leishmaniae. The moist type (*L. t. major*) has a short incubation period, a short duration and few leishmaniae occur in the lesion. Ulcers form rapidly and heal spontaneously.

Immunity to Old World Cutaneous Leishmaniasis. This is reviewed by Adler (1963), Stauber (1963) and Zuckerman (1962). In the absence of treatment the local lesion of *L. tropica* runs its full course of reaction and proliferation of local histiocytes with intracellular multiplication of organisms. With the invasion of the lesion by lymphocytes and plasma cells the macrocytic proliferation diminishes, as do the organisms, until finally they completely disappear, spontaneous cure having taken place. The process may take up to 2 years in some cases (Adler, 1963). Spontaneous cure is followed by immunity which may persist more than 20 years after the disappearance of the lesion.

Immunisation of susceptible persons, using material from sores, has been practised for many years in the Middle East and Central Asia. A portion of the body hidden from view is infected, to prevent facial disfigurement from the active infection. A more modern approach to this consists of using living leptomonads from cultures of *L. tropica* (Berberian, 1939). Immunity is slow to develop and is not complete until the lesions have healed and the leishmaniae are no longer present. The process may take 4–6 months (Berberian, 1944). If the local lesion is surgically removed before spontaneous cure has taken place the patient remains susceptible to infection.

The immunological relationship between the various biological strains has yet to be clarified. With the Russian strains it has been stated that *L. t. minor* (the dry form) does not protect against *L. t. major* (the wet form) (Manson Bahr, 1963). However, Kozhevnikov (1959) was able to immunise against the dry form with the wet form and he also showed that immunisation with leptomonads from cultures of *L. t. major* isolated from gerbils give good protection against both forms. Ansari & Mofidi (1950), in Iran, obtained partial immunity against the wet form, using the dry type infection.

Diagnosis of Old World Cutaneous Leishmaniasis. Microscopic examination of material from the edge of an ulcer or a local lymph node will show the organisms in the epithelial and mononuclear cells. Culture of materials in NNN medium should also be made.

Treatment and Control. The pentavalent antimony compounds used for the visceral leishmaniasis are effective against the dermal infection.

Control measures include treatment and control and/or elimination of dogs. The destruction of gerbils greatly reduces the incidence of the wet form of infection. Vaccination with leptomonads from cultures obtained from experimentally infected animals has been widely practised in the Middle East, but the increasing elimination of sandflies due to mosquito and malarial control measures has greatly decreased the necessity for immunisation in urban areas. It is still applicable in rural communities.

Leishmania braziliensis Vianna, 1911 (syn. *L. tropica* var. *americana*). The organism is morphologically identical with the other species. It is the cause of American leishmaniasis, Espundia, Uta and mucocutaneous leishmaniasis, etc. The organisms are found in endothelial and mononuclear cells of the skin and mucous membranes of the nose, mouth, pharynx and elsewhere.

Man is the primary host for the parasite. Though dogs, cats, the spiny pocket mouse, the white-footed mouse and the tree rat have been found naturally infected, there is some doubt that these animals are the main reservoir hosts and it is probable that there are some wild jungle animals, as yet unknown, which serve as this. The disease is restricted to hot, humid forest areas usually under 2,500 feet altitude though the Uta form can occur up to 9,000 feet.

There is confusion about the identity of the forms or strains which cause cutaneous leishmaniasis in the New World. Floch (1954) considers that all forms of cutaneous leishmaniasis are caused by *Leishmania tropica* and that three sub-species occur in South America, namely *L. tropica braziliensis, L. tropica mexicana* and *L. tropica guyanensis.*

Pessôa (1961) considers that all forms of South American cutaneous and mucocutaneous leishmaniasis are caused by *L. braziliensis* and he distinguishes five distinct varieties. This subject is considered in detail by Adler (1964).

Leishmania braziliensis braziliensis Vianna, 1911. This causes the classical espundia of the Brazilian rain forest, metastases occurring in the oropharynx in 80 per cent of cases. The skin lesions are chronic and invasion of the mucous membrane sometimes causes great disfigurement by erosion of the soft and cartilaginous tissues. The disease may last for many years and spontaneous recovery is rare. Death may occur due to septicaemia or bronchial pneumonia. The vectors are *P. intermedius, P. migonei* and *P. whitmani*, etc.

Leishmania braziliensis guyanensis Floch, 1953. Floch (1954) gave this name to the leishmania of French Guinea which causes a similar condition to that in Panama, Costa Rica, and other parts of northern South America. Levine (1963) equates this type with American forest leishmaniasis, pian bois or buba of northern South America. The skin ulcerations tend to show spontaneous healing and only in about 5 per cent of cases do metastases occur in the nasal mucosa. Dogs may be naturally infected; the important animal reservoirs are unknown. *L. b. guyanensis* is transmitted by *P. evansi, P. migonei, P. parasinensis, P. anduzei* and *P. suis.*

Leishmania braziliensis mexicana Biagi, 1953. This is a cause of Chiclero ulcer or Bay sore of Mexico, Guatemala and Honduras. The primary lesion may be small and heal within a few weeks. This strain also characteristically attacks the ear, causing a granulomatous lesion which grossly deforms the earlobe. Metastases are rare. No animal reservoir infection has yet been found. Transmission is by *P. cruciatus* (Mexico), *P. panamensis, P. ylephytar,* and *P. shannoni.*

Leishmania braziliensis peruviana Velez, 1913. This is the cause of Uta in the mountains of Peru. It is a benign form of the disease showing numerous small skin lesions which generally resemble the Old World form of leishmaniasis in its clinical course. The distribution of Uta in Peru coincides with the distribution of *P. noguchi*; animal reservoirs are not known.

Leishmania braziliensis pifano Medina and Romero, 1957. This name was created for the parasite associated with the rare form of cutaneous leishmaniasis known as leishmaniasis tegumentaria diffusa which is a chronic diffuse form.

Pathogenesis of American Cutaneous Leishmaniasis. Though there are a number of different strains of organisms generally the disease process can be divided into the metastasising form (*L. b. braziliensis*) and the non-metastasising forms (others). In the non-metastasising form the initial papule gives way to ulceration with induration which heals in 6 to 18 months. The classical espundia shows metastases which may take several years to develop. The nasal septum, nasopharynx and even the larynx may be involved with appalling disfigurement.

Immunity to American Cutaneous Leishmaniasis. Recovery is followed by a relatively solid immunity to reinfection in the non-metastasising form, and it thus resembles the Old World form of cutaneous leishmaniasis. With espundia there is less evidence of spontaneous recovery though the cellular reaction apparently reduces the number of organisms in the lesions to a minimum. Adler (1963) has reported that two volunteers previously infected with *L. tropica* were immune to *L. b. mexicana.*

Cutaneous and mucocutaneous leishmaniases give a delayed skin reaction. This is utilised in the 'Montenegro' test for which organisms obtained from culture serve as antigen. Pelligreno (1951) used a polysaccharide antigen of *L. braziliensis.*

Diagnosis of *L. braziliensis* infection is much the same as for *L. tropica.*

In long-standing infections, where organisms are few, immunodiagnostic tests such as the Montenegro reaction can be employed.

Treatment consists of using antimony compounds but where metastases have occurred treatment may have to be prolonged.

Control. American cutaneous leishmaniasis is principally an infection of persons working in forests. Personal protection against sandflies by using repellents is of immediate but limited value; the long-term control must depend on wide-scale sandfly control.

ORDER: POLYMASTIGIDA BLOCHMAN, 1895

Organisms of this order are characterised by possessing three to six flagella, one of which may be a trailing flagellum, frequently attached to an undulating membrane. They may have one or two nuclei and reproduction is asexual, usually by binary fission. In a few cases it may be sexual. Cysts may be produced in some forms.

The majority of the forms are nonpathogenic and a large variety of species is found in the alimentary canal of animals.

From time to time pathological changes have been ascribed to a number of species, since they may be found in large numbers in the faeces or in samples from the digestive tract. However, this is not conclusive evidence of a disease relationship, especially since many species multiply readily in a fluid environment. There are, however, some pathogenic forms, these being found in the genera *Tritrichomonas, Trichomonas, Giardia* and *Hexamita*.

FAMILY TRICHOMONADIDAE WENYON, 1926

These are the trichomonads occurring usually in the digestive tract but they may also be found in the reproductive system and elsewhere.

They are pyriform in shape, have a rounded anterior end and a somewhat pointed posterior end. There is a single nucleus in the anterior part of the body and anterior to this is the blepharoplast which is associated with a number of basal granules. Arising from the blepharoplast are the anterior flagella and a posterior flagellum, which runs along the edge of an undulating membrane and often extends posteriorly from the body. A deeply staining costa extends along the base of the undulating membrane and, especially characteristic, is a rod-like axostyle which runs through the body arising from the blepharoplast and emerging from the posterior end. Several genera occur in the family and the speciation is largely dependent on the number of anterior flagella. Those with three anterior flagella belong to the genus *Tritrichomonas*, those with four to *Trichomonas* and those with five to the genus *Pentatrichomonas*.

Genus: Tritrichomonas Kofoid, 1920

Members have three anterior flagella. Details of the many species which occur may be obtained from Grassé (1952), Kudo (1954) and Levine (1961). The following are the species of major interest.

Tritrichomonas foetus (Riedmuller, 1928) Weinrich and Emmerson, 1933. This is a parasite of cattle. It may also occur in the zebu, pig, horse and deer but pathogenic effects are seen only in the bovine, in which it causes the specific venereal disease, bovine trichomoniasis.

The organism is world wide in distribution and at one time was of major economic importance especially in dairy herds. Its incidence in cattle is now very much less than formerly due to the widespread use of artificial insemination and to the decrease in the number of bulls kept on small dairy farms. It is still of importance in beef herds, and in a 7-year survey made in the Rocky Mountain States of the U.S.A. Johnson (1964) found it in 62 of 828 beef bulls tested in thirty-four separate herds, nine herds being infected, giving a herd infection rate of 26 per cent.

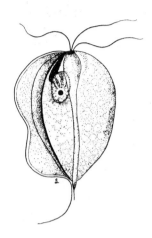

FIG. 269. *Tritrichomonas foetus* (Original)

Morphology. The organism is roughly pear-shaped, 10–25 μ long by 3–15 μ wide. It moves with a characteristic vigorous jerky movement. The nucleus is anterior, there is a cytosome which is difficult to discern and a sausage-shaped parabasal body. Three anterior flagella are present and the posterior flagellum extends back along the undulating membrane and trails behind the organism. The undulating membrane runs the full length of the body, the costa is prominent, the axostyle is well developed and it emerges from the end of the body through a chromatic ring.

Multiplication is by longitudinal binary fission. No sexual process or encystation has been observed.

The organism can be readily cultured on a variety of media. For immunological work a 'diphasic' glucose-broth-serum medium (Kerr & Robertson, 1953) has been used while a trypticase yeast extract, maltose cysteine and serum medium has been used by Diamond (1957). A detailed discussion of the nutritional requirements of the species is given by Shorb (1964).

Two serologically distinct strains of organism have so far been found; these are the 'Belfast' and 'Manley' strains (Kerr & Robertson, 1945). The Belfast strain is the predominant strain, occurring in Europe, Africa and the U.S.A. The number of outbreaks of disease due to the Manley strain are few. The two strains have been maintained in culture for more than 20 years and still retain their immunological distinctness (Kerr, 1964).

Transmission. Under natural conditions the infection is transmitted during coitus. It may also be transmitted by artificial insemination and by gynaecological examination of cows.

Pathogenesis. In the bull the most common infection site is the preputial cavity. Commonly the infection does not cause any apparent clinical condition, however in the early stages of the infection an inflammatory balanitis may occur with pain on micturition and a disinclination to serve cows. A mucoid to mucopurulent discharge may be present along with small reddish papules on the mucous membrane of the prepuce and the glans penis. These signs disappear in 1–2 weeks but infection may remain in the prepuce for a considerable period of time. Occasionally the testes, epididymus and seminal vesicles become infected and undergo inflammation. Spontaneous recovery is uncommon and generally, once a bull is infected he is to be regarded as a permanent source of the infection. Usually the infection does not affect the fertility of the bull or the viability of the spermatozoa.

In the female, natural infection is introduced into the vagina during coitus. The initial lesion is a vaginitis of varying intensity; it may be so slight as to pass unnoticed or it may produce a mucopurulent discharge. The maximum number of organisms are present in the vagina 14 to 18 days after service (Hammond & Bartlett, 1945) and from this site they invade the uterus through the cervix. They may then completely disappear from the vagina, or a low level of infection may remain, producing catarrh and roughness of the vaginal mucosa.

The sequelae to the invasion of the uterus are several. In some cases, despite the infection, the animal may conceive normally, carry the calf to full term, and give birth to a normal healthy calf. The number of infections where this happens is, however, small.

Frequently a placentitis results with detachment of the placental membranes and death of the foetus. This leads to an abortion, which is characteristically early, usually 8–16 weeks after the infected service. Later abortions (i.e. after 6 months) are rare and only a few verified cases have been reported (Morgan & Hawkins, 1952). If abortion occurs very early (e.g. 1–2 weeks) the foetus and membranes frequently pass out unnoticed and this may lead to the belief that there has been an irregular oestrus cycle. Following the abortion there may be a uterine discharge and where this persists, the animal may show a series of irregular heat periods. In some animals the foetus and membranes are not completely eliminated and maceration occurs leading to a chronic catarrhal and sometimes purulent endometritis. This causes more prolonged, and at times permanent, sterility. There is anoestrus, and a persistent uterine discharge occurs, which may be especially noticeable when the animal lies down.

At times the cervix is closed and, in the presence of a retained corpus luteum, a closed pyometra results. Fluid accumulates over several weeks and ultimately the uterus contains a large volume of thin, greyish-white, odourless material swarming with trichomonads. There is associated anoestrus and the owner may consider the animal to be pregnant during this period.

Immunology of Trichomoniasis in Cattle. There is little evidence that bulls become immune to infection. Usually the organism persists in them for life and the animal is a continuous source of infection for cows.

In the cow, immunity to reinfection commonly follows abortion and it is unusual for more than one abortion to take place; however, a recovered cow may not always be cleared of the organism. Despite the development of immunity to the parasite permanent sterility may result if there has been extensive involvement of the uterine mucosa.

Reviews of the immunology of *T. foetus* infection have been given by Levine (1961), Robertson (1963) and Kerr (1964). Robertson (1963) tabulates the antibodies produced in *T. foetus* infection as:

(a) Circulating humoral antibody stimulated by antigen which reaches the systemic circulation from the uterus.

(b) Uterine antibody developing *in situ.*

(c) Vaginal antibody developing locally.

These antibodies are most readily detected by an agglutination technique (Kerr & Robertson, 1941; 1943). A capillary agglutination test has been described by Feinberg (1952).

A normal agglutinin for *T. foetus* has been detected in cattle, being at a fairly constant titre of 1–48 to 1–96. It is absent from the serum of unsuckled calves at birth and is acquired with other antibodies in collostrum. It persists in a calf for 17–55 days (Kerr & Robertson, 1954).

The circulating humoral antibody is developed in field infections only when there is an adequate degree of infection with large numbers of ·trichomonads in the uterus. This occurs in cases of abortion or pyometra (Pierce, 1949). Circulating antibody can also be induced by intramuscular injection of lyophilised organisms, but this does not pass to the lumen of the uterus. Circulating antibody sensitises the skin of the animal and the development of this can be followed by the interdermal injection of a diethylene glycol extract of lyophilised *T. foetus* (Feinberg & Morgan, 1953). The skin reaction is of the immediate type hypersensitivity, producing a local oedema which reaches its maximum in 20–30 minutes and disappears within 2–3 hours.

Sensitisation of the uterus occurs as a result of antibody being produced by the uterus. Repeated introduction of antigen into the uterus results in a local anaphylactic reaction, which, at times, may become general in nature. The free antibody in the uterus, which can be obtained by irrigating the uterus with saline, is induced only by trichomonads in the uterus or by the injection into this site of freeze-dried organisms

(Robertson, 1963). She considers this local antibody to be responsible for the disappearance of *T. foetus* from the uterus in mild infections, especially where pregnancy is not interrupted.

Pierce (1953, 1959) demonstrated that vaginal antibody could occur before there was circulating antibody in the serum and he also found that a high titre of antibody could exist in the vaginal mucus while trichomonads were numerous in the uterine discharge. He concluded that the vaginal mucosa was producing antibody locally, independently of the uterine and circulating antibodies. The protective effects of the vaginal antibody are suggested by Robertson (1963) to be a local control of parasites in the vagina.

Epidemiology. Under natural conditions trichomoniasis of the bovine is spread by the bull. Once infected he must be regarded as being a permanent source of infection, whereas in the female the infection is self-limiting and the parasites gradually disappear. Following recovery from infection a cow will usually conceive and undergo gestation without any danger of abortion. A cow may, however, also serve as a carrier of the infection.

Of the other methods of infection, artificial insemination is the most common, though gynaecological examinations of cows may be responsible for local spread. The use of fresh semen from an infected bull in artificial insemination may lead to widespread outbreaks of disease, however this danger has been recognised early in the development of artificial insemination and strict examination of bulls in artificial insemination centres avoids this. The development of techniques for preserving bovine semen has also assisted in the control of *T. foetus* infection. A number of investigators have reported, variously, that *T. foetus* does or does not survive, when freezing in the presence of glycerol. The organisms are killed by glycerol at 37°C or at ordinary refrigeration temperatures but below this, survival depends on the diluting fluids used to preserve the semen and the stage of the population growth of *T. foetus*. The subject is reviewed by Levine, Mizell & Houlahan (1958). A detailed study on the survival of *T. foetus* under extended storage conditions in the presence of glycerol has been carried out by Levine et al. (1962). These authors found that the organisms survived much better at −95°C than at −28°C in the presence of 1 M glycerol. At the lower temperature trichomonads remained viable for up to 256 days.

The importance of other animals in the transmission of *T. foetus* to cattle has received attention. Organisms similar to *T. foetus* have been found in the genital tract and aborted foetuses of horses (Schoop & Oehlikers, 1939), and Schoop & Stolz (1939) have found trichomonads resembling *T. foetus* in the genital organs of roe deer in Germany. There is little evidence however that these play any part in the epidemiology of the bovine infection. The relationship of *Tritrichomonas foetus* of cattle to the swine form *Tritrichomonas suis* remains to be determined. Switzer

(1951) reported that the inoculation of cultures of trichomonads from the nasal and digestive tract of swine into the vagina of cattle produced infections. Fitzgerald *et al.* (1958) infected a series of heifers with tri-chomonads from the nose, stomach or caecum of pigs. Infections lasted up to 133 days with the nasal forms, 88 days with the stomach forms, and 2 infections with caecal trichomonads lasted 84 and 33 days. In one experiment the intrauterine inoculation of swine caecal trichomonads into a 4 months pregnant heifer was followed 20 days later by an abortion and trichomonads were found in the foetal fluids and in the foetus. Such work confirms the idea that swine trichomonads can become established in the reproductive tract of cattle but it is not known whether they play any part in the naturally occurring disease. The spontaneous recovery which is seen with the swine trichomonad infection, especially in the male bovine, would suggest that infection is of a temporary nature. However, Robertson (1960) studied the antigenic relationships between bovine and swine trichomonads and found cross-reactions between them. Two strains of *T. suis* were more closely related to the Belfast strain of *T. foetus* than to the Manley strain and she concluded that the serological distinction between the organisms did not justify separate speciation. She proposed that they all be called *T. foetus*.

Diagnosis. Presumptive evidence of trichomonas in a herd can be obtained from a history of early abortions, an increased incidence of cows returning to service and a failure of animals to become pregnant except after repeated service. There may also be an increase in the prevalence of vaginal discharge and pyometra in a herd, all of which may be related to the importation of new stock, especially a new bull.

Confirmation of a diagnosis is based on the demonstration of the organisms in the vaginal or uterine discharges or in the foetus, and on serological tests. Trichomonads are found most readily in the stomach of an aborted foetus, in the amniotic and allantoic fluids and in the uterine discharges after abortion. Where such material is not available uterine discharges may be collected from the cow and this is best done 2–3 days before the expected time of the next oestrus. Samples may also be obtained by washing the vagina with physiological saline or by irrigation of the uterus with saline. In the bull, preputial washings are the best source of material. In all sampling procedures, however, it is important to avoid contamination with faecal material since this may introduce intestinal protozoa into the sample and these may readily be confused with *T. foetus*. In heavily infected material, especially purulent mucus, the organism may be observed directly, the sample being examined on a slide under a coverslip. In less grossly infected samples the material may be allowed to sediment and be centrifuged before examination. The sample should be kept warm throughout and warm saline added before examination. The main feature of *T. foetus* is its characteristic motility, but old material, or that which has become cold may show very sluggish organisms and careful observation is required to detect the parasites. In sluggish forms the undulating membrane is seen but care should be taken not to confuse the organism with the many other species of protozoa that may be present in samples, especially if these have been obtained carelessly.

Where organisms are too few to allow an accurate diagnosis the preparation should be stained or, more satisfactorily, cultures should be prepared from the material. Several media are available for cultivation purposes and have been mentioned previously. These should be examined at 24 and 48 hours and also 4 days. The cervical mucus agglutination test is the most satisfactory immuno-diagnostic test (Pierce, 1949a). Mucus samples are collected from the vagina of the cow, using a sterile glass tube 50 cm. in length and 9 mm. in diameter and bent at an angle of 150° about 9 cm. from one end. The other end is plugged with cotton wool. Mucus is obtained preferably a few days after oestrus, from the anterior end of the vagina by suction. The mucus is mixed with glucose saline and serially diluted or the antibody in the mucus allowed to diffuse into saline which is then diluted. The test organisms consist of a suspension of *in vitro* cultured *T. foetus*, a density of 100,000 organisms per ml. being satisfactory. Though the mucus agglutination test is considerably superior to the serum agglutination test (Pierce, 1949b), it is essentially a herd test since the status of the sexual cycle of the cow may affect the reaction. Unsatisfactory results are obtained with mucus samples taken during the oestrus period, or shortly after it and mucus from pregnant animals may give false reactions.

An interdermal test developed by Kerr (1944) gives inconsistent results. Thus Morgan (1948) obtained negative results with it and other workers have found that animals may be desensitised to the skin test during acute uterine infections with *T. foetus* or by the injection of antigen intramuscularly.

It is important with any diagnostic method to conduct several examinations before an animal is declared uninfected. Even after a satisfactory gestation and the birth of a normal calf an animal should be bred by artificial insemination to avoid the risk of infecting bulls. In the bull more lengthy testing is necessary before he can be considered free from infection. It is useful to breed the bull to 2 or more virgin heifers to assess his freedom from infection.

Treatment. A vast number of compounds have been used in the treatment of trichomoniasis in the cow, but since the infection is essentially a self-limiting one, and leads to an adequate immunity, treatment should be aimed at giving the animals a breeding rest and, subsequently, artificial insemination should be used to avoid infecting clean bulls.

Infected bulls are much more difficult to treat since trichomonicidal agents must be introduced to all parts of the preputial cavity. Since treatment is tedious, time consuming, and must be repeated on several occasions, it is frequently better to slaughter the bull. Of the compounds which have been used in treatment trypaflavine and acriflavine have been most commonly employed (Bartlett, 1948; and Hammond et al., 1953).

In the treatment of the bull, pudendal anaesthesia (Larson, 1953) is used to relax the retractor penis muscle. The penis is washed with a weak solution of detergent, dried and flavine ointment introduced into the preputial cavity and massaged in for 15–20 minutes. A solution of acriflavine is also injected into the urethra to kill any organisms which may be there. Fitzgerald et al. (1963) demonstrated that acriflavine ointment was effective in eliminating infection in the majority of treated bulls, however, the use of more than 1 per cent of acriflavine may result in tissue damage. Several treatments may be necessary to eliminate infection but if the epididymis or testes are affected treatment is of little use.

Fitzgerald et al. (1963) reported that berenil (4,4-diamidinodiazo-aminobenzene aceturate), which is used for the treatment of trypanoso-miasis, is also a useful therapeutic agent for bovine trichomoniasis. One hundred to 150 ml. of 1 per cent solution of berenil is injected into the prepuce and is retained there for 15 minutes while the penis and the prepuce are thoroughly massaged. Five successive daily treatments usually eliminate an infection.

Control. The major control measure for trichomoniasis in cattle is the use of artificial insemination. The practice of using communal bulls is to be discouraged since it leads to the spread of the disease. In an overall policy it is also wise to eliminate cows which have been infected since, though they may breed satisfactorily, their freedom from infection cannot be assumed.

Tritrichomonas suis (Gruby & Delafond, 1843). This is the largest of the pig trichomonads, occurring chiefly in the stomach, but also in the nasal passages, caecum, and small intestine. The trichomonad parasites of pigs have been studied in detail by Hibler et al. (1960), who concluded that three forms were present, namely the large *T. suis* and two small forms, *Tritrichomonas rotunda* and *T. buttreyi* (see later).

T. suis is world wide in distribution. It is elongate or spindle shaped, $11 \cdot 19\,\mu$–$14 \cdot 44\,\mu$ by $3 \cdot 3\,\mu$–$3 \cdot 5\,\mu$. Forms as small as $9\,\mu$ and up to $16\,\mu$ in length may be found. The three anterior flagella are equal in length, each ending in a small round knob. The undulating membrane and the costa run the full length of the body and the axostyle extends $0 \cdot 6\,\mu$–$1 \cdot 7\,\mu$ beyond the body as a cone-shaped projection narrowing sharply to a short tip.

In the past, the association of *T. suis* with a high percentage of cases of atrophic rhinitis has led to the belief that this organism is responsible for that condition. The disease has been produced in young pigs with nasal washings containing trichomonads but when *T. suis* is grown axenically it is no longer able to produce the disease. It is now generally known that atrophic rhinitis is due to another agent. Consequently *T. suis* is regarded as nonpathogenic.

Tritrichomonas rotunda Hibler, Hammond, Caskey, Johnson and Fitzgerald, 1960. This is the medium-sized trichomonad of pigs, occurring principally in the caecum and colon. It was recognised as a new species by Hibler *et al.* (1960) as a result of their extensive study of the trichomonads of swine, it being found in the caecum of 10·5 per cent of approximately 500 pigs in Utah. Up to the present it has been recognised only in North America but it is presumed that it has a similar distribution to that of *T. suis.*

It is broadly pyriform in shape measuring 8·59 μ by 5·8 μ with a range of 7–11 μ and 5–7 μ. The three anterior flagella are equal in length and terminate in small knob-like structures; the undulating membrane is low, the costa extends only $\frac{1}{2}$ to $\frac{2}{3}$ the length of the body and the posterior free flagellum is shorter than the body. There is no evidence that this organism is pathogenic.

Tritrichomonas buttreyi Hibler, Hammond, Caskey, Johnson, and Fitzgerald, 1960. This is the small trichomonad of pigs, occurring in the caecum and colon. So far it has been recognised only in the United States but it is presumed that its distribution is similar to the other two in swine. Hibler *et al.* (1960) found it in 25 per cent of 496 pigs in Utah. It measures a mean of 5·92 μ by 3·44 μ; there are three or four anterior flagella; the undulating membrane runs the full length of the body and the axostyle is narrow and protrudes 3–6 μ posteriorly from the body. There is no evidence that *T. buttreyi* is pathogenic.

Tritrichomonas equi (Fantham, 1921). This species has been found in the caecum and colon of horses. It is probably world wide in distribution though it has been specifically reported only from South Africa and the United States. It measures 11 μ by 6 μ and has three anterior flagella and an undulating membrane with a slender axostyle. There is no evidence that this organism is associated with any pathogenic entity, though its association with a persistent diarrhoea of horses has been reported.

Tritrichomonas eberthi (Martin & Robertson, 1911) Kofoid, 1920. This is a common trichomonad occurring in the caecum of the chicken, turkey and duck. It is world wide in distribution and appears to be common, McDowell (1953) finding it in 35 per cent of chickens in Pennsylvania. It is broadly crescent-shaped, 8 μ–14 μ by 4 μ–7 μ, there are three anterior flagella, the undulating membrane is prominent, extending the full length of the body. The costa and axostyle are distinct.

There is no evidence that this species is pathogenic.

Several other species of *Tritrichomonas* are found in various animals. These include the two species *Tritrichomonas enteris* (Christl, 1954), which has been reported from the caecum and colon of the ox and zebu in

Germany and in the East, and *Tritrichomonas fecalis* (Cleveland, 1928), isolated from human faeces. Neither form is associated with any pathogenic effects.

Genus: Trichomonas Donne, 1837

Members of this genus are pyriform and typically have four free anterior flagella. Numerous species exist (Grasse, 1952).

Trichomonas gallinae (Rivolta, 1878) Stabler, 1938 (syn. *Trichomonas columbae*, *T. hepaticum*, *T. halli*, etc.). *Trichomonas gallinae* is the cause of avian trichomoniasis of the upper digestive tract and is found particularly in pigeons, but the turkey, chicken, hawk, mourning dove, golden eagle etc. may be infected (Levine, 1961).

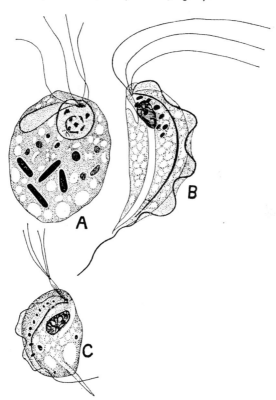

FIG. 270. Flagellates from the Caecum of the Fowl (×4000). (From Wenyon, 1926.)
A. *Chilomastix gallinarum*. B. *Tritrichomonas eberthi*. C. *Trichomonas gallinarum*

The organism is pyriform in shape, usually small, and measures 10 μ by 5 μ, however, it may range in size from 6 μ–19 μ by 2 μ–9 μ. There are 4 anterior flagella each up to 13 μ in length. The axostyle is narrow and protrudes a short distance posteriorly from the body, the undulating membrane extends about ⅔ of the total length of the body and does not terminate in a trailing flagellum. A cytosome is present.

T. gallinae is extremely common in the domestic pigeon in which it may cause serious disease. It is also fairly common in the turkey and chicken and it may be responsible for disease in mourning doves (Stabler & Herman, 1951). Hawks may be infected when they feed on pigeons.

Pathogenesis. Avian trichomoniasis caused by *T. gallinae* is a disease of young birds. Eighty to 90 per cent, or more, of adult pigeons are infected but show no evidence of disease, but infected pigeon squabs may die within 10 days. A difference in the pathogenicity of strains of *T. gallinae* has been reported by Stabler. The most virulent is the Jones' Barn (J.B.) strain which has maintained its pathogenicity through three hundred serial passages in pigeons (Stabler, 1953; 1957). Honigberg (1961) found that the growth rate of three strains of *T. gallinae* was positively correlated to the virulence for pigeons and mice. Thus the virulent J.B. strain had a generation time of $3\frac{1}{2}$ hours, a T.G. strain one of 3 hours 50 minutes, and a less virulent (Y.G.) strain one of 5 hours 50 minutes.

With a virulent strain the earliest lesions appear as small yellowish circumscribed areas in the mouth cavity, especially the soft palate, 3–14 days after infection. These increase in size and number and extend to the oesophagus, crop and proventriculus; the liver may also be involved and there may be extension to the lungs and the serous surfaces of the intestine, the pancreas and the heart. The lesions of the digestive tract do not extend beyond the proventriculus. Histologically the lesions consist of inflammation and ulceration of the oropharyngeal mucosa associated with a palisading of the parasites on the mucous surface (Mesa *et al.*, 1961). The organisms invade the pharyngeal glands, penetrate the underlying tissues and reach the liver. It is considered that the abscesses in the liver are the cause of death. Mesa *et al.* (1961) suggested that the J.B. strain of *T. gallinae* produces a hepato-toxin.

In the turkey and chicken the lesions most commonly occur in the crop, oesophagus and pharynx and are uncommon in the mouth. Lesions in the mourning dove are similar to those seen in the pigeon.

The pathogenicity of *T. gallinae* in experimental hosts has been studied by various authors (Frost & Honigberg, 1962). In studies with mice, only the J.B. strain was significantly pathogenic while a mild strain of *T. gallinae* produced a minor effect.

Honigberg *et al.* (1964), using, chicken liver cell cultures, found that the parasites caused degeneration of epithelial and fibroblast cells and stimulated activity of macrophages. Organisms multiplied mainly within macrophages but some invasion of the epithelial cells and fibroblasts occurred. Subsequent work by Abraham & Honigberg (1965) demonstrated a reduction of RNA in chick liver cell cultures from the 8th hour after inoculation with the parasites, this effect becoming pronounced with time. The DNA in such cultures remained unchanged.

Clinical Signs. Infected pigeon squabs show an initial depression with ruffled feathers and later they become weak and emaciated. There is an accumulation of a greenish fluid, or cheesy, material in the mouth and crop and this may exude from the beak. In turkey poults and chickens, drowsiness and a pendulous crop are usually observed and there is a foul odour from the mouth. On post mortem yellowish to greyish necrotic lesions are evident in the mouth, crop, and oesophagus with extension to the bones of the skull, the liver, and elsewhere. Organisms are usually very numerous in the mouth and crop contents.

Immunity. Recovered birds are immune to reinfection but survive as symptomless carriers. Infection with a nonvirulent strain produces immunity against the more virulent strains (Stabler, 1951). Certain breeds of birds may be more susceptible than others and Miessner & Hansen (1936) considered that Roller and Tumbler pigeons were the most susceptible.

Epidemiology. In pigeons the organism is transmitted directly from carrier older birds to the newly hatched pigeon squab via the 'pigeon's milk' from the crop. This may occur within a few minutes of hatching. Adult birds may remain infected for a year or more and are a constant source of infection for their young. The mode of infection of turkeys and chickens is most likely to be through drinking water contaminated by trichomonads from the mouths of infected birds (Stabler, 1954) but since the organism does not survive readily almost direct contamination is necessary. Wild pigeons and other birds probably play an important role in introducing the infection to domestic birds.

Diagnosis. Diagnosis is based on the characteristic lesions in the oral cavity, oesophagus and crop, and usually the organism is readily demonstrated in the greenish fluid material or in the lesions. It is also readily cultured on a variety of media including a glucose–broth–serum medium (Richardson & Kendall, 1963) or a trypticase–yeast extract–maltose–cysteine–serum medium (Diamond, 1957).

Treatment

2-amino-5-nitrothiazole. Homing pigeons—30 mg. per kg. daily for 7 days; other birds—45 mg. per kg. Carrier birds may also be treated with this drug (Stabler & Mellentin, 1953).

Furazolidone. 25–30 mg. per day for 7 days, given in gelatin capsules (Stabler, 1957).

Control. Control is readily obtained by treatment with 2-amino-5-nitrothiazole. The introduction of infection from wild pigeons and other birds may be prevented by shielding the drinking places.

Trichomonas gallinarum Martin and Robertson, 1911. This organism is found in the lower digestive tract and sometimes the liver of turkey, domestic fowl, and guinea fowl. It has also been found in quail, pheasant and partridge, and forms very similar to it have been found in the Canada goose by Diamond (1957). It is cosmopolitan in distribution.

The organism is pear-shaped, 9 μ–15 μ by 5 μ–9 μ, the axostyle is long and slender and projects from the posterior part of the body. The original form described by Martin & Robertson (1911) had four anterior flagella and one posterior flagellum which extended behind the body. A form with five anterior flagella has been described by Allen (1940), and Mc-Dowell (1953) reports that occasionally three or five anterior flagella may occur but four is the most usual number.

Pathogenesis. *T. gallinarum* has been found in turkeys in liver lesions resembling those due to histomoniasis (Allen, 1936; 1941; Walker, 1948). These authors consider *T. gallinarum* capable of causing a disease similar to enterohepatitis.

The liver lesions are said to differ from those produced by *Histomonas meleagridis* by having a more irregular outline and by being raised above the liver surface instead of being depressed below it, as in the case of *H. meleagridis*. Allen (1941) reported that the administration to young turkeys of cultures of an organism resembling *T. gallinarum* produced entero-hepatitis; however, this finding has not been confirmed and in fact Delappe (1957) was unable to produce any lesions with a strain of *T. gallinarum* isolated from the liver lesions of a turkey with enterohepatitis.

Infection is by the ingestion of trichomonads in contaminated feed or water. McLoughlin (1957) found that *T. gallinarum* could survive for 24 hours in caecal droppings kept at 37°C and for 120 hours when they were kept at 6°C.

Other trichomonads of domestic birds include *Trichomonas anseri* (Hegner, 1929) of the caecum of geese (8 μ × 4·7 μ) and *Trichomonas anatis* (Kotlan, 1923) from the duck (13 μ–27 μ × 8 μ–18 μ). Neither are known to be pathogenic.

Trichomonas ovis (Robertson, 1932) Morgan, 1946. This organism was found in the caeca of 12 out of 16 domestic sheep in Illinois and Utah by Anderson *et al.* (1962). It is pyriform, 6 μ–9 μ by 4 μ–8 μ, with an anterior nucleus and a slender tapering axostyle which protrudes 5 μ beyond the body. There are four anterior flagella of unequal length and a prominent undulating membrane which extends beyond the body. There is no evidence that this species is pathogenic in sheep.

Other species of the genus *Trichomonas* which occur in domestic animals are *Trichomonas felistomae*, Hegner & Ratcliffe, 1927, which occurs in the mouth of cats in the United States. It is a nonpathogenic form 6 μ–11 μ by 3 μ–4 μ. It is possibly the same as *Trichomonas canistomae*, Hegner & Ratcliffe, 1927, which occurs in the mouth of the dog. *Trichomonas equibuccalis*, Simitch, 1939, occurs in the mouth and around the teeth of the horse in Central Europe. It is a nonpathogenic form 7 μ–10 μ in length. *Trichomonas macacovaginae*, Hegner & Ratcliffe, 1927, has been found in the vagina of the rhesus monkey.

In the human, two species of the genus are of importance, *T. vaginalis* and *T. tenax*.

Trichomonas vaginalis Donné, 1837. This form occurs in the vagina, prostate and urethra of man. Experimentally the golden hamster can be infected intravaginally and the mouse subcutaneously.

This is the largest of the human trichomonads, being 7μ–23μ by 5μ–12μ (mean $17\mu \times 7\mu$). There is an oval nucleus at the anterior end; the undulating membrane extends $\frac{1}{3}$ to $\frac{2}{3}$ of the body length; there is no free posterior flagellum and the axostyle is slender and projects from the posterior end as a pointed rod.

Trichomonas vaginalis is world wide in distribution and various surveys have shown prevalencies of from 2 per cent to 90 per cent in various areas. It is more common in females aged 30 to 49; it is uncommon in preadolescent girls, and Faust & Russell (1964) give an overall prevalence in child-bearing women of 25 per cent and in men of 4 per cent or more. The infection is venereal in origin, the organism being transmitted during sexual intercourse. In exceptional cases transmission may occur through contaminated towels, clothing, and toilet seats.

Pathogenesis. Very frequently *T. vaginalis* infection is asymptomatic, especially so in the male. Definite clinical signs may develop, however, the organism causing degeneration and desquamation of the vaginal epithelium. This is followed by inflammation of the vagina and vulva and a leucocytic discharge may be evident. There may be tendency for the condition to flare up after each menstrual period. The differences in the intensity of the clinical condition possibly relate to different strains of the organism, since Kott & Adler (1961) demonstrated nineteen different serotypes of *T. vaginalis.*

In the male the infection is usually latent and symptomless, however, occasionally it may be responsible for a urethritis which may be persistent or recurrent. In both males and females bacterial and/or fungal infection may accentuate the local inflammatory reaction. Invasion of the tissues by *T. vaginalis* has been reported by Frost *et al.* (1961) who found the organism in the cytoplasm of the columnar epithelial cells at the squamo-columnar junction in endocervical biopsy material. The pathogenicity of *T. vaginalis* in experimental hosts such as mice has been studied by Honigberg (1961).

The diagnosis of *T. vaginalis* infection may be made microscopically by the examination of vaginal secretions or urine and in the male by examination of urine or prostatic secretions. The organism can be readily cultured on several media used for other trichomonads. A specific fluorescent antibody technique was introduced by McEntegart *et al.* (1958) and this method was assessed by Hayes & Kotcher (1960). These authors found that fluorescent antibody staining gave approximately the same positive diagnosis as the culture method but because it required much less time to perform it was very satisfactory in diagnosis.

The infection may be difficult to cure. In the male oxytetracycline ointment is introduced into the urethra and this is irrigated with other antibiotics or sulphonamides. In the female lactic acid douches may be used but diodoquin or oxytetracycline, etc. are more satisfactory.

Trichomonas tenax (Müller, 1773) Dobell, 1939. This is a non-pathogenic trichomonad of man and monkeys occurring in the mouth. It is more common in persons with oral disease or dental disorders. It is world wide in distribution and may be found in up to 26 per cent of persons with dental caries or pyorrhoea and in up to 11 per cent of those with apparently normal, healthy mouths.

The organism is pyriform in outline, 5 μ–12 μ in length, the undulating membrane extends almost to the posterior end of the body but there is no free portion to the posterior flagellum. The axostyle is slender and extends from the posterior part of the body as a pointed rod.

There is no evidence that *T. tenax* is pathogenic. Transmission is probably direct, from droplet spray from the mouth, kissing, or the use of contaminated dishes and drinking water. The organism will survive at normal temperatures in drinking water for several hours.

Though no specific treatment is required, an improvement in oral hygiene will reduce the infection.

Genus: Pentatrichomonas Mesnil, 1914

Members of this genus have five anterior flagella.

Pentatrichomonas hominis (Davaine, 1860) (syn. *Trichomonas hominis, T. intestinalis* etc.). This is a common intestinal flagellate of man and of other primate species which have been detailed by Flick (1954). It can be transmitted experimentally to a number of laboratory animals including the rat, cat, dog, hamster, guinea pig, and chicken (Levine, 1961).

The body is oval to pear-shaped, 5 μ–20 μ by 3 μ–14 μ; the oval nucleus lies in the anterior half of the body, and there are usually five free anterior flagella though some forms may possess only three or four; rarely the number is six or more. The sixth flagellum runs along the undulating membrane and extends behind the body. The undulating membrane extends the full length of the body, a costa is present and the axostyle is thick, hyaline and protrudes outside the body as a pointed process.

Transmission is direct by ingestion, though it has been suggested that flies may serve as mechanical vectors.

There is no evidence that the organism is pathogenic or causes intestinal disturbance. It may be present in large numbers in loose or diarrhoeic faeces.

Genus: Monocercomonas Grassi, 1897

Members of this genus have a pyriform body, three anterior flagella, a trailing flagellum but no undulating membrane. The axostyle is rod-like and protrudes from the posterior end of the body. A list of species is given by Morgan (1944).

Monocercomonas ruminantium (Braune, 1914) Levine, 1961, occurs in the rumen of cattle, *M. cuniculi* (Tanabe, 1926) in the caecum of rabbits and *M. gallinarum* (Martin & Robertson, 1911) Morgan & Hawkins, 1948, in the caecum of the chicken. No pathogenic effects are ascribable to these species.

Genus: Chilomastix Alexeieff, 1912

Members of this genus are pyriform organisms with a large cytostomal cleft at the anterior end, near the nucleus. There are three anteriorly directed flagella and a short fourth flagellum that lies in the oral groove. Cysts are produced.

Chilomastix mesnili (Wenyon, 1910) Alexeieff, 1912. This is a nonpathogenic flagellate of the human intestine and is one of the largest flagellates found in man. It is pear-shaped, 5 μ–20 μ in length (commonly 10 μ–15 μ) and the posterior end of the body is drawn out into a long point. The well defined cytostomal groove is 6 μ– 8 μ in length by 2 μ wide and the lateral margins of the cystostome are supported by two fibrils. The cysts are pyriform, 7 μ–10 μ in length, contain a single nucleus and the cystome is readily visible being almost as long as the organisms.

C. mesnili occurs in the caecum and colon and sometimes the small intestine of man, the prevalence of infection varying from 2–25 per cent in various parts of the world. It has also been found in monkeys and the pig. Transmission is via the cysts. Generally, *C. mesnili* is considered to be a nonpathogenic commensal; however, Mueller(1959) has reported diarrhoea in children and in himself to be associated with very large numbers of organism.

Other species of *Chilomastix* include:

Chilomastix gallinarum Martin and Robertson, 1911 (caecum of chickens and turkey).

Chilomastix caprae da Fonseca, 1915 (rumen of goats in Brazil and India).

Chilomastix cuniculi da Fonseca, 1915 (caecum of rabbits).

Chilomastix intestinalis Kuezynski, 1914 (caecum of guinea pigs).

Genus: Cochlosoma Kotlan, 1923

Members of this genus have an oval body which is broad anteriorly and narrow posteriorly. Six flagella of unequal length arise from a complex of blepharoplasts, two of which are trailing flagella. On the anterior ventral surface of the body there is a large sucker.

Cochlosoma anatis Kotlan, 1923. This occurs in the posterior large intestine and caeca of domestic and wild ducks. A similar form has been found in turkeys and Campbell (1945) considers it to be identical with the duck form. It is probably world wide in distribution. The organism is

6 μ–10 μ in length by 4 μ–6·5 μ, the ventral sucker is about half the body length. Ovoid cysts, with four or more nuclei, occur in the faeces of infected ducks.

The importance of the parasite in ducks is unknown. Campbell (1945) described a disease entity of catarrhal enteritis in turkeys associated with large numbers of *C. anatis*; however the exact relationship of *C. anatis* to enteritis in turkeys needs further investigation since this organism is usually found associated with *Hexamita meleagridis*, a known pathogen for turkeys.

Genus: Hexamita Dujardin, 1838

Members of this genus have a pyriform body with two nuclei. Near the anterior end there arise six anterior and two posterior flagella, and there are two axostyles. Some members of the genus form cysts. A number of

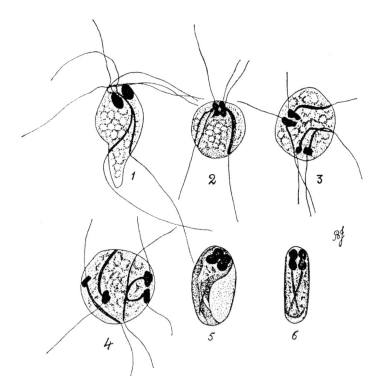

FIG. 271. *Hexamitus muris* from the Intestine of the Mouse (× ca. 3000). (From Wenyon, 1926)

1. Ordinary free form. 2–4. Dividing forms. 5, 6. Encysted forms, showing division of nuclei

free-living species are found in stagnant water whereas others are parasitic in insects, fish, and frogs. The principal species of importance is *Hexamita meleagridis* which occurs in turkeys.

Hexamita meleagridis McNeil, Hinshaw and Kofoid, 1941. This is found principally in the turkey, but organisms morphologically identical with it have been found in quail, partridge, pheasant etc. *H. meleagridis* has been transmitted experimentally from the turkey to the chicken, quail, domestic duck, etc. (Levine, 1961). *H. meleagridis* occurs in the duodenum and small intestine of young turkeys; it has been reported from North and South America, Great Britain, Europe and is probably world wide in distribution. It is associated with an infectious catarrhal enteritis of turkeys which appears to occur in all the major turkey producing areas in the Western world.

Morphology. The organism is bilaterally symmetrical, pear-shaped and 6 μ–12 μ in length by 2 μ–5 μ broad. The six anteriorly directed flagella arise in two groups of three each from distinct blepharoplasts which lie anterior to the two nuclei. The caudal flagella arise on each side from a distinct blepharoplast posterior to the larger anterior blepharoplast and pass posteriorly, emerging at the posterior end of the body.

Life-cycle. Multiplication is by longitudinal binary fission and transmission is through contaminated feed and drinking water. Slavin & Wilson (1953) stated that the life-cycle consisted of the formation of the binucleate cysts and the production of invasive forms which penetrated the reticulo-endothelial cells. In this site the authors described the developments of schizonts, merozoites, and eventually mature flagellates. This description was severely criticised by Hoare (1955) who pointed out that insufficient evidence had been produced to support the statements regarding the life-cycle of the organism and further stated that the figures presented were unconvincing and unacceptable. Subsequently Slavin & Wilson (1960) published a more detailed account of the life-cycle of *H. meleagridis* accompanying this by numerous micro-photographs of the life-cycle and the morphology of the flagellate.

Pathogenesis. Young turkey poults up to the age of about 2 months are the most susceptible. Death may occur within a week of infection in some cases, and the mortality in the flock may reach up to 80 per cent. The essential lesion is a catarrhal enteritis of the upper digestive tract and this produces a marked lack of tone in the duodenum and jejunum so that distended bulbous areas containing watery contents appear. The small intestine is inflamed and oedematous; there is congestion of the glandular tissue of the caecum, and myriads of *Hexamita* are found in the bulbous areas.

Clinically, the affected poults become nervous and show a foamy, watery diarrhoea. They usually continue to eat but in the later stages of the disease they become listless, lose weight rapidly and finally die. Recovered birds grow poorly and may act as carriers since large numbers of organisms may persist in the lower jejunum, ileum and bursa of Fabricius.

Epidemiology. The chief source of infection are carrier adult birds, and Hinshaw & McNeil (1941) found that the prevalence of *H. meleagridis* in adult turkeys may be as high as 32 per cent. Clinical disease may not occur until several batches of turkey poults have been processed through an infected area and this may indicate that the virulence of the organism needs to be increased by passage. Hinshaw (1959) indicated that this was necessary with some strains from carrier turkeys. Studies by McNeil & Hinshaw (1941) showed that *H. meleagridis* could be transmitted to chickens and that the organism could persist in the bursa of Fabricius and the caecal tonsils of these for at least 22 weeks. Clinical disease was not found in infected chickens, but if turkey poults were placed with infected chickens, the turkeys developed the disease. Thus the chicken must be regarded as a potential carrier of *H. meleagridis*. Quail, pheasant, and partridge may also be a source of infection for turkeys. A species in pigeons, *Hexamita columbae*, is not transmissible to turkeys.

Diagnosis. This is most satisfactorily made by the demonstration of the living organisms in a drop of the contents of the small intestine, especially from the bulbous regions. It is important that the preparation should be examined fresh since within an hour or two of death of the bird the organisms are dead and extremely difficult to recognise. Impression smears can be made from cross-sections of the fresh small intestine and stained with Giemsa. The organism has not been cultured in artificial medium, however, Hughes & Zander (1954) were able to obtain axenic cultures in the allantoic cavity of chick embryos with the use of streptomycin and bacitracin.

Treatment

Wilson & Slavin (1955) reported that therapeutic treatment proved disappointing but found that 2-amino-5-nitrothiazole was 50 per cent effective in artificially infected turkeys. The effectiveness of furazolidone for the control of *H. meleagridis* infection was investigated by Mangrum *et al.* (1955). A rate of 50 mg. per pound, 2 days prior to experimental infection, reduced the mortality from between 56 per cent to 66 per cent to 10 per cent, and where treatment was begun at the time of the first death after inoculation, the mortality in treated groups was 26 per cent. Subsequently Briggs (1959) reported that *H. meleagridis* in turkeys could be prevented by the continuous feeding of furazolidone. Fogg (1957) reported that nithiazide [1-ethyl-3-(5-nitro-2-thiazolyl)urea] at a concentration of 0·02 per cent in drinking water controlled fatal outbreaks due to *Hexamita* and *Histomonas* either singly, or in mixed infections.

Prevention and Control. This is based on general hygienic measures. Poults should be reared away from adult turkeys and chickens, overcrowding should be avoided and adequate housing and ventilation should be provided. If possible, separate equipment should be used for the young birds and attendants should disinfect themselves when entering the pens of young poults.

Other species of the genus *Hexamita* include *Hexamita columbae* (Nöller

& Buttgereit, 1923), which occurs in the small intestine of pigeons. It is a small form, 5 μ–9 μ by 2·5 μ–7 μ, and it may be pathogenic for pigeons, causing a catarrhal enteritis (Nöller & Buttgereit, 1923). It is not transmissible to turkeys.

Hexamita muris (Grassi, 1888) is found in the posterior intestine and caecum of rats, mice and hamsters.

Genus: Giardia Kunstler, 1882

Species of this genus are pyriform to elliptical in outline and are bilaterally symmetrical. The anterior end is broadly rounded and the posterior drawn out and somewhat pointed. The dorsal side is convex and the ventral side concave with a large sucking disc in the anterior half. There

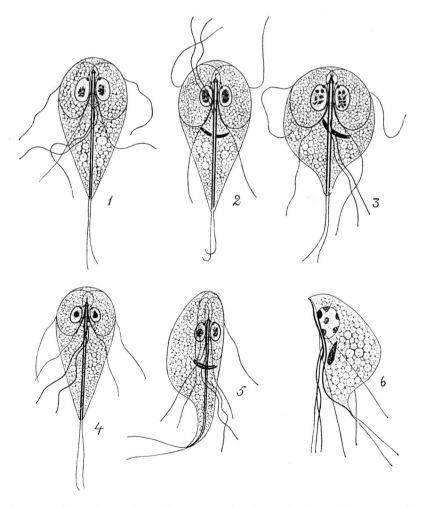

FIG. 272. *Giardia lamblia* from Human Intestine (×5000). (From Wenyon, 1926) 1–4. Variations in size and shape of body. 5. Partial side view. 6. Side view

are two nuclei, two axostyles, eight flagella arranged in four pairs, and a pair of darkly staining bodies placed medially. Cysts are produced which are oval or elliptical and possess two or four nuclei.

The members of the genus which occur in vertebrates are all morphologically similar, but it is customary to give them different names which indicate the host in which they are found. However, Filice (1952) has suggested that only two species occur in mammals, namely *Giardia muris* and *Giardia duodenalis*, the latter occurring in a wide range of animals including man, ox, dog, and cat. The necessary cross-transmission experiments to verify this opinion have not been conducted and for convenience, if nothing else, the more conventional method of describing the various species of the genus will be adopted here.

Giardia lamblia Stiles, 1915 (syn. *G. (Lamblia) intestinalis*, etc.). The organism is found in the duodenum, other parts of the small intestine and occasionally in the colon of man. It has also been found in monkeys and pigs, and experimentally it is transmissible to laboratory rats (*Rattus norvegicus*) but *Rattus rattus* and the laboratory mouse cannot be infected (Haiba, 1956). It is world wide in distribution, the prevalence varying from 2 per cent–60 per cent or more. It is more common in children and is considered to be the most common flagellate of the human.

It is 9μ–20μ (commonly 10μ–18μ) by 5μ–10μ, and essentially the body of the parasite resembles a pear which has been cut in half longitudinally, the flat side representing the ventral surface of the organism and the convex side the dorsal. The cysts are ovoid and refractile, 8μ–14μ by 6μ–10μ in size. The cyst wall is thin and the organism does not fill the entire cyst. The most prominent structures seen in the cysts are the two, or later four, nuclei and the comma-shaped body.

Reproduction is by binary fission.

Transmission is by the ingestion of cyst-contaminated food and drink. The cyst may remain viable in moist surroundings for up to 2 weeks.

Pathogenesis. There has been considerable debate over the years concerning the significance of *G. lamblia* in the human. Probably the majority of infections are symptomless, but some, especially in children, are associated with sub-acute to chronic diarrhoea and duodenal irritation with an excess of mucus production. In a review of the pathogenicity of *G. lamblia*, Pizzi (1957) indicated that an upset fat metabolism may result in a deficiency in fat-soluble vitamins.

There is no evidence that *G. lamblia* has any pathogenic significance in the monkey or in the pig.

Diagnosis of *G. lamblia* is based on the microscopic demonstration of the cysts in faecal material. Usually only cysts are passed but in cases of acute diarrhoea, the free flagellates may be found. The cysts are most satisfactorily concentrated by a 33 per cent zinc sulphate flotation technique, and a small amount of iodine solution may be added to aid in the recognition of the cysts.

Giardia infections in human can be successfully treated with quina-crine, chloroquine, or diodoquin (di-iodo-hydroxyquinoline).

Giardia canis Hegner, 1922. This occurs in the duodenum and jeju-num of the dog, principally in the United States. The trophozoite form is 12 μ–17 μ long by 7·6 μ–10 μ wide, and the cysts are oval, measuring 9 μ–13 μ by 7 μ–9 μ.

Various surveys on the incidence of infection in dogs have been carried out in the United States. Craige (1948) reported 8·8 per cent of 160 dogs infected in California, and Bemrick (1961) found 7·5 per cent of 2063 dogs infected in the Minnesota area. It is likely that the organism is cosmopolitan in its distribution and if searched for, a wide prevalence would be evident.

Pathogenesis. The controversy on the significance of *Giardia* in the human is equalled by a similar controversy about the dog. Many clini-cians subscribe to the view that the organism has a definite pathologic significance producing diarrhoea and dysentery. This opinion is streng-thened by the fact that therapy usually eliminates the organisms and alleviates clinical signs. Craige (1948) found *Giardia* in seventeen of seventy-one dogs with dysentery, however, it is certain that the organism may be found in large numbers in apparently completely healthy dogs. Several thousand cysts may be present in the stools of dogs which are perfectly healthy.

Diagnosis of the infection is the same as for the human species. Quina-crine has been found an effective treatment being given at the rate of 50–100 mg. twice daily for 2–3 days (Craige, 1949); chloroquine and diodoquin have also been found effective. Control measures consist of an improvement in the hygiene of dog kennels.

Giardia cati Deschiens, 1925 (*Giardia felis*), occurs in the small in-testine of the cat in the United States and Europe. It is very similar to *G. canis* with which it may be synonymous. There is no evidence that this form is pathogenic.

Giardia chinchillae Filice, 1952, occurs in the small intestine, especially the duodenum of the chinchilla. The trophozoite stage is 10 μ to 20 μ by 6 μ to 12 μ.

This organism has been incriminated as the cause of severe blood-stained diarrhoea and death in the chinchilla. The clinical picture is an intense mucoid diarrhoea, and Shelton (1954) has reported a 38 per cent mortal-ity in experimentally induced infections in chinchillas. Severe infections have occurred on chinchilla ranches.

For treatment, 6–9 mg. of quinacrine for 5–7 days has been recom-mended (Hagan, 1950) while diodoquin, diluted in water and sprayed on the hay until the food material is damp, has also been used.

Control consists of the segregation and treatment of sick animals, and an improvement of the hygiene of the ranch.

Giardia bovis Fantham, 1921, occurs in the small intestine of the ox in North America, Europe, and South Africa. The trophozoite stage is 11 μ–19 μ by 7 μ–10 μ and the cysts 7 μ–16 μ by 4 μ–10 μ. There is no good evidence that *G. bovis* is pathogenic.

Other species of *Giardia* include *G. caprae* (goat), *G. equi* (horse), *G. duodenalis* (rabbit), *G. muris* (mouse, rat) and *G. caviae* (guinea pig). There is no unequivocal evidence that any of these are pathogenic forms.

ORDER RHIZOMASTIGIDA BÜTSCHLI

These are forms which possess pseudopodia as well as flagella. The family of interest in this order is *Mastigamoebidae*, the forms possessing one to three flagella and the only genus of interest is *Histomonas*.

Genus: Histomonas Tyzzer, 1920

Members of this genus are amoeboid with a single nucleus. Flagella number one, two, or four, according to species.

Histomonas meleagridis (Smith, 1895) Tyzzer, 1920. This is found in the caeca and liver and is the cause of histomoniasis, infectious enterohepatitis, or 'blackhead', in the turkey. It may also occur in the

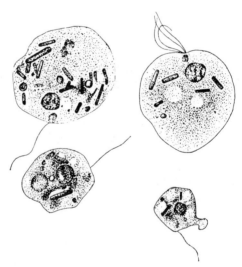

Fig. 273. Various Forms of *Histomonas meleagridis* (×2000). (From Wenyon, 1926)

chicken, peafowl, guinea fowl, pheasant, partridge, and quail. It is world wide in distribution and is an important disease entity in turkeys, assuming great economic importance where turkeys are kept in large numbers. It is probably ubiquitous also in chickens, though the incidence of disease in these is low.

Morphology. The organism is somewhat pleomorphic, the morphology

PLATE XXIII

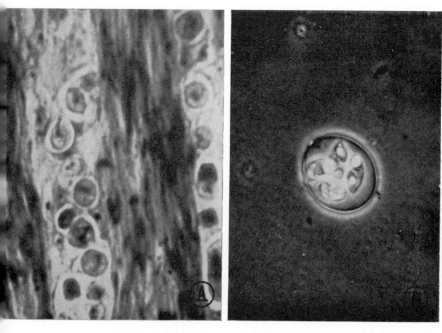

A. *Histomonas meleagridis* in wall of caecum of turkey poult. (× 1200)

B. Sporulated oocyst of *Eimeria* sp. (× 600)

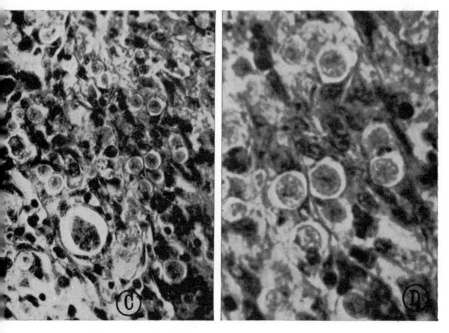

C. Section of turkey liver infected with *Histomonas meleagridis*. (× 750)

D. *Histomonas meleagridis* organisms in liver tissue of turkey poult. (× 1200)

depending on the organ location and the stage of the disease. Tyzzer (1919) described three stages of the parasite, an invasive stage of the early caecal and liver lesions, a vegetative stage occurring near the centre of lesions, and a resistance phase. A more recent study by Farmer *et al.* (1951) failed to identify the different forms described by Tyzzer.

The stage which occurs in the lumen of the intestine, and in culture, is 5 μ–30 μ in diameter, amoeboid, has a clear ectoplasm, and a granular endoplasm. The latter may contain food vacuoles with bacteria, starch grains etc. The nucleus is vesicular and a flagellum arises from a small blepharoplast near the nucleus. Occasionally two flagella may be present. A related form, *Histomonas wenrichi*, occurs in the pheasant and this possesses four flagella (see below).

In the tissues the organism is found singly or in clusters and is 8 μ–15 μ in diameter. It is amoeboid, the flagellum being absent.

Though Tyzzer described a 'resistant' stage of the parasite, there is no evidence that any stage is more resistant than another and cysts are not formed.

Cultivation. The organism was first cultivated by Drbohlav (1924) who found that coagulated white of egg covered with bouillon with 1 per cent peptone was the most satisfactory medium. In culture the organism feeds on bacteria or red blood cells, and until recently it could not be grown axenically. However, Lesser (1960) utilised tissue culture medium 199 supplemented with sterilised cream and a nutrient broth culture of mixed bacterial flora from turkey caecal droppings which had been subjected for at least 1 hour to the action of high concentrations of penicillin and streptomycin. Histomonads were maintained for more than forty consecutive sub-cultures without evidence of bacterial growth. Organisms failed to mutiply if the bacterial nutrient cultures also failed to support histomonad growth. Lesser concluded that a heat-labile intracellular factor, present in turkey caecal bacteria, was required for the successful growth and reproduction of *H. meleagridis*.

Life-history and Transmission. Reproduction of the organism is by binary fission.

Primary infection occurs in the caecum, and under natural conditions the main route of infection is by the ingestion of the embryonated eggs of the caecal worm *Heterakis gallinarum* (Graybill & Smith, 1920). This mode of transmission has been fully confirmed by numerous workers and it is the method of choice for inducing experimental infections. However, despite the abundant circumstantial evidence that the egg of the caecal nematode is responsible for transmission, the organism itself has been demonstrated in *Heterakis* in only a few instances. It has never been observed in infective eggs, but Tyzzer (1926) found a protozoan in half grown *Heterakis* larvae and later (in 1934) in the cells of the intestinal wall of 10–20 day old worms from experimentally infected birds. Connell (1950) observed abnormalities in a proportion of second stage larvae of

H. gallinarum obtained from blackhead-infected birds. These included cuticular swellings and diffuse thickenings in the intestinal and oesophageal regions. Kendall (1959) observed what he believed to be *H. meleagridis* in the gut cells of young larvae of *H. gallinarum* obtained from poults killed on the 4th day after infection.

Despite the fact that infection of *H. gallinarum* eggs is widespread and blackhead infection can be induced with batches of eggs taken from a high percentage of turkeys, or almost any chicken, the rate of infection of eggs is low. Lund & Burtner (1957) reported that less than 0·5 per cent of embryonated eggs of *H. gallinarum* from experimentally infected chickens contained the protozoan.

Under certain circumstances the protozoan discharged from acutely infected turkeys may produce infection if it is ingested at once (Tyzzer & Collier, 1925). The acidity of the gizzard is important in such direct infection, and Horton-Smith & Long (1956) found that infection could be created with the free forms when chickens were starved or had received an alkaline diet to raise the pH of the gizzard from a level of 2·9–3·3 to one of 6·2–7·6. Blackhead may also be induced by the rectal injection of cultures of *H. meleagridis* or ground-up infective tissues (Farmer & Stephenson, 1949).

Pathogenesis. Histomoniasis is essentially a disease of young turkeys, and, in the absence of treatment, the birds die. The chicken is much more resistant to the pathogenic effects of the infection.

The histomonads are released from the larvae of *H. gallinarum* and they enter the wall of the caecum and multiply.

One or both caeca may be involved and the earliest lesions consist of small, raised, pin-point ulcers in which the organisms are plentiful. These become much enlarged and may involve the whole of the caecal mucosa. The mucosa becomes greatly thickened and its surface necrotic and eventually the caecum contains a hard caseous, adherent core. Macroscopically the caeca are enlarged and haemorrhagic. The histomonads further invade the mucosa and 'stream' to the deeper layers of the organ. They gain entry to the hepatic portal system and are carried by this to the liver. The liver lesion is a focal necrosis which increases by peripheral extension to produce characteristic circular depressed lesions. These consist of a yellow to yellowish green area of necrosis with a greyish peripheral region with radiating streaks of necrosis. The lesions vary in diameter, being up to 1 cm. or more in size; they may be confluent and extend deeply into the liver. They are not encapsulated and in older birds a repair process may be seen with the initiation of a fibrinous and lymphoid tissue reaction.

The detailed pathology of experimentally induced histomoniasis has been studied by Malewitz *et al.* (1958). Lesions occur in the caeca and liver and also in the spleen, kidney, and lungs. Lesions in which the parasites could be readily demonstrated were characterised by hyperaemia, haemorrhage, an infiltration of lymphocytes and macrophages, multi-nucleated giant cells, necrosis, and usually a serous exudate. Areas of hyperaemia and exudate occurred in the lungs, pancreas and heart, but parasites were not demonstrated in such lesions; a lymphocytic infiltration was seen in the lungs.

The organisms disappear from the tissues of birds which recover, and the necrotic lesions are repaired by an invasion of lymphocytic cells and fibroblasts. A firm caecal plug is produced, this becomes contracted and is finally ejected, and then the caeca eventually return to normal size, though much scarring may remain. Extensive scarring may remain in the liver for a very long time.

The relationship between the bacterial flora of the turkey and *H. mele-agridis* and the production of lesions in the liver has been studied by Harrison *et al.* (1954). These workers produced bacteria-free lesions in the liver by the intrahepatic injection of infected liver homogenates. However, this study utilised conventional turkeys and a number of normal, unidentified, bacterial factors may have contributed to the pathogenesis. Doll & Franker (1963) studied the pathogenicity of histomoniasis in gnotobiotic turkeys. Of twelve gnotobiotic turkeys infected with sterile *H. gallinarum* eggs, only one showed signs of histomoniasis and none died of the disease; but of twelve conventional turkeys, 11 developed histomoniasis and died. The results suggest a synergism may exist between the host flora and either *H. meleagridis* or *H. gallinarum* since nematode infection was absent in the germ-free group of animals. Subsequent work by Franker & Doll (1964) showed in germ-free turkeys that surface-sterilised embryonated *H. gallinarum* eggs mono-contaminated with either *Escherichia intermedia* or *Streptococcus faecalis* produced lesions of histo-moniasis. Similar work by Bradley *et al.* (1964) demonstrated typical enterohepatitis in gnotobiotic turkeys inoculated with *H. meleagridis* plus *Escherichia coli* or *Clostridium perfringens*.

Under field conditions the most severe disease occurs in young poults between the age of 3–12 weeks, losses ranging from 50–100 per cent of the flock. Birds may die within a few days of showing the first clinical signs. In older birds the disease runs a more chronic course and recovery may occur, to be followed by immunity (Kendall, 1957). Nevertheless, mature birds may sustain acute infections and die. On a general flock basis the overall mortality may vary from 0–90 per cent.

Immunity. Birds which have recovered from infection do not develop any clinical signs on reinfection; they may, however, harbour the organisms in the caeca (Kendall, 1957). Early studies by Tyzzer (1933) demonstrated that an attenuated strain of *H. meleagridis* protected against virulent strains which were almost 100 per cent fatal to unprotected birds. He suggested that the attenuated strains produced a slight and transient invasion of the host tissue but were not sufficient to produce a progressive disease. Continuous culture of *H. meleagridis* produces initially a loss of the invasive properties and later a loss of immunising properties, and Tyzzer (1934, 1936) was able to demonstrate good protection against newly isolated virulent strains with forms which had lost all virulence in culture. Lund (1957, 1959) reported that the administration of a non-pathogenic strain of *Histomonas* by infected *Heterakis* eggs did not protect turkeys against pathogenic strains of the organism. However, immunisation by rectal inoculation gave, after 3 weeks, some protection against a rectal challenge of 10,000 pathogenic histomonads. Though this was almost complete after 6 weeks, typical enterohepatitis could be produced with *Heterakis* egg-induced infection. Lund believed that the immune barrier was limited to the surface of the caecal mucosa and that the failure to protect against histomonads introduced by *Heterakis* was due to the larval worms penetrating the mucosal barrier to liberate the histomonads into the tissues. The failure to immunise by the introduction of nonpathogenic histomonads with *Heterakis* eggs was probably due to the low numbers of organism which would be introduced by this method.

Epidemiology. Heterakis gallinarum is a common nematode parasite of the domestic turkey and chicken, and usually it is possible to produce histomoniasis in turkeys with any batch of eggs from domestic chickens. Consequently, the chicken is the principal reservoir of infection for turkeys and outbreaks of histomoniasis are likely to occur when turkeys are reared with domestic fowls or when they are placed on ground recently vacated by domestic poultry. The unprotected blackhead organism dies within a few hours outside the avian host and its survival on pasture is due to the protection afforded by the *Heterakis* egg. Farr (1956) has shown that eggs may retain both helminth and protozoan infectivity for 66 weeks in the soil. In further work Farr (1961) found that *H. meleagridis* in *Heterakis* eggs was infective as late as the 151st week after exposure on soil out of doors.

In addition to the domestic chicken, various wild gallinaceous birds such as the pheasant, grouse, partridge, quail, and wild turkey may serve as reservoir of infection for domestic turkeys.

Outbreaks of disease vary very much in severity, this probably being an effect of the virulence of the strain. With continued use of infected land, it is likely that the incidence and severity of the disease will increase as time goes by.

Clinical Signs of Enterohepatitis. The clinical signs of blackhead appear 8 or more days after infection. The first evidence of the infection in a flock is a noticeable decline in the feed consumption; this is followed by depression, drooping wings, ruffled feathers, and especially characteristic in the turkey, the appearance of sulphur-yellow coloured droppings. Yellow droppings are not a common sign in the chicken. A few birds may show a darkened or cyanotic discoloration of the skin of the head and wattles (from which the name 'blackhead' arises), however, this is by no means a constant feature of the disease, nor is it a significant clinical sign since it may occur in other disease entities. Occasionally, the disease may be peracute in nature with no marked clinical signs, the birds dying within 24 hours. In older birds a chronic wasting form of the disease is seen; this may be followed by death or recovery.

Diagnosis. In living birds, the characteristic sulphur yellow droppings are suggestive of enterohepatitis, while at post-mortem the necrotic lesions of the liver are pathognomonic. Histological examination of stained sections of the liver shows necrosis and colonies of the organism. The latter appear like punched out holes in the necrotic tissue, each hole containing a fragment of protoplasm which represents the parasite. The caecal lesions may be confused with those due to *Eimeria tenella* but this infection may readily be eliminated by a microscopic examination of the mucosa when the characteristic developmental stages of the sporozoan are missing.

Treatment

The literature on the chemotherapy of enterohepatitis has been reviewed by Wehr *et al.* (1958).

2-amino-5-nitrothiazole [Enheptin-T (U.S.A.), Entramin (U.K.)]. This compound can be given in the food or in drinking water. It is recommended in the food at a concentration of 0·05 per cent as a preventative or of 0·1 per cent for curative purposes. It will prevent mortality completely when given over a period of 14 days provided this is begun not later than 72 hours after a single oral infection. When treatment is started as late as 13 days after infection mortality is reduced and few deaths occur until more than one week after withdrawal of the drug.

2-acetylamino-5-nitrothiazole [Enheptin-A (U.S.A.), Entramin A (U.K.)]. As efficient as Enheptin-T for prophylaxis. It is less soluble than Enheptin-T and is given in the food at a concentration of 0·025 per cent.

Nithiazide [1-ethyl-3-(5-nitro-2-thiazolyl)urea]. This compound is more potent and less toxic than 2-amino-5-nitrothiazole for the treatment of enterohepatitis. It is most effective when given prior to, or 3–7 days after, infection. It is equally effective administered in the feed or water. Field trials have shown that 0·02 per cent of the drug in drinking water controlled field outbreaks of both histomoniasis and hexamitiasis; 0·025 per cent in the feed controlled outbreaks of histomoniasis in chickens and turkeys, and 0·0125 per cent in the feed provided effective field prophylaxis against blackhead in turkeys (Fogg, 1957; Craig *et al.* 1959).

Furazolidone (NF-180) [N-(5-nitro-2-furfurylidone)-3-amino-2-oxazolidinone]. At concentrations of 0·01 per cent–0·02 per cent in the food, furazolidone is almost wholly effective in preventing histomoniasis when continuous medication is commenced before infection takes place. A suitable concentration for preventive medication is 0·015 per cent and for the treatment of established histomoniasis, 0·04 per cent is satisfactory. However, even with the higher doses, the histomonads are only inhibited and they continue to multiply if medication is withdrawn. Consequently, relapses may result if this occurs.

Dimetridazole (1,2-dimethyl-5-nitroimidazole). This compound was investigated by Lucas (1961) who found that concentrations of 0·0125 per cent in the food were effective against *H. meleagridis*.

Control of Enterohepatitis. Control consists of a combination of good husbandry and preventive medication.

It is essential to avoid contact between turkeys and domestic chickens and where the two are kept on the same farm a separate area should be allocated to each of them. The use of hens for incubating and rearing turkey poults should be avoided and young turkeys should not be placed on land that has carried poultry, unless the land has been rested for at least 2 years. Regular treatment of all birds with phenothiazine to reduce the incidence of *Heterakis gallinarum* infection is of benefit in reducing the overall incidence of histomoniasis. The eggs of worms passed following phenothiazine therapy are still capable of hatching and releasing histomonads and consequently ground should be regarded as a potential source of infection for some time after anthelmintic treatment.

Where large-scale turkey raising is in operation, young turkeys should be raised on wire floors which are out of contact with the ground. If possible separate attendants should be used for turkeys and other domestic poultry, but if not, attendants should change footwear and clothing before going from the chicken flock to the turkey flock. Unnecessary visitors should be discouraged. Pens and equipment should be regularly sterilised, especially prior to the introduction of new birds.

Where young turkeys are reared on open ground, clean ground should be reserved for this. Light, sandy soil is more satisfactory, thus allowing less survival of *Heterakis* eggs than heavy, damp soil. Low-lying areas and ponds and streams should be avoided and these should be drained or fenced off from poultry.

In large-scale turkey rearing establishments, continuous medication with one or other of the above therapeutic agents is often practised.

Histomonas wenrichi Lund, 1963. This species is a nonpathogenic form of gallinaceous birds, chiefly of pheasant. It is about 1·5 times larger than *H. meleagridis* and has four flagella instead of the one or two of the latter species. It does not multiply in the host tissues nor does it produce any visible pathological change. *Histomonas wenrichi* may occur along with *H. meleagridis* and it is transmitted by the embryonated eggs of *Heterakis gallinarum*. It does not grow in media which support the growth of *H. meleagridis* nor has it been grown in media which supports growth of trichomonads, amoeba or other parasitic protozoa (Lund, 1963).

CLASS: SARCODINA HERTWIG AND LESSER, 1874

Members of this class do not possess a thick pellicle, they move by means of pseudopodia, and only rarely do they have flagella. The cytoplasm is usually differentiated into ectoplasm and endoplasm but this is not constant. With few exceptions reproduction is asexual by binary fission. Nutrition is holozoic, the forms being predatory on bacteria, protozoa and small metozoa. Only a few are parasitic and of direct interest in this book.

The *Sarcodina* are divided into two sub-classes, the *Rhizopoda* Siebold, which contains the organisms of interest in the medical field and the sub-class *Actinopoda* Calkins. The latter sub-class contains the *Radiolaria*, which occur in the oceans, and vast areas of the ocean floor are covered with ooze made up of the skeletons of such radiolarians. In addition to being of geological interest, these protozoa are at times extremely exquisite and beautiful.

FAMILY: ENDAMOEBIDAE CALKINS, 1926

This family contains, exclusively, the parasitic amoebae which occur in the digestive tract of vertebrates and invertebrates. Multiplication is by binary fission and encystment is common. This family should be differentiated from the family *Amoebidae* Brown, which contains the free-living amoeba of water, soil, etc. The well-known *Amoeba proteus* occurs in the latter family.

Genus: Entamoeba Casagrandi and Barbagallo, 1895

Members of this genus have a vesicular nucleus with a comparatively small endosome at or near the centre of the nucleus. A varying number of chromatin granules occur in the peri-endosomal region and attached to the nuclear membrane. Cysts containing one to eight nuclei are produced.

This genus should be differentiated from the genus *Endamoeba* Leidy, 1897, the latter lacking a defined central endosome. Members of the *Endamoeba* occur in the intestine of invertebrates.

A large number of species of *Entamoeba* occur in a wide range of animals, and a check list of species has been given by Hoare (1959). The forms can be conveniently grouped according to the trophozoite and cyst morphology and Hoare (1959) recognises 4 such groups. Levine (1961) adopted a similar grouping.

1. *Entamoebae with 8-nucleate cysts* (e.g. *E. coli, E. wenyoni, E. muris* etc.).
2. *Entamoebae with 4-nucleate cysts* (e.g. *E. histolytica, E. hartmanni, E. equi* etc.).
3. *Entamoebae with 1-nucleate cysts* (e.g. *E. bovis, E. bubalis, E. suis* etc.).
4. *Entamoebae in which cysts are unknown* (e.g. *E. gingivalis, E. canibuccalis, E. equibuccalis* etc.).

The only species of importance as a pathogen is *E. histolytica*.

Entamoeba histolytica Schaudinn, 1903. This is the cause of amoebic dysentery of man. It has also been found in many species of monkey and in the dog, cat, rat, and pig. Experimentally, the rat, mouse, guinea pig and rabbit can be infected. Geographically, it is world wide in distribution occurring in countries with temperate, sub-tropical or tropical climates. It is, however, more prevalent in the tropics and sub-tropics than in cooler climates, though surveys in countries such as Great Britain and the United States have shown a substantial level of infection. The prevalance in various countries is detailed by Hoare (1950), and the results of various other surveys are quoted by Levine (1961).

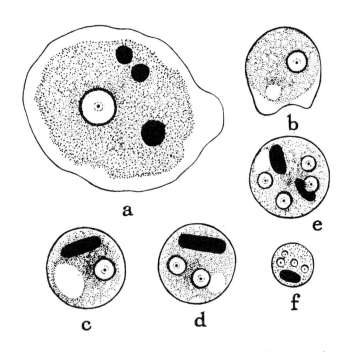

Fig. 274. *Entamoeba histolytica* (× 2000). (From Hoare, 1950)
a. Active (tropic) amoeba with ingested red blood corpuscles; b. Precystic amoeba; c–f. Cysts; c. 1-nucleate with chromatoid body and glycogen vacuole; d. 2-nucleate with chromatoid body and small glycogen vacuole; e. 4-nucleate (mature) with 2 chromatoids and small glycogen vacuole; f. Mature cyst of small race, with chromatoid body

Morphology. The active trophozoite of *E. histolytica* ranges in size from 10 μ–60 μ. It has finely granular endoplasm and the ectoplasm is hyaline in appearance and well differentiated from the inner endoplasm. A characteristic of the organism is its active movements, pseudopodia, which are long and finger-like, appearing suddenly and the endoplasm flowing rapidly into them. There is a single spherical nucleus 4 μ–7 μ in diameter and it contains a distinct central endosome about 0·5 μ in diameter. The endosome is surrounded by a clear zone or halo. The nuclear membrane is lined with fine chromatin granules giving the appearance that the nucleus is outlined by a ring of small beads. Active tropho-zoites also possess food vacuoles which contain red blood cells in the process of digestion. This feature is one which differentiates *E. histolytica* from the nonpathogenic forms.

The cysts of *E. histolytica* are spherical, occasionally ovoid, and measure 5 μ–20 μ in diameter. The cyst wall, visible in living specimens, but not seen in stained preparations, is about 0·5 μ in thickness. Initially the cysts are uninucleate but finally a four-nucleate cyst is produced. The nuclei are comparable to those seen in the vegetative form though smaller, moreover the cysts contain chromatoid bodies and glycogen. The chromatoid bodies appear as refractile rods with rounded ends and stain deeply with chromatin stains. Glycogen vacuoles are seen most clearly

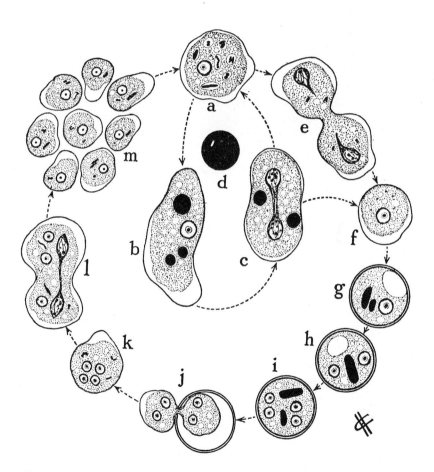

FIG. 275. Life-cycle of *Entamoeba histolytica* (×1300). (From Hoare, 1950) a, e–m. Development in lumen of intestine; a. Amoeba with ingested bacteria; e. Division of amoeba; f. Precystic amoeba; g, h, i. uni-, bi- and quadri-nucleate cysts, with glycogen vacuole and chromatoid bodies; j. Excystation of quadrinucleate amoeba; k–m. Metacystic stages; k. Excysted quadrinucleate amoeba; l. Division of metacystic amoeba; m. Eight uninucleate amoebulae, resulting from divisions of metacystic amoeba; b–c. Development in intestinal wall; b. Tissue-invading amoeba with ingested erythrocytes; c. Division of tissue-invading amoeba; d. Normal red blood corpuscle

in young cysts and stain brown when treated with iodine solution. The glycogen disappears from the cysts when they reach the 4-nucleate stage, though the chromatin rods may persist longer. Ultimately, they too disappear, being used up as reserve food supply.

Differences in the morphology, pathogenicity and culture characteristics of *E. histolytica* have been recognised for many years. A small and large form of the organism are recognised. The small form, or race, is nonpathogenic and has been named *Entamoeba hartmanni* by Brumpt (1925), while the large forms may be divided into an avirulent race and a virulent race (Hoare, 1957). More recently, Faust & Russell (1964) have suggested the compromise that the large forms be designated *E. histolytica histolytica* and the small forms *E. histolytica hartmanni*.

Developmental Cycle. In the trophozoite phase, the organism multiplies by binary fission, this taking place solely in the vertebrate host. The cystic form is passed in the faeces of the host, encystation occurring in the lumen of the bowel. Prior to encystment, the active amoebae divide producing smaller forms which expel food particles, round up, and cease to feed. The cysts are at first uninucleate but later the nucleus divides into two and each then further divides so that a 4-nucleate cyst is produced. Cysts are passed in the faeces in all stages of development, but apparently only the quadrinucleate forms, which represent the mature stage, remain viable and are capable of inducing new infection.

On subsequent infection of a human, or animal, the mature 4-nucleate cyst excysts in the small or large intestine. The newly released metacystic form undergoes a series of nuclear and cytoplasmic divisions resulting in the production of 8 uninucleate amoebae. These then pass to the large bowel where they grow into the larger forms which may remain in the lumen of the bowel or may invade the tissues.

Pathogenesis. Only the large forms of *E. histolytica* are considered to be pathogenic. The mechanism of tissue invasion by the parasite is by no means clearly understood and the various factors of the pathogenesis and pathogenic mechanisms of *E. histolytica* have recently been considered by Maegraith (1961). The penetration of the intestinal epithelium is probably brought about by lysis of the epithelium by proteolytic enzymes; and trypsin and pepsin, but not chymotrypsin, have been found in *E. histolytica*. However, these enzymes have been found in both pathogenic and nonpathogenic strains, and it is not possible at present to differentiate the two on the basis of enzymes. Nevertheless, the presence of the enzymes may be an indication of the mode of invasion. Maegraith (1961) suggests that the ability or otherwise to invade may be determined more by the host than the parasite.

The relationship between bacteria and amoebae may be of importance since experiments in germ-free guinea pigs have shown that it was impossible to infect these animals with *E. histolytica* without the addition of intestinal bacteria. Two species of bacteria (*Aerobacter aerogenes* and

Escherichia coli) permitted the protozoans to become established and invade the tissues (Phillips *et al.* 1955).

Following invasion of the epithelium the amoebae multiply, forming small colonies, and then penetrate into the deeper tissues and reach the submucosa where they spread laterally. They undermine the mucous membrane and produce a flask-shaped ulcer, which has a narrow canal or neck leading to the lumen of the bowel and a dilated distal part in the submucosa.

The initial lesions, which occur principally in the caecum and the ascending colon, show little cellular reaction or bacterial invasion, the process being exclusively one of lytic necrosis. The lesions may remain confined to the mucosa and repair may keep pace with the disease process, resulting in spontaneous elimination of the organism. In other cases, the amoebae penetrate more deeply into the intestinal wall, invasion by bacteria occurs and there is associated hyperaemia, inflammation, and an infiltration of neutrophils. Amoebae are found chiefly at the periphery of the ulcer, in contact with healthy tissue into which they gradually penetrate, leaving the cavity of the ulcer filled with necrotic tissue. Maegraith (1963) tested several potentially pathogenic strains of *E. histolytica* for the presence of hyaluronidase but he was unable to equate the presence of this enzyme with pathogenicity. It was absent from nonpathogenic forms and was also absent from two of the potentially pathogenic forms.

Amoebae may pass into the lymphatics or the mesenteric venules and invade other tissues of the body. They have been found in almost all soft tissue of the body but the commonest location is the liver, especially the right lobe. Amoebae are trapped in thrombi in the interlobular veins and here produce lytic necrosis of the walls of the vessels. They then enter the sinusoids, and secondary colonies produce lytic necrosis. The lesions increase in size, with considerable cell infiltration, and one or more may enlarge to produce a hepatic amoebic abscess. In rapidly forming abscesses there may be no limiting capsule, but in the more chronic types a fibrous wall is produced. Abscesses may occur elsewhere such as in the lungs and brain, and rarely they may occur on the skin.

Pathogenesis of E. histolytica in Animals. Dogs, kittens, monkeys, guinea pigs, hamsters, rats, rabbits, and pigs have been infected experimentally. The kitten is especially susceptible and when infected orally with cysts, or per rectum with the trophozoites, an acute amoebic dysentery results with extensive ulceration of the bowel wall. The organisms appear unable to encyst in the cat and natural cat-derived infections are therefore rare. Kessel (1928) reported the organism in kittens in China.

In the dog, natural infections have been recorded from many parts of the world. These have usually been sporadic infections and probably acquired from human contacts. The majority of cases have been reported from the Far East (Levine, 1961; Hoare, 1959), but in the United States the organism has been found in association with diarrhoea in a dog in Baltimore (Andrews, 1932); and Thorson *et al.* (1956) recorded a systemic infection in a puppy, organisms being found in large numbers in the lungs, liver, kidneys, and spleen.

A prevalance of 8·4 per cent in dogs in Tennessee detected by cultural methods was reported by Eyles *et al.* (1954) which may indicate that canine infection with *E. histolytica* is more extensive than has been thought. In the dog, the infection is chiefly localised in the caecum and usually runs a symptomless course. Occasionally, however, the organism invades the tissues and produces clinical signs of acute or chronic amoebiasis.

An outbreak of dysentery in cattle associated with *E. histolytica* has been recorded by Walkiers (1930); this occurred in an area in which there was an epidemic of amoebiasis in Africans. The organism has also been found in the lungs of zebu cow in Dakar by Thiéry & Morel (1956).

Natural infections with *E. histolytica* are common in a wide range of monkeys, and the human and simian strains are interchangeable as demonstrated by cross infections. The parasites correspond to the small form of man and occur as commensals in the monkey gut, infections usually being symptomless. Nevertheless, they are potentially pathogenic since they can produce typical amoebic dysentery when inoculated into kittens and also when cysts of these forms are fed to humans. Furthermore, Fremming *et al.* (1955) have reported a fatal case of amoebiasis in the chimpanzee.

Monkey infection may be of public health importance, especially since large numbers of these animals are imported into different countries for experimental purposes.

Wild rats may harbour an *Entamoeba* which is indistinguishable from *E. histolytica*, and it is generally assumed that such infections are derived from humans. The pathology of *E. histolytica* infection in the rat varies greatly; the organism may occur as a harmless commensal in the large bowel or it may invade the mucosa producing typical signs of amoebic dysentery.

Epidemiology. E. histolytica is primarily a parasite of man, infected and carrier humans forming the reservoir of infection. Man is also the reservoir host for animal infections. Infection is by the ingestion of the mature cysts, and trophozoites do not survive long outside the host. The cysts are relatively resistant to adverse conditions; they may remain viable for at least 2 weeks in a stool sample kept at room temperature and for about 2 months in a refrigerator. In water, they may remain viable for up to 5 weeks at room temperature. The thermal death point is 50°C, and desiccation is rapidly fatal. Generally, the cysts are transmitted in food or water, and raw vegetables may also be a source of infection. Various flies (*Musca, Lucilia* etc.) have been shown capable of transmitting cysts in their vomitus (Pipkin, 1949). The major outbreaks of amoebiasis in man are usually caused by faulty water supply, and several major outbreaks have been traced to the contamination of drinking water with sewage.

Diagnosis. This is based on the demonstration of the trophozoite or the cyst in the faeces. In a normally formed stool, usually only cysts are found, but in diarrhoeic stools the trophozoite is also seen. Actively motile organisms may be seen in warm, freshly passed, diarrhoeic faeces; but at other times the cysts may be seen more readily if a drop of iodine solution (a saturated solution of iodine in 1 per cent potassium iodine) is added. Cysts may be concentrated by a zinc sulphate flotation solution, but other flotation solutions such as salt and sugar should be avoided since these cause undue distortion. A specific diagnosis is more satisfactory, made from a permanent preparation fixed in Schaudinn's solution and stained by the iron haematoxylin method.

Immunological diagnosis of amoebiasis has been advanced by the fluorescent antibody technique introduced by Goldman (1954, 1960). Originally, Goldman reported that fluorescein conjugated antiserum could readily distinguish the small form of *E. histolytica* and other amoebae of man from the large form of *E. histolytica*; however, more recently Goldman *et al.* (1960) reported that there was a spectrum of antigenic relationships between *E. histolytica* and *E. hartmanni*. A preliminary study by Maddison & Elsdon-Dew (1961) indicated the possible value of gel diffusion precipitin tests in the diagnosis of amoebiasis, and subsequently Maddison (1965) found that precipitin antibodies, directed against specific amoebic components, were detected in a high proportion of patients with invasive amoebiasis.

In the diagnosis of *E. histolytica*, it is, of course, necessary to differentiate the nonpathogenic entamoebae which may occur.

Treatment. The therapy of amoebiasis in animals is based on that applicable to humans. Several compounds are available for the treatment of the intestinal form. Penicillin and streptomycin have an indirect action by their effect on associated bacteria; the tetracyclines affect both the bacteria and the amoebae while fumagillin has an exclusively antiamoebic effect.

The iodohydroxyquinolines include diodoquin (diodohydroxyquin) which is used commonly for asymptomatic and carrier cases, and vioform (iodochlorhydroxyquin) has been used extensively for several years. Of the arsenilic acid derivatives, carbarsone has been used for several years and bismuth glycoarsanilate has been introduced recently. Carbarsone and fumagillin have been used successfully in chimpanzees by Fremming *et al.* (1955) at a dose of 0·25 g. twice daily for 10 days and 20–30 mg. twice daily for 10 days, respectively.

Control. The control of *E. histolytica* infection is essentially a question of good sanitation, improved sewage disposal, the avoidance of faecal contamination of food, and an improvement in personal hygiene.

Entamoeba coli (Grassi, 1879) Casagrandi and Barbagallo, 1895.

This is a nonpathogenic form in humans, and its importance lies in the fact that it must be distinguished from the pathogenic *E. histolytica*. It is found in the caecum and colon, and up to 30 per cent of some populations may be infected. It is world wide in distribution, being commoner in warm, moist climates.

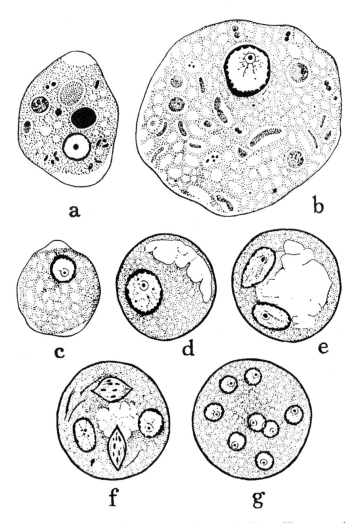

FIG. 276. Nonpathogenic Entamoebae (×2000). (From Hoare, 1950) a. *Entamoeba gingivalis*, from human mouth; b–g. *E. coli*, from human intestine; b. Active (trophic) amoeba with ingested bacteria, etc.; c. Precystic amoeba; d–g. Cysts: d.1-nucleate with glycogen vacuole; e. 2-nucleate with large glycogen vacuole; f. 4-nucleate (2 nuclei dividing), with filamentar chromatoids; g. 8-nucleate (mature).

Morphology. The active trophozoite is 20 μ–30 μ in diameter with a range of 15 μ–50 μ. The ectoplasm is thin and the cytoplasm possesses food vacuoles containing bacteria, yeast, starch grains, and vegetable debris. The nucleus differs from that of *E. histolytica* in having a larger endosome, which is also eccentric in position. The endosome is surrounded by a halo, and the peripheral chromatin of the nucleus is composed of coarser granules than in *E. histolytica*. Chromatin granules also appear on a network between the nuclear membrane and the endosome. The movements of *E. coli* are sluggish, and finger-like pseudopodia are not formed.

The cysts are 10 μ–30 μ in diameter, most frequently 15 μ–20 μ. When newly formed, the cyst is uninucleate but eventually eight nuclei are produced, this representing the mature infective stage. The chromatoid bodies are splinter-like; a glycogen vacuole is present in young cysts but it has generally disappeared by the 4-nucleate stage and is usually absent in the 8-nucleated cyst.

Entamoeba coli may occur in some monkeys, and the simian strain is transmissible to man. Many simian infections are acquired from humans, and the monkey does not form a major source of human infection. Natural infections with an entamoeba resembling *E. coli* have been found in the dog (Simic, 1933) and in the pig (Kessel, 1928).

Entamoeba gingivalis (Gros, 1849) Brumpt, 1914. This species is commonly found in the mouth of man, occasionally in the gingival tissue around the teeth, especially if inflammation, suppuration, or pyorrhoea is present. It is a harmless species, being more common in unhygienic mouths, though it can also be found in those which are well kept.

Only the trophozoite stage is known; encystment apparently does not occur. The trophozoite is 5 μ–35 μ in diameter (usually 10 μ–20 μ), and it has a clear ectoplasm and a granular endoplasm in which food vacuoles containing leucocytes, epithelial debris, bacteria etc. may be seen. The nucleus is nearly spherical, 2 μ–4 μ in diameter, with a small endosome and a distinct nuclear membrane lined by closely packed chromatin granules.

A form indistinguishable from *E. gingivalis* has been found in the mouths of dogs and cats, and this has been referred to as *Entamoeba canibuccalis* Simitch, 1938. *Entamoeba equibuccalis* Simitch, 1938, and *Entamoeba suigingivalis* Tumka, 1959, occur in horses and pigs, respectively.

Other Entamoeba

A large number of other species of the genus occur in domestic and other animals. These have been reviewed by Noble & Noble (1952, 1961), Hoare (1959), and Levine (1961).

Of those which occur, the following are of more interest. All are non-pathogenic.

Entamoeba moshkovskii Chalaya, 1941. In sewage. This resembles *E. histolytica* and may lead to confusion in diagnosis. Attempts to transmit it to kittens, rats and other animals have failed.

Entamoeba bovis Liebetanz, 1905. In cattle. Trophozoites 5 μ–20 μ, cytoplasm filled with vacuoles; nucleus large with a large central endosome made up of a compact mass of granules. Cysts uninucleate, 4 μ–15 μ.

Entamoeba ovis Swellengrebel, 1914. In sheep. Trophozoites 13 μ–14 μ, endosome of the nucleus large and composed of several granules. Cysts uninucleate, 4 μ–13 μ.

Entamoeba gedoelsti Hsiung, 1930. Colon and caecum of horses. Trophozoites 7 μ–13 μ, nucleus resembles that of *E. coli*, endosome is eccentric. No cyst formation.

Entamoeba equi Fantham, 1921. In horse in South America. Trophozoite 40 μ–50 μ by 23 μ–29 μ, nucleus oval. Cysts 15 μ by 24 μ, contain four nuclei.

Entamoeba suis Hartmann, 1913. In swine. Trophozoite 5 μ–25 μ, cysts uninucleate, 4 μ–17 μ.

Entamoeba muris (Grassi, 1879), **Entamoeba caviae** Chatton, 1918, and **Entamoeba cuniculi** Brug, 1918, occur in the caecum and colon of rats and mice, guinea pigs, and rabbits, respectively.

Genus: Endolimax Kuenen and Swellengrebel, 1917

These are small amoebae with a vesicular nucleus and an irregularly shaped, fairly large endosome composed of chromatin granules embedded in an achromatic ground substance. Achromatic threads connect the endosome with the nuclear membrane. Members of the genus are found in the hind gut of man and other animals. As far as is known, they are all nonpathogenic.

Endolimax nana (Wenyon and O'Conner, 1917) Brug, 1918. This is a nonpathogenic form of man and monkeys. The trophozoite is about 9 μ in diameter, the cytoplasm is pale and vacuolated, and the pseudopodia are short and broad. The nucleus contains a large endosome which is often eccentric in position and may even lie against the nuclear membrane. The cysts are oval, thin walled and measure 8 μ–10 μ. The mature cyst contains four nuclei. Chromatoid bodies are absent.

Endolimax caviae Hegner, 1926, occurs in the caecum of guinea pigs; only the trophozoites are known, these being 5 μ–11 μ.

Endolimax ratti Chiang, 1925, occurs in the caecum and colon of laboratory and wild rats. It closely resembles *E. nana* and may be a synonym of it.

Genus: Iodamoeba Dobell, 1919

Amoeba of this genus have a vesicular nucleus with a large endosome rich in chromatin. The cysts are uninucleate and contain a large glycogen vacuole which stains darkly with iodine. The genus occurs in the intestinal tract of man and animals.

Iodamoeba bütschlii (Von Prowazek, 1912) Dobell, 1919. This species occurs in the lower digestive tract of pig, man, a variety of monkeys, and baboons. It is world wide in distribution. The trophozoite is

6 μ–25 μ (average 8 μ–15 μ), the ectoplasm is not clearly differentiated and the endoplasm contains bacteria and yeast cells in food vacuoles. The nucleus has a dense endosome about half the diameter of the nucleus. The cysts are uninucleate, irregular, 6 μ–15 μ in diameter and contain a conspicuous glycogen vacuole which stains deeply with iodine.

Though generally regarded as nonpathogenic, Derrick (1948) has associated the trophozoite with ulceration of the stomach, small intestine, large intestine etc. of man.

Genus: Dientamoeba Jepps and Dobell, 1918

These are small amoebae frequently showing a binucleate character. The nuclear membrane is delicate, and the endosome consists of several chromatin granules connected to the nuclear membrane by delicate strands.

Dientamoeba fragilis Jepps and Dobell, 1918. This has been found in the caecum and colon of man and monkeys. It is nonpathogenic. The trophozoite is actively amoeboid, 4 μ–18 μ in diameter, and usually there are two nuclei. Encystation has not been observed.

CLASS: SPOROZOA LEUCKART, 1879

Members of the *Sporozoa* are parasitic and produce spores. They possess no organs of locomotion such as cilia or flagella except in the gamete stage. Reproduction is asexual by binary or multiple fission (schizogony) or sexual (gametogony). Gametogony leads to the formation of a zygote which in turn initiates the process of sporogony or spore formation.

The classification of the class *Sporozoa* has occasioned much discussion, but for the purposes of this book, that proposed by Schaudinn (1900) and adopted by Kudo (1954) will be used. An alternative approach is used by Levine (1961).

Kudo (1954) has divided the sporozoa into three subclasses:

Subclass *Telosporidia* Schaudinn; spores without a polar filament and each spore may contain one to many sporozoites.

Subclass *Acnidosporidia* Cepede; spores without polar filaments and containing 1 sporozoite.

Subclass *Cnidosporidia* Dolfein; spores with polar filament.

Only the subclass *Telosporidia* is of interest in this book.

The subclass *Telosporidia* is further divided into three orders: *Gregarinida* Lankester, in which the mature trophozoite is extracellular, *Coccodia* Leuckart and *Haemosporidia* Danilewsky, in both of which the mature trophozoite is intracellular and small. The *Coccidia* and *Haemosporidia* are of interest in this volume.

ORDER: COCCIDIA LEUCKART, 1879

Several classifications have been proposed for the order *Coccidia*. In the strict zoological sense, it is necessary to consider the division of the order into suborders, families etc. This is dealt with in detail by Pellerdy (1965). The majority of organisms of medical or veterinary importance belong to the family *Eimeriidae*.

FAMILY: EIMERIIDAE POCHE, 1913

These organisms are, with a few exceptions, intracellular parasites of the epithelial cells of the intestine. They have a single host in which they undergo asexual (schizogony) and sexual (gametogony) multiplication. The macro- and microgametocytes develop independently, the latter producing many gametes. A zygote results from the union of these, and by a process of *sporogony*, a variable number of spores (*sporocysts*) containing one or more *sporozoites* are formed. At present, twenty-five genera are recognised in the family *Eimeriidae*, and these are illustrated diagrammatically by Levine (1961) and in tabular form by Pellerdy (1965). The following genera are of importance in this book:

Cryptosporidium Tyzzer, 1910; no sporocysts, four sporozoites in the oocyst. *Tyzzeria* Allen, 1936; no sporocysts, eight sporozoites in the oocyst. *Isospora* Schneider, 1881; two sporocysts each containing four sporozoites. *Eimeria* Schneider, 1881; four sporocysts each containing two sporozoites.

The majority of the coccidia of importance in domestic animals belong to the genus *Eimeria*. The following account of the morphology and life-cycle of the coccidia of veterinary importance is based principally on this genus.

Life-cycle and Morphological Stages of Coccidia

Oocyst. The oocyst, which contains a zygote, is extruded from the host tissues and passed to the exterior in the faeces. This is the resistant stage of the life-cycle, and under appropriate conditions it forms the mature infective oocyst.

The most common shapes for oocysts are spherical, sub-spherical, ovoid or ellipsoidal, and they vary in size according to species. The oocyst wall is composed of two layers and is generally clear and transparent with a well defined double outline, in some species, however, it may be yellowish or even green in colour. Other species possess striations or punctations. The outer layer of the oocyst wall is a quinine-tanned protein while the inner layer is in fact two further layers, one showing an accumulation of lipids firmly associated with a protein lamella (Monné & Hönig, 1954). Several species of coccidia possess a micropyle at one extremity, this usually being the pointed end. The micropyle may be covered by a micropyle cap, and occasionally there may be a dome shaped projection of the cyst wall to the exterior in the form of a polar cap.

In the sporulated oocyst there are, according to genus, four sporocysts (*Eimeria*) or two sporocysts (*Isospora*). The sporocysts in *Eimeria* are more or less elongate ovoid forms with one end more pointed than the other. At the more pointed end is the Stieda body, and in some forms a micropyle may occur at the same place. An oocystic residual body and a polar granule may also be present in the oocyst. Each sporocyst contains two sporozoites, each having a granular cytoplasm and a distinctly placed central nucleus. Typically, the sporozoites are bent and comma-shaped and contain a round homogeneous vacuole at one end. A secondary, or sporocystic, residual body may be present.

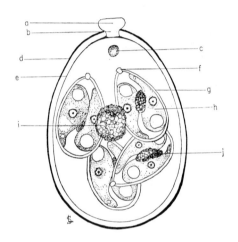

FIG. 277. Sporulated Oocyst of *Eimeria*
a. Polar cap; b. Micropyle; c. Polar granule; d. Outer layer of oocyst wall; e. Inner layer of oocyst wall; f. Stieda body; g. Sporocyst wall; h. Sporozoite; i. Oocyst residual body; j. Sporocyst residual body (Original)

The parasitic life-cycle of the coccidia is initiated when the infective oocyst is ingested by the appropriate host. Excystation releases the contained sporozoites.

The factors which induce excystation have not been fully clarified. Smetana (1933) suggested that trypsin was the specific enzyme which induced excystation of *Eimeria stiedae*, but this was not confirmed by Itagaki & Tsubokura (1958) nor by Landers (1960). However, more recently Ikeda (1960) restated that trypsin was necessary for excystation. Oocysts kept in trypsin in hanging drop preparations at 39–40°C showed movement of sporozoites within sporocysts and these then actively moved through the sporocyst micropyle into the oocyst; eventually they migrated through the micropyle of the oocyst.

Liberated sporozoites measure 10 μ by 1·5 μ and are transparent, fusiform organisms which show contraction and elongation and rapid gliding movements. The mode of entry of the sporozoites into the tissues is not known for all species. In the case of *Eimeria necatrix* Van Doorninck & Becker (1957) have shown that, initially, the sporozoites invade the intestinal epithelium at the tips of the villi and are there engulfed by macrophages and carried by them through the lamina propria of the villi to reach the epithelium in the depths of the glands of Lieberkühn. Here they leave the macrophages and enter the epithelial cells to undergo further development. A similar form of development has been demonstrated for *Eimeria tenella* (Pattillo, 1959; Challey & Burns, 1959) and for *E. meleagrimitis* (Clarkson, 1959).

Asexual Reproduction or Schizogony. This process is initiated when the sporozoite enters the epithelial cell and becomes rounded up. In many forms development occurs above the nucleus of the epithelial cell, in a few below it, and in one bovine species, within the nucleus. The rounded up sporozoite is, at this stage, known as a *trophozoite*, and within a few hours the nucleus of the trophozoite divides by schizogony to become a schizont. This is the first generation of schizogony or the first generation schizont. The nuclear division in schizogony is considered to be of the mitotic type (Pellerdy, 1965).

Initially the cytoplasm is undivided but later the daughter nuclei are each surrounded by a clear zone of cytoplasm, and eventually a number of elongate fusiform organisms are produced: the first generation *merozoites*. These, according to species, measure approximately 5 μ–10 μ by 1·5 μ. They have a granular cytoplasm with a centrally placed round nucleus. The mature schizont is surrounded by a distinct wall and the parasitised host cell is generally enlarged and distorted and protudes into the lumen of the gut, etc.

The number of merozoites which are formed in the first generation schizont varies according to species. In some of the large forms, e.g. *Eimeria bovis* more than 100,000 first generation merozoites may occur, but in *Isospora bigemina* only sixteen may be formed.

When the schizont is mature the first generation merozoites are released, and they then enter other epithelial cells in the area and continue the cycle of asexual development. In some species this results in 'colonies' of second generation schizonts, but in others the second generation forms are spread widely in the tissues. In the new host cell the merozoite first rounds up to become a trophozoite and then undergoes multiple fission as before. In some species the second generation schizont is much larger than the first, whereas in others it is much smaller. The number of merozoites produced also varies according to the species.

The second generation merozoites may proceed to a third or more generation of asexual reproduction or they may differentiate into sexual or gametogonous forms.

Sexual Reproduction or Gametogony. The factors which are responsible for determining the initiation of the gametogonous cycle are poorly understood.

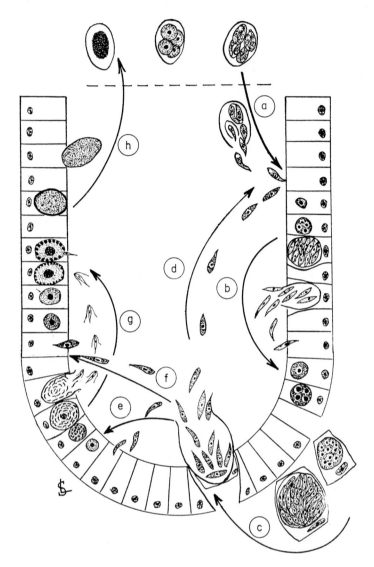

FIG. 278. Diagrammatic Representation of the Life-cycle of *Eimeria Tenella*
a. Ingestion of sporulated oocyst and liberation of sporozoites; b. First generation of
schizogony; c. Second generation of schizogony with migration of schizonts to sub-
epithelial tissues; d. Second generation merozoites initiate third generation of schizogony;
e. Second generation merozoites initiate microgametocyte formation; f. Second generation merozoites initiate macrogametocyte formation; g. Microgametes fertilise macrogametes with formation of zygote; h. Oocyst is shed from cell and passes to exterior
to undergo sporogony (Original)

In some forms of coccidia the merozoites destined for the sexual process
(telomerozoites) may show sexual dimorphism. Rutherford (1943)
found with rabbit *Eimeria* species th*t* two distinct types of schizonts and
merozoites of both the first and secoٖd generation were formed. A type 'A'

schizont was small in size, contained fewer merozoites and occurred in that part of the intestine where male or microgametocytic forms developed; another form, type 'B', consisted of large schizonts which developed where female gametes were usually found. There is at present no indication that such forms occur in the coccidia of domestic animals nor in fact is there any evidence that the different-sized schizonts have any relationship to the subsequent sexual cycle. An increase in resistance of the host to the infection has been claimed to initiate the sexual cycle but there is no adequate experimental proof of this. On the other hand, Levine (1940) transferred merozoites which would ordinarily have become sexual forms in one host to another fully susceptible host and produced the sexual cycle in the second host. In this case, at least, resistance was not a factor in the initiation of the sexual cycle.

In general the number of microgametes (male forms) greatly exceeds the number of macrogametes (female forms), the former being very much smaller than the latter. However, the macrogametocytes greatly outnumber the microgametocytes.

The young macrogametocyte is initially morphologically indistinguishable from the asexual trophozoite. Later, however, it is readily distinguished from it since the nucleus of the macrogametocyte does not divide. The macrogametocyte is round and roughly equivalent to the size of the oocyst which will result from it. The nucleus is clearly seen, and in stained preparations a karyosome is visible. Pattillo & Becker (1955) and Cheissin (1959) failed to find DNA in the nucleus of macrogametocytes of various poultry and rabbit coccidia. However, the method used (Feulgen stain) possibly was inadequate to detect small quantities of DNA in the nucleus. Subsequently, however, Horton-Smith & Long (1963) reported a weak Feulgen reaction in the macrogametocyte nucleus of *Eimeria maxima*.

In the young macrogamete small granules are initially found in the vicinity of the nucleus; later these enlarge and become scattered over the cytoplasm, the larger granules being found on the periphery of the cell. These are 'plastic granules' which Pattillo & Becker (1955) describe as composed largely of muco-protein; they are assumed to form the wall of the oocyst following fertilisation of the macrogamete. A detailed consideration of the histochemistry of the plastic granules and also of the macrogametocyte is given by Horton-Smith & Long (1963). Fertilisation by the microgamete may occur at any point on the surface of the macrogamete: a zygote is formed and the oocyst wall is laid down around it. When the cyst wall is complete the oocyst is extruded from the tissues and passed to the exterior.

The microgametocyte arises in the same way as the macrogametocyte, but as it enlarges the nucleus undergoes multiple division with the production of a large number of microgametes. Initially, the nuclei are scattered over the cytoplasm of the microgametocyte, but later they assume a comma shape and accumulate on the periphery of the cell leaving a residual mass of cytoplasm in the cell. The microgametes are slender, slightly bent, and the anterior end is pointed with two flagella for loco-motion. They measure about 5 μ in length, stain intensely with haema-toxylin and give strong reaction for DNA by the Feulgen reaction (Cheis-sin, 1959).

Rupture of the microgametocyte liberates the microgametes which fertilise the macrogametes.

Sporogony. With few exceptions, sporulation does not occur until the oocyst is shed to the exterior of the body. Initially, the zygote almost fills the oocyst cavity, but within a few hours outside the host the protoplasm contracts from the wall of the oocyst to form a *sporont* and leaves a clear space between it and the wall. The sporont divides into four sporoblasts, any remaining cytoplasm being left as an oocystic residual body. The sporoblasts are, initially, more or less spherical, but later they elongate into ovoid or ellipsoid bodies which then become sporocysts by the laying down of a wall of refractile material around each sporoblast. The proto-plasm inside each sporocyst further divides to form two sporozoites. Protoplasm remaining from the division is left as a sporocystic residual body.

The time required for sporulation to the infective stage is a specific feature of each species of coccidium and is used as a characteristic in identification. Oxygen and adequate moisture are necessary for the sporulation, and at constant temperatures an increasing percentage of oocysts are killed as relative humidity decreases. Temperature also has an important influence on sporulation. The optimum temperature for sporulation is about 30°C. In general sporulated oocysts are more resistant to desiccation and cold and may survive for up to two weeks at temperatures of -12 to -20°C. Unsporulated forms are killed in 96 hours at these temperatures. The survival of oocysts under natural condi-tions has received substantial consideration from various workers over the years. Factors such as soil types, exposure to direct sunlight or otherwise, the amount of humus in soil, moisture etc. are important in the longevity of oocysts.

General. Coccidial infections are self-limiting, and asexual reproduction does not continue indefinitely. In the absence of re-infection, therefore, only one cycle of development can take place. Under natural conditions, however, repeated infection usually occurs. As a result of repeated infec-tion, the host may develop immunity and with certain species of coccidia immunity may be marked following a single infection. One of the effects of immunity is to reduce the biotic potential of the coccidium. Whereas an initial infection may produce a maximum number of oocysts, as immunity supervenes the life-cycle is progressively inhibited, so that at one level only a few oocysts may be produced, and at another the infective sporozoites may fail to get further than the initial penetration of the host cell.

PLATE XXIV

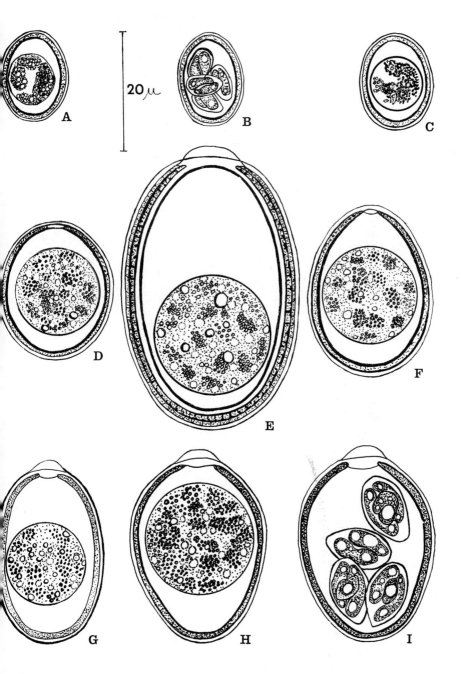

Coccidia of sheep. A. *Eimeria pallida;* B. *E. pallida* (sporulated); C. *E. parva;* D. *E. ninakohlyakimovi;* E. *E. intricata;* F. *E. faurei;* G. *E. arloingi;* H. *E. granulosa;* I. *E. granulosa* (sporulated).

(Plates XXIV and XXV redrawn with kind permission from Christensen, J. F. (1938). 'Species differentation in the coccidia from the domestic sheep'. *J. Parasit.*, **24,** 453–467)

PLATE XXV

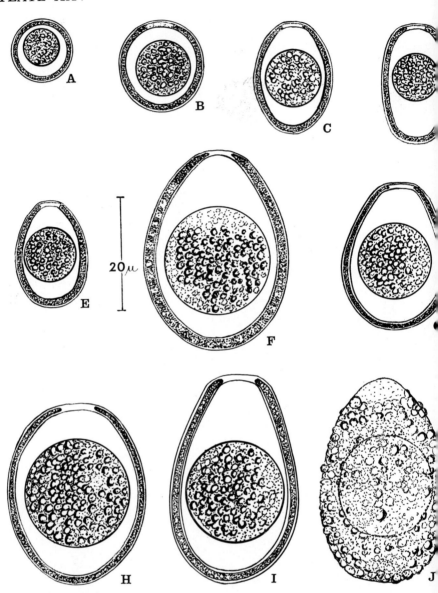

Coccidia of cattle. A. *Eimeria subspherica;* B. *E. zurnii;* C. *E. ellipsoidalis;* D. *E. cyli‐
drica;* E. *E. alabamensis;* F. *E. bukidnonensis;* G. *E. bovis;* H. *E. canadensis;* I. *E.
auburnensis* (with homogeneous wall); J. *E. auburnensis* (with mammillated wall)

PLATE XXVI

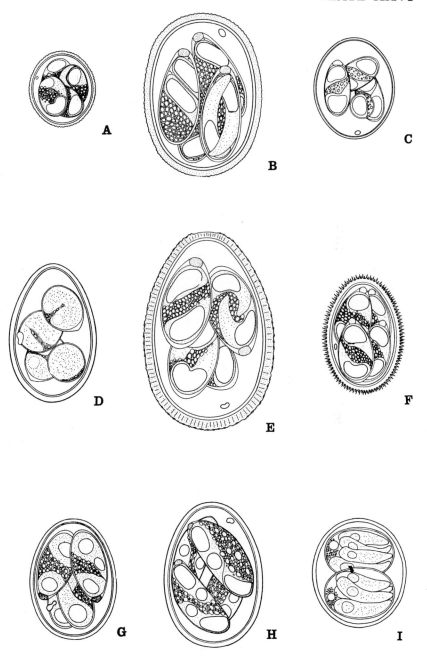

Coccidia of swine. A. *Eimeria perminuta*; B. *E. cerdonis*; C. *E. suis*; D. *E. porci*; E. *E. scabra*; F. *E. spinosa*; G. *E. neodebliecki*; H. *E. debliecki*; I. *Isospora suis*

(Reproduced with kind permission from Vetterling, J. M. (1965). 'Coccidia (Protozoa: Eimeriidae) of swine', *J. Parasit.*, **51**, 897–912)

PLATE XXVII

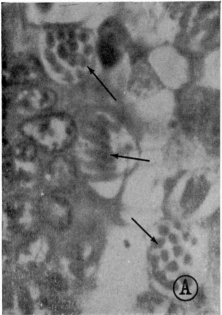

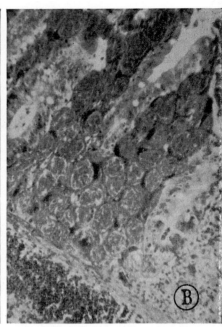

A. Bile duct epithelium of rabbit infected with *Eimeria stiedae*. Three schizonts are visible. (× 1200)

B. Caecal mucosa of chicken infected with *Eimeria tenella*. A colony of second generation schizonts is visible in a sub-epithelial position. (× 300)

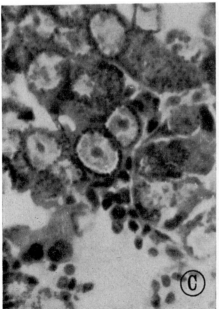

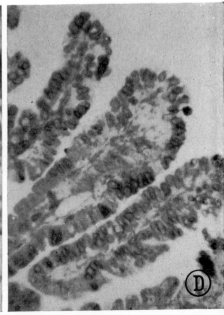

C. Small intestinal mucosa of chicken infected with *Eimeria acervulina*. Macro-gametocytes are visible, central field. (× 800)

D. Small intestinal mucosa of sheep infected with *Eimeria arloingi*. Gametogonous stages are visible in the epithelial cells of the villi which have undergone marked hypertrophy. (× 300)

Coccidia of Sheep and Goats

It is generally stated that the coccidia of sheep and goats are inter-changeable. It may be presumptuous to claim this for all the species, and further clarification on this is necessary.

Eimeria ahsata Honess, 1942
Eimeria arkhari Yakimoff and Matschoulsky, 1937
Eimeria arloingi (Marotel, 1905) Martin, 1909
Eimeria christenseni Levine, Ivens and Fritz, 1962
Eimeria crandallis Honess, 1942
Eimeria faurei (Moussu and Marotel, 1902) Martin, 1909
Eimeria gilruthi (Chatton, 1910) Reichenow and Carini, 1937
Eimeria granulosa Christensen, 1938
Eimeria intricati Spiegl, 1925
Eimeria ninakohlyakimovae Yakimoff and Rastegaieff, 1930
Eimeria pallida Christensen, 1938
Eimeria parva Kotlan, Mocsy, and Vajda, 1929
Eimeria punctata Landers, 1955

Eimeria ahsata. *Hosts:* Domestic sheep, Rocky Mountain big horn sheep, Moufflon (*Ovis musimon*), Siberian ibex (*Capra ibex siberica*). At one time this species was considered to be a form of *E. arloingi* (Lotze, 1953), recently however Smith *et al.* (1960) confirmed its validity. *Oocyst;* ellipsoidal, wall smooth, pinkish-yellow, a dome-shaped polar cap over the micropyle, $32 \cdot 7 \mu$ by $23 \cdot 7 \mu$ in forms from the big horn sheep, $33 \cdot 4 \mu$ by $22 \cdot 6 \mu$ in forms from domestic sheep (Levine, 1961). Prepatent period, 18–20 days (Smith *et al.*, 1960). Smith *et al.* (1960) consider *E. ahsata* to be the most pathogenic coccidium in sheep. Lambs, infected with from 100,000 to 800,000 oocysts showed severe disease; four out of nine lambs, 1 to 3 months of age, being killed by the lower dose. Clinical signs consisted of diarrhoea and loss of body weight and ability. At autopsy the wall of the ileum was thickened, especially in the anterior part, and there was inflammation of Peyer's patches.

Eimeria arkhari. *Hosts:* wild sheep in the Soviet Union. *Oocyst:* ellipsoidal to oval, $22 \cdot 4 \mu$ by $17 \cdot 4 \mu$, double contoured oocyst wall with a yellowish tint, micropyle absent.

Eimeria arloingi. *Hosts:* domestic sheep and goat, the Rocky Mountain big horn sheep, Moufflon, Ibex, angora (also in chamois, red deer and roe deer, though Pellerdy (1965) doubts that these are true records). *Oocyst;* 27μ by 18μ, but a wide range occurs, 17μ–42μ by 13μ–31μ (Christensen, 1938). Levine *et al.* (1962) give a range of 22μ–31μ by 17μ–22μ with a mean of 28μ by 20μ. Oocysts predominantly ellipsoidal, ovoid ones may occur, micropyle 2μ–3μ in width with a distinct polar cap. Sporulation time 48–72 hours.

Eimeria arloingi is probably the most common coccidium of sheep. Christensen (1938) found it in 90 per cent of sheep examined in the United

States and a similar finding was made by Richardson (1939) in Great Britain.

Developmental Cycle. The liberated sporozoites may be found for several days free in the lumen of the intestine; later they penetrate the epithelial layer and enter the endothelial cells lining the central lacteals of the villi. Only one generation of schizonts occurs, and schizonts become mature 13–21 days after infection. They reach a size of 122 μ–146 μ in diameter and contain several million merozoites, each about 9 μ in length. Merozoites are released from the giant schizonts about 19 days after infection, and they enter the epithelial cells of the small intestine. In heavy infections large numbers of epithelial cells are parasitised and the affected villus may greatly enlarge to form a papillomatous growth. The macrogametocytes are markedly granular and there is a preponderance of these forms in the infection. The prepatent period is about 20 days (Lotze, 1953).

Pathogenicity. Lotze (1952) found, in 3-month-old lambs, that no clinical signs were seen in lambs receiving less than 1 million oocysts. With higher doses clinical signs of soft, watery faeces appeared on the 13th day. The majority of animals had returned to normal by the 20th day. Slight haemorrhages occurred in the small intestine up to the 13th day, and by the 13th and 19th days the small intestine was oedematous and thickened, the villi distended with schizonts, and there was a loss of epithelium.

Eimeria christenseni. *Hosts:* Domestic goat (*Capra hircus*). *Oocyst:* ovoid and slightly flattened at one end, 38 μ by 25 μ, range 34 μ–41 μ by 23 μ–28 μ, micropyle covered by a prominent dome-shaped micropylar cap. Not known to be pathogenic.

Eimeria crandallis. *Hosts:* Rocky Mountain big horn sheep, domestic sheep, Moufflon, Siberian ibex. *Oocyst:* spherical to broadly ellipsoidal, 23 μ by 19 μ, range 20 μ–27 μ by 17 μ–20 μ, visible micropylar cap. *Distribution:* North America, Soviet Union. Life-cycle and pathogenicity unknown.

Eimeria faurei. *Hosts:* sheep, goat, Rocky Mountain big horn sheep, chamois, ibex, Siberian ibex, Moufflon, aoudad or barbary sheep (*Ammotragus lervia = Ovis tragelapus*) and various wild sheep. World wide in distribution and relatively common. *Oocyst:* ovoidal, micropyle distinct, no polar cap, wall transparent, brownish-yellow to salmon pink, 28·9 μ by 21 μ, range 25 μ–33 μ by 18 μ–24 μ (Christensen, 1938). Sporulation time 1–2 days.

Developmental Cycle. Not known in detail. Lotze (1953) described schizonts which measured up to 100 μ in diameter and contained thousands of merozoites.

Pathogenicity. At the most, the species is only mildly pathogenic. Lotze (1954) reported that infection of 3-month-old lambs with 5 million oocysts produced only a slight softening of the faeces, and infections of 50 million oocysts failed to cause death.

Eimeria gilruthi. *Hosts:* sheep and goat. World wide in distribution. Occurs principally in the abomasum, rarely seen in the small intestine. Only the schizonts have been described, and these occur in the abomasal wall. They are large (giant schizonts), up to 700 μ in length, and are readily visible to the naked eye; many thousands of merozoites fill the schizont.

This species was originally described by Maske (1893) from the abomasum of a sheep. It was later found by Gilruth (1910) and studied in detail by Chatton (1910), who named it *Gastrocystis gilruthi*. Since that time it has been found in various parts of the world; Alicata (1930) found it in up to 11 per cent of sheep in the United States; Sarwar (1951) found it in 32 per cent of sheep and 40 per cent of goats in the Sudan.

Virtually nothing is known of its endogenous developmental cycle. Several species of sheep coccidia have giant schizonts in their life-cycle (e.g. *E. arloingi, E. parva*), and there seems little doubt that it represents the schizont of some species of coccidium. Until further evidence is available about it, it would seem wise to follow the suggestion of Levine (1961) that as a temporary measure it be called *Eimeria gilruthi*.

Eimeria granulosa. *Hosts:* domestic sheep, Rocky Mountain sheep. North America and Germany. Location inside the host is not known, only the oocysts having been found in the faeces. *Oocyst:* urn-shaped, distinct micropyle, 3 μ–5 μ in diameter, with a micropylar cap. Oocyst wall transparent, brownish to yellowish in colour. Mean size 29·4 μ by 20·9 μ, range 22 μ–35 μ by 17 μ–25 μ. Sporulation time 3–4 days.

Eimeria intricata. *Hosts:* domestic sheep, Rocky Mountain big horn sheep, other members of the genus *Ovis*. Relatively common and world wide in distribution. *Oocyst:* largest of the species of *Eimeria* in sheep, 47 μ by 32 μ, range 39 μ–53 μ by 27 μ–34 μ, ellipsoidal, well developed micropyle, 6 μ–10 μ in diameter, with a distinct light-coloured polar cap. Sporulation time 3–5 days. Endogenous development of this species is not known with certainty. Reichenow (1940) considered the forms of globidium to be giant schizonts of *E. intricata*.

Eimeria ninakohlyakimovae. *Hosts:* domestic sheep, Rocky Mountain big horn sheep, Barbary sheep, Siberian ibex, Moufflon, other wild sheep, and also in Persian gazelle, roe deer and red deer. World wide in distribution. Occurs in posterior part of small intestine and caecum and colon. *Prevalence:* 52 per cent of sheep and 31 per cent of goats were found infected in Kazakhstan (Svanbaev, 1957); 5 per cent of sheep in Germany (Jacob, 1943); 3 per cent of sheep in the U.S.A. (Christensen, 1938). *Oocyst:* ellipsoidal, sometimes ovoid; 23·1 μ by 18·3 μ, range 20 μ to 28 μ by 15 μ to 22 μ (Christensen, 1938). Variations in the size of oocysts from other host species have been recorded, thus those from the moufflon measure an average 25·2 μ by 19·5 μ (Yakimoff *et al.*, 1933). Generally no micropyle, no polar cap. Cyst wall thin, smooth and transparent, slightly brownish yellow. Sporulation 1–2 days.

The endogenous development of this species was described by Lotze (1954). Sporozoites entered the epithelial cells at the base of the villi in the crypts of Lieberkühn of the small intestine where they developed to giant schizonts (up to 300 μ in diameter) containing many thousands of merozoites. Following rupture of the schizonts, the gametogonous stages are found in the epithelial cells of the ileum, caecum and upper part of the large intestine. The prepatent period is 15 days (Shumard, 1957).

Lotze (1954) considered this species to be the most pathogenic of sheep coccidia. As few as 50,000 oocysts caused diarrhoea in a 3-month-old lamb, half a million causing death. Profused diarrhoea occurred in a 2-year-old sheep given a million oocysts. Faeces became soft 12–17 days after infection, remaining in this state for a week or more: in heavily infected animals the faeces were mixed with blood. Haemorrhages were found in the posterior part of the small intestine of severely affected animals by the 15th day, and the wall of the intestine was thickened and inflamed. During the gametogonous part of the cycle the caecum and colon were thickened, oedematous and haemorrhagic by the 19th day, and large areas of the small intestine were denuded of epithelium. In contrast to these findings, Shumard (1957), using an obviously less pathogenic strain, found that only slight diarrhoea and lowered food consumption occurred with an infection of 7 million oocysts.

Eimeria pallida. *Hosts:* domestic sheep in North America. Site of development in the host is not known. *Oocyst:* ellipsoidal, 14·2 μ by 10 μ, range 12 μ–20 μ by 8 μ–15 μ (Christensen, 1938). Micropyle imperceptible, no polar cap, oocyst wall thin, pale yellow to yellowish-green and appearing fragile. Sporulation time 24 hours.

The developmental cycle of this species is unknown and no pathogenesis is ascribed to it.

Not all authors agree that this is a valid species, for example Kotlan *et al.* (1951) consider it a synonym of *Eimeria parva*.

Eimeria parva. *Hosts:* domestic sheep and goat; also Siberian ibex, Rocky Mountain big horn sheep, Barbary sheep. World wide in distribution. Asexual stages in the small intestine, gametogonous stages in the caecum, colon and small intestine. *Prevalence:* 50 per cent of sheep infected in U.S.A. (Christensen, 1938), 52 per cent of sheep and 9 per cent of goats infected in Germany (Jacob, 1943). *Oocyst:* sub-spherical to spherical, 16·5 μ by 14·1 μ, range 12 μ–22 μ and 10 μ–18 μ (Christensen, 1938). Oocyst wall smooth with a uniform thickness, no visible micropyle, no polar cap; pale yellow to yellowish-green. Sporulation time, 1–2 days.

The endogenous development has been described by Kotlan *et al.* (1950). Giant schizonts of the globidial type occur in the small intestine.

Two types of schizonts were recognised, smaller ones measuring 60 μ by 40 μ and large sub-spherical forms 185 μ by 179 μ; the latter sometimes became elongate, reaching lengths of up to 256 μ. The larger schizonts were visible as whitish bodies in the mucosa, being found over the entire length of the small intestine. The schizonts reach maturity in 12–14 days, and there appears to be only one asexual generation. The gametocytic stages occur in epithelial cells of the mucous membrane of the caecum and colon. Prepatent period, 16–17 days.

This species is not markedly pathogenic. Massive infections produce a catarrhal inflammation with loss of epithelium; faeces are dark and mixed with blood. The large intestine may become necrotic and infiltrated with leucocytes and neutrophils.

Eimeria punctata. *Hosts:* domestic sheep in North America (Wyoming). Site of development in the host is unknown. *Oocyst:* sub-spherical to spherical, 21·2 μ by 17·7 μ, range 17·8 μ–25·1 μ by 16·2 μ to 21·1 μ (Landers, 1952); micropyle present, small polar cap present. Wall of oocyst covered by an even distribution of cone-shaped pits about 0·5 μ in depth, inner part of the wall with a greenish tint. Sporulation time 36–48 hours. The developmental cycle is unknown, and no pathogenesis has been ascribed to the parasite.

Coccidiosis in Sheep and Goats

Coccidiosis in sheep and goats is chiefly confined to young animals up to 4–6 months of age. Mixed infections are usual and the species of clinical importance are *E. arloingi*, *E. parva* and *E. ninakohlyakimovae*.

In the United States coccidiosis is primarily a disease of feed lot lambs, outbreaks of disease occurring when range-reared lambs are moved to intensive conditions of husbandry. The disease frequently appears 2–3 weeks after the lambs are placed in the feed lot. Though the feed lot may become relatively free of infection during the time it is left vacant, infection is introduced by the range lambs, and as a result of crowding and poor hygienic conditions the output of oocysts in the faeces rises markedly. Oocyst output reaches a peak about 1 month after lambs enter the feed lot; it remains at a high level for a further 1–3 weeks and then falls quickly so that at the end of the feeding period only a few oocysts are passed in the faeces (Christensen, 1940).

A mortality of 10 per cent due to *E. arloingi* and *E. ninakohlyakimovae* has been reported in lambs in Georgia by Becklund (1957); a similar outbreak was recorded by Davies *et al.* (1957) in a flock which had been corralled nightly for 3 weeks to guard against attacks of dogs. Coccidiosis has been reported as a cause of morbidity and mortality in lambs in other countries. Salisbury & Whitten (1953) considered coccidiosis the cause of unthriftiness and death in lambs aged 4–6 months in New Zealand; Favati & Guerrieri (1961) reported the disease to be common in Italy, and Rao

& Hiregaudar (1954) stated that the coccidiosis was a severe parasitic disease among sheep and goats in India.

In Great Britain, infections of coccidia with a high morbidity and a low mortality have been observed by the author in young lambs, aged 2–3 months, in flocks where nursing ewes were fed grain and concentrates in open troughs in fields. The same area was used continuously for feeding and the environment of the troughs was heavily contaminated with sporulated oocysts. The pathogenic process was largely due to *E. arloingi*.

The seasonal incidence of coccidiosis is determined by the availability of young animals for the development of the parasite (older animals being immune) and by the survival of oocysts from one season to the next. Freezing conditions either kill oocysts or prevent them from sporulating; consequently, pastures, or feed lots, are usually relatively free of coccidia at the time of the new season's crop of lambs.

The Clinical Signs and Pathology of Coccidiosis. These consist of a brownish to yellowish-green diarrhoea, which may be streaked with blood especially when caused by those species which undergo gametogony in the large intestine. Abdominal pain, some anaemia, inappetence, weakness and loss of weight may occur. The diarrhoea may continue for up to 2 weeks, and though lambs may die from it or the consequent dehydration, the majority recover, and it is unusual to see a mortality exceeding about 10 per cent. Nevertheless, the setback in growth and production may be economically important. Shumard (1957) found that eighty lambs, experimentally infected with a mixture of *E. ninakohlyakimovae* and *E. arloingi*, lost an average of 0·205 pounds per pound of feed consumed over a 24 day period as compared with a gain of 0·062 pounds per pound of feed consumed in a group of control lambs. The severity of the clinical entity is dependent on the size of the initial infection. Where this is low, clinical disease may never appear, rather the animal develops immunity but it may continue to shed small numbers of oocysts for the rest of its life.

The pathological changes vary with the species concerned. With *E. arloingi*, lesions occur in the posterior part of the small intestine, the giant schizonts and the gametogonous stages producing enlargement of the villi, so much so that these may be visible to the naked eye. Where groups of villi have enlarged, a papillomatous-like growth may be readily visible on the mucosa of the small intestine. In more acute cases the wall of the intestine is thickened, oedematous, and it may be haemorrhagic. Scrapings of the mucosa show large numbers of schizonts and oocysts. With *E. parva* infection, the mucosae of the caecum and colon are thickened, oedematous, and haemorrhagic. Necrotic areas may occur on the mucosa, and the contents of the bowel are fluid and dark brown to haemorrhagic in colour. With *E. ninakohlyakimovae* infection, the intestinal mucosa is covered with petechial haemorrhages, and the wall is thickened and inflamed.

Diagnosis. This is based on the history of the outbreak (there is usually evidence of poor hygiene either in feed lots or in grazing management), the lesions seen at post-mortem and by an examination of the faeces. Usually very large numbers of oocysts are found in the faeces (several thousand oocysts per g. of faeces). However, in peracute infections clinical signs may arise before oocysts are shed. It should be recognised that coccidia probably are present in all sheep, and the mere presence of oocysts in the faeces is not grounds for a diagnosis of coccidiosis. It is advisable therefore to conduct a post-mortem examination on a representative member of the flock before a definite diagnosis is reached.

Treatment

Sulphonamides. Foster *et al.* (1941) reported that sulphaguanidine at a dose of 2 g. per day for 6 days suppressed oocyst output in sub-clinical infections and prevented the acquisition of natural infections. In field studies in New Zealand, Whitten (1953) reported no growth response following treatment with sodium sulphadimidine (2 g. on the first day followed by 1 g. daily for the next 2 days), sulphanilamide, sulphaguanidine, or a triple sulphonamide formulation (2 g. followed by 1 g. daily for the next 2 days), sulphaquinoxaline (0.7 g. daily for 3 days), or a single dose of 4 g. of sulphadimidine.

Nitrofurazone. This has been shown to be effective against *E. faurei* at a dose of 7–10 mg. per kg. daily for 7 days (Tarlatzis, *et al.*, 1955). It may be given in the feed at a level of 0·0165 per cent (Shumard, 1959). Shumard (1959) also demonstrated that 0·008 per cent, 0·01 per cent and 0·0133 per cent of nitrofurazone in the drinking water prevented mortality and reduced morbidity resulting from experimental infections produced with 10 million oocysts consisting of a mixture of *E. ninakohly-akimovae*, *E. arloingi*, *E. intricata*, *E. parva*, *E. faurei* and *E. pallida*.

No information is available on the usefulness in sheep of the more recent coccidiocidal and coccidiostatic agents used for poultry. It is possible that they may be of value in sheep.

Prevention and Control. Feed lots should be kept dry and clean, the feed troughs should be constructed so that there is no wastage from them and so that they are not contaminated by faeces. Proper drainage of the feed lot is necessary.

Where nursing ewes are fed concentrates at pasture, the feeding area should be changed regularly. If inclement weather necessitates that lambs and ewes be kept in yards or barns, then the bedding should be changed regularly to avoid an accumulation of large numbers of sporulated oocysts.

Coccidia of Cattle

Bovine coccidiosis occurs in all parts of the world and serious outbreaks may occur in dairy herds where young stock are kept in large numbers.

The following species have been described from cattle:
Eimeria alabamensis Christensen, 1941
Eimeria auburnensis Christensen and Porter, 1939
Eimeria bovis (Züblin, 1908) Fiebiger, 1912
Eimeria braziliensis Torres and Ramos, 1939
Eimeria bukidnonensis Tubangui, 1931
Eimeria canadensis Bruce, 1921
Eimeria cylindrica Wilson, 1931
Eimeria ellipsoidalis Becker and Frye, 1929
Eimeria mundaragi Hiregaudar, 1956
Eimeria pellita Supperer, 1952
Eimeria subspherica Christensen, 1941
Eimeria wyomingensis Huizinga and Winger, 1942
Eimeria zürnii (Rivolta, 1878) Martin, 1909

Eimeria alabamensis. *Hosts:* domestic cattle, North America. Davis *et al.* (1955) found this species in 93 per cent of 102 dairy calves examined and subsequent reports indicate that it is a common coccidium of cattle in the United States. The developmental stages occur in the posterior part of the ileum and may extend to the caecum and colon. *Oocysts:* predominantly pear-shaped, some ellipsoidal, sub-cylindrical or asymmetrical; $18·9\,\mu$ by $13·4\,\mu$, range $13\,\mu–24\,\mu$ by $11\,\mu–16\,\mu$ (Christensen, 1941). Oocyst wall thin, homogeneous, transparent and generally colourless, no micropyle. Sporulation time, 96–120 hours.

Life-cycle. The endogenous developmental cycle was reinvestigated by Davis *et al.* (1957). It is unusual in that the developmental stages occur in the nucleus of the epithelial cell. Sporozoites penetrate the intestinal cells as early as the 2nd day after infection, and schizonts are visible in the nucleus 2 to 8 days after infection. The cells usually parasitised are those at the tips of the villi. Multiple invasion of the nucleus may occur, and schizonts may reach a size of $12·6\,\mu$ by $9·7\,\mu$ by 6 days. They produce fifteen to thirty-two merozoites, and free merozoites may be found in the small intestine as early as 4 days after infection. Davis *et al.* (1957) consider that more than one asexual generation occurs.

Gametocytes are found in the posterior third of the small intestine, but they may also occur in the mucous membrane of the caecum and colon in heavy infections. Oocysts may be seen in the tissues of the lower part of the ileum as early as 6 days after infection, but the average prepatent period is 8·6 days with a range of 6–11 days. The duration of oocyst production from a single infection is 1–10 days with an average of 4·6 days for low-grade infections and 1–13 days with an average of 7·2 days for heavy infections.

The Pathogenicity of E. alabamensis. It is low under field conditions and is generally considered to be unimportant in clinical bovine coccidiosis. Disease may be produced if large numbers of oocysts are given to young calves. Thus Boughton (1943) fed 200 million oocysts to young calves and produced severe diarrhoea; two of five animals died. Davis *et al.* (1955) found that 140 million oocysts produced a yellowish-green diarrhoea, admixed with blood, in 14-month-old animals. The small intestine showed hyperaemia, destruction of the epithelium, a leukocytic infiltration and oedema.

Eimeria auburnensis. *Hosts:* domestic cattle. *E. auburnensis* is one of the most common coccidia in cattle in North America; reports generally indicate that it is widespread elsewhere in the world. *Oocysts:* ovoidal, varying from ellipsoidal to tapering, 38·4 μ by 23·1 μ, range 32 μ–46 μ by 20 μ to 25 μ (Christensen & Porter, 1939; Christensen, 1931). Oocyst wall smooth and homogeneous, transparent, yellowish-brown in colour; occasionally it may have a coarsely granulated surface and at times be heavily mammillated. Micropyle appears as a pale area at narrow end. Sporulation time, 48 to 72 hours.

Life-cycle. The endogenous developmental cycle of *E. auburnensis* was investigated by Hammond *et al.* (1961) and Davis & Bowman (1962). The sporozoites invade the endothelial cells of the lacteals of villi in the posterior part of the small intestine. Giant schizonts, resembling those of *E. bovis* are produced. The number of asexual generations has not been determined.

The sexual stages occur in cells of mesodermal origin, especially those lying beneath the epithelium of the villi of the small intestine. The microgametocytes are unusually large and may be seen with the naked eye, each producing several thousand microgametes. More than one gametocyte may be seen in an individual cell in heavy infections, and both male and female forms may occur in the same cell. Oocyst production is complete in about 18 days after infection, however, the epithelium needs to be broken before the oocysts can be shed. The prepatent period is 24 days, oocysts being discharged in maximal numbers for 3 days (Christensen & Porter, 1939).

The Pathogenic Effect of E. auburnensis. It is low under field conditions. A profused green diarrhoea was produced in a 2-week-old calf given 8000 oocysts by Christensen & Porter (1939), clinical signs appearing between the 9th and 15th day of infection. Davis & Bowman (1952) reported the passage of blood and mucus, with straining, in artificial infections with large numbers of oocysts and in natural outbreaks.

Eimeria bombayansis. *Hosts:* zebu, India. This species has been recognised from oocysts in faeces, and Rao & Hiregaudar (1954) indicated it was common in dairy calves near Bombay. *Oocysts:* ellipsoidal, 37 μ by 22·4 μ, range 32 μ–40 μ by 20 μ–25 μ. Oocyst wall smooth, transparent and homogeneous. Pellerdy (1965) considers this species to be identical with *E. auburnensis.*

Eimeria bovis. *Hosts:* cattle, zebu, water buffalo. Together with *Eimeria zürnii,* this species is most commonly involved in clinical coccidiosis of cattle. World wide in distribution. The asexual stages occur in the small intestine, the gametogonous stages in the terminal part of the ileum and in the caecum and colon. *Oocysts:* ovoidal, blunted across the narrow end; in massive infections a variation in shape of oocysts may occur: $27 \cdot 7 \mu$ by $20 \cdot 3 \mu$, range $23 \mu - 34 \mu$ by $17 \mu - 23 \mu$. Oocyst wall smooth, homogeneous, transparent, greenish-brown in colour, micropyle present appearing as a lighter area of the wall. Sporulation time, 48–72 hours at room temperature.

Life-cycle. The endogenous developmental cycle was investigated by Hammond *et al.* (1946). The sporozoites invade the endothelial cells of the central lacteals of villi in the posterior half of the small intestine. Schizonts appear as early as 5 days after infection, and swollen cells may become detached from the lacteal cavity. These forms grow to mature giant (globidial) schizonts, and by 14–18 days after infection they may measure up to 400 μ in diameter, the mean size being 281 μ by 303 μ. Each schizont contains an average of 120,000 merozoites, each about 11 μ in length. A second generation schizont has been reported by Hammond *et al.* (1963), this being smaller than the first (about 100 μ) and occurring in the epithelial cells of the caecum and colon. The second schizont produces 30–36 merozoites and takes $1 \cdot 5$ to 2 days to develop. Merozoites from the second generation schizonts invade the epithelial cells chiefly of the caecum and colon, though in heavy infections they may be found also in the terminal 3 ft of the small intestine. The gametogonous cycle is initiated about 15–16 days after infection (Hammond *et al.*, 1960a), and the gametes are mature 3 days later. Oocysts are formed in a minimum of 18 days and peak numbers of oocysts are discharged 19–22 days after infection. Small numbers of oocysts continue to be discharged for 2–3 weeks after the initial major discharge.

Pathogenesis. *Eimeria bovis* is one of the most common coccidia of cattle. Forty per cent or more of cattle have been reported infected in various parts of the world; Boughton (1945) found it in 41 per cent of more than 2000 bovine faecal samples in the south-eastern U.S.A.; similar figures have been reported by Hasche & Todd (1959) in the U.S.A., by Supperer (1952) in Austria and Rao & Hiregaudar (1954) in India.

Though the later stages of the development of the first stage schizont cause distortion of the villi and disruption when the merozoites escape (as is also the case with the second schizonts), it is the gametocytic stages which cause the greatest pathogenic effect. Hammond (1964) has estimated that if the full potential of *E. bovis* were to be realized, 1000 oocysts could result in the destruction of 24 billion intestinal cells. In experimental infections Hammond *et al.* (1944) found that an infective dose of 125,000 oocysts or more caused marked signs of illness with diarrhoea occurring on the 18th day when the faeces were streaked with blood. A calf given 125,000 oocysts became moribund, and with higher doses animals became moribund or died within 3–4 weeks of infection.

In severe infections the majority of the crypts of the large intestine, and sometimes of the terminal part of the small intestine, are destroyed, the epithelial layer denuded and the lumen of the intestine filled with blood. The mucosa is necrotic and sloughed and this damage may extend to the sub-mucosa; the wall of the intestine is congested and oedematous, and large numbers of gametocytes and oocysts are visible microscopically.

Immunity. A resistance to re-infection with *E. bovis*, lasting at least 3–6 months and possibly longer, was demonstrated by Senger *et al.* (1959). Infections of 10 to 100,000 oocysts induced a rapid immunity, and animals became resistant 14 days after initial infection. Schizonts and merozoites of the first generation, second generation schizonts and merozoites and the gametocytes were affected by the immune reaction, the immune response affecting the numbers but not the timing of the various stages of the life cycle (Hammond *et al.*, 1963). In other studies Hammond *et al.* (1964) reported that the invasion of the epithelial cells by first generation merozoites of *E. bovis* was inhibited in immune calves, and merozoites were lysed when placed in immune serum (Anderson *et al.*, 1965). A similar effect was seen with normal serum but not at the dilutions which caused the effect with immune serum.

Eimeria brasiliensis. *Hosts:* cattle, zebu, in North and South America, Europe (Austria), Nigeria and the Soviet Union. Marquardt (1959), following a comparison of *E. brasiliensis* with *Eimeria böhmi* Supperer, 1952, considered the two were synonymous. This species is known from the oocysts only. *Oocysts:* oval, 37·5 μ by 27·1 μ, range 34·2 –42·7 μ by 24·2 μ–29·9 μ (Torres & Ramos, 1939). Oocysts wall, colourless to yellow, smooth, with a distinct micropyle and a polar cap. Sporulation time, 6–7 days (Lee & Armour, 1958).

The endogenous developmental cycle is unknown, and no pathogenesis is ascribed to it. Prevalence generally low, though Lee & Armour (1958) reported it a frequent parasite in cattle in Nigeria.

Eimeria bukidnonensis. *Hosts:* domestic cattle, buffalo, and zebu. Found originally in the Phillipines but subsequently in North and South America, Africa and the Soviet Union. This species is known from the oocysts only. *Oocysts:* pear-shaped to oval, yellowish-brown to dark brown in colour, 44 μ by 31·1 μ (Lee, 1954), micropyle at the narrower end, oocyst wall shows radial striations. Sporulation time, about 17 days (Lee, 1954).

The endogenous developmental cycle is unknown. Baker (1939) stated the prepatent period to be about 10 days and observed diarrhoea in an experimentally infected calf.

Eimeria canadensis. *Hosts:* bovine and zebu, North America and Soviet Union. This species is known only from oocysts in the faeces. *Oocysts:* ellipsoidal, occasionally cylindrical, 32·5 μ by 23·4 μ, range 28 μ–37 μ by 20 μ–27 μ (Christensen, 1941). Oocyst wall, smooth, transparent, slightly yellowish-brown in colour, micropyle present. Sporulation time, 72–96 hours.

The developmental cycle is unknown, as is the pathogenicity. The species is relatively common in the United States, 35 per cent of cattle being found infected in Wisconsin (Hasche & Todd, 1959).

Eimeria cylindrica. *Hosts:* bovine and zebu, North America and India. It is known only from its oocyst. *Oocysts:* cylindrical, some may be narrow cylinders, 23·3 μ by 13·3 μ, range 16 μ–27 μ by 12 μ–15 μ. Oocyst wall, thin, colourless, smooth, no micropyle. Sporulation time, 2 days. The endogenous developmental cycle is not known. The prevalence of this species is quite high, Hasch & Todd (1959) finding it in 20 per cent of cattle in Wisconsin. Rao & Hiregaudar (1954) found it quite prevalent in zebu calves in Bombay.

Eimeria ellipsoidalis. *Hosts:* bovine, zebu, European bison and water buffalo; North America, Europe and Soviet Union. Developmental stages occur in the small intestine. *Oocysts:* ellipsoidal, occasionally spherical or cylindrical, 16·9 μ by 13 μ, range 12 μ–27 μ by 10 μ–18 μ. Oocyst wall, thin, homogeneous, and transparent, no micropyle. Sporulation time, 48–72 hours.

The endogenous developmental cycle has been studied by Hammond *et al.* (1963). Schizonts occur in the epithelial cells of the crypts of the ileum and colon. They are fairly small, 10·6 μ by 9·4 μ and contain 24–26 merozoites, 8 μ–11 μ in length. The number of generations of the asexual cycle is not known. Gametocytes and oocysts occur in the lower parts of the small intestine, mature oocysts being formed 10 days after infection.

Boughton (1945) reported that *E. ellipsoidalis* may cause diarrhoea in young calves 3 months of age, and Hammond *et al.* (1963), in addition to demonstrating pathogenesis, showed that a varying degree of immunity developed after infection with 50,000 to 1 million oocysts.

This species is common in cattle, Boughton (1945) finding it in 45 per cent of more than 2000 bovine faecal samples in the south-eastern U.S.A. Christensen (1941) reported it to be more frequent than any other species in healthy cattle in Alabama, and similar incidences have been found in other countries.

Eimeria pellita. *Hosts:* bovine, Austria (Supperer, 1952). It is known only from the oocysts. *Oocysts:* egg-shaped, 39·48 μ by 28·4 μ, range 36·1 μ–40·9 μ by 26·5 μ–30·2 μ. Oocyst wall, relatively thick, dark brown, uniformly placed protuberances give it a velvety appearance, micropyle present. Sporulation time, 10–12 days. The developmental cycle is unknown, as is its pathogenicity.

Eimeria mundaragi. *Hosts:* bovine and zebu, India. Known only from the oocysts. *Oocysts:* oval to egg-shaped, 36 μ–38 μ by 25 μ–28 μ. Oocyst wall, thin, smooth, transparent, and yellowish in colour, distinct micropyle. Sporulation time, 1–2 days. Developmental cycle and pathogenicity unknown.

Eimeria subspherica. *Hosts:* bovine, North America. Known only from the oocysts. *Oocysts:* smallest of all of the bovine *Eimeria* spp., 11 μ by 10·4 μ, range 9 μ–11 μ by 8 μ–12 μ, ellipsoidal to sub-spherical. Oocyst wall, uniformly thin, smooth and transparent, no visible micropyle. Sporulation time, 4–5 days. The developmental cycle is unknown; the organism is not known to be pathogenic.

Eimeria wyomingensis. *Hosts:* bovine, Wyoming. This species is similar to *E. bukidnonensis* but the oocysts are slightly smaller. Becker (1956) suggested the two species may be synonymous. *Oocysts:* ovoidal, 40·3 μ by 28·1 μ, range 37 μ–44·9 μ by 26·4 μ–30·8 μ. Oocyst wall, yellowish-brown to greenish-brown, slightly speckled, micropyle present. Sporulation time, 5–7 days (Huizinga & Winger, 1942). The developmental cycle and the pathogenicity are unknown.

Eimeria zürnii. *Hosts:* cattle, zebu, and water buffalo, world wide in distribution. This species is the most common and also the most pathogenic of the bovine coccidia. Boughton (1945) found it in 42 per cent of more than 2000 bovine faecal samples in the south-eastern U.S.A.; Hasche & Todd (1959) reported a prevalence of 26 per cent in cattle in Wisconsin, and figures of 10–30 per cent prevalence have been reported from other parts of the world. Developmental stages occur in the small intestine, caecum, colon and rectum. *Oocysts:* spherical, sub-spherical to ellipsoidal, 17·8 μ by 15·6 μ, range 15 μ–22 μ by 13 μ–18 μ (Christensen, 1941). Oocyst wall, thin, homogeneous, transparent, colourless to pale yellow, no visible micropyle. Sporulation time, 3 days at 20°C, 9–10 days at 12°C, 23–24 hours at 30–32·5°C (Marquardt *et al.*, 1960).

Life-cycle. The endogenous developmental cycle has been described by Davis & Bowman (1957). By the 2nd and 3rd day of infection, trophozoites are found in the mucosa, some penetrating as far as muscularis mucosa. By the 6th day schizonts are found in the epithelial cells of the upper and lower part of the small intestine, the parasites lying distally to the cell nucleus. Schizonts may still be present up to the 19th day, and by this time occur throughout the small intestine and also in the caecum and colon. Mature schizonts measure up to 7 μ–9·8 μ and produce twenty-four to twenty-six merozoites. Davis & Bowman (1957) suggested that more than one asexual generation occurred, there is however no definite evidence for multiple generations of the asexual stages. The earliest sexual stage is the macrogametocyte, first seen 12 days after infection in the epithelial cells of the villi of the lower small intestine and in the caecum, colon and rectum. The microgametocytes are seen first on the 15th day, being found in the lower colon and rectum. They are much fewer than the macrogametocytes. Oocysts may be found in the tissues of the caecum and colon as early as 12 days after infection, but oocyst production is highest 19–20 days after infection.

Pathogenesis. Eimeria zürnii is the major pathogenic coccidium of cattle. In Europe it is the most frequent cause of bovine coccidiosis. The acute disease is characterised by haemorrhagic diarrhoea, and the condition may become so intense that the faeces are frank blood. Tenesmus is marked, there is anaemia, weakness and emaciation. In severe infections death may occur as early as 7 days after the onset of clinical signs. At post mortem the major lesions occur in the large intestine, though general catarrhal enteritis may be present in both the small and large intestine. In severe cases the caecum and colon may be filled with semifluid haemorrhagic material or even frank blood with fibrinous clots. The epithelium may slough away leaving large denuded areas which are infiltrated with lymphocytes and leucocytes. In less acute cases the mucous membrane is roughened and spotted with petechial haemorrhages. Smears from the mucosa show very large numbers of developmental stages and oocysts.

Immunity. Wilson & Morley (1933) reported that resistance to re-infection developed in 2 calves which they studied. However Davis & Bowman (1954) were able to re-infect animals and induce transient clinical signs, indicating that immunity was not complete.

Coccidiosis in Cattle

Foster (1949) has estimated that the annual loss in the United States from coccidiosis is 10 million dollars. The two major pathogenic species are *E. zürnii* and *E. bovis*, the former being the principal parasite in Europe. Other species, such as *E. auburnensis*, may, at times, contribute to the general clinical picture. In general the infection occurs in animals 3 weeks to 6 months of age, but occasionally clinical disease occurs in yearlings and even adults, especially if massive infections are acquired. The most serious losses are seen in dairy herds where large numbers of calves are kept; nevertheless, appreciable losses can also occur in range cattle, and occasionally severe outbreaks may occur in stabled or yarded animals, especially with *E. zürnii*. The latter entity is frequently referred to as 'winter coccidiosis', and it is assumed that the bedding provides enough warmth and moisture for sporulation of oocyst even in sub-zero temperatures. In other parts of the world also infection may be severe, and Biswal (1948) considered bovine coccidiosis to be the primary disease in buffalo herds in India.

Older cattle are carriers of coccidia and though immune, continue to pass oocysts in the faeces. Successive passage of the parasites in young animals results in a build up of infection in yards, barns and on pasture so that severe and fatal coccidiosis may result when a new batch of calves is placed on a pasture or in a yard which hitherto has appeared perfectly safe. Outbreaks of coccidiosis sometimes reach epidemic proportions amongst calves in the autumn and winter months in the U.S.A. In Great Britain, coccidiosis is an important disease in the late summer and autumn in the South-west of England and in Northern Ireland. In the latter area, it is seen particularly in animals at pasture which graze, following a dry summer, around pools, ponds or damp areas, such sites being grossly contaminated with sporulated oocysts.

Diagnosis of coccidiosis in cattle is based on the clinical signs, especially the haemorrhagic diarrhoea in acute cases and the demonstration of large numbers of oocysts in the faeces. Boughton (1943) reported that 5000 to 10,000 oocysts per g. of faeces may occur in clinical cases. In peracute cases, especially those due to *E. zürnii*, oocysts may be few, the marked pathogenic effects being produced by the developmental stages prior to the shedding of the oocysts. It is important to distinguish this condition from the intestinal form of anthrax.

Where a post-mortem examination is possible, scrapings of the small and large intestinal mucosae should be examined for the developmental stages of *Eimeria* spp.

Treatment

The clinical signs of coccidiosis appear usually only when the life cycle of the parasite is advanced and marked destruction of the mucosa may already have taken place. Consequently, treatment of clinically affected animals cannot be expected to induce a radical cure. Nevertheless, coccidiosis is usually a herd problem, and treatment of the whole group of animals, including those which are not showing clinical signs, will be beneficial.

Sulphonamides

Sulphamezathine (Sulfamethazine). Davis & Bowman (1954) found this compound reduced the severity of experimental *E. zürnii* or mixed species infections, the drug being given at the rate of 7·25 g. per 100 lb. body weight on the 1st day, followed by 3·6 g. daily for 3 days. Three such courses of treatment were given on the 1st, 2nd and 4th week after infection. Hammond *et al.* (1959) found that 0·215 g. per kg. given 13 days after infection controlled the disease and also that a 10 to 18 day course of 0·0215 g. per kg. given on alternate days was effective.

Sulphaguanidine. Boughton (1943) reported 0·1 g. per kg. produced successful results in experimental infections, but Arthur (1944) failed to confirm these results in clinical cases.

Sulphaquinoxaline and *sulphamerazine.* Both these are effective when given at the rate of 0·143 g. per kg. for 2 days, when treatment is begun 13 days after experimental infection (Hammond *et al.*, 1956).

Phthalylsulphathiazole. This has been reported to be effective in doses of 5 to 7·5 g. per 100 lb. body weight daily for 3 to 4 days (Henning, 1956).

Nicarbazin and *nitrofurazone.* Neither of these compounds are of value in the treatment or control of bovine coccidiosis (Hammond *et al.*, 1958; Hammond *et al.*, 1960b).

4,4 diaminodiphenyl sulphone. Horton-Smith (1958) reported this to be an effective drug for *E. bovis* and *E. zürnii* infection in cattle. It was given at the rate of 4 g. per 100 lb. body weight every 24 hours for 6 days.

Mepacrine hydrochloride, at the rate of 1 g. per 200 lb. body weight, has been reported effective (Horton-Smith, 1958).

Amprolium. Hammond (1964) has indicated that this compound, normally used for chicken coccidia, will control *E. bovis* coccidiosis in calves when given in milk for 3 weeks beginning on the day before infection or for 5 days beginning 13 days after infection. It is not effective when given as a single dose 13 days after infection.

In studies on six compounds, Peardon *et al.* (1963) found that sulfaquinidine, sulfamethazine, glycarbylamid, nitrofurazone, framycetin sulphate, and zoalene, when administered orally or in capsules or mixed in the food, were neither coccidiostatic nor coccidiocidal, even when administered to near the toxic dose.

Prevention and Control. The prevention of bovine coccidiosis is based on treatment and good sanitation. In feed lots the feeding troughs and water containers should be high enough to prevent faecal contamination and wastage of fodder. The feed lot should also be kept dry and well drained and be cleaned out regularly. Where dairy calves are reared in yards, the bedding should be kept dry, well drained, and should be cleaned out regularly. When outbreaks occur at pasture, water holes and ditches should be fenced off and young calves denied access to them. Bedding and soil may be sterilised by 1·25 per cent sodium hypochloride, 0·5 per cent cresol or phenol or by fumigation with formaldehyde.

Coccidia of Swine

Low grade infections of coccidia are common in pigs. However, the prevalence of clinical disease attributable to coccidiosis is low, and it is possible that many of the disease entities ascribed to coccidiosis have been based on an uncritical assessment of the illness and the presence of oocysts in faeces of pigs. The following species have been described from the pig:

Eimeria debleicki Douwes, 1921
Eimeria perminuta Henry, 1931
Eimeria polita Pellerdy, 1949
Eimeria scabra Henry, 1931
Eimeria scrofae Galli-Valerio, 1935
Eimeria spinosa Henry, 1931
Isospora suis Biester and Murray, 1934
Isospora almaataensis Paichuk, 1951

Eimeria debliecki. *Hosts:* pig. World wide in distribution. Small intestine and occasionally the large intestine. Probably the most common species in the pig. *Oocysts:* ovoid to sub-spherical, 21·8 μ–28·8 μ by 12·8 μ–19·2 μ. Oocyst wall; smooth, no visible micropyle. Sporulation time; 4–9 days.

Life-cycle: Morgan & Hawkins (1948) described migration of sporozoites to the large intestine and schizogony in the epithelial cells at that site. However, Wiesenhütter (1962b) found schizogony stages in the jejunum and ileum. The number of asexual generations is not known. The prepatent period varies from 4–7 days in experimental infections, according to the age of the animal.

The Pathogenic Effects of E. debliecki. These are confined to young pigs; older animals are seldom, if ever, clinically affected. Biester & Murray (1934) observed diarrhoea, loss of appetite, emaciation and stunting of growth when young pigs were fed large numbers of sporulated oocysts. Some pigs died from the infection. Using mixed infections, Alicata & Willet (1946) confirmed that heavy infections (20 to 30 million oocysts) produced diarrhoea and anorexia on the 7th day after infection, this lasting 2–15 days. More recent work by Wiesenhütter (1962b) and Boch & Wiesenhütter (1963) demonstrated that infections of 10,000 oocysts or more of *E. debliecki* produced diarrhoea and emaciation in young pigs.

The pathological changes consist of catarrhal inflammation of the small and large intestine in association with large numbers of oocysts. The wall of the large intestine may be greatly thickened, a muco-fibrinous exudate may be adherent to the wall, and a marked necrotic enteritis may occur. However, in view of the preponderance of enteritic conditions in the young pig, it would seem wise to exercise caution in attributing pathological changes of the intestine in pigs to coccidiosis unless there is overwhelming evidence of massive numbers of organisms in the intestinal mucosa.

Eimeria perminuta. *Hosts:* pig, probably world wide in distribution. This species is known only by the oocysts in the faeces. *Oocysts:* ovoid, occasionally spherical, 11·2 μ–16 μ by 9·6 μ–12·8 μ. Oocyst wall, rough, frequently yellowish in colour, no visible micropyle. Sporulation time, 11 days. No information is available on the endogenous developmental cycle or the pathogenesis.

Eimeria polita. *Hosts:* domestic pig, wild boar. Hungary and U.S.A. (Alabama). This species is known only from oocysts in the faeces. *Oocysts:* ellipsoidal, occasionally broad to oval, 23·8 μ by 17·9 μ, range 23 μ–27 μ by 10 μ–21 μ (Pellerdy, 1949). (Boch et al. (1961) state a range of 24·5 μ–40 μ by 20 μ–26·8 μ.) Oocyst wall, generally smooth and yellowish-brown to pinkish-brown in colour, occasionally roughened, no micropyle present. Pellerdy (1965) states that oocysts of *E. polita* may be confused with those of *E. scabra* and *E. debliecki*. They may be distinguished from *E. scabra* by the smooth wall and from *E. debliecki* by size differences. Sporulation time, 8–9 days.

The endogenous developmental cycle is unknown. Pellerdy (1949) reported a prepatent period of 8–9 days in experimental infections which were followed by mild diarrhoea and the production of large numbers of oocysts.

Eimeria scabra. *Hosts:* domestic pig and wild boar. Probably world wide in distribution. Developmental stages occur in the epithelial cells of the large intestine. *Oocysts:* ellipsoidal to ovoid, 25 μ–35·5 μ by 16·8 μ–25·5 μ (Kutzer, 1960). Oocyst wall, yellowish-brown and rough,

22

micropyle is present at the narrower end. Sporulation time, 9–12 days.

Life-cycle. The endogenous developmental cycle has been partially described by Pellerdy (1949), who found the prepatent period to be 9–10 days following artificial infection. The output of oocysts lasted for 4–6 days. Schizogonous and gametogonous forms occurred in the epithelial cells of the large intestine.

Pathogenicity. Alicata & Willett (1946) infected pigs experimentally with 20 to 30 million mixed oocysts (*E. scabra* and *E. debliecki*) and produced profuse diarrhoea which lasted 2–15 days. Pellerdy (1965) reported on the death of a single piglet weighing 50–60 kg. in which large numbers of developmental stages of *E. scabra* were found in the intestinal mucosa. The pathological changes consisted of marked reddening of the mucous membrane of the large intestine especially the caecum and colon.

Eimeria scrofae. *Hosts:* domestic pig, Lausanne, Switzerland. This species is known only from oocysts in the faeces. *Oocysts:* cylindrical, one end flattened, 24 μ by 15 μ, distinct micropyle. The endogenous developmental cycle and pathogenesis of this species are unknown. Pellerdy (1949, 1965) suggests that *E. scrofae* may be a form of *E. debliecki*.

Eimeria spinosa. *Hosts:* domestic pig, U.S.A., Hawaii and Soviet Union. Uncommon. *Oocysts:* ellipsoidal to ovoid, 16 μ–22·4 μ by 12·8 μ–16 μ. Oocyst wall, brown, opaque, and its entire surface is covered with spines approximately 1 μ in height and 1 μ apart; no micropyle. Sporulation time, 15 days (Kitzer, 1960).

Life-cycle. The endogenous developmental cycle has been described by Wiesenhütter (1962a), who reported a prepatent period of 7 days. The developmental stages were found in the epithelial cells of the small intestine. Mature schizonts, 8 μ–10 μ; macrogametocytes, 7 μ–9 μ; microgametocytes, 6 μ–8 μ.

Pathogenicity. Wiesenhütter (1962a) reported that experimental infections of 12,000 oocysts caused severe diarrhoea and slight fever in young pigs. One 8 week old pig died of coccidiosis on the 11th day. Lesions consisted of a marked inflammation of the small intestine with destruction and desquamation of the epithelium. Andrews & Spindler (1952) found this species was only slightly pathogenic. No clinical signs were observed in a pig which passed as many as 7 million oocysts per g. of faeces.

Isospora suis. *Hosts:* domestic pig, U.S.A. (Iowa) and Soviet Union (Kazakhstan). Developmental stages in the small intestine. *Oocysts:* sub-spherical, 20 μ–24 μ by 18 μ–21 μ. Oocyst wall, light yellow in colour, micropyle absent. Sporulation time, 4 days. Two ellipsoidal sporocysts produced, 16 μ–18 μ by 10 μ–12 μ, each containing four sporozoites.

Pellerdy (1965) has suggested that *Isospora suis* is an *Isospora* species from a wild bird, e.g. the sparrow, since these birds are frequent cohabitants of pig pens and pig feeding areas. However, Biester & Murray (1934) described the endogenous developmental cycle of this species, indicating the prepatent period to be 6–8 days. Developmental stages occurred in the small intestine, especially the jejunum and ileum, the parasitised epithelial cells migrating sub-epithelially. A catarrhal enteritis was produced on infection, with a diarrhoea which lasted 3–4 days.

Isospora almaataensis. *Hosts:* domestic pig, Kazakhstan, U.S.S.R. This species is known only by the oocysts in the faeces. *Oocysts:* large, oval to spherical, dark grey in colour, 27·9 μ by 25·9 μ, range 24·6 μ– 31·9 μ by 23·2 μ–29 μ. Sporulation time, 5 days. The endogenous developmental cycle and the pathogenicity of this species are unknown.

A recent evaluation of the coccidia of swine in the United States has been made by Vetterling (1965). He considers that the various species can be placed in 2 major groups; the first is the *debliecki* group in which the oocysts have a smooth, colourless oocyst wall, no distinct micropyle, and range in size from 12 μ–40 μ; the second group is the rough-walled group, being a heterogeneous group with a rough, yellow to brownish oocyst wall. Within these groups Vetterling has recognised the following species, *Eimeria debliecki* (synonyms of which are *E. scrofae* and *E. polita*), *Eimeria suis* (which was previously regarded as a synonym of *E. debliecki* and is re-instated as a valid species), *Eimeria scabra, Eimeria perminuta, Eimeria spinosa, Eimeria neodebliecki* Vetterling, 1965, a new species, *Eimeria porci* Vetterling, 1965, a new species, and *Eimeria cerdonis* Vetterling, 1965, also a new species. *Isospora suis* and *Isospora almaataensis* remain as valid species.

Coccidiosis of Pigs

There is relatively little information on the clinical entity in swine. The disease is primarily a disease of the young animal, older pigs being carriers. *Eimeria debliecki* is probably the most pathogenic species, but *E. scabra* and *I. suis* have also been incriminated in disease. Swanson & Kates (1940) briefly reported details of an outbreak of coccidiosis in a litter of 4½ month old pigs in which up to 145,000 oocysts per g. of faeces were found, the condition being one of a profuse diarrhoea. In the Belgian Congo, Deom & Mortelmans (1954) reported that considerable losses may occur in young pigs due to *E. debliecki*. The clinical signs consisted of diarrhoea, emaciation and constipation in the final stages.

Diagnosis of coccidiosis. It is based on the clinical signs and, preferably, the demonstration of large numbers of endogenous developmental stages in the intestine. Since coccidia and enteritic conditions are common in swine, diagnosis by a faecal examination alone, unless oocysts are present in very large numbers, is unsound.

Treatment. Alicata and Willett (1946) found that sulphaguanidine given at the rate of 1 g. per 10 pounds body weight in the feed from 2 days before infection and until 10 days after infection prevented clinical disease when piglets were experimentally infected with 20 to 30 million oocysts of *E. scabra* mixed with *E. debliecki*. Deom & Mortelmans (1954) found that 0·44 per cent of nitrofurazone in the feed for 7 days was an effective treatment in two pigs infected with *E. debliecki*. In a review of the therapy of coccidiosis in domestic animals, Horton-Smith (1958) suggested that, in addition to sulphamethazine, various other sulphonamides, mepacrine hydrochloride and diaminodiphenyl sulphone might be effective against coccidiosis of pigs.

Control of Coccidiosis of Swine: This is based on improved hygiene; overcrowding of young piglets should be avoided, pens cleaned out regularly and feeding facilities improved.

Coccidia of Horses

Little information is available on the coccidia of equines, and this group of organisms in horses is in need of drastic re-examination. The species which have been reported are as follows:

Eimeria leuckarti (Flesch, 1883) Reichenow, 1940

Eimeria solipedum Gousseff, 1934

Eimeria uniungulati Gousseff, 1934

Renal coccidiosis, without specific identification of the organism, has been described by Zulinski (1957). Asexual development occurred in the epithelial cells of the renal tubules. No further information is available on this form, and confirmation of its existence is necessary.

Eimeria leuckarti. Known also as *Globidium leuckarti*, this species is found in the small intestine of horses and asses in Europe and the Indian sub-continent. Its prevalence is unknown. *Oocysts:* some of the largest in the genus *Eimeria*, 80 μ–87·5 μ by 55 μ–59 μ, oval, flattened at the narrower end, oocyst wall thick, 6·5 μ–7 μ, dark brown, distinct micropyle. Sporulation time, prolonged, 20–22 days at 20°C.

Life-cycle. Various stages in the endogenous developmental cycle have been described from natural cases of parasitism but there is disagreement as to what these represent. Hemmert-Halswick (1943) reported sexual stages beneath the epithelium in the villi of the small intestine, but Pellerdy (1965) maintains that Hemmert-Halswick's illustrations are of schizonts. Consequently, *E. leuckarti* possesses the 'giant schizont' type of development comparable to that seen in *E. bovis* of cattle and *E. arloingi* of sheep.

Pathogenesis. Hemmert-Halswick (1943) described marked inflammatory changes in the intestine. In diagnosis of the infection, it is to be noted that the oocysts are heavy and do not rise to the surface of normal flotation solutions. They must be looked for by sedimentation techniques.

Eimeria solipedum. *Hosts:* domestic horse, mule, and donkey, Soviet Union. It is known only from the oocysts in the faeces. *Oocysts:* spherical, double contoured wall, 15 μ–28 μ. Distinctively orange-red or yellowish-brown in colour with no micropyle. No information is available regarding endogenous developmental cycle or pathogenicity.

Eimeria uniungulati. *Hosts:* domestic horse and mule, Soviet Union. It is known only by oocysts found in the faeces. *Oocysts:* oval to ellipsoidal, bright orange in colour, 15·5 μ–24 μ by 12·4 μ–17 μ. The developmental cycle and pathogenesis are unknown.

Coccidia of Dogs and Cats

These two host animals are considered together since the more pathogenic species of the genus *Isospora* are to some extent interchangeable between the hosts.

The species which have been reported in dogs and cats are as follows:

Eimeria canis Wenyon, 1923
Eimeria felina Nieschulz, 1924
Eimeria cati Yakimoff, 1933
Isospora canis Nemeseri, 1959
Isospora bigeminia (Stiles, 1891) Lühe, 1906
Isospora rivolta (Grassi, 1879) Wenyon, 1923
Isospora felis Wenyon, 1923

Eimeria canis. *Hosts:* dog and cat, Europe and North America, dingo, Australia. It is known only from the oocysts in faeces. The validity of this species is doubted. Levine (1961) and Pellerdy (1965) suggest it may be a coccidium of the rabbit (e.g. *E. stiedae*). *Oocysts:* ovoid to ellipsoidal, 18 μ–45 μ by 11 μ–28 μ. Oocyst wall, fairly thick, visible micropyle, pinkish to red in colour or colourless. Sporulation time, 3–4 days.

Eimeria cati. *Hosts:* dog and cat, Soviet Union. Rare. The validity of this species is doubted (Pellerdy, 1965). *Oocysts:* elongate, ovoid to spherical, 21 μ–25·3 μ by 12·6 μ–14·7 μ, mean 21 μ by 17 μ, no micropyle. No information is available regarding its life cycle or its pathogenicity.

Eimeria felina. *Hosts:* domestic cat, lion, Europe (Holland). Rare. It is known only from the oocysts in the faeces. *Oocysts:* ellipsoidal, 21 μ–26 μ by 13 μ–17 μ wide. Oocyst wall, smooth, colourless, micropyle absent. The developmental cycle and the pathogenicity are unknown.

Isospora canis. *Hosts:* dog. Probably world wide in distribution. For many years this species in the dog has been referred to as *Isospora felis*, which it was thought occurred in both cat and dog. Nemeseri (1960) was unable to transmit the canine form to the cat and concluded that *I. canis* was a valid species. *Oocysts:* broadly ovoid, 39 μ by 32 μ, range 44 μ by 29 μ to 36 μ. Oocyst wall, colourless, micropyle absent. Sporulation time, 4 days. Prepatent period, 11 days. Endogenous developmental cycle and pathogenesis not known.

Isospora bigemina. *Hosts:* domestic dog, cat, red fox (*Canis vulpes*), polecat (*Putorius putorius*), mink (*Mustela vison*), and probably other members of the *Canidae* and *Felidae*. World wide in distribution. Developmental stages occur in the small intestine.

In general this parasite is rare in cats. Gassner (1940) found it in 74 per cent of dogs examined in Colorado; Catcott (1946) reported an incidence of only 3 per cent in more than 100 dogs in Ohio, and Levine & Ivens (1965) found it in only one of 139 in Illinois. In the Netherlands Laarman found it in 50 per cent of eighty dogs. *Oocysts:* two sizes have been reported, one small, 10 μ–16 μ by 7·5 μ–10 μ, spherical to oval; the smaller oocyst is more common and occurs both in cats and dogs; larger type oocyst, 18 μ–20 μ by 14 μ–16 μ, spherical to oval, occurs in the dog only. In both cases the oocyst wall is thin and there is no evidence of a micropyle. Under normal circumstances the oocysts are sporulated when passed in the faeces, but in acute infections oocysts may be passed in the unsporulated state; in these circumstances the sporulation time is 4 days. Sporocysts may rupture from the oocyst and appear in the faeces so that bodies containing four sporozoites are found on faecal examination.

Life-cycle. The endogenous developmental cycle has been described by Wenyon & Sheather (1925) and Wenyon (1926b). Developmental stages are found throughout the small intestine. In acute infections parasitic development occurs in the epithelial cells, schizonts containing eight merozoites, gametocytic stages and oocysts being found there. In chronic infections schizonts may appear in the sub-epithelial cells; in this case schizonts produced twelve merozoites, and the sexual stages occur both epithelially and in the sub-epithelial tissues. Oocysts from acute infections are unsporulated, but when oocysts are produced in the sub-epithelial tissues they leave the body in a sporulated stage. Gassner (1940) observed sporocyst formation in the tunica propria of the villi. The prepatent period for the infection is 6–7 days, and oocyst production ceases about the 28th day of infection (Lee, 1934).

Pathogenesis. This species is one of the more pathogenic forms for dogs and cats, and the clinical picture has been studied by Lee (1934). Younger animals are most seriously affected, older dogs serving as carriers. In experimental infections of cats and dogs, diarrhoea is seen on the 3rd day and blood is found in the faeces between the 4th and 6th day. In severe natural cases, a catarrhal enteritis leads to a haemorrhagic enteritis in which the faeces may be frank blood. This is associated with dehydration, general anaemia, emaciation, weakness and, ultimately, death. If the animal survives the acute phase, the bloody diarrhoea gives place to a gelatinous mucous discharge, the dog or cat showing signs of recovery 7–10 days after the onset of clinical signs. At post mortem there is an haemorrhagic enteritis throughout the small intestine, especially in the lower small intestine. In light infections petechiae are present, there may also be ulcers, and the mucosa is thickened.

Isospora felis. *Hosts:* cat, also lion, lynx and tiger; possibly other *Felidae.* World wide in distribution. Developmental stages occur in the small intestine and occasionally the large intestine.

For many years it has been accepted that *I. felis* occurs in both cat and dog. Work by Nemeseri (1960) indicated that the dog form of *I. felis* could not be transmitted to the cat and consequently he suggests it be renamed *I. canis* (see above). Levine & Ivens (1965) concur with this view. *Oocysts:* ovoidal, largest of the *Isospora* species in cats, 39 μ–48 μ by 26 μ–37 μ (Wenyon, 1923). Oocyst wall, smooth, possibly pinkish in colour, no micropyle. Sporulation time, 72 hours.

Life-cycle. The endogenous developmental cycle has been studied by Hitchcock (1955), Lickfeld (1959), and Tomimura (1957). Early stages are found above or alongside the nuclei of the superficial epithelial cells of the small intestine; occasionally they occur in the sub-epithelial tissues. First generation schizonts appear 2–4 days after infection and when mature are about 20 μ in diameter. The number of merozoites produced is unclear: thus Wenyon (1923) stated two, four or six; Hitchcock (1955) forty to sixty; whereas Lickfeld (1959) stated twelve or less. Second generation schizonts are found on the 5th–6th day, principally in the epithelial cells of the small intestine but occasionally in the large intestine. Up to twenty-four merozoites are produced though Lickfeld (1959) stated that thirty to a hundred may occur. Sexual stages occur on the 7th–8th day of infection, mainly in the small intestine but some also are found in the caecum. The prepatent period is 7–8 days (Hitchcock, 1955; Nemeseri, 1960).

Pathogenesis. Isospora felis appears to be fairly benign under natural circumstances. Andrews (1926) was able to kill young cats by feeding 100,000 sporulated oocysts, but Hitchcock (1955) was unable to produce severe clinical signs in 4–9 week old kittens with 100,000 oocysts. Using heavy infections, Tomimura (1957) reported diarrhoea, anorexia, emaciation and death in experimental cats. The pathological changes consist of a catarrhal enteritis in mild cases, to a haemorrhagic enteritis with heavy infections.

Isospora rivolta. *Hosts:* domestic dog and cat, also dingo (*Canis dingo*), and probably occurs in a number of other *Canidae* and *Felidae*. World wide in distribution. Prevalence rates of 13–70 per cent have been recorded from various areas. Developmental stages occur in the small intestine. *Oocysts:* ellipsoidal, 20 μ–25 μ by 15 μ–20 μ, micropyle present. Sporulation time, 4 days.

Life-cycle. The endogenous developmental cycle has been studied by Zapfe (1921) and Wenyon & Sheather (1925). Schizonts and gametocytic stages occur principally in the epithelial cells of the small intestine but may occasionally be found in the sub-epithelial tissues. The prepatent period is 7 days.

Pathogenicity. Under natural circumstances it would appear that this is not a serious pathogen of dogs and cats. No experimental work has been conducted with this species.

Coccidiosis of Dogs and Cats

Though coccidial infection of dogs is quite common, there is no general agreement as to the pathogenic significance of the infections. Thus, Pellerdy (1965) states that, despite the frequent occurrence of coccidia, they cannot be said to produce serious disease. Such a statement is not borne out by clinical experience, and severe outbreaks of coccidiosis may be seen especially in breeding or boarding kennels where sanitation is poor and animals are crowded together. Profuse and sometimes frank haemorrhagic diarrhoea may occur, and kennel conditions may be so bad that all puppies go through an episode of coccidiosis, some dying from it. The condition is less common in cats, however isolated outbreaks do occur.

Diagnosis of coccidiosis is based on the clinical signs and the presence of very large numbers of oocysts in the faeces. Since young puppies and kittens are prone to various enteritides, care should be taken in the diagnosis of a condition as 'coccidiosis', especially since an enteritis due to other causes may release oocysts from the sub-epithelial tissues (e.g. *I. bigeminia*). Undoubtedly, a post-mortem examination is the most adequate diagnostic method at which large numbers of developmental stages can be demonstrated in the mucosa.

Treatment. There has been little critical work in the treatment of canine and feline coccidiosis. The activity of the various sulphonamides against the genus *Isospora* is low, though McGee (1950) used sulphamethazine, and Brumpt (1943) found mepacrine at a dose of 0·01 g. per kg. effective for cats. Altman (1951) reported satisfactory results with aureomycin, and Parkin (1943) used an enema of 1 per cent sodium sulphanilyl sulphanilate at the rate of 10 ml. per kg. repeated after 24 hours. Smith & Edmonds (1959) used nitrofurazone at the rate of 2 mg. per pound body weight 3 times a day for 10 days. Duberman (1960) gave three equally divided daily doses of 4–10 mg. per lb. b.w. of nitrofurazone for an average of 9·3 days to twenty dogs, these being compared with twenty other dogs treated with a combination of sulphonamides consisting of 0·166 g. of sulphamezathine, 0·166 g. of sulphathiazole, and 0·166 g. of sulphamezazine per lb. b.w. Though nitrofurazone was effective for *I. felis* (*sic*), it did not show any significant advantage over the combined sulphonamides. To some extent both these treatments may well be considered ineffective since some dogs took as long as 25 days to recover from the infection.

Coccidia of the Domestic Fowl

The coccidia of the domestic fowl are responsible for substantial losses to the poultry industry in various countries of the world. The following species have been reported from the domestic chicken:

Eimeria acervulina Tyzzer, 1929
Eimeria brunetti Levine, 1942
Eimeria hagani Levine, 1938

Eimeria maxima Tyzzer, 1929
Eimeria mivati Edgar and Siebold, 1964
Eimeria mitis Tyzzer, 1929
Eimeria necatrix Johnson, 1930
Eimeria praecox Johnson, 1930
Eimeria tenella (Railliet and Lucet, 1891) Fantham, 1909
Cryptosporidium tyzzeri Levine, 1961
Wenyonella gallinae Ray, 1945

Eimeria tenella and *E. necatrix* are the most pathogenic and important species in domestic poultry. Other species may be present in birds as part of a mixed infection, but death is frequently due to the pathogenic effects of one of these main species. *Eimeria acervulina* and *E. maxima* are common and slightly to moderately pathogenic, *E. brunetti* is uncommon, though markedly pathogenic when it does occur and both *E. mitis* and *E. praecox* are relatively nonpathogenic and common. *Eimeria hagani* is only slightly pathogenic and is rare.

Eimeria tenella. One of the most common and pathogenic coccidia of domestic poultry. World wide in distribution. Developmental stages occur in the caecum. *Oocysts:* broadly ovoidal, $22 \cdot 9 \, \mu$ by $19 \cdot 16 \, \mu$, range $14 \cdot 2 \, \mu$–$31 \cdot 2 \, \mu$ by $9 \cdot 5 \, \mu$–$24 \cdot 8 \, \mu$. Oocyst wall, smooth, no micropyle. Sporulation time, 18 hours at 29°C; 21 hours, 26°C–28°C; 24 hours, 20°C–24°C; 24–48 hours at room temperature; no sporulation below 8°C (Edgar, 1955).

Life-cycle. Ikeda (1960) reported that excystation of sporulated oocysts was induced by pancreatic juice, trypsin being the enzyme concerned in the mechanism. (However, Jackson, 1962, found that oocysts of sheep coccidia would excyst if treated with CO_2 under anaerobic conditions in the presence of a reducing agent. It is possible that the stimulus for excystation in coccidia is comparable to that for exsheathment of nematode larvae.) The liberated sporozoites invade the surface epithelium of the caecum, Pattilo (1959) having observed 'penetration tubes' in the striated border of the epithelium through which the sporozoites passed. They are engulfed by macrophages in the lamina propria and are transported in these to the glands of Lieberkühn. Here they leave the macrophages and enter the epithelial cells lining the glands, developmental forms being found distal to the host cell nucleus (Challey & Burns, 1959).

In the epithelial cell the sporozoite rounds up and becomes a trophozoite. Subsequent development has been described by Tyzzer (1929), and numerous authors have confirmed his original description of the life cycle.

Mature first generation schizonts are found at the bottom of the crypts of the caecal glands; they measure $24 \, \mu$ by $17 \, \mu$ and the host cell is hypertrophied to several times its normal size so that it bulges into the lumen of the gland. Approximately 900 first generation merozoites, each $2 \mu–4 \mu$ in length by $1 \mu–1\cdot5 \mu$, are produced. The first generation schizonts rupture into the lumen of the gland about 60–72 hours after infection, and the merozoites penetrate other epithelial cells, round up and form the young second generation schizonts. These are found proximal to the host cell nucleus. The parasitised cell increases in size, breaks loose from its epithelial position and migrates to the sub-epithelial tissues where the mature second generation schizonts are produced. Colonies of second generation schizonts are first apparent by 72 hours, and by 96 hours mature schizonts, up to 50μ in diameter, but commonly $21–31 \mu$, are found. These contain 200 to 350 second generation merozoites, 16μ by 2μ. Disruption of the second generation schizonts and the overlying epithelium releases the merozoites into the lumen of the caecum, and when large numbers of second generation schizonts do this, a massive haemorrhage into the caecal lumen may be evident at about the 96th hour of infection.

Second generation merozoites penetrate new epithelial cells and initiate either a third generation of schizonts or the gametogonous cycle; the majority undertaking the latter process. Third generation schizonts lie distally to the cell nucleus; they are smaller than the previous stages, 9μ by $7\cdot6 \mu$, and produce four to thirty merozoites each $6\cdot8 \mu$ by 1μ. Pellerdy (1965) suggests it is possible that more than three asexual cycles are undertaken.

The gametogonous stages appear initially as rounded trophozoites. Repeated nuclear division indicates the formation of the microgametocytes which lie distal to the cell nucleus, as do the macrogametocytes. The prepatent period is 7 days, oocyst production rising to a peak by the 10th day and then rapidly decreasing.

In vitro cultivation of *E. tenella* has been achieved by Patton (1965), who succeeded in obtaining asexual development in monolayer cultures of mammalian fibroplasts, epithelial cells and avian fibroplasts maintained under various media at $41°C$. All the stages in one complete asexual generation of *E. tenella* were demonstrated, merozoites being ready for release from host cells 4–6 days after inoculation of the monolayer. This compares with the 3 days required for the first generation in the chicken. Sexual stages of the parasite were not seen. The incubation temperature had a decisive effect on the development; cultures incubated at $41°C$ supported a complete asexual generation in bovine kidney cell cultures, whereas those held at $37°C$ showed only a few immature schizonts which failed to develop further.

Pathogenesis. Caecal coccidiosis due to *E. tenella* most frequently occurs in young birds, those aged 4 weeks being most susceptible. Gardiner (1955) reported that chicks of 1–2 weeks of age were more resistant. Nevertheless, it is possible to infect day old chicks. Older birds are generally immune as a result of previous infection. In general, clinical caecal coccidiosis is produced only when heavy infections are acquired

)ver a relatively short period of time, not exceeding 72 hours (Davies *t al.*, 1963). Resistance to reinfection may be demonstrable by the 96th 1our following infection, and in the absence of a pathogenic burden in he early stages, an adequate resistance may be acquired to prevent 'atal effects (Kendall & McCullough, 1952). The number of oocysts 'equired to produce clinical disease has been investigated by Gardiner 1955) and others. In chickens, aged 1–2 weeks, 200,000 oocysts were 'equired to produce mortality, while 50,000 to 100,000 produced mortality n birds a few weeks older.

On a flock basis coccidiosis first becomes noticeable about the 72nd 1our after infection. Chickens droop, cease feeding, huddle to keep varm, and by the 96th hour blood appears in the droppings. The greatest 1aemorrhage occurs on the 5th–6th day of infection, and by the 8th or)th day the bird is either dead or on the way to recovery. Mortality is 1ighest between the 4th and 6th day, death sometimes occurring un-expectedly due to excessive loss of blood. In birds recovered from the 1cute disease, a chronic illness may develop as a result of a persistent :aecal core; however, this is usually expelled about 14 days after nfection.

The pathological changes are mainly due to the second generation chizonts. Petechial haemorrhages occur during the first 3 days, and 1oticeable lesions consisting of marked haemorrhagic spots appear on the 4th day. By the 5th–6th days the caeca are dilated, the contents containing 1nclotted and partly clotted blood, schizonts and merozoites; from the 7th day onwards gametogonous stages are found in the mucosa. By this .ime, too, the caecal contents have become more consolidated and caseous 1nd adherent to the mucous membrane, and by the 8th day the consoli-lated caseous plug completely fills the lumen of the caecum. The caecal :ore detaches from the mucous membrane by 8–10 days and may be shed n the faeces. At this time the caecal wall is still thickened but it has lost ts intense haemorrhagic appearance, and following shedding of the :ore regeneration of the mucosa occurs and the wall contracts, though a legree of fibrosis may remain for some time.

Immunity. The genetic aspects of resistance to caecal coccidiosis have)een investigated by Champion (1954) and Rosenberg *et al.* (1954), 1mongst others. Experimental matings involving resistant and susceptible F1 and F2 individuals showed that selective breeding was effective in :stablishing lines of chickens resistant or susceptible to caecal coccidiosis. 3ex linkage, maternal effect or cytoplasmic inheritance did not play a .ignificant role in this, and it was concluded that resistance or suscepti-)ility to caecal coccidiosis is controlled in a large part by multiple gene-:ic factors which do not exhibit dominance and presumably act in an 1dditive manner.

A striking feature of the acquired immunity to *E. tenella* is its specificity;)irds immune to *E. tenella* are completely susceptible to other *Eimeria* spp. The second generation schizonts are the principal stages responsible for the induction of the immunity. Various techniques have been used to determine this including abbreviated infections using therapeutic agents and the manipulation of the developmental cycle. Thus, Horton-Smith *et al.* (1963) found that the introduction of sporozoites into the rectum to produce second generation schizonts and the sexual cycle induced a high degree of resistance but the introduction of second generation merozoites to produce sexual stages and oocysts induced a much lower level of immunity.

The degree of immunity induced is proportional to the intensity of the initial infection. Repeated small doses of *E. tenella* oocysts will produce satisfactory immunity. Under field conditions, repeated small infections maintain the immune status of the bird so that for practical purposes it is immune for the rest of its life.

Basic studies on the immunity to *E. tennella* indicate that the sporozoite is affected by the immune response very shortly after penetration of the epithelium and few or no first generation schizonts develop from a challenge infection in resistant birds (Pierce *et al.* 1962). Protective substances are not present in the lumen of the caecum in sufficient concentration to affect the free sporozoites. A similar immune mechanism probably operates against the second generation merozoites as against the sporozoites. Merozoites may be found deep in the glands, but they fail to develop to gametocytes.

Circulating antibodies in chickens immune to *E. tenella* were first demonstrated by McDermott & Stauber (1954), who found agglutinins for merozoites in the serum of infected chickens. Since then precipitins have been demonstrated using antigens prepared from second generation schizonts (Pierce *et al.*, 1962; Rose & Long, 1962). The role of circulating antibody in immunity to *E. tenella* was investigated by Burns & Challey (1959) and Horton-Smith *et al.* (1961). An infection of *E. tenella* was allowed to develop in one caecum while the other was kept in an isolated and uninfected state. On challenge, the previously uninfected caecum was shown to be immune, this suggesting that a factor (or factors) was responsible for transferring immunity from one caecum to the other. Attempts to induce passive immunity to *E. tenella* infections have met with no success even though large amounts of immune serum were used (Pierce *et al.*, 1963). However, if the challenge infection of sporozoites is given intravenously, a substantial protective effect can be demonstrated in passive immunity (Rose, 1963).

Epidemiology. Caecal coccidiosis is primarily a disease of young chickens older birds, though immune, act as carriers. Under ordinary farm or poultry rearing conditions, it is likely that all birds are exposed to infection, but the severity of disease is dependent, very largely, on the number of oocysts ingested. Clinical disease arises only when heavy infection, in relation to previous experience, is acquired over a period of time not exceeding 72 hours (Davies *et al.*, 1963). Infections acquired more slowly than this tend to result in resistance rather than clinical disease. Consequently, the majority of a flock is likely to acquire a clinical infection over a short period of time, and Davies & Kendall (1954) estimate this period to be 10 days.

Diagnosis, treatment and control of *E. tenella* coccidiosis will be dealt with later under the heading 'Coccidiosis of Poultry'.

Eimeria necatrix. *Host:* domestic fowl. World wide in distribution, extremely common. Asexual development in the small intestine, gametogony cycle in the caecum. This species is one of the most important pathogens of the small intestine of poultry. *Oocysts:* similar to those of *E. tenella*, ovoidal, 16·7 μ by 14·2 μ, range 13·2 μ–22·7 μ by 11·3 μ–18·3 μ. (Davies, 1956, gives a mean of 20·5 μ by 16·8 μ, range 15·5 μ–25·3 μ by 13·6 μ–20·4 μ.) Oocyst wall, smooth, colourless, no micropyle. Sporulation time, 2 days, but may be 18 hours at 29°C (Edgar, 1955).

Life-cycle. The initial behaviour of sporozoites is similar to those of *E. tenella*. Van Doorninck & Becker (1957) observed that sporozoites passed through the epithelium of the tips of villi into the lamina propria and migrated towards the muscularis mucosa. During this migration most of the sporozoites were engulfed by macrophages and were carried in them to the epithelial cells of the fundus of the crypts of Lieberkühn. The first generation schizonts occur proximal to the host cell nucleus; merozoites appear in the gland lumen 2–3 days after infection, and they enter adjacent epithelial cells and develop into second generation schizonts. This stage of *E. necatrix* is relatively large, and the epithelial cells containing the developing schizont leave their epithelial position and migrate into the sub-epithelial tissues and sometimes into the submucosa. They are evident here from the 4th day of infection onwards, developing in a colonial manner (Tyzzer *et al.*, 1932). The second generation schizonts of *E. necatrix* are relatively large, 63 μ by 49 μ, this serving to differentiate them from the schizonts of the other species of coccidia which occur in the small intestine. The second generation merozoites are liberated on the 5th–8th day of infection, though a few may be released for several days thereafter. They are then carried by the peristaltic action of the small intestine to the caecum. Here they penetrate the epithelial cells and may undergo a further generation of schizogony or differentiate to the gametogonous cycle. The third generation schizonts are small, and multiple infection of cells may occur, 3 or 4 third generation schizonts being found in a single host cell. Gametogonous stages may arise from either second or third generation merozoites. They lie distal to the host cell nucleus, displacing it and they may also grossly distort it.

The prepatent period, according to Tyzzer *et al.* (1932), is 7 days, and to Davies (1956), 6 days. The peak of oocyst production occurs from the 8th to the 10th day.

Pathogenesis. Next to *E. tenella*, *E. necatrix* is considered to be the most common pathogenic species of *Eimeria* in domestic poultry. It tends to cause a more chronic disease than the former and affects older birds, however, disease can be produced in young chickens. The age at which chickens suffer coccidiosis due to *E. necatrix* depends on the biotic potential of the parasite (it is a poor producer of oocysts, and a longer time is necessary for a high level of environmental contamination to occur) and on the degree of immunity which results from light infections, this being less marked than that which is seen in *E. tenella* (Tyzzer *et al.*, 1932).

The principal lesions are found in the middle third of the small intestine. In acute cases a severe sub-mucosal haemorrhage occurs on the 5th and 6th day, the wall of the small intestine is markedly swollen, haemorrhagic and the contents filled with unclotted blood. The haemorrhages are associated with the large, deeply seated, second generation schizonts, and at times these may be seen as white, opaque foci surrounded by a zone of haemorrhage. Where there has been excessive haemorrhage, blood may also be found in the caeca so that the condition may be confused with *E. tenella* infection, though dual infections may be seen in natural outbreaks.

In mild infections, scattered white spots indicating the colonies of schizonts are surrounded by a zone of petechial haemorrhage, but there is no evidence of gross haemorrhage into the lumen. In contrast to *E. tenella* infection, birds which recover may remain emaciated for several weeks or months afterwards. The chronic form of the infection is a marked contrast to the acute type of disease seen in caecal coccidiosis.

Immunity. Chickens surviving a severe infection with *E. necatrix* become sufficiently resistant to withstand a new fatal infection; however, this immunity is not as strong as that seen in *E. tenella* infection. Experimentally, it is possible, by repeated exposure, to immunize birds to the level where parasitism is prevented. The developmental stages associated with the induction of immunity are the asexual phases in the small intestine; the gametogonous stages having little immunising power. Horton-Smith *et al.* (1963) showed that the intrarectal inoculation of second generation merozoites causes no diminution in oocyst production with successive inoculations, and when such birds were challenged with oocysts, little or no immunity was demonstrated.

Eimeria acervulina. *Hosts:* domestic poultry, quail; world wide in distribution. Very common. It is less pathogenic than the two previous species and is responsible for sub-acute or chronic intestinal coccidiosis in older birds and chickens at the point of lay. Development stages occur in the anterior part of the small intestine. *Oocysts:* ovoid, $19 \cdot 5 \ \mu$ by $14 \cdot 3 \ \mu$, range $17 \cdot 7 \ \mu$–$22 \cdot 2 \ \mu$ by $13 \cdot 7 \ \mu$–$16 \cdot 3 \ \mu$ (Tyzzer, 1929). Becker (1956) recorded a mean size of $16 \cdot 4 \ \mu$ by $12 \cdot 7 \ \mu$. Oocyst wall, smooth, thinner at narrow end, inconspicuous micropyle present. Sporulation time, 25 hours at room temperature, 17 hours at 28°C (Edgar, 1955).

Life-cycle. The asexual stages of *E. acervulina* are found proximal to the nucleus in the epithelial cells of the anterior small intestine. More than one parasite may be found within a single cell. Mature schizonts containing merozoites are seen by the 3rd day of infection. Such schizonts produce sixteen to thirty-two merozoites, each 6 μ by 0·8 μ, and these initiate another asexual cycle of development. More asexual cycles may occur before the gametogonous stages are produced. Gametogony occurs in the anterior small intestine from the 4th day of infection onwards. The prepatent period is 4 days, and oocyst production continues for a longer period than for the other chicken coccidia.

Pathogenesis. Tyzzer (1929) originally regarded this species as a producer of chronic inflammation of the small intestine; later (1932), however, he concluded that it was of little or no pathogenic significance. Brackett & Bliznick (1950) were unable to kill chickens with any level of infection but found 500,000 oocysts reduced weight gains of 2 week old chickens; Morehouse & McGuire (1958), using chickens of 4–10 weeks, found that single or multiple doses of 5 million or more sporulated oocysts produced a 75 per cent mortality, and this was confirmed by Horton-Smith & Long (1959), who produced deaths in 8 day old chickens with a total of 10 million oocysts in three doses over 3 successive days. Within recent years, especially in large poultry establishments, the significance of *E. acervulina* as a pathogen has increased steadily. The biotic potential of this species is great, the prepatent and sporulation periods are short, and very large numbers of oocysts may accumulate in the environment.

The clinical signs consist of weight loss and a watery, whitish diarrhoea. At post mortem greyish-white, pin-point foci or transversely elongated areas are visible from the serous surface of the duodenum; these consist of dense foci of oocysts and gametogonous stages, and when examined microscopically excessive numbers of sexual stages and unsporulated oocysts are present. The intestinal wall and mucosa are thickened and may be covered with catarrhal exudate, but haemorrhage is rare except when excessive numbers (several million) of oocysts are administered.

Immunity. Repeated infections with *E. acervulina* are necessary to induce a good degree of immunity (Peterson & Munro, 1949).

Eimeria maxima. *Hosts:* domestic poultry. World wide in distribution. Common. Developmental stages in the small intestine. *Oocysts:* large ovoidal, 29 μ by 23 μ, range 21·4 μ–42·5 μ by 16·5 μ–29·8 μ. Oocyst wall, slightly yellow, some may be roughened, micropyle absent. Sporulation time, 2 days.

Life-cycle. Accounts of the developmental cycle have been given by Tyzzer (1929), Long (1959) and Scholtyseck (1959, 1963). Sporozoites enter the epithelial cells of the tips of the villi in the duodenum and schizonts develop proximal to the nucleus. The schizonts are small, 10 μ by 8 μ, and produce 8–16 merozoites by the 4th day. Tyzzer and Long considered there to be only one schizogonous generation, but

Scholtyseck suggested that two occurred, being indistinguishable morphologically. Gametogonous stages are found distal to the epithelial cell nucleus; they are larger than the asexual stages, and as they enlarge the parasitised cell may move to a sub-epithelial position, some reaching the muscularis mucosa. The first oocysts may appear 120 to 121 hours after infection, but large numbers usually occur between the 123rd and the 136th hour of infection (Long, 1959). Oocyst output lasts for a few days.

Pathogenesis. This species is moderately pathogenic, the most serious effects being due to the sexual stages. Few marked changes occur in the small intestine until the 5th day after infection, and then in severe infections numerous petechial haemorrhages occur on the intestinal wall. There is a marked production of mucus, the mucosa is thickened, there may be a loss of tone and the intestine becomes flaccid and dilated. The mucosal surface is inflamed and the intestinal contents consist of a pinkish mucoid exudate. Microscopic examination of scrapings of the mucosa reveals large numbers of oocysts.

Immunity. The onset of immunity in *E. maxima* infection is quick, resulting in a rapid termination of the infection. Of the poultry species studied by Rose & Long (1962), *E. maxima* possessed the major immunising power. No information is available on developmental stages which are responsible for the immunising effect.

Eimeria mivati. *Hosts:* domestic fowl. U.S.A. and Canada. Developmental stages in small intestine but may extend from duodenum to rectum. *Oocysts:* ellipsoidal to broadly ovoidal, $15 \cdot 6 \, \mu$ by $13 \cdot 4 \, \mu$, range $10 \cdot 7 \, \mu$ to $20 \cdot 0 \, \mu$ by $10 \cdot 1 \, \mu$ to $15 \cdot 3 \, \mu$. Oocyst wall, colourless, smooth, micropyle present. Sporulation time, 11 to 12 hours ($29 °C$).

Life-cycle. The developmental cycle was described by Edgar & Siebold (1964). Three and possibly four asexual generations are undergone. Sporozoites develop in the epithelial cells at the bases of villi, particularly of the duodenum. They are located just below the surface and well above the nucleus of the host cell. Mature first generation schizonts, measuring $10 \cdot 4 \, \mu$ by $10 \cdot 1 \, \mu$, are produced about 36 hours after infection. Ten to thirty merozoites are produced. Second generation schizonts develop in a similar situation and are mature by the 55th–65th hour after infection. These are $9 \cdot 2 \, \mu$ by $7 \cdot 2 \, \mu$ and produce sixteen to twenty merozoites. The second generation merozoites parasitise cells of the jejunum, ileum, caeca and rectum in addition to those of the anterior small intestine. Mature third generation schizonts are produced about 80 hours after infection. Some third generation merozoites develop into sexual stages, but others may develop into 4th generation schizonts (Edgar & Siebold, 1964). Peak oocyst production occurs during the 5th to 7th day after infection.

Pathogenesis. Marked changes of the anterior small intestine appear by the 4th day when chickens show listlessness, anorexia and a watery diarrhoea. The affected area of the intestine is swollen, oedematous and shows scattered petiechiae. Death, if it occurs, takes place on the 6th–7th day. Depression of growth, a drop in egg production and impaired food conversion are seen in growing and laying birds.

Immunity. A strong immunity is developed with *E. mivati* which is species specific. This can persist for at least 3 months.

Eimeria mitis. *Hosts:* domestic poultry. World wide in distribution. Common. Developmental stages occur in the anterior small intestine, occasionally also in the posterior small intestine and caecum. *Oocysts:* sub-spherical, slightly tapering, $15\cdot8\,\mu$ by $13\cdot83\,\mu$, range $11\cdot5\,\mu$–$20\cdot7\,\mu$ by $10\cdot35\,\mu$–$18\cdot4\,\mu$ (Joyner, 1958), (Tyzzer, 1929, gives $16\cdot2\,\mu$ by $15\cdot5\,\mu$). Sporulation time, 2 days at room temperature, 18 hours at $29°C$ (Edgar, 1955).

Life-cycle. This has been studied by Tyzzer (1929) and Joyner (1958). The early stages in the life cycle have yet to be determined. Schizonts are demonstrable 67 hours after infection, being superficially situated in the epithelial cells throughout the length of the small intestine. Merozoites are found in the intestinal contents about 4 days after infection.

Gametocyte formation is increasingly present from the 5th day of infection onwards, and sexual stages are numerous by the 8th day. Both the asexual and the sexual stages of the cycle occur together. The prepatent period is about 100 hours.

Pathogenesis. Under normal conditions, the species is, at the most, only a mild pathogen. Tyzzer (1929) was unable to produce clinical signs or lesions in chickens with large doses of sporulated oocysts. However, Joyner (1958) produced 38 per cent mortality in 6 day old chicks following the administration of $2\cdot5$ million oocysts. Half a million oocysts reduced weight gains of chickens aged 6–26 days. The pathological changes associated with *E. mitis* are minimal and are not characterised by any visible haemorrhage.

The immunity developed to this parasite is of a low order. Both Tyzzer (1929) and Joyner (1958) noted that chickens could be infected several times before a decrease in the susceptibility of the host occurred.

Eimeria brunetti. *Hosts:* domestic poultry. U.S.A., Europe. Sporadic. Developmental stages in the small intestine, caecum and cloaca. *Oocysts:* ovoid, $26\cdot8\,\mu$ by $21\cdot7\,\mu$, range $20\cdot7\,\mu$–$30\cdot3\,\mu$ by $18\cdot1\,\mu$–$24\cdot2\,\mu$ (Levine, 1942) (Becker *et al.*, 1955, record $23\cdot4\,\mu$ by $19\cdot7\,\mu$, range $13\cdot8\,\mu$–$33\cdot7\,\mu$ by $12\cdot4\,\mu$–$28\cdot3\,\mu$). Oocyst wall, smooth, micropyle absent. Sporulation time, 1–2 days at room temperature, 18 hours at $24°C$ (Edgar, 1955).

Life-cycle. The endogenous development has been described by Boles & Becker (1954), Pellerdy (1960) and Davies (1963). First generation schizonts develop in the epithelium cells of the villi, especially at points in contact with, or close to, the basement membrane. The upper small intestine is the major site of parasitism, but stages may also occur in the lower part and even in the caeca. Mature first generation schizonts, $30\,\mu$ by $20\,\mu$, containing approximately 200 merozoites, are found 50–76 hours after infection. By the 4th day second generation schizonts occur in the posterior part of the small intestine, the rectum, the caecum and the cloaca. Two types of second generation schizonts have been described; large ones, 29·6 μ by 16·2 μ, containing fifty to sixty merozoites, are usually found at the tips of the villi at the 95th hour, and a smaller type, 9·8 μ by 8·8 μ, containing twelve merozoites, may also be seen. Boles & Becker (1954) suggest that the size difference may be caused by crowding; alternatively it may indicate a third generation of schizonts or sexual dimorphism. Schizonts may enter the sub-epithelial tissues in heavy infections, but usually they are confined to the epithelium of the villus. Gametocytes occur in the epithelial cells of the lower intestine, caecum, rectum and cloaca. The prepatent period is 5 days.

Pathogenesis. Eimeria brunetti usually causes disease in chickens between 4–9 weeks of age. The lesions are characteristically confined to the posterior part of the small intestine, between the yolk stalk and the caeca, and the condition is typically a rectal coccidiosis. In severe infections the gut wall is thickened, there is a haemorrhagic catarrhal exudate, which appears 4–5 days after experimental infection, and the droppings are fluid and may be blood-stained. The haemorrhagic condition may become necrotic due principally to asexual stages developing in the sub-epithelial tissues.

Eimeria hagani. *Hosts:* domestic poultry. North America, India. This species was differentiated from the other species of the chicken by cross immunity tests. Developmental stages in the small intestine. Generally regarded as of little or no pathogenicity. *Oocysts:* broadly ovoid, 19 μ by 18 μ, range 16 μ–21 μ by 14 μ–19 μ (Levine, 1938) (Edgar, 1955, reported a mean of 18·1 μ by 16·5 μ). No micropyle. Sporulation time, 1 to 2 days (Edgar, 1955).

Life-cycle. The endogenous developmental cycle is not known in detail but occurs in the anterior part of the small intestine. The developing stages cause small petechial haemorrhages which are visible from the serous surface. The prepatent period is 6 days (Edgar, 1955).

Levine (1942) fed large numbers of *E. hagani* to 10 week old chickens and reported a catarrhal inflammation of the duodenum on the 6th day of infection.

Eimeria praecox. *Hosts:* domestic poultry. Probably world wide. Developmental stages in the upper part of the small intestine. *Oocysts:* ovoid, 21·2 μ by 17 μ, range 19·7 μ–24·7 μ by 15·6 μ–19·7 μ. Oocyst wall, smooth, colourless, no micropyle. Sporulation time, 2 days at room temperature.

Life-cycle. The endogenous developmental cycle has been studied by Tyzzer *et al.* (1932). Two schizogonic generations occur distal to the nuclei of the epithelial cells of the villi of the small intestine. Sporozoites are found in the epithelial cells 8 hours after infection, and second generation schizonts may occur as early as 32 hours; subsequently, both schizonts and gametogonous stages may appear together. The prepatent period is 4 days, and the infection remains patent for about 4 days.

The pathogenicity of this species is low, it being regarded as a non-pathogenic form. Tyzzer *et al.* (1932) were unable to produce gross changes in the intestines with heavy infections of oocysts. Nevertheless, despite the lack of marked pathogenesis, immunity to infection develops quickly.

Cryptosporidium tyzzeri. *Hosts:* domestic chicken. North America (Massachusetts). Rare. All developmental stages occur extra-cellularly on the microvilli of the epithelial cells of the tubular part of the caecum. There is no obvious pathogenicity associated with this form. *Oocysts:* ovoid, small, $4\,\mu$ to $5\,\mu$ by $3\,\mu$. Contain four naked sporozoites. During the life cycle minute schizonts $3\,\mu$–$5\,\mu$ in diameter are attached to the surface of the cell; these produce 8 merozoites which then produce small microgametocytes and macrogametocytes.

Wenyonella gallinae. *Hosts:* domestic poultry. India. This species was reported by Ray (1945) from the intestine and caecal contents of 4–6 week old chickens which had died of an outbreak of coccidiosis in India. Developmental stages occur in the terminal part of the intestine. *Oocysts:* oval, $29\cdot4\,\mu$–$33\cdot5\,\mu$ by $19\cdot8\,\mu$–$22\cdot7\,\mu$. Oocyst wall, thick, the outer layer having a rough coat. Sporulation time, 4–6 days.

Life-cycle. The endogenous developmental cycle is unknown. In experimental infections Ray (1945) found the prepatent period to be 7–8 days, oocyst production continuing for 3 days.

Infected chickens passed blackish-green semi-fluid faeces, but no marked lesions were noted except in the natural outbreak.

Coccidiosis of Poultry

Details of the pathogenic effects of the various species of poultry coccidia have been described under the individual species. Infections with a single species of coccidium are rare in natural conditions, mixed infections being the rule; nevertheless, in many outbreaks the clinical entity can be ascribed principally to one species, or occasionally a combination of two or three. *Eimeria tenella* is the most pathogenic and important species, followed by *Eimeria necatrix.* Many coccidiostatic drugs have been directed against *E. tenella,* with the result that other species are increasingly incriminated as a cause of poultry coccidiosis. *Eimeria brunetti* may be markedly pathogenic but is uncommon. *E. maxima* and *E. acervulina* are increasingly common but are of moderate pathogenicity and *E. mitis* and *E. praecox* are considered to be nonpathogenic.

Coccidiosis should be regarded as ubiquitous in poultry management, since even under the extreme conditions of experimental work, it is difficult to avoid infection completely for any length of time. Essentially, the clinical disease entity is dependent on the number of oocysts ingested by individual birds. If the environmental hygiene is poor, this number may be very large and this is particularly so with *E. tenella* which has a high biotic potential. Where young birds are placed on heavily contaminated litter, deaths may occur within a few days and up to 100 per cent of the flock of chickens may die. In order to produce severe and fatal caecal coccidiosis, the intake of the pathogenic level of oocysts must take place within 72 hours, otherwise a rapidly developing immune response will protect against a fatal infection. Such conditions frequently obtain in poorly maintained litter houses and in broiler systems. However, caecal coccidiosis may also occur in 'free range' birds, especially if they frequent shaded and damp areas to feed.

The environment is being contaminated continuously, even from immune birds, and the initiation of an outbreak depends upon factors which allow oocysts to sporulate and remain viable. For sporulation oocysts require moisture and warmth and survive best in shaded, moist conditions. Poorly maintained litter houses may well supply such needs, and excessive numbers of sporulated oocysts may be found in poorly kept quarters.

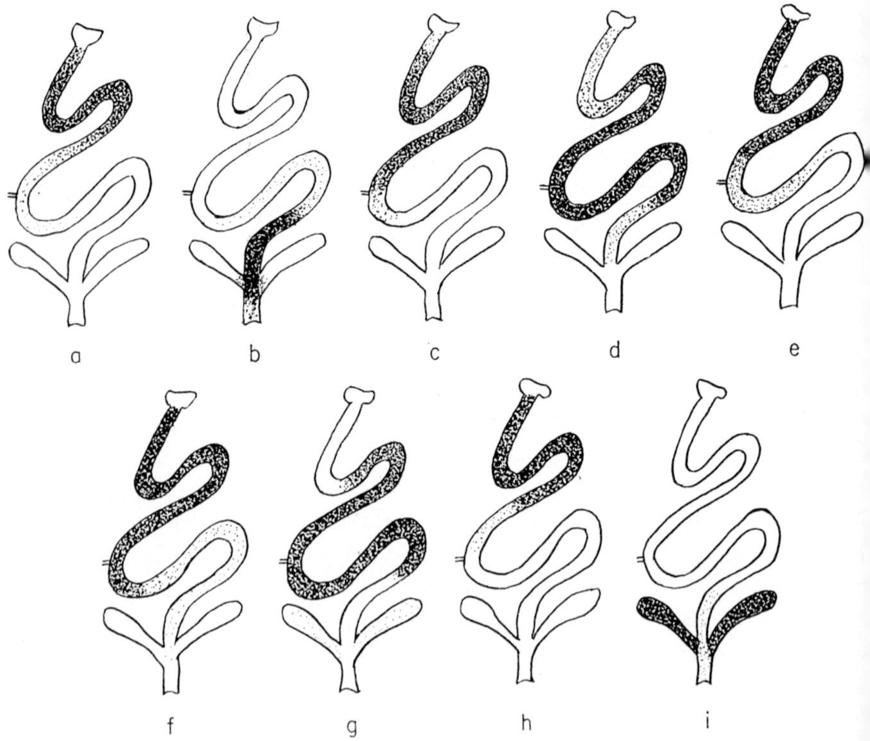

FIG. 279. Diagrammatic Representation of the Location of Lesions for 9 Species of Poultry Coccidia

a. *E. acervulina*; b. *E. brunetti*; c. *E. hagani*; d. *E. maxima*; e. *E. mivati*; f. *E. mitis*; g. *E. necatrix*; h. *E. praecox*; i. *E. tenella*

(Adapted from Redi, W. M. (1964). A diagnostic chart of nine species of fowl coccidia. *Georgia agric. exp. Stat. Bull.*, N.S. 39)

The resistance which is developed from a previous infection will protect birds from subsequent exposure to that species, but it is a specific resistance and does not induce immunity to another species. Thus, for example, an attack of caecal coccidiosis does not preclude subsequent disease caused by *E. necatrix* or any of the other species.

Various measures can be adopted to avoid the intake of large numbers of oocysts by susceptible poultry. In litter houses the removal of the litter may be timed so that the majority of oocysts are removed before they have sporulated (e.g. every 2 days); however, under modern conditions of poultry husbandry, this is completely uneconomical and impossible. Steps may be taken to keep litter dry so that oocysts do not sporulate, and litter may be redistributed frequently to avoid concentrations of oocysts at places such as feeding troughs, watering troughs etc. It is important that watering appliances should be effective and do not allow localised areas of dampness to occur. When broiler houses are emptied for a new batch of chickens, the litter should be stacked so that the heat evolved is sufficient to kill oocysts. Heaped litter, left for 12 hours or more, will normally generate a temperature of about $51\,°C$, which is sufficient to destroy the oocysts. Poultry in outside pens should be moved regularly to other pens and the contaminated pen left vacant, or better still, brought under cultivation.

Diagnosis. Diagnosis of coccidiosis in chickens is best accomplished by a post-mortem examination of a representative number of birds. Diagnosis by faecal examination may lead to quite erroneous results. In some instances the major pathology is produced before oocysts are shed in the faeces (e.g. *E. tenella*), and conversely, the presence of large numbers of oocysts may not necessarily indicate a serious pathogenic condition. Thus, with *E. acervulina*, which has a high biotic potential, comparatively larger numbers of oocysts are shed per oocyst given than, for example, with *E. necatrix*. Furthermore, the accurate identification of the oocysts of various poultry coccidia is not easy.

All this may be avoided by a post-mortem examination. The location of the major lesions gives a good indication of the species of coccidia concerned. Thus, haemorrhagic lesions in the central part of the small intestine would suggest *E. necatrix;* those in the caecum, *E. tenella;* those in the rectum, *E. brunetti*. It is not sufficient to look for oocysts only, since these may be found with regularity in the small intestine or caecum of chickens, rather, it is necessary to determine if large numbers of schizonts are present in the sub-epithelial tissues for the major pathogens, and in an epithelial position for the other species.

Treatment and Control of Poultry Coccidiosis

A formidable and extensive literature exists on the treatment of coccidiosis in poultry: it is possible only to give a brief outline of it here. The majority of the research which has been done has been concerned with *E. tenella* and to a lesser extent with *E. necatrix*, and it is only in recent years that the other species of coccidia of poultry have been considered with regard to coccidial therapy and prophylaxis.

A major advance in the therapy of coccidiosis was the introduction of sulphanilamide by Levine (1939). Since then, several other sulpha compounds have been used, and these include the sodium salt of sulphaquinoxaline, the soluble sodium salt of sulphadimidine (sulphamezathine, sulfamethazine) and a combination of sulphaquinoxaline and pyrimethamine. Other compounds available are nitrofurazone, furazolidone, amprolium etc. These are discussed below.

Curative treatment should be instituted immediately after a diagnosis of coccidiosis is made. An interrupted form of treatment is more satisfactory with the sulpha drugs than continuous treatment, the aim of which is to avoid undue concentrations of the compounds which inhibit the earlier developmental stages of the parasite and thus interfere with the acquisition of immunity. To avoid this, Davies & Kendall (1954a, b) have suggested that sodium sulphadimidine be given at a concentration of 0·2 per cent in drinking water for two periods of 3 days separated by 2 days without treatment. Sodium sulphaquinoxaline is given in the feed at the rate of 0·5 per cent. Nitrofurazone, with furazolidone, to a final concentration of 0·0126 per cent, is given over a 7 day treatment, and this may be repeated after a 5 day interval.

The sulphonamides have a coccidiostatic action rather than a coccidiocidal effect. Consequently, they have no direct curative effect, but rather their value lies in halting the onset of disease in other members of the flock. They are active against the schizontal stages and especially the second generation schizonts of *E. tenella* and *E. necatrix*. Increased concentrations affect the first generation schizonts of these species, but much higher doses are required to affect the gametocytic stages.

Preventive medication consists of prolonged or continuous use of coccidiostatic compounds in the feed or water. These include amprolium (0·0125 per cent in the feed), nitrofurazone (0·005–0·01 per cent), nicabazin (0·0125 per cent), sulphaquinoxaline (0·0125 per cent) and zoalene (0·0125 per cent).

Details of the action, indications, modes of use and toxicities of these compounds are dealt with below.

Sulphadimidine (Sulphadimethylpyrimidine: 4,6-dimethyl-2-sulphanilamidopyrimidine: 'sulfamethazine,' 'sulphamezathine'). This compound is used in Europe as a curative drug; however, it is not commonly used in the United States. It is given in the food at the rate of 0·4 per cent or in the drinking water as a 0·2 per cent solution of the sodium salt. It has been used most satisfactorily for many years in the control of clinical outbreaks of coccidiosis. Active against *E. tenella*, *E. necatrix* and the other species of coccidia.

Toxicity. Prolongation of blood coagulation time, probably due to an interference with the vitamin K synthesis in the intestine. Male birds given excessive doses show hyperplasia of the seminiferous tubules of the testicles; reduced egg production in laying hens.

Sulphaguanidine (*p*-aminobenzenesulphonylguanidine). The first of the sulphonamides to show good activity against coccidia. Used as a 1 per cent mixture in the food. It has now been superseded by more effective drugs.

Sulphamerazine (4-methyl-2-sulphanilamidopyrimidine: 'sulphamethyl-pyrimidine'). May be mixed in the feed or given in the drinking water at a level of 0·25 per cent. The compound has fallen into general disuse because of toxicity, especially in birds 6–7 weeks of age, these showing haemorrhagic and necrotic spleen lesions when concentrations higher than 0·125 per cent are given.

Sulphaquinoxaline (2-sulphanilamidoquinoxaline). An important, effective and commonly used coccidiostat, in general use throughout the world. For preventive medication, doses ranging from 0·0125 per cent–0·033 per cent may be given over fairly long periods. For therapeutic purposes a dose of 0·043 per cent in the water given for two treatments each for 2 days with a 3–5 day interval between them is satisfactory. Sulphaquinoxaline has been used primarily for *E. tenella* and *E. necatrix* infection, but it is also active against *E. acervulina*. It exerts a marked inhibitory effect on schizogony, and Cuckler & Ott (1947) stated that a level of 0·1 per cent in the ration inhibited invasion by the sporozoites.

Toxicity of sulphaquinoxaline has been demonstrated. A level of 0·1 per cent in the ration for a few days has no adverse effect on chickens, but when this concentration is fed for a longer time (e.g. 30 days) or when lower percentages are incorporated in the ration over a long period of time, toxic manifestations may be seen. These consist of a haemorrhagic syndrome characterised by multiple haemorrhages in many of the organs sometimes accompanied by necrotic lesions in the spleen. There is also hypoplasia of the bone marrow and an agranulocytosis (Sadek *et al.* 1955). There are indications that toxicity is associated with an interference with vitamin K metabolism.

Amprolium [1-(4-amino-2-*n*-propyl-5-pyrimidinylmethyl)-2-picolinium chloride hydrochloride]. This quaternised derivative of pyrimidine, which is a thiamine antagonist, has been introduced within recent years, and it is highly active against *E. tenella*, *E. necatrix* and *E. acervulina*.

It is available as a premix and is given prophylactically to birds in a final concentration of 0·0125 per cent. A combination of Amprolium and sulphaquinoxaline at levels of 0·006 per cent of each in the food is more effective against poultry coccidia than either of the two drugs used alone (Long, 1963).

Zoalene (2-methyl-3,5-dinitrobenzamine). Very good results have been reported for this compound. It is given prophylactically at a level of 0·01 per cent–0·015 per cent in the food and is active against both the caecal and intestinal form of coccidiosis (Arundel, 1960; Hymas & Stevenson, 1960). Peterson (1960) conducted a comparative study of various anti-coccidial drugs against infection with *E. tenella* and *E. necatrix* and found that Zoalene, at the recommended level, was completely protective against *E. tenella* and was even more active against *E. necatrix* since full protection was achieved at a level of 0·005 per cent of the active ingredient in the feed. Zoalene inhibits the development of the second generation schizont but does not inhibit the development of immunity under field conditions.

Nitrofurazone (5-nitro-2-furfuraldehydesemicarbazone) (Furacin, Furazol). As well as being a coccidiostat, it also possesses bacteriostatic properties, being active against both Gram-positive and Gram-negative organisms. For preventive medication, nitrofurazone is recommended at levels of 0·0005–0·001 per cent in the food or drinking water. Harwood & Stunz (1949) suggest that newly hatched chickens be placed on such a concentration continuously until they are marketed about 12 weeks of age. For therapeutic purposes it is used at a concentration of 0·022 per cent, but if this level is continued for more than 10 days, toxic effects may be seen, these being manifest by nervous signs. When 0·0055 per cent of nitrofurazone is combined with 0·0008 per cent of furazolidone (Bifuran), there is a marked coccidiostatic effect against *E. tenella* and *E. necatrix* (Harwood *et al.* 1956).

Furazolidone [N-(5-nitro-furfurylidene)-3-amino-2-oxazolidinone]. This compound has been used for infections due to the enteric bacteria, and it is also of value against *E. tenella* at a dose of 0·011 or 0·0055 per cent in the feed. However, it is usually employed in combination with nitrofurazone (Bifuran) at the doses mentioned above and is chiefly used against *E. tenella* infections. Horton-Smith & Long (1959) found it effective against *E. necatrix* if fed at twice the recommended level.

Nicarbazin (aryl derivative having an equimolecular complex of 4,4-dinitrocarbanilide and 2-hydroxy-4,6-dimethylpyrimidine). This compound is used principally as a prophylactic; the therapeutic dose lies near the toxic dose. Nicarbazin is usually available as a 22·5 per cent premix, and it is incorporated into the food to give a final concentration of 0·0125 per cent. It is effective against *E. tenella*, *E. necatrix* and *E. acervulina* and does not interfere with the acquisition of immunity (Horton-Smith & Long, 1959). McLoughlin & Wehr (1960) confirmed that it has a marked inhibitory effect on the second generation schizonts, and they also reported a moderate action on the asexual stages prior to this.

The drug is eminently suitable for administration to broiler flocks, and it is usually given for the first 12 weeks of the chicken's life. It is unsuitable for laying or breeding stock because of the effect on egg colour and hatchability.

Toxicity may be seen at the level of 0·03 per cent or above in the ration. There is interruption of egg laying, eggs are depigmented, and yoke mottled, and the hatchability is reduced. Ataxia has been seen at feed levels of 0·05 to 0·1 per cent for 3 weeks (Newberne & Buck, 1956). Where death is due to toxicity, there is degeneration of the epithelium of the renal tubules and liver cells.

Nitrophenide (3,3-di-nitrodiphenyldisulphide). This is used under field conditions at the level of 0·025 per cent in the feed. Horton-Smith & Long (1959) reported good coccidiostatic effect against both *E. tenella* and *E. necatrix*. Its maximum effect occurs at the 49th–96th hour of infection, which suggests that the drug inhibits the development of second generation schizonts. The difference between the toxic and therapeutic dose is small, and deaths may occur with a level of 0·16 per cent in the feed. At levels of 0·04 per cent in the feed, administered continuously for 4–12 weeks, there was no effect on growth or egg production or egg hatchability (Waletsky *et al.* 1949).

Unistat. This is a mixture consisting of 30 per cent N_4-acetyl-N_1-p-nitrophenyl sulphanilamide, 25 per cent of 3,5-dinitrobenzamide and 5 per cent 4-hydroxy-3-nitrophenylarsonic acid. At a level of 0·1 per cent in the feed it prevents death and allows more or less normal weight gains with heavy infections of *E. tenella*, *E. necatrix* and *E. acervulina*.

Trithiadol. A formulation of bithionol [2,2-dihydroxy-3,3,5,5-tetra-chlorodiphenyl sulphide] and methiotriazamine [4,6-diamino-1-(4-methylmercaptophenyl)-1,2-dihydro-2,2-dimethyl-1,3,5-trizaine] in the proportion of 5 parts bithionol to 1 part the latter. It is active against *E. tenella*, *E. necatrix*, *E. maxima* and *E. acervulina* at the rate of 0·06 per cent–0·09 per cent in the diet. Good immunity develops to coccidia at these levels. It is not harmful to growing chicks and has no effect on egg production, colour or quality, but hatchability may be affected, and hence it is not recommended for breeding birds.

Polystat. A formulation active against *E. tenella* and *E. necatrix* given at the rate of 0·02 per cent in the feed. When so presented, it contains 0·03 per cent of acetyl-(paranitrophenyl)-sulphanilamide, 0·002 per cent of dibutylin dilaurate, 0·02 per cent of dinitrodiphenylsulphonylethylene diamine and 0·0075 per cent of 4-hydroxy-3-nitro phenylarsonic acid.

Glycamide (4,5-imidazoledicarboxamide). This acts against the stages prior to the second generation schizont though birds develop an immunity when receiving the drug. It is given at the rate of 0·003 per cent in the feed.

Pyrimethamine [2,4-diamino-5(p-chlorophenyl)-6-ethyl pyrimidine] (Daraprim). This is an antimalarial drug which Joyner & Kendall (1955) found to act as a synergist when added to sulphonamides. With sulphamezathine, the dose of sulphonamide for *E. tenella* could be reduced to $\frac{1}{8}$ to $\frac{1}{16}$ of that normally required. It is a folic acid antagonist.

Antibiotics. Ball (1959) re-examined several antibiotics and found that aureomycin, chloramphenicol, erythromycin, spiromycin and terramycin were all active against *E. tenella* infections, spiromycin giving the most satisfactory effect.

PROTOZOA

Resistance of Coccidia to Drugs. Because of the extensive and continued use of therapeutic and prophylactic compounds in poultry feed over a period of many years, it might be expected that resistant strains of coccidia would develop. This was initially reported for sulphaquinoxaline and sulphamezathine with a field strain of *E. tenella* (Waletsky, *et al.* 1954). Subsequently, Cuckler & Malanga (1955) studied forty field strains of allegedly resistant coccidia, finding that 43 per cent were sensitive to one or more of the drugs studied, while 43 per cent were resistant to nitrophenide, 45 per cent to sulphaquinoxaline and 57 per cent to nitrofurazone. Some of the strains were resistant to all the anti-coccidial drugs while others were resistant to two of the compounds, cross resistance occurred more frequently than specific resistance. Joyner (1957) showed that it was possible to induce drug resistance to nitrofurazone in a laboratory strain of *E. tenella*, this being obtained by nine passages through chicks treated continuously with 0·01 per cent of nitrofurazone in the food. However, the disease entity which resulted from this drug resistant strain was adequately controlled by sulphaquinoxaline at the rate of 0·0645 per cent in the water for 2–5 days or sulphamezathine at the level of 0·2 per cent in water. Glycamide appears especially vulnerable to the development of resistant strains, and Gardiner & McLoughlin (1963) have shown that resistance to this drug can be maintained when the resistant strain of coccidium was serially propagated in the absence of the drug. Reciprocal cross resistance may occur with other compounds, thus resistance to zoalene involves cross resistance to nitrofurazone, and reverse reciprocal resistance also occurs. However, coccidia with cross resistance between nitrofurazone and zoalene are affected by arsenoso-benzene, glycarbylamide, nicarbazin, trithiadol or unistat.

Vaccination Against Coccidia. The high degree of immunity which occurs with several species of poultry coccidia would suggest that artificial immunisation would be an advantageous method of controlling these infections. An application of this principle was developed by Edgar (1958). Small doses of oocysts are given to young birds which are then allowed to run on litter, but the infection is controlled by a low level of prophylactic coccidiostat. Two types of vaccine are marketed: one for broilers which contains *E. tenella*, *E. necatrix* and *E. acervulina* oocysts, and one for laying birds which contains 5 species, *E. hagani* and *E. maxima* being added to the previous three (Edgar *et al.*, 1956). Birds are 'inoculated' at 3 days of age, and low level medication is started about the 13th day of age and continued until the birds are 5½–6 weeks of age. Edgar *et al.* (1956) have reported that inoculated chickens usually develop a solid immunity to three or five types of coccidiosis by 4 weeks of age even when fed continuous prophylactic levels of certain coccidio-static drugs. The choice of drug is important, and those which are satisfactory and compatible with immunisation include 0·0125 per cent nitro-phenide, 0·0125 per cent sulphaquinoxaline, 0·000325 per cent 2-sulphanilamido-6-chloropyrazine, 0·0055 per cent nitrofurazone, 0·5 pounds per ton of feed of bifuran, and 2 pounds per ton of feed of trithiadol or polystat. Nicarbazin at a level of 0·0125 per cent was not compatible with the development of immunity to three or more species of coccidia, birds being susceptible at 12–16 weeks of age. Stuart *et al.* (1963), who carried out a comparative trial of 0·1 per cent of trithiadol and 0·0083 per cent of zoalene given to chickens in the feed for 35 days, demonstrated that vaccinated chickens, fed trithiadol, were immune to *E. tenella*, *E. maxima*, and *E. acervulina* and partially immune to *E. necatrix*; however, those which received zoalene were fully immune only to *E. acervulina* and partially immune to *E. maxima*.

The use of such a vaccine has been criticised by several people. For example, it is difficult to control the vaccine and more especially the factors on which the vaccine depends for immunisation; thus an unsatisfactory environment for the sporulation of oocysts from the initial infection may provide the chickens with little or no immunising infection from the litter. Nevertheless, the method has been used extensively in several parts of the United States, and despite the theoretical objections to it, it would appear to be a practical method of control in many areas.

Methods of attenuating sporulated oocysts so that a nonpathogenic but immunising infection may be produced in chickens have been investigated with special reference to the use of X-rays. Waxler (1941) reported that the exposure of oocysts to X-rays at the rate of 450 roentgen per minute to provide a total exposure of 4500, 9000 and 13,500 r. produced a progressive attenuation, which was indicated by a decrease in the severity of infection. More recently, Hein (1963) has demonstrated that the attenuation of oocysts of *E. tenella* can result in the production of a useful vaccine against this species.

Coccidia of the Turkey

Seven species of coccidia occur in the turkey, but only two of these, *Eimeria adenoeides* and *Eimeria meleagrimitis*, are considered to be of pathogenic significance. The species which have been described are as follows:

Eimeria adenoeides Moore and Brown, 1951
Eimeria dispersa Tyzzer, 1929
Eimeria gallopavonis Hawkins, 1950
Eimeria innocua Moore and Brown, 1952
Eimeria meleagridis Tyzzer, 1927
Eimeria meleagrimitis Tyzzer, 1929
Eimeria subrotunda Moore, Brown and Carter, 1954
Cryptosporidium meleagridis Slavin, 1955

Eimeria adenoeides. *Hosts:* domestic turkey. North America, Great Britain. Developmental stages occur in the small intestine, large intestine and caecum. *Oocysts:* ellipsoidal, but show a wide variation in shape and size; 25·6 μ–16·25 μ, range 21·5 μ–30 μ by 13·5 μ–19·8 μ.

Oocyst wall, double contoured with a smooth surface, a micropyle may or may not be present. Sporulation time, 24 hours at room temperature (Edgar, 1955).

Life-cycle. The endogenous developmental cycle has been investigated in great detail by Clarkson (1956, 1958). First generation schizonts occur in the epithelial cells of the tubular part of the caeca and the terminal part of the ileum as early as 6 hours. These mature about 60 hours after infection and at this stage measure 30 μ by 18 μ and contain approximately 700 merozoites. Second generation schizonts are distributed proximal to the nucleus in the epithelial cells throughout the small intestine and rectum. They are mature at 96 to 108 hours after infection, measure 10 μ by 10 μ and produce 12–24 merozoites. Sexual stages appear by the 5th day of infection, and the prepatent period is 114 to 132 hours. Patency lasts for about 2 weeks.

Pathogenicity. Eimeria adenoeides is one of the most pathogenic species of coccidia in turkeys; young poults are particularly susceptible, but even older turkeys may be seriously affected if they have not had immunising infections in earlier life. Moore & Brown (1951) produced 100 per cent mortality in poults up to 5 weeks of age with large doses of sporulated oocysts. Clarkson (1956) found that 200,000 oocysts invariably resulted in death of 3 week old poults, whereas 100,000 oocysts caused a mortality of 45 per cent. Lower doses of 30,000 and 10,000 oocysts failed to produce death, though in poults less than 5 weeks they caused severe disease associated with anorexia and blood in the droppings. On the other hand, 6 week old turkeys given 1 million oocysts suffered a mortality of 33 per cent and 11 week old poults given 3 million oocysts showed no mortality (Clarkson, 1958; Clarkson & Gentles, 1958).

The clinical signs commence on the 4th day of infection, consisting of loss of appetite, droopiness and ruffled feathers. Deaths begin on the 5th or 6th day when the droppings are liquid and contain mucus and blood. The main lesions are confined to the posterior small intestine, caecum and rectum, the walls of these being swollen and oedematous; petechial haemorrhages are visible, and the contents of the lower digestive tract are white or grey in colour and contain mucus or blood at a later stage.

Immunity. Immunity induced by *E. adenoeides* is specific, and Clarkson (1959) found no cross immunity to *E. meleagridis.*

Eimeria dispersa. *Hosts*: domestic turkey; possibly also Bobwhite quail, Hungarian partridge, pheasant. The developmental stages occur in the small intestine. *Oocysts*: broadly ovoid, 26·1 μ by 21·04 μ, range 21·8 μ–31·1 μ by 17·7 μ–23·9 μ (Hawkins, 1952). Oocyst wall, no double contoured appearance, no micropyle. Sporulation time, 2 days at room temperature. (Differences in sizes of oocysts from different hosts have been reported by Tyzzer (1929). Oocysts from the turkey were smaller than those from the quail, the latter measuring 22·7 μ by 18·8 μ, range 17·6 μ–26·4 μ by 15·4 μ–22·4 μ.)

Life-cycle. The parasites develop in the epithelial cells of the tips of the villi. Two types of first generation schizonts have been described (Tyzzer, 1929; Hawkins, 1952). One form appears about the 55th hour of infection and reaches a size of 6 μ and produces fifteen merozoites; the other is larger, measuring 24 μ by 18 μ and producing fifty merozoites. First generation schizonts are mature by 48 hours, and second generation forms are mature 4 days after infection. The latter measure 11 μ–13 μ and produce eighteen to twenty-three merozoites. The gametocytic stages are observed from the 4th day onwards, and oocysts appear in the faeces from the 5th to the 6th day after infection.

Pathogenesis. This species is only mildly pathogenic for the turkey. Hawkins (1952) with experimental infections, produced only a slight tendency to liquid faeces and a mild depression in weight gains. He also reported that infection with a few thousand oocysts daily would immunise birds so that massive infections are resisted after the 2nd week.

Eimeria gallopavonis. *Hosts:* domestic turkey. North America, India. Developmental stages in the lower small intestine, rectum and caecum. *Oocysts:* ellipsoidal, 27·1 μ by 17·2 μ, range 22·2 μ–32·7 μ by 15·2 μ–19·4 μ, difficult to distinguish from *E. meleagridis.* Oocyst wall, double contoured, no micropyle. Sporulation time, 24 hours.

Life-cycle. The endogenous developmental cycle has been studied by Hawkins (1952). Schizonts occur proximal to the nucleus in the epithelial cells of the tips of the villi of the ileum and the rectum 3 days after infection. Second generation schizonts are found in a similar situation. Two types of second generation schizont occur: a small form producing ten to twelve large merozoites and a large form producing many small merozoites. A few scattered third generation schizonts may occur, but the majority of second generation merozoites give rise to the sexual cycle. This is first apparent on the 4th day, epithelial cells of the ileum, caecum and, mainly, the rectum being affected. The prepatent period is 6 days.

Pathogenicity. Generally thought to be nonpathogenic. Hawkins (1952) reported oedema, sloughing of the mucosa and lymphocytic infiltration of the intestine in experimental infections. Hawkins (1952) also reported a strong, specific immunity. Turkeys immune to *E. meleagridis, E. meleagrimitis* and *E. dispersa* could be readily infected with oocysts of *E. gallopavonis.*

Eimeria innocua. *Hosts:* domestic turkey, U.S.A. (New York). As its name suggests, it is nonpathogenic. *Oocysts:* sub-spherical, 22·4 μ by 10·9 μ, range 18·6 μ–25·9 μ by 17·3 μ–24·5 μ. No micropyle. Sporulation time, 24–48 hours.

The endogenous developmental cycle takes place in the epithelial cells of the tips of the villi of the small intestine. The prepatent period is 5 days, and patency lasts for no longer than 14 days.

Moore & Brown (1952) found this species to be nonpathogenic, and they could observe no microscopic lesions even in heavy experimental infections.

Eimeria meleagridis. *Hosts:* domestic and wild turkey. Probably cosmopolitan. At one time it was thought that this species was pathogenic for young turkeys; however, it is probable that earlier reports of its pathogenicity should rightly be ascribed to *E. adenoeides*. It is now generally considered that *E. meleagridis* is, at the most, only a mild pathogen. The developmental stages occur initially in the small intestine and later in the caecum and rectum. *Oocysts:* ellipsoidal, 23·8 μ by 17·3 μ (Tyzzer, 1927) (Clarkson (1959b) gives 22·5 μ by 16·25 μ). Oocyst wall, smooth, micropyle absent. Sporulation time, 24 hours.

Life-cycle. First generation schizonts develop in the epithelial cells of the small intestine in the region of the rudimentary yoke stalk; merozoites from this generation are found at the 54th hour of infection (Clarkson, 1959b). Second generation schizonts and gametocytes occur in the caeca, but some gametogonous stages may be found in the lower ileum and the rectum. Second generation schizonts are found in their greatest number 84 hours after infection; they measure 9 μ in diameter and contain eight to sixteen merozoites. A third generation of schizogony has been reported by Hawkins (1952), but Clarkson makes no mention of this in his description of the life cycle. Gametocytes are found from the 91st hour of infection onwards, and the average prepatent period is 110 hours.

Pathogenicity. This is minimal. Clarkson (1959b) failed to produce disease in 2 week old turkey poults with doses of up to 1 million oocysts, and Hawkins (1952) observed only a minor weight loss in poults infected with half a million to a million oocysts.

Eimeria meleagrimitis. *Hosts:* domestic turkey. Probably world wide in distribution. Common. Developmental stages occur in the small intestine. *Oocysts:* sub-spherical, 18·1 μ by 15·3 μ, range 16·2 μ–20·5 μ by 13·2 μ–17·2 μ (Tyzzer, 1929). (Hawkins (1952) states 19·2 μ by 16·3 μ and Clarkson (1959a) 20·1 μ by 17·3 μ, range 16 μ–25·5 μ by 13·7 μ–22 μ.) Oocyst wall, double contoured, smooth surface, no micropyle. Sporulation time, 24 hours.

Life-cycle. The endogenous developmental cycle has been studied by Hawkins (1952), Clarkson (1959a) and Horton-Smith & Long (1961). Hawkins described two generations of schizonts, Clarkson described three, the latter being confirmed by Horton-Smith & Long. The earliest trophozoites appear in the epithelial cells lining the glands of the small intestine 24 hours after infection. First generation schizonts are mature by the 48th hour, reaching 17 μ by 13 μ and containing eighty to one hundred merozoites. Second generation schizonts occur in the epithelial cells of the glands in the same vicinity and form further colonies of schizonts. These are mature by the 66th hour of infection, are smaller than the first generation forms, being 8 μ by 7 μ and contain eight to sixteen merozoites. A third generation schizont occurs prior to the gametogonous cycle. Forms of this generation occur as early as 72 hours after infection, and they reach maturity by the 96th hour. They are small, 8 μ by 7 μ and produce eight to sixteen merozoites. Gametogonous stages are seen in the epithelial cells 4–5 days after infection, occurring in the jejunum, mainly in the epithelial cells at the tips of the villi. The prepatent period is 114–118 days.

Pathogenicity. Peterson (1949) reported 70–90 per cent mortality in turkey poults aged 4–5 weeks due to this parasite. Clarkson (1959a) and Clarkson & Gentles (1958) produced heavy mortality in poults aged 1·5–3 weeks by feeding 100,000 oocysts. Poults aged 4 weeks fed 400,000 oocysts suffered 100 per cent mortality. Birds aged 5–10 weeks showed no mortality when fed 200,000 to 2 million oocysts.

Clinical signs appear on the 5th day, birds cease to eat, huddle together, and the droppings become fluid and may be brown or blood-tinged. Deaths commence about the 6th day in severe infections and continue for the next few days.

Thickening and dilation of the intestinal wall is seen on the 4th day, and from the 5th day onwards the duodenal mucosa is greyish-white, the blood vessels engorged and the contents fluid, containing caseous mucous threads. Sometimes the contents are reddish due to haemorrhage, though excessive haemorrhage is not a feature of the condition. Sometimes the duodenum may be plugged with a core of reddish-brown material which is firmly adherent to the mucosa, later it becomes detached, recedes and is eventually discharged.

Eimeria subrotunda. *Hosts:* domestic turkey. U.S.A. This species, which was isolated by Moore *et al.* (1954) on the basis of immunological studies and cross transmission, is essentially nonpathogenic. The developmental stages occur in the small intestine. *Oocysts:* very similar to those of *E. innocua*, subspherical, 21·8 μ by 19·8 μ, range 16·5 μ–24·4 μ by 14·2 μ–22·4 μ. Oocyst wall, smooth, no micropyle. Sporulation time, 48 hours.

Life-cycle. The endogenous developmental cycle is unknown, though material from 2 infected turkey poults has been examined by Moore *et al.* (1954), and they describe developmental stages in the epithelial cells of the tips of the villi especially in the duodenum, the jejunum and the upper part of the ileum. The prepatent period is 96 hours, and patency continues for 12–13 days.

Pathogenicity. Moore *et al.* (1954) regarded *E. subrotunda* as a harmless parasite, and even massive infections of poults aged 5 weeks failed to induce any departure from the normal. Recovery from *E. subrotunda* infection results in immunity. This is specific.

Cryptosporidium meleagridis. *Hosts:* domestic turkey. Great Britain. This organism has been reported by Slavin (1955) as a cause of diarrhoea and moderate mortality in turkey poults in the first 2 weeks of life in Scotland. As far as can be ascertained, it is the only report of a species of this genus causing trouble in turkeys. In the outbreak reported by Slavin, six different parasites were identified in the turkeys; however, he considered that *C. meleagridis* was responsible for the diarrhoea and the mortality. The parasitic forms are found on the epithelium of the intestine and do not invade the tissues. *Oocysts:* small, oval, 4·5 μ by 4 μ, cytoplasm foamy in consistency, nucleus stains poorly, located eccentrically. Sporulated oocysts and sporozoites have not been described.

The endogenous developmental cycle includes an asexual generation with the production of schizonts and merozoites. Young schizonts are attached to the epithelium of the villi, sometimes in enormous numbers. Slavin (1955) described an organ of attachment which penetrated distal to the microvilli of the epithelial cells; developmental forms were also seen in goblet cells and between the epithelial cells as far down as the basement membrane. Mature schizonts measure 5 μ by 4 μ and contain eight merozoites, though sometimes only two or four occur. Microgametocytes are about 4 μ in diameter and produce sixteen rod-shaped microgametes; the macrogametes measure 4·5 μ–5 μ by 3·5 μ–4 μ. Slavin suggested that the microgametes were not motile, and the process of fertilisation consisted of the male and female forms attaching themselves closely to one another. Oocysts may be found in the faeces in large numbers, but sporulated oocysts were not detected (Slavin, 1955).

The pathogenic entity produced by this parasite consisted of diarrhoea and moderate mortality in turkey poults 10 to 14 days of age. The terminal third of the small intestine was especially affected; however, since the organisms occur on the surface of the epithelial cells, gross microscopic or histopathological lesions were absent.

Coccidiosis of Turkeys

Coccidiosis may be responsible for severe disease and heavy economic loss in the turkey industry, the organisms of especial importance being *E. adenoeides* and *E. meleagrimitis*. It is primarily a disease of young turkey poults, though older birds serve as carriers, and it has been suggested by Skamser (1947) that turkeys beyond the age of 8 weeks are not seriously affected. The increased importance of coccidiosis in turkeys has derived in part from intensive production systems which are now used to rear turkeys. Where overcrowding and poor sanitation are present, the prevalence of coccidiosis may be very high. This is especially so when turkeys are kept in open yards since these often are damp and provide ideal conditions for the sporulation of oocysts.

Diagnosis of Coccidiosis in Turkeys. This is similar to that for coccidiosis of the chicken. The finding of large numbers of oocysts in the faeces is not an infallible guide, and diagnosis is more satisfactorily done at post-mortem examination.

Treatment of Turkey Coccidiosis. Essentially the same compounds are used for turkeys as for chickens with the exception that the sulphonamides are generally more effective against the turkey coccidia. Thus, Boyler & Brown (1953) found that sulphamezathine and sulphaquinoxaline in the feed, or 0·1 per cent–0·05 per cent sulphamezathine in the water, was effective against *E. adenoeides, E. gallopavonis, E. meleagridis, E. innocua, E. subrotunda, E. dispersa* and *E. meleagrimitis*. This was confirmed by Horton-Smith & Long (1959). Warren & Ball (1963) have demonstrated that both sulphaquinoxaline and amprolium, at the rate of 0·0125 per cent and 0·008 per cent in the food, controlled *E. adenoeides* and *E. meleagrimitis* in turkeys. Some evidence that amprolium may interfere with the acquisition of immunity was produced in that when poults were challenged with a severe infection 14 days after cessation of the drug, those treated with sulphaquinoxaline were less susceptible than those treated with amprolium. Some doubt exists as to the effectiveness of nicarbazin against *E. meleagrimitis*. Cuckler, *et al.* (1955) reported it to be ineffective; in addition, they found nitrofurazone and glycarbylamid also ineffective against this pathogenic species.

Coccidiosis of Geese and Ducks

Eight species of coccidia have been reported from domestic geese and ducks, and some of these have been associated with severe disease and death. A much larger number of species has been recorded from wild ducks and geese, a brief list of these is given on p. 673.

The species of importance in domestic geese and ducks are:
Eimeria anatis Scholtyseck, 1955
Eimeria anseris Kotlan, 1932
Eimeria nocens Kotlan, 1933
Eimeria parvula Kotlan, 1933
Eimeria stigmosa Klimes, 1933
Eimeria truncata (Railliet and Lucet, 1891) Wasielewski, 1904
Tyzzeria anseris Nieschulz, 1947
Tyzzeria perniciosa Allen, 1936

Eimeria anatis. *Hosts:* domestic duck, mallard. Europe (Germany and United Kingdom). This species is principally a parasite of the mallard (*Anas platyrhynchos platyrhynchos*); however, a species of *Eimeria* with oocysts similar to those of *E. anatis* was found by Davies (1956) in domestic ducks in Britain, and he has shown that this species will develop both in the domestic duck and the mallard. In all probability, the infection of domestic ducks is derived from wild ducks which may frequent the pasture on which the domestic ducks graze. *Oocysts:* ovoid, 16·8 μ by 14·1 μ, range 14·4 μ–19·2 μ by 10·8 μ–15·6 μ. Oocyst wall, smooth, uniform thickness, distinct micropyle at the more pointed end and a distinct ring shaped projection of the wall forming shoulders round the micropyle. Sporulation time, 4 days at 20°C (Scholtyseck, 1955).

The endogenous developmental cycle is unknown, but it is assumed that both schizogony and gametogony occur in the small intestine.

As far as is known, this species is nonpathogenic. Davies (1957) was unable to induce pathogenic effects in experimental studies.

23

Eimeria anseris. *Hosts:* domestic goose, blue and lesser snow goose and Richardson's Canada goose. Europe and North America. Prevalence in these geese is generally low. *Oocysts:* oval to pear-shaped, $21 \cdot 7 \mu$ by $17 \cdot 2 \mu$, range $20 \mu – 24 \mu$ by $16 \mu – 19 \mu$. Oocyst wall, narrow part has a distinct truncated cone, micropyle present, smooth and colourless, slightly thickened in the area of the micropyle and incised sharply to form a plate or shelf across the micropyle. Sporulation time, 24–48 hours.

Life-cycle. The endogenous developmental cycle has been described by Kotlan (1933). Only one schizogonous cycle occurs, developmental stages being found in compact clumps in the epithelial cells of the villi of the posterior part of the small intestine. Some stages may penetrate to near the muscularis mucosa. Mature schizonts measure $12 \mu – 20 \mu$ and produce fifteen to twenty-five sickle-shaped merozoites. Gametogenous stages occur in the sub-epithelial tissues of the villi in heavy infections, but in milder infection they often occur superficially. The prepatent period is 7 days, and patency lasts from 2–8 days.

Pathogenicity. Kotlan (1933) considered the pathogenicity low; however, Klimes (1963) and Pellerdy (1956) indicated that this species may produce a haemorrhagic enteritis which may terminate fatally in geese as old as 9 months. Klimes (1963) also observed that immunity developed rapidly after infection.

Eimeria nocens. *Hosts:* domestic goose, blue and lesser snow goose (*Anser coerulescens coerulescens*). Europe and North America. Uncommon. *Oocysts:* ovoidal to ellipsoidal, flattened at the micropyle end, 31μ by $21 \cdot 6 \mu$, range $29 \mu – 33 \mu$ by $10 \mu – 24 \mu$ (Hanson *et al.*, 1957). (Kotlan, 1933, quotes a range of $25 \mu – 33 \mu$ by $17 \mu – 24 \mu$.) Oocyst wall, smooth, green to pale yellow, micropyle present, but covered by the outer layer of the oocyst wall. Sporulation time, unknown.

Life-cycle. Developmental stages occur in the epithelial cells of the tips of the villi in the posterior part of the small intestine. The nucleus of the host cell may be displaced or destroyed by the developing forms, and they may also pass to the sub-epithelial tissues. Mature schizonts measure $15 \mu – 30 \mu$ and produce fifteen to thirty-five merozoites. No information is available on the time sequence of these developmental stages.

Eimeria nocens is infrequently found in domestic geese. Kotlan (1933) described two outbreaks of intestinal coccidiosis in goslings in Hungary, but the infection consisted of *E. nocens* and *E. anseris.* Klimes (1963) considers it affects mainly young geese and that it may be pathogenic in these.

Eimeria parvula. *Hosts:* domestic geese. Hungary. Developmental stages occur in the small intestine. *Oocysts:* spherical to sub-globular, 13μ by 10μ, range $10 \mu – 15 \mu$ by $10 \mu – 14 \mu$. Oocyst wall, smooth, colourless, no micropyle. Klimes (1963) has suggested that the species described by Kotlan (1933) is, in fact, a member of the genus *Tyzzeria*, and proposes it be called *Tyzzeria parvula.* Klimes noted that sporulation took 24 hours and resulted in the formation of 8 sporozoites but no sporocysts.

The endogenous developmental cycle occurs in the epithelial cells of the villi in the posterior part of the small intestine. The prepatent period is about 5 days, and the output of oocysts may continue for several months. Pellerdy (1965) suggests this may indicate a lack of immunity on the part of the host to the organism.

Eimeria parvula appears to be of little or no pathogenic significance.

Eimeria truncata. *Hosts:* domestic goose, Graylag goose (*Anser cinereus*), Ross's goose (*Anser rossi*), Canada goose (*Branta canadensis*) etc. World wide in distribution. Developmental stages occur in the kidney tubules. *Oocysts:* ovoid to ellipsoidal, truncated narrower end, 14·3 μ– 23·5 μ by 11·7 μ–16·3 μ (Becker, 1934). Oocyst wall, smooth, micropyle present. Sporulation time, 24 hours to 5 days.

Life-cycle. Schizonts occur in the epithelial cells of the kidney tubules. When fully grown, they measure approximately 13 μ in diameter and contain twenty to thirty merozoites. The infected epithelial cells are destroyed, and the adjacent cells show pressure atrophy and destruction. No information is available at present on the route which sporozoites take to reach the epithelial cells of the kidney tubules. Macrogametocytes stain intensely blue and reach a size of 15 μ–17 μ, while the micro-gametocytes are smaller, reaching a size of 7 μ by 13 μ. The prepatent period is 5 days.

Pathogenesis. This species is a highly pathogenic form for goslings, occasionally causing 100 per cent mortality within a few days of the onset of clinical conditions. However, under natural conditions, and especially in wild geese, there may be a high rate of infection with apparently low mortality. Affected birds show marked weakness and emaciation, and the condition may be so acute as to kill goslings within a day or so. Birds drink water copiously and may show muscular incoordination and a staggering gait.

The pathological changes consist of markedly enlarged kidneys, these being light in colour, and show numerous small, white nodules, streaks and lines on the surface and in the substance (Stubbs, 1957). There is destruction of the epithelial cells of the kidney tubules, and the affected tubules are packed with urates, oocysts and gametogonous stages in various stages of development. A marked and general infiltration of round cells occurs.

Eimeria truncata occurs as a sporadic parasite in domestic geese, and it is most likely to occur when geese are kept crowded together in unsanitary surroundings. Contact with wild geese may be responsible for the intro-duction of the infection. The organism has been associated with losses in the Canada goose in its winter quarters at Pea Island, North Carolina (Critcher, 1950); however, the true incidence of the species in wild geese is not known.

Eimeria stigmosa. *Hosts:* domestic goose. Czechoslovakia. A nonpathogenic coccidium of young geese. *Oocysts:* oval, 23 μ by 16·7 μ, thickenings at the poles. Oocyst wall, markedly striated transversely, dark brown in colour, micropyle present. Sporulation time, 48 hours at room temperature.

Klimes (1963) found the prepatent period to be 5 days, the developmental stages occurring in the epithelial cells of the villi in the anterior part of the small intestine.

Tyzzeria anseris. *Hosts:* domestic goose, white fronted goose, snow goose, Ross's goose, Canada goose and several other forms. North America and Europe. Developmental stages in the small intestine. *Oocysts:* ellipsoidal, 13 μ by 11 μ, range 10 μ–16 μ by 9 μ–12 μ (Levine, 1952), no micropyle. When sporulated, the oocysts contain eight banana-shaped sporozoites, there being no sporocysts, this being characteristic of the genus. The endogenous developmental cycle is unknown.

Tyzzeria perniciosa. *Hosts:* domestic duck. U.S.A., Britain, Holland. Developmental stages occur in the small intestine. *Oocysts:* ellipsoidal, 10 μ–13·3 μ by 9 μ–10·8 μ. Oocyst wall, colourless, no micropyle. When passed in the faeces, the oocyst space is completely filled with granular material. Sporulation time, 24 hours, 8 sporozoites being formed without any sporocyss.

Life-cycle. The endogenous developmental cycle has been described by Allen (1936). Sporozoites invading the mucosa and sub-mucosa throughout the whole length of the small intestine; first generation schizonts appear 24 hours after infection, these measure 11·6 μ by 9·3 μ and contain four small merozoites. At least three asexual generations have been reported, schizonts of the third generation being large, 16 μ by 15 μ, and completely fill many of the tissue cells. They also contain a large number of merozoites. Gametocytic stages appear about 48 hours after infection, and oocysts first appear in the faeces 6 days after infection.

Pathogenesis. This species is fairly pathogenic, especially in young ducks, and mortality may reach 10 per cent in acute outbreaks. The clinical signs consist of anorexia, there is marked loss of weight, difficulty in standing, and it is reported that baby ducklings cry continuously. The lesions consist of a markedly thickened intestinal wall with haemorrhagic spots and areas showing greyish-white nodules. In severe cases there may be sloughing of the mucosa and plugging of the lumen with a haemorrhagic or cheesey exudate. The parasitic stages may penetrate as far as the muscular layer and here produce massive destruction of tissue; Allen (1936), on occasion, noticed penetration of the muscular layer.

Coccidiosis of Geese and Ducks

There is scant information about the clinical importance of coccidia in ducks and geese and still less about the economic importance of the disease. With the exception of *E. truncata*, which may cause 100 per cent mortality in acute cases of renal occidiosis, the other species appear to be important only in sporadic outbreaks, presumably where the environment is overcrowded and unhygienic.

Treatment of coccidiosis of geese and ducks has been little studied. McGregor (1952) found that sodium sulphamezathine was satisfactory for *E. truncata* infections, and Davies *et al.* (1963) report that a 0·1 per cent solution of sodium sulphamezathine in the water, given in the form of an interrupted treatment for two periods of 3 days separated by 2 days, was successful for acute coccidiosis in ducks.

Prevention and control depends on the same considerations as have been discussed with regard to the chicken and turkey coccidioses.

Coccidia of Wild Ducks and Geese

A large number of species are found in wild ducks and geese, and the list, presented below, indicates some of the more common species.

Eimeria boschadis Waldén, 1961 (Mallard, *Anas platyrhynchos platyrhynchos*) (Sweden)

Eimeria brantae Levine, 1953 (Hutchins goose, *Branta canadensis hutchinsi*; Lesser Canada goose, *Branta canadensis parvipes*) (North America)

Eimeria bucephalae Christiansen and Madsen, 1948 (Golden Eye, *Bucephala clangula clangula*) (Denmark)

Eimeria christianseni Waldén, 1961 (Mute swan, *Cygnus olor*) (Sweden)

Eimeria clarkei Hanson, Levine and Ivens, 1957 (Lesser snow goose, *Anser coerulescens coerulescens*) (North America)

Eimeria farri Hanson, Levine and Ivens, 1957 (White fronted goose, *Anser albifrons frontalis*) (North America)

Eimeria fulva Farr, 1953 (Lesser snow goose; Canada goose, *Branta canadensis canadensis*) (U.S.A.)

Eimeria hermani Farr, 1953 (Lesser snow goose; Canada goose and cackling goose, *Branta canadensis minima*) (North America)

Eimeria magnalabia Levine, 1951 (White fronted goose; lesser snow goose; Hutchins goose; Canada goose and cackling goose) (North America)

Eimeria somateriae Christiansen, 1952 (Long tailed duck, *Clangula hymenalis*; eider duck, *Somateria mollissima mollissima*) (Developmental stages in kidney) (Europe)

Eimeria striata Farr, 1953 (Canada goose) (Hanson *et al.*, 1957, considered this synonymous with *Eimeria magnalabia*) (North America)

Tyzzeria alleni Chakravarty and Basu, 1947 (Cotton teal, *Chenicus coromandelianus*) (India)

Coccidia of Guinea Fowl

One species is of importance in this host, namely *Eimeria numidae*, which may be a severe pathogen of young guinea fowl chicks.

Eimeria numidae Pellerdy, 1962. *Hosts:* guinea fowl. Europe. *Oocysts:* elliptical, 19 μ by 15 μ, range 15 μ–21 μ by 12 μ–17 μ. Oocyst wall, smooth, no visible micropyle. Sporulation time, 1–2 days.

The endogenous developmental cycle occurs in the small and large intestines. First generation schizonts are found in the epithelial cells of the duodenum and jejunum from the 2nd day onwards; they measure 4 μ–5 μ and produce two to ten merozoites. Second generation schizonts are larger, 12 μ–14 μ, producing six to fourteen merozoites and occur in the jejunum, ileum and rectum. The prepatent period is 5 days.

Severe clinical signs appear on the 4th–5th day of infection, a dose of 50,000 oocyts being sufficient to kill young birds. This is a parasite specific for the guinea fowl since Pellerdy (1956) reported failure to infect the chicken with this species, or the guinea fowl with chicken coccidia.

Coccidia of Pigeons

Coccidiosis of the pigeon may occasionally be seen in young squabs, especially where these are reared intensively and when conditions of hygiene are poor. Older birds serve as carriers and remain apparently healthy. Three species have been reported in the pigeon:

Eimeria columbae Mitra and DasGupta, 1937
Eimeria columbarum Nieschulz, 1935
Eimeria labbeana (Labbé, 1896) Pinto, 1928

Eimeria columbae. This occurs in the pigeon (*Columba livia intermedia*) in India. *Oocysts:* 16·4 μ by 14·3 μ and have a thin wall. Sporulation time, 4–5 days at room temperature.

Eimeria columbarum. This has been found in the rock dove (*Columba livia livia*); however, Levine (1961) considers this species a synonym of *Eimeria labbeana*. As described by Nieschulz (1935) the oocysts are spherical, colourless, 20 μ by 18·7 μ and have no micropyle.

Eimeria labbeana. *Hosts:* domestic pigeon (*Columba domestica*); rock dove; ring dove (*Columba palumbus*) and the turtle dove (*Streptopelia turtur*). World wide in distribution. *Oocysts:* spherical or sub-spherical, 16·7 μ by 15·3 μ, range 15 μ–18 μ by 14 μ–16 μ (Nieschulz, 1935). (Levine, 1961, gives a size of 13 μ–24 μ by 12 μ–23 μ.) Oocyst wall, an inner dark and outer lighter layer, no micropyle. Sporulation time, 24 hours at room temperature.

The endogenous developmental cycle has been studied by Nieschulz (1925). Developmental stages occur in the epithelial cells of the intestine from the anterior region down to the rectum. Mature first generation schizonts are produced in about 3 days, and second generation forms may penetrate into the deeper tissues. The prepatent period is 6 to 7 days. Oocyst production may show periodicity, most oocysts being passed from 9 a.m. to 3 p.m.

Pathogenicity. In young pigeons severe clinical signs commence 4–5 days after artificial infection. Infected squabs show inappetence, diarrhoea and thirst; the droppings may be markedly green and may even be blood-tinged. In severe infections there is a high mortality, and the major lesion is a marked inflammation of the intestinal mucosa, the lumen being filled with a haemorrhagic exudate.

For treatment Morini (1950) reported that sulphaguanidine was satisfactory, while Hauser (1959) commented that nitrofurazone was effective for the infection.

Prevention consists of an improvement in hygiene of the pigeon loft and, in general, of following the procedures for the control of coccidiosis in the domestic chicken.

Coccidia and Coccidiosis of Game Birds

Pheasant. Coccidiosis may be a problem in the young pheasant, especially in rearing establishments, resulting in serious disease and high mortality.

Eimeria dispersa Tyzzer, 1929. This species is primarily a parasite of the turkey, but Tyzzer believed that a pheasant-adapted strain existed which could pass from the pheasant to the bobwhite quail. More recent work has indicated that a turkey strain transmitted to the bobwhite may not subsequently infect the pheasant (Moore, 1954).

Eimeria langeroni Yakimoff and Matschoulsky, 1937. Occurs in the pheasants *Phasianus colchicus chrysomelas* and *P. colchicus tschardynensis*. *Oocysts:* 32·5 μ by 18·4 μ, range 30 μ–36 μ by 16 μ–20 μ. Oocyst wall, double contoured, pinkish-yellow with no micropyle. No information is available on the endogenous life cycle or pathogenicity.

Eimeria megalostromata Ormsbee, 1939. Occurs in the ring-necked pheasant (*P. colchicus torquatus*). *Oocysts:* ovoid, 24 μ by 19 μ, range 21 μ–29 μ by 16 μ–22 μ. Oocyst wall, smooth, bright yellow to brown, micropyle present. Sporulation time, 48 hours. No information is available regarding developmental time or pathogenicity.

Eimeria pacifica Ormsbee, 1939. Occurs in the ring-necked pheasant. *Oocysts:* ovoid, 23 μ by 18 μ, range 17 μ–26 μ by 14 μ–20 μ. Oocyst wall, double contoured, bright yellow in colour, no micropyle. Sporulation time, 48 hours. Development occurs in the anterior part of the small intestine, schizonts developing proximal to the cell nucleus. Apparently of low pathogenicity.

Eimeria phasiani Tyzzer, 1929. Occurs in the ring-necked pheasant. *Oocysts:* ellipsoidal, 23 μ by 16 μ, range 19.8 μ–26·4 μ by 13·2 μ–17·8 μ. Oocyst wall, brownish-yellow, no micropyle. Sporulation time, 24 hours. Endogenous development occurs in the epithelial cells of the villi of the small intestine, developmental stages occurring distal to the cell nucleus. Prepatent period, 5 days. Tyzzer (1929) considered that severe disease could be produced in young pheasants by this species.

Sodium sulphamezathine can be used for treatment and control.

Partridge, Quail etc. A few studies have indicated that infection rates may be high in these hosts. Madsen (1941) indicated an incidence of 48 per cent in adults and 62 per cent in young birds in Denmark, and Herman *et al.* (1942) reported a high infection rate in both wild and domesticated birds.

Eimeria dispersa. The turkey form of this species has been transmitted to the bobwhite quail *(Colinus virginianus)*.

Eimeria coturnicus Chakravarty and Kar, 1947. Occurs in grey quail *(Coturnix coturnix coturnix)* in India. *Oocysts:* 26·4 µ–38·8 µ by 19·8 µ–26·4 µ. No micropyle.

Eimeria kofoidi Yakimoff and Matikaschwili, 1936. Occurs in stone partridge and grey partridge *(Perdix perdix perdix)*. *Oocysts:* 20 µ by 17·6 µ.

Eimeria lyruri Galli-Valerio, 1927. This species occurs in the red-legged partridge *(Perdix ruber)*, the black grouse *(Lyrurus tetrix tetrix)* and the capercaillie *(Tetrao urogallus aquitanicus)*. *Oocysts:* 24 µ–27 µ by 15 µ, cylindrical in outline.

Eimeria procera Haase, 1939. This occurs in the grey partridge. *Oocysts:* 28·8 µ–31·2 µ by 16·4 µ–17·2 µ, no micropyle, oocysts elliptical.

Eimeria tetricis Haase, 1939. Occurs in black grouse. *Oocysts:* 29·8 µ–31·4 µ by 14·2 µ–15·4 µ, micropyle present, wall smooth.

Eimeria nadsoni Yakimoff and Gousseff, 1936. Occurs in the black grouse. *Oocysts:* 24·9 µ by 21·3 µ, spherical, no micropyle.

Eimeria augusta Allen, 1934. This occurs in the spruce grouse *(Canachites canadensis)*, sharp-tailed grouse *(Pediocetes phasianellus campestris)* and the ruffed grouse *(Bonsar umbellus)* in the United States. *Oocysts:* 29·6 µ by 18·8 µ, range 25 µ–33·9 µ by 16 µ–27·1 µ. Developmental stages occur in the caecum.

Eimeria bonasae Allen, 1934. Occurs in the spruce grouse, willow grouse or ptarmigan *(Lagopus lagopus)*, a sharp-tailed grouse and hazel hen in Canada. *Oocysts:* 21 µ in diameter and spherical. No micropyle. Parasite of caecum.

Eimeria lagopodi Galli-Vallerio, 1929. Occurs in ptarmigan. *Oocysts:* 24 µ by 15 µ, sub-cylindrical. Micropyle present.

Eimeria brinkmanni Levine, 1953. Occurs in rock ptarmigan *(Lagopus mutus rupestris)* in Canada. *Oocysts:* 28·6 µ by 18·8 µ, ellipsoidal, micropyle present. Oocyst wall, brownish-yellow, slightly roughened.

Eimeria fanthami Levine, 1953. Occurs in rock ptarmigan in Canada. *Oocysts:* 28·3 µ by 18·8 µ, ellipsoidal, no micropyle.

Coccidia of the Rabbit

Coccidial infection in the rabbit may, at times, cause serious disease and death especially in young rabbits in intensive breeding establishments for fur, flesh or experimental purposes. One of the most severe is *Eimeria stiedae*, the cause of hepatic coccidiosis. In addition, the intestinal species may be responsible for severe ill health and death. At one time it was thought that the coccidia of rabbits were similar to those of hares (*Lepus* species); however, after extensive studies, Pellerdy (1956) concluded that the majority of the species from domestic and cottontail rabbits were specific for these animals and were not found in hares or jackrabbits. However, the host lists of many of the species of coccidia of the rabbit still contain hosts which Pellerdy would invalidate, and it is clear that further studies on cross transmission are necessary.

The species of coccidia which occur in rabbits are detailed below:

Eimeria coecicola Cheissin, 1947
Eimeria exigua Yakimoff, 1934
Eimeria intestinalis Cheissin, 1948
Eimeria irresidua Kessel and Jankiewicz, 1931
Eimeria magna Pérard, 1925
Eimeria matsubayashii Tsunoda, 1952
Eimeria media Kessel, 1929
Eimeria neoleporis Carvalho, 1942
Eimeria perforans (Leuckart, 1897) Sluiter and Swellengrebel, 1912
Eimeria piriformis Kotlán and Pospesch, 1934
Eimeria stiedae (Lindemann, 1865) Kisskalt and Hartmann, 1907

Eimeria coecicola. *Hosts:* domestic and wild rabbit. Hungary, Soviet Union. Development occurs in the posterior ileum and caecum. *Oocysts:* ovoid, 25 μ–40 μ by 15 μ–21 μ. Oocyst wall, smooth, light yellow in colour, micropyle present. Sporulation time, 3 days at room temperature. The developmental cycle has been described by Cheissin (1947). Asexual development occurs in the epithelial cells of the villi of the posterior small intestine, and the gametogonous stages are found in the cells of the crypts of the caecum. The prepatent period is 9 days. This species has negligible pathogenicity. Pellerdy (1965) maintains that this species is synonymous with *Eimeria neoleporis* Carvalho, 1942.

Eimeria exigua. *Hosts:* tame rabbit, Greenland hare and the cottontail rabbit. *Oocysts:* small, more or less sub-spherical, 14·5 μ by 12·7 μ. Oocyst wall, smooth, no visible micropyle. No information is available on the endogenous developmental cycle, and as far as is known, there is no pathogenicity associated with this species.

Eimeria intestinalis. *Hosts:* domestic rabbit (*Oryctolagus cuniculus*). Hungary and the Soviet Union. Relatively uncommon. Developmental stages occur in the small intestine. *Oocysts:* pyriform, 27 μ by 18 μ, range 23 μ–30 μ by 15 μ–20 μ. Oocyst wall, yellowish, smooth, micropyle present. Sporulation time, 1–2 days at room temperature.

Life-cycle. First generation schizonts are found in epithelial cells of the distal portion of the ileum, developing in a colonial manner at the base of the villi. Up to three generations of schizonts have been reported (Pellerdy, 1965). Gametocytes are visible as early as 7–8 days after infection, and the prepatent period is 10 days.

Artificial infection of young rabbits produced moderate to severe intestinal inflammation, associated with diarrhoea and at times death.

Eimeria irresidua. *Hosts:* domestic rabbit; cottontail rabbit (*Sylvilagus floridanus*); California jackrabbit (*Lepus ruficaudatus*) and the white-tailed jackrabbit (*Lepus townsendii*). World wide in distribution. *Oocysts:* ovoid, 38·3 μ by 25·6 μ, range 31 μ–43 μ by 22 μ–27 μ. Oocyst wall, smooth, light yellow in colour, distinct micropyle. Sporulation time, 50 hours at room temperature.

The endogenous development of *E. irresidua* has been studied by Rutherford (1943). Developmental stages occur in the epithelium of the villi of the whole of the small intestine. Two types of schizonts occur, a smaller form which produces two to ten merozoites and a larger type which produces thirty-six to forty-eight merozoites. Gametocytic stages are apparent from the 8th day of infection, and the prepatent period is 9–10 days (Rutherford, 1943). However, Cheissin (1946) reported that the endogenous development required 7–7·5 days, and he also maintained that sexual stages developed from the third and fourth generation merozoites.

Pathogenesis. Heavy infections produce destruction of large numbers of epithelial cells with associated inflammation of the mucosa. In severe infections there may be haemorrhage into the intestinal lumen with marked diarrhoea and high mortality.

Eimeria magna. *Hosts:* domestic rabbit, California jackrabbit, cottontail, also in two species of hare (*Lepus timidus, Lepus europaeus*). World wide in distribution. Common. Developmental stages in jejunum and ileum. *Oocysts:* broadly ovoidal, 35 μ by 24 μ, range 31 μ–40 μ by 22 μ–26 μ. Oocyst wall, yellow to yellowish-brown, area around the micropyle especially prominent, with a shoulder-like or collar-like protrusion formed by the outer oocyst wall. The outer wall may become detached, especially during sporulation, and then the distinct collar-like protrusion is absent. Sporulation time, 2–3 days.

Developmental stages occur distal to the nuclei of the epithelial cells, and parasitised epithelial cells migrate into the sub-mucosal tissues. Rutherford (1943) recognised two types of schizonts which reached up to 10 μ–20 μ in diameter. The larger schizonts produced fewer merozoites and appeared earlier than the second schizontal stages. Gametocytes appear from the 5th day after infection onwards, and these, too, may become sub-epithelial in position. The prepatent period is 7–8 days, and patency persists for 15–19 days.

Pathogenicity. Rutherford (1943) considered *E. magna* as a marked pathogen for the domestic rabbit, probably the sub-epithelial location of developmental stages contributing to this. Lund (1949) observed that 300,000 oocysts of some strains may lead to death of young rabbits, whereas other strains were less pathogenic and up to 1 million oocysts failed to cause death. Clinical signs consist of progressive emaciation and diarrhoea with mucoid faeces.

Eimeria matsubayashii. *Hosts:* domestic rabbit, Japan. *Oocysts:* broadly ovoidal, 24·8 μ by 18·2 μ, range 22 μ–29 μ by 16 μ–22 μ. Oocyst wall, smooth, light yellow, micropyle present. Sporulation time, 32–40 hours. The endogenous developmental cycle is not known in detail. Tsumoda (1952) reported it to be similar to *E. magna*, developmental stages occurring in the epithelial cells of the ileum. The prepatent period is 7 days.

No detailed information is available on the pathogenesis of this species, though following heavy infection a diphtheritic enteritis may occur in the ileum with the clinical signs of diarrhoea.

Eimeria media. *Hosts:* domestic rabbit, cottontail, jackrabbit. World wide in distribution. *Oocysts:* ellipsoidal, 31·2 μ by 18·5 μ, range 27 μ–36 μ by 15 μ–22 μ. Oocyst wall, smooth, light pinkish in colour, well defined micropyle. Sporulation time, 2 days.

Life-cycle. The endogenous developmental cycle has been studied by Rutherford (1943) and Pellerdy & Babos (1953). Early developmental stages occur in the epithelial cells of the villi but later are found in a subepithelial position. First generation schizonts are mature by the 4th day. Two forms have been reported, a type 'A' schizont which produces two to ten merozoites, and a type 'B', smaller than the first, which produces twelve to thirty-six merozoites. Second generation schizonts appear on the 6th day of infection, and again two types of schizonts are seen. Gametocytic stages may be present on the 5th–6th day after infection, and the prepatent period is 6–7 days (Rutherford, 1943).

Pathogenicity. Pellerdy & Babos (1953) reported that 50,000 oocysts were fatal to young rabbits, these producing a severe enteritis with excessive destruction of the intestinal epithelium. On post mortem, lesions occur in the small intestine and frequently extend into the large intestine. The wall of the caecum may be markedly thickened and greyish-white in colour due to the accumulation of large numbers of developmental stages.

Eimeria neoleporis. *Hosts:* cottontail, domestic rabbit (experimentally). U.S.A., Europe, U.S.S.R. *Oocysts:* sub-cylindrical to ellipsoidal, 38·8 μ by 19·8 μ, range 32·8 μ–44·3 μ by 15·7 μ–22·8 μ. Oocyst wall, smooth, yellowish, distinct micropyle. Sporulation time, 2–3 days.

Life-cycle. The endogenous developmental cycle occurs in the posterior part of the small intestine and the caecum. Carvalho (1943) described four types of schizonts resulting in an endogenous developmental cycle of 12 days. The first schizonts develop in the epithelial cells lining the crypts of Lieberkühn and produce forty to forty-eight merozoites which are released about the 5th day. The second generation schizonts are produced on the 7th day, and they contain sixty to seventy merozoites. The third generation schizont is mature by the 9th day; two types occur, a small form producing fourteen merozoites and a larger form producing sixty to eighty-six merozoites. Gametogony is detectable on the 10th day, and the prepatent period is approximately 12 days. Patency continues for a further 10 days.

Pathogenicity. This species is moderately pathogenic. It is more pathogenic in the cottontail than the domestic rabbit. Pellerdy (1954) found that doses of 50,000 to 100,000 oocysts produced death in young rabbits by the 10th day of infection. Pathologic changes occurred mainly in the region of the ileocaecal valve and in the vermiform appendix; there was thickening of the intestinal wall, which was whitish-grey in colour due to the large number of developmental stages. Severe infections produced necrosis of the superficial mucosa.

Eimeria perforans. *Hosts:* domestic rabbit, jackrabbit, cottontail, also reported from hare (*Lepus europaeus*), Greenland hare (*L. articus groenlandicus*). World wide in distribution. Developmental stages occur in duodenum and ileum. *Oocysts:* ovoid to ellipsoidal, 22·7 μ by 14·2 μ, range 15 μ–29 μ by 11 μ–7 μ. Oocyst wall, smooth, colourless to lightish pink, micropyle not readily distinguishable. Sporulation time, 30–56 hours at room temperature.

Life-cycle. The endogenous developmental cycle has been described by Rutherford (1943). Two types of first generation schizonts have been observed: type 'A' forms produce four to eight merozoites and type 'B' up to twenty-four merozoites. Second generation schizonts occur on the 5th day of infection, and gametocytic stages are first evident on the 4th–5th day. The prepatent period is 5–6 days, this being the shortest endogenous cycle of the rabbit coccidia.

Eimeria perforans is of low pathogenicity. In young rabbits it may cause mild to moderate diarrhoea. On post mortem the wall of the anterior small intestine is thickened and whitish in colour due to the accumulation of developmental stages.

Eimeria piriformis. *Hosts:* domestic rabbit; France and Hungary. *Oocysts:* pyriform, 29 μ by 18 μ, range 26 μ–32 μ by 17 μ–21 μ. Oocyst wall, smooth, double contoured, yellowish-brown in colour, prominent micropyle visible at the tapering end. Sporulation time, 24–48 hours.

Life-cycle. This has been described by Pellerdy (1953); however, Levine (1961) maintains that his description refers to *E. intestinalis* and not *E. piriformis.*

Parasites develop in the jejunum and ileum proximal to the nucleus of the epithelial cell. Two types of schizont are reported, type 'A' producing up to twelve merozoites and type 'B' producing a large number of slender forms. The majority of the first generation merozoites appear to be of the type 'A' form. In the second generation schizogony, the type 'B' merozoites (long, slender) predominate. Gametogonous stages are seen on the 7th day, and the prepatent period is 9–10 days.

Pellerdy (1965) states that an infection of 30,000 oocysts may produce death in animals, irrespective of age. The pathological lesions consist of a catarrhal inflammation of the small intestine.

Eimeria stiedae. *Hosts:* domestic rabbit, cottontail, various hares (*L. europaeus, L. americanus, L. timidus*). Developmental stages occur in the liver. *Oocysts:* ovoidal to ellipsoidal, 36·9 μ by 19·9 μ, range 28 μ–40 μ by 16 μ–25 μ. Oocyst wall, smooth, yellowish-orange or salmon coloured, distinct micropyle. Sporulation time, 3 days at room temperature, 58 hours at 22°C.

Life-cycle. Smetana (1933a, b, c) provided the first extensive account of the life cycle. Excystation occurs in the small intestine, and sporozoites penetrate the intestinal mucosa and pass *via* the hepatic-portal blood system to the liver and enter the epithelial cells of the bile ducts. Developmental stages are normally found here 5-6 days after infection, but in heavy infections stages may be seen at 72 hours. Development occurs proximal to the nucleus of the epithelial cell. Mature schizonts measure 15 μ–18 μ, and there is no definite information concerning the number of asexual generations which take place. Gametogony is observed as early as the 11th day after infection, but large numbers of gametocytes are not evident until several days later. Both schizogony and gametogony can be observed in the later stages of infection. The prepatent period is 18 days, excessive numbers of oocysts are shed about the 23rd day and patency lasts until about the 37th day after infection.

Pathogenesis. In mild infections little or no clinical signs are evident, but in heavy infections severe liver involvement produces progressive emaciation, an enormous enlargement of the liver, and death. When several hundred oocysts are given to young rabbits, death may be expected from 3 weeks onwards. Animals lose appetite, there is progressive emaciation and diarrhoea, and there is an enormous distention of the abdomen in which the enlarged liver can be felt; this is also associated with ascites.

In fatal cases the liver may be 5 to 10 times its normal size. It is pale and shows a mass of yellow hepatic lesions filled with pus-like material. Petechial haemorrhages occur on the liver, in the kidneys and elsewhere in the body; oedema is seen in the peritoneal cavity, and the whole body may be oedematous.

The liver lesions are due essentially to an extensive enlargement of the bile ducts caused by a proliferation of the bile duct epithelium, this being thrown into a very large number of folds. The epithelial covering is filled with developmental stages of the parasite. The pus-like material in the bile ducts consists of desquamated epithelial cells, gametogonous stages and oocysts. There is a massive infiltration of lymphocytes, plasma cells, eosinophils and a smaller number of neutrophils. If the animal survives, an invasion of the lesions by fibrous tissue occurs, new bile ducts proliferate, and large areas of the liver are transformed into fibrous tissue.

Coccidiosis in Rabbits

Coccidiosis is essentially a disease of the young rabbit and is seen especially in breeding and rearing establishments where sanitation is poor. However, outbreaks of disease are not uncommon under natural conditions, especially where the warren type of habitat is found. The important species are *E. stiedae* of the liver and *E. irresidua* and *E. magna* of the intestine.

A diagnosis of coccidiosis may be made on the demonstration of very large numbers of oocysts in the faeces; however, since coccidia are frequently present in rabbits and may be present in large numbers without any serious clinical signs, the most satisfactory diagnosis is made at a post-mortem examination. With liver coccidiosis only massive infection is associated with ill health, and there is no evidence that a small number of lesions cause ill health.

The most effective compounds for treatment are the sulphonamides. Davies *et al.* (1963) state that sodium sulphamezathine in the drinking water, at a concentration of 0·2 per cent, is highly effective for hepatic coccidiosis and can be given for a long time without danger of toxicity. Other compounds for hepatic coccidiosis are sulphaguanidine, succinyl sulphathiazole at the rate of 0·5 per cent in the feed (Horton-Smith, 1947) and sulphaquinoxaline at the rate of 0·03 per cent in the feed (Lund, 1954). The nitrofurans are unsatisfactory for hepatic coccidiosis. Nitrofurazone has been recommended for intestinal coccidiosis by Boch (1957) at a dose of 0·5–1 g. per kg. The author found that zoalene and amprolium had no protective action when they were fed at various levels in the food to rabbits experimentally infected with *E. stiedae*.

Control of rabbit coccidiosis is based on the improvement of hygiene in breeding and rearing establishments. Cages, hutches or pens should be cleaned out regularly, preferably every day; proper facilities should be made for feeding animals, and food should not be thrown on the floor for the animals. Feeding and watering troughs should be so placed that they are not contaminated with droppings. In large establishments a periodical post-mortem examination on a few animals is a valuable check on the status of the infection.

ORDER: HAEMOSPORIDIA DANILESKY, 1886

The development of the Haemosporidia is similar to that of the Coccidia; however, in the former the life cycle is shared by two hosts, schizogony occurring in vertebrates, and gametogony and sporogony occurring in blood-sucking invertebrates.

The order is divided by Kudo (1966) into three families, namely:

Plasmodiidae, schizogony in the peripheral blood of vertebrates. Pigment present.

Haemoproteidae, schizogony in the endothelial cells of inner organs; only gametocytes appear in the peripheral blood. Pigment present.

Babesiidae, small, non-pigmented parasites of erythrocytes.

Levine (1961) has suggested that the family *Plasmodiidae* should embrace the *Haemoproteidae*, while the *Babesiidae* should be placed in a separate class, the *Piroplasmasida*, in which an order *Piroplasmorida* would include the forms originally included in the *Babesiidae*. For the purposes of this volume, however, it is convenient to retain in part the classification proposed by Kudo (1966). A modification of Kudo's classification has been adopted for the *Babesiidae*.

FAMILY: PLASMODIIDAE MESNIL, 1903

This family contains one genus of importance, *Plasmodium*.

Genus: Plasmodium Marchiafava and Celli, 1885

This genus contains the malarial organisms of man, other mammals and vertebrates. Schizogony occurs in the red blood cells and also in endothelial cells of inner organs, while the sexual phase of the cycle occurs in blood-sucking insects; for mammalian forms these are anopheline mosquitoes and for the avian forms, culicine mosquitoes.

Extensive accounts of the malarial organisms have been given by numerous authors, and a detailed account of malaria and malariology with a consideration of the taxonomy, morphology, life cycle, vector and other aspects may be found in the textbook *Practical Malariology* by Russell *et al.* (1963).

Although mammalian malaria is of no immediate concern to the veterinarian, it is, nevertheless, of considerable importance as a global disease, and no text of protozoology would be complete without reference to it. The major consideration is devoted to avian malaria.

AVIAN MALARIA

An extensive, general review of avian malaria is given by Hewitt (1940), and a catalogue of the plasmodia of birds is given by Coatney & Roundbush (1949). Levine & Hanson (1953) list the species which occur in waterfowl, and Levine & Kantor (1959) list those which are found in columbiform birds. The more recent information on avian malaria is reviewed by Huff (1963).

The more common species of avian malarial organisms are listed below (after Russel *et al.*, 1963):

Species with Round or Irregular Gametocytes which Displace the Nucleus of the Host Cell:

Plasmodium cathemerium Hartman, 1927; *Plasmodium gallinaceum* Brumpt, 1935; *Plasmodium juxtanucleare* Versiani and Gomes, 1941; *Plasmodium relictum* (Grassi and Feletti, 1891).

Species with Elongate Gametocytes which Do Not Usually Displace the Host Cell Nucleus:

Plasmodium circumflexum Kikuth, 1931; *Plasmodium turae* Herman, 1941; *Plasmodium elongatum* Hugg, 1930; *Plasmodium fallax* Schwetz, 1930; *Plasmodium hexamerium* Huff, 1935; *Plasmodium lophurae* Coggeshall, 1938; *Plasmodium polare* Manwell, 1935; *Plasmodium rouxi* Sergent and Catanei, 1928; *Plasmodium vaughani* Novy and MacNeal, 1904.

Developmental Cycle of Avian Plasmodia. A major advance in the understanding of the life cycle of the malarial organism was made by the demonstration that the infective sporozoites did not enter erythrocytes directly, but rather developed as exoerythrocytic forms in cells of the reticulo-endothelial system prior to invasion of the erythrocytes.

Following the introduction of the sporozoites from infected culicine mosquitoes, numerous pre-erythrocytic schizonts are found in the macrophages and fibroblasts of the skin near the point of entry. These are referred to as cryptozoites. Merozoites from this first generation of pre-erythrocytic schizonts form a second generation of pre-erythrocytic schizonts, the metacryptozoites. Merozoites from the metacryptozoites enter erythrocytes and other cells of the body and in the latter form exoerythrocytic schizonts. In the case of *P. gallinaceum*, *P. relictum* and *P. cathemerium*, these other cells are endothelial cells, but in the case of *P. elongatum* and *P. vaughani* they are cells of the haemopoietic system. In some species of avian plasmodia, e.g. *P. gallinaceum* and *P. elongatum*, the exoerythrocytic developmental stages may be added to by forms which are derived from the erythrocytic cycle. These are known as phanerozoites, being derived from the merozoites of the schizonts in the erythrocytic cycle.

The erythrocytic cycle is initiated 7 to 10 days after infection by merozoites from metacryptozoites and at other times by merozoites from exoerythrocytic schizonts located, according to species, in the endothelial or haemopoietic cells. On entering the red blood cell, the merozoite rounds up to form a trophozoite. This is a small rounded form containing a large vacuole which displaces the cytoplasm of the parasite to the periphery of the cell. The nucleus is situated at one of the poles, giving the young form a 'signet ring' appearance when stained by the Romanowsky stains. The early trophozoites undergo schizogony to

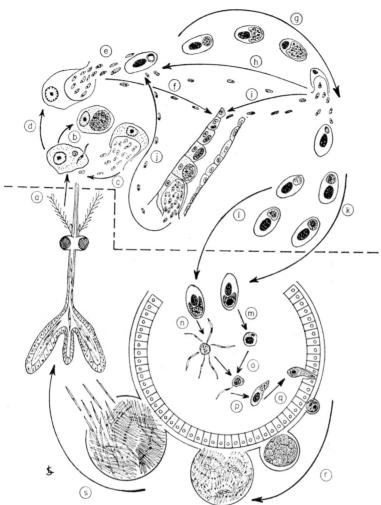

FIG. 280. Diagrammatic Representation of the Life Cycle of *Plasmodium gallinaceum*
a. Introduction of sporozoites by infected culicine mosquito; b. Development of pre-
erythrocytic schizonts (cryptozoites) in skin macrophages; c. Release of merozoites from
cryptozoites which enter other macrophages of skin; d. Formation of metacryptozoites;
e. Entry of merozoites from metacryptozoites into erthyrocytes; f. Entry of merozoites
from metacryptozoites into endothelial cells to form exoerythrocytic schizonts; g. Erythrocytic schizogony; h. Erythrocytic merozoites initiate further erythrocytic schizogony;
i. Erythrocytic merozoites initiate further exoerthyrocytic schizonts (phanerozoites);
j. Merozoites from exoerythrocytic schizonts initiate further erythrocytic stages; k.
Development of macrogametocytes; l. Development of microgametocytes; m. Maturation of macrogamete in mosquito midgut; n. Maturation and exflagellation of microgamete in mosquito midgut; o. Syngamy; p. Formation of motile zygote (oökinete);
q. Penetration of oökinete to outside wall of midgut; r. Sporogony; s. Rupture of oocyst
and migration of sporozoites to salivary glands of mosquito. (Original)

produce merozoites, the number produced depending on the species of parasite. During the process of schizogony, the parasite takes in host cell cytoplasm by invagination, haemoglobin is digested and the residual haematin pigment is deposited in granules within the food vacuoles. Apparently, schizogony may continue indefinitely, the length of each cycle of schizogony depending on the species of parasite. The release of merozoites from the schizonts occurs synchronously in the host, and in human malaria this is associated with a paroxysm of fever. Fever does not appear to be a significant part of the syndrome in avian hosts (Russell *et al.*, 1963).

After a number of asexual generations has occurred, some merozoites undergo sexual development with the formation of microgametocytes and macrogametocytes. Levine (1961) claims that the female forms should be referred to as macrogametes since they possess a haploid number of chromosomes. The haploid nature is maintained throughout the whole of the life cycle of the malarial parasite, except that a diploid state is found following fertilisation and zygote formation. The female forms are generally more numerous than the male forms, and they stain more intensely blue with Romanowsky stains than do the male forms. In addition, of course, the nucleus of the microgametocyte is more diffuse than in the female cell. Further development of the gametocytic stages can take place only when the blood is ingested by a suitable mosquito.

Development in the mosquito is rapid. Within 10 to 15 minutes the nucleus of the microgametocyte divides, and through a process of exflagellation, six to eight long, thin, flagella-like microgametes are extruded from the parent cell. These remain attached to the parent cell for a few minutes, lashing actively; they then become detached and swim away to find, and fertilise, the macrogamete. The zygote resulting from fertilisation is motile and is called an oökinete. This oökinete penetrates the midgut mucosa and comes to lie on the outer surface of the stomach, forming an early oocyst about 50 μ–60 μ in diameter. The nucleus of the oocyst divides repeatedly to produce a very large number of sporozoites. These are about 15 μ in length with a central nucleus. Maturation of the oocyst takes a variable period of time depending on the species of parasite, temperature and the species of mosquito; but in general, it is 10–20 days. When mature, the oocyst ruptures, liberating the sporozoites into the body cavity of the mosquito, and these then migrate all over the body of the mosquito but eventually reach the salivary glands. Here they may lie intracellularly, extracellularly or in the ducts of the salivary glands. They are now infective to a new host, infection occurring when the mosquito takes a blood meal. A mosquito remains infected for its life span, transmitting malarial parasites every time it takes a blood meal.

More detailed information on the exoerythrocytic and erythrocytic cycles of malarial organisms may be found in Bray (1957), Bishop (1955) and in the account of the life cycle of *P. gallinaceum* given by Huff & Coulston (1944).

Plasmodium cathemerium. *Hosts:* Common in passerine birds, e.g. English sparrow, red-winged blackbird etc. It has been extensively used for experimental work in canaries, in which it causes an acute fatal disease. Gametocytes are rounded, with rod-shaped rather coarse pigment granules, and displace the nucleus of the cell. Gametocytes and schizonts, about 7 μ–8 μ in diameter; schizogony, 24 hour cycle with a peak of segmentation about 6–10 p.m.; six to twenty-four merozoites produced. Transmitted by several species of *Culex* and *Aedes*. Developmental cycle is comparable to that already described and has been investigated by Bray (1957).

Splenic infarcts occur in experimentally infected canaries, and there is marked enlargement of the spleen and liver with anaemia and subcutaneous haemorrhages.

Plasmodium gallinaceum. *Hosts:* Primarily a parasite of the domestic fowl in India. Other birds, pheasant, goose, partridge and peacock, can be infected experimentally; however, the canary, duck, guinea fowl, pigeon and English sparrow are resistant to infection. Gametocytes, round and possessing pigment granules of relatively large size and few in number; schizonts, round to irregular, produce eight to thirty merozoites. Both developmental stages cause displacement of the host cell nucleus. Schizogony, 36 hour cycle, peak of segmentation noon and midnight, alternatively.

The developmental cycle is comparable to that described above. Exoerythrocytic stages occur in the endothelial cells, and the reticulo-endothelial cells of the spleen, brain and liver.

The natural vectors have not been identified. Experimentally, the parasite will develop in species of the genus *Aedes*, *Armigeres* etc.

Pathogenesis. The chicken is particularly susceptible, and even adult birds may suffer a mortality of up to 80 per cent in some areas. Birds become progressively emaciated as the disease progresses, there is anaemia and spleen and liver enlargement. Paralysis may occur due to massive numbers of exoerythrocytic forms in the endothelial cells of the brain capillaries.

Plasmodium juxtanucleare. *Hosts:* Domestic chicken, South and Central America. Turkeys have been infected experimentally but not ducks, guinea fowl, pigeon or canary. Gametocytes, round to irregular, relatively small, parasites tend to be in contact with the host cell nucleus, host erythrocyte is often distorted. Schizogony, 24 hour cycle; three to seven, usually four, merozoites produced. Developmental cycle poorly known.

The species is highly pathogenic, Brazilian strains appearing to be especially so. Chickens become listless, weak with anaemia, and occasionally central nervous system involvement may be seen (Al-Dabagh, 1961).

Plasmodium relictum. *Hosts:* Pigeon, mourning dove, a number of Anatidae and various passerines. Experimentally transmissible to canary, duck, chicken and other birds. World wide in distribution. Gametocytes, round to irregular, displace the host cell nucleus, which may be expelled from the erythrocyte, pigment fine and pin-point. Schizogony, from 12 hour to 36 hour cycle; merozoites produced, eight to thirty-two depending on the strain.

The developmental cycle of this species has been studied extensively by Bray (1957), who demonstrated exoerythrocytic stages in the endo-thelial cells. Several species of *Culex, Anopheles, Aedes* etc. serve as vectors.

This parasite is highly pathogenic for pigeons. Young birds become weak and anaemic, the anaemia being the principal cause of death. On post mortem there is a markedly enlarged spleen and pigmented liver.

Plasmodium circumflexum. *Hosts:* Wide variety of hosts, e.g. passerine birds, ruffed grouse and Canada goose (Levine & Hanson, 1953). A large species, both the schizonts and gametocytes are elongate and tend to encircle the erythrocyte nucleus though they are not in contact with it; nor do they displace it. Schizogony, 48 hour cycle, twelve to thirty merozoites produced.

Life cycle, similar to above, exoerythrocytic stages occurring in the endothelial cells.

Plasmodium durae. *Hosts:* Turkey, Africa. Transmissible to ducks. Gametocytes, elongate, nucleus of the host cell frequently displaced; pigment granules usually large and stain intensely. Schizogony, 24 hour cycle, six to fourteen merozoites produced.

Exoerythrocytic stages of *P. durae* have been found in the endothelial cells of the liver, spleen, lungs and brain of turkeys. Cerebral involvement may occur, and other clinical signs are emaciation and oedema. In young turkeys the disease takes an acute course (Purchase, 1942). At post mortem there is congestion of the liver, spleen, kidneys and the capil-laries of the brain and meninges.

Plasmodium elongatum. *Hosts:* English sparrow, canaries and ducks experimentally. Gametocytes, elongate.

Plasmodium fallax. *Hosts:* Owl, African guinea fowl; chickens and pigeons experimentally. Gametocytes, large, resembling those of *Haemo-proteus,* tending to surround the nucleus of the host cell without displacing it.

Plasmodium hexamerium. *Hosts:* Passerine birds. Gametocytes and schizonts, elongate. Four to eight merozoites produced.

Plasmodium lophurae. *Hosts:* Originally found in fire-back pheasant *(Lophura igniti)*; chickens and ducklings are susceptible experi-mentally, but canaries are not. Gametocytes, large, elongate, host cell nucleus not displaced. Eight to eighteen merozoites produced. Schizo-gony, 24 hour cycle.

Plasmodium rouxi. *Hosts:* Sparrows, finches, Near East. Gametocytes, elongate, host cell nucleus not displaced. The schizonts have a cycle of 24 hours and produce four merozoites.

Plasmodium vaughani. *Hosts:* American robbin (*Turdus migratorius migratorius*), starling (*Sturnus vulgaris vulgaris*), also other birds. Gameto-cyte, elongate, host cell nucleus not displaced. Schizogony, 24 hour cycle, four merozoites produced.

Therapy of Avian Malaria. Many of the compounds which are used for the treatment of human malaria have been developed, initially, against avian species. Reviews of the compounds which may be used, their mode of action and the development of resistant forms are given by Rollo (1964) and Bishop (1962). Chloroquin at the rate of 5 mg. per kg., paludrine at 7·5 mg. per kg. and pyrimethamine at 0·3 mg. per kg. are all effective against *P. gallinaceum*.

Malarial Parasites of Man

The species of the Plasmodia of man are:
Plasmodium falciparum Welch, 1897
Plasmodium malariae (Laveran, 1881) Grassi and Felletti, 1890
Plasmodium ovale Stephens, 1922
Plasmodium vivax (Grassi and Felletti, 1890) Labbé, 1899
These four species are those which are considered to be natural para-sites of man. However, recent evidence has indicated that under certain circumstances man may be infected also with simian malaria. Accidental laboratory infection of two humans with *Plasmodium cynomolgi bastianelli* has been reported by Eyles *et al.* (1960) and Boye *et al.* (1961). It has also been realised that *Plasmodium malariae* is apparently common to man and chimpanzee, previously being known in the latter as *Plasmodium rodhaini* (Manwell, 1963). *Plasmodium knowlesi* of *Macaca irus* is experimentally transmissible to man by blood inoculation, but mosquito-induced infec-tions are not yet known. *Plasmodium vivax* can produce mild infections in chimpanzees when human infected blood is inoculated, but mosquito infections fail since sporozoites seem unable to develop in chimpanzees. Jeffery (1961) failed to find any pre-erythrocytic forms in monkeys inoculated with sporozoites of *P. vivax*.

Endogenous Developmental Cycle of Human Malaria. Although exoerythro-cytic schizogony has been known in avian malaria for a number of years, it is only within the recent decade that this has been established for the human forms. Detailed accounts of the life cycle of each species may be found in Russell *et al.* (1963) and Faust & Russell (1964).

Following the bite of the infected mosquito the sporozoites remain in the blood for a short time, but after an hour the blood is no longer infective for another host. Sporozoites enter the parenchyma cells of the liver and here develop into pre-erythrocytic schizonts (cryptozoites). The exoery-throcytic forms are confined to the liver in mammalian malaria and, unlike the avian forms, are sparse. The hepatic form grows to become a large schizont, the time for this and the size of the mature form depending on the species of parasite. Thus, in *P. falciparum* pre-erythrocytic growth is rapid, taking 5·5–6 days, and schizonts measure 60 microns when mature and contain about 40,000 merozoites. There appears to be only a single generation of cryptozoites in *P. falciparum* and a one way passage of merozoites from the exoerythrocytic cycle. With *Plasmodium cynomolgi* pre-erythrocytic schizogony is observed from the second day onwards, and by the 8th day schizonts measure thirty-eight microns in diameter and contain about 10,000 merozoites. The majority of the merozoites from this schizogony enter the erythrocytic cycle, but some may return to the liver parenchyma cells and continue exoerythrocytic schizogony, these being a constant source of infection for the erythrocytes. Details of the exoerythrocytic development of other species may be found in Faust & Russell (1964).

Following exoerythrocytic development, merozoites invade the erythrocytes, and the cycle of development in the blood and subsequently in the mosquito is comparable to that described previously for avian malaria.

Plasmodium falciparum. The cause of malignant tertian malaria, falciparum malaria or subtertian malaria. There is a tendency for infected erythrocytes to clump, and consequently the schizonts and merozoites are found almost exclusively in the capillaries of the inner organs. Eight to eighteen (eight to thirty-two) merozoites are produced per schizont, the pigment granules are dark brown or black and usually occur in a compact mass. The gametocytes are sausage- or crescent-shaped and appear in the peripheral blood. Macrogametes stain blue and the pigment granules are grouped around the nucleus, whereas the microgametes stain bluish to reddish and have scattered pigment granules. This parasite differs from the other species of human Plasmodia in that normally only the ring forms of trophozoites and gametocytes are seen in the peripheral blood.

The parasite is widely distributed in the tropics and is relatively uncommon in temperate zones. It is generally regarded as the most malignant form of malaria in the human.

Plasmodium malariae. The cause of quartan malaria. The schizonts appear in the circulating blood and frequently assume a band form across the erythrocytes; when mature they almost fill the host cell. Six to twelve merozoites are produced per schizont, and these may be arranged around a mass of pigment granules. The gametocytes are round, the macrogametes stain more deeply than the male forms and they have a smaller, more deeply staining nucleus and coarse pigment granules. Microgametocytes possess a larger, lightly staining nucleus and finer and more numerous pigment granules.

This species is less common than the other three species and occurs in tropical and sub-tropical areas. Though widely distributed, it has a low prevalence.

Plasmodium ovale. The cause of mild tertian malaria. A distinctive feature of the parasitised red cell is the appearance of Schuffner's dots, and the host cell is often fimbriated. Schizonts produce eight to ten merozoites. The gametocytes resemble those of *P. malariae*, and the host cells are markedly affected with Schuffner's dots and slightly enlarged. Pigment is evenly distributed. This species has a limited distribution, being confined to Africa, the Philippines and India.

Plasmodium vivax. The cause of benign tertian or vivax malaria. The developing schizonts are irregular, amoeboid and active and extend over the cell which is enlarged, pale and contains Schuffner's dots. Mature schizonts almost fill the host cell and produce eight to twenty-four merozoites (usually twelve to eighteen). The macrogametes are $9\ \mu$–$10\ \mu$ in diameter, more or less fill the host cell, stain deeply and contain a compact nucleus with evenly distributed pigment granules. The microgametocytes are a little smaller, have a paler blue cytoplasm with a larger nucleus that stains less deeply than the female form.

Benign tertian malaria is the commonest and the most widely distributed malarial infection in the world; it extends into the temperate zones and occurs in North America and the more northern parts of Europe.

Therapy and Control of Malaria. A detailed account of malaria therapy and drug prophylaxis, a consideration of the action of different compounds on various developmental stages and a list of trade, proprietary and national names of the existing malarial compounds is given by Russell *et al.* (1963). A review of the chemotherapy of malaria is given by Rollo (1964). The control of malaria by use of insecticides, drainage and other control measures are discussed by Russell *et al.* (1963).

FAMILY: HAEMOPROTEIDAE DOFLEIN, 1916

Two genera of interest, *Haemoproteus* and *Leucocytozoon*, occur in this family. Schizogony occurs in the endothelial cells of the inner organs, and only gametocytes appear in the circulating blood. Subsequent development occurs in blood-sucking insects, the developmental stages being comparable to those found in the genus *Plasmodium*.

Genus: Haemoproteus Kruse, 1819

Gametocytes occur in the erythrocytes and possess a halter-shaped appearance encircling the nucleus (synonym *Halteridium*). Pigment granules also occur. Schizogony occurs in the endothelial cells of the blood vessels, especially in the lungs. The parasites are transmitted by hippoboscid flies and in some cases by members of the genus *Culicoides*. The genus is widespread in birds and also occurs in reptiles. The following species have been recorded from birds:

Haemoproteus columbae Celli and Sanfelice, 1891
Haemoproteus lophortyx O'Roke, 1930

Haemoproteus meleagridis Levine, 1961
Haemoproteus nettionis (Johnston and Cleland, 1909) Coatney, 1936
Haemoproteus sacharovi Novy and MacNeal, 1904
A check list and a host list of the species of the genus *Haemoproteus* has been prepared by Coatney (1936), and Herman (1944) has prepared a check list of the species in North American birds.

Haemoproteus columbae. *Hosts:* Domestic and wild pigeons; also in mourning doves, turtle doves and a number of other wild birds. World wide in distribution.

The only forms which occur in erythrocytes are the gametocytic stages. These may range from tiny ring forms to elongate, crescent-shaped gametocytes which partially encircle the nucleus of the host cell in the form of a halter. The nucleus may be displaced but not to the edge of the cell. Macrogametes stain dark blue with Romanowsky stains, the nucleus is compact, staining dark purple to red, and the pigment granules are dispersed throughout the cytoplasm. Microgametocytes stain pale blue to pinkish, the nucleus is pale pink and diffuse, and pigment granules are collected into a spherical mass.

Life-cycle. The endogenous developmental cycle, which has been described by Aragao (1908) and Huff (1942), is initiated when sporozoites are injected by an infected hippoboscid fly. Sporozoites enter the blood stream, penetrate endothelial cells of blood vessels and here develop into early schizonts. The early stages are minute cytoplasmic bodies with a single nucleus, but by growth and nuclear division fifteen or more small, unpigmented masses, or cytomeres, each with a single nucleus, are produced. Each cytomere continues to grow, and its nucleus undergoes repeated division until the now greatly enlarged endothelial cell is filled with a large number of multi-nucleate bodies, or cytomeres, surrounded by a fine cyst wall. Each cytomere produces an enormous number of minute merozoites. Subsequently, the endothelial cell breaks down and the cytomeres are liberated, these accumulate in the capillaries which they may block, but soon after liberation, the cytomeres rupture and the merozoites escape into the blood stream. The development to this stage takes about 4 weeks.

The merozoites enter red blood cells and become gametocytes, though it is probable that others enter further endothelial cells and repeat the asexual cycle, this being carried on for several generations. The young gametocytes first appear in the blood about 30 days after infection. Though multiple infections of erythrocytes with trophozoites may occur, it is rare for more than one mature gametocyte to exist in a cell.

Subsequent development occurs in hippoboscid flies. The only proven vector is *Pseudolynchia canariensis*. Baker (1957), in England, showed that *Ornithomyia avicularia* could support sporogony, but he was unable to infect domestic pigeons with infected hippoboscid flies. Levine (1961) suggests that hippoboscids are probably not the only vectors for *H. columbae*, and since *Haemoproteus nettionis* is transmitted by *Culicoides*, it is possible that these insects are also concerned in the life cycle of *H. columbae*. Development in the hippoboscid fly is comparable to that of the genus *Plasmodium* in the mosquito. Exflagellation of the male gametocytes occurs in the midgut of the fly, and the motile zygote (oökinete) migrates to the outer surface of the midgut. Here sporogony takes place with the production of sporozoites. These are liberated in the body cavity of the insect and pass to the salivary glands to await injection into a new host.

Pathogenicity. The pathogenicity of *H. columbae* is generally low, and adult birds usually show no evidence of disease. However, an acute form of the infection has been reported in pigeon nestlings, in which heavy mortality has been recorded. The clinical signs consist of anorexia and anaemia, and on post mortem the liver and spleen are enlarged and dark in colour.

Diagnosis of *H. columbae* infection is based on the demonstration of the gametocytic stages in blood smears and the presence of large numbers of schizonts in the endothelial cells of the blood vessels of the lungs. Schizonts may also be found in the liver, spleen and kidneys.

Little is known regarding treatment. Coatney (1935) has indicated that quinacrine is effective against the young gametocytic stages, but no information is available regarding treatment against the schizontal stages. Prevention and control is dependent upon the control of the insect vector.

Haemoproteus lophortyx. *Hosts:* California valley quail, Gambel quail and Catalina Island quail. The mature gametocytes are halter-shaped and contain numerous pigment granules, and the schizonts are found in the liver, lungs and spleen. Though the fly *Lynchia hirsuta* has been incriminated as a vector for this parasite, attempts to obtain transmission by fly-bite have been negative. On the other hand, Tarshis (1955) has successfully transmitted *H. lophortyx* from quail to quail by *Stilometopa impressa*.

Haemoproteus meleagridis. *Hosts:* Domestic and wild turkeys, North America. Relatively rare. Gametocytes are elongate and sausage-shaped, partially encircling the host cell nucleus, and frequently in close contact with it. The life cycle is unknown. No pathogenesis has been ascribed to it.

Haemoproteus nettionis. *Hosts:* Domestic duck and goose, and other wild ducks, geese and swans. Lists of species which may be infected have been given by Herman (1954) and Fallis & Wood (1957). World wide in distribution and reasonably common. A survey by Bennett & Fallis (1960) of 3000 birds in Algonquin Park, Canada, showed *Haemoproteus* in 26 per cent of them.

Gametocytes are elongate and sausage-shaped, partially, and in some cases almost completely, encircling the host cell nucleus. The cell nucleus may also be displaced. Pigment granules are usually coarse and tend to be grouped at the poles of the parasite.

Life-cycle. Fallis and Wood (1957) demonstrated that *Culicoides* (possibly *piliferus*) could transmit the infection. Oökinetes, oocysts and sporozoites were found 14–21 days later. Fallis & Bennett (1960) also demonstrated that *Haemoproteus canachites* of the spruce grouse developed in the biting midge *Culicoides spagnumensis*.

Haemoproteus nettionis is only slightly, if at all, pathogenic.

Haemoproteus sacharovi. *Hosts:* Domestic pigeon, mourning dove and turtle dove; North America and Europe.

Gametocytes are distinctive in that they completely fill the host cell when they are mature; they distort it and push the host cell nucleus to one side. They also possess little pigment compared with the other species of *Haemoproteus.* The natural vectors of this species are not known. It has been transmitted by *Pseudolynchia canarensis,* though Levine (1961) suggests that a species of *Culicoides* may also be concerned.

The pathogenic effect of *H. sacharovi* is low, though it is reported to cause hepatomegaly in pigeon squabs.

Genus: Leucocytozoon Danilewsky, 1890

Parasites of this genus undergo schizogony in the endothelial and parenchymatous cells of the liver, heart, kidney and other organs of avian hosts. Large schizonts are produced. The gametogonous stages occur in the circulating blood, and the infected host cells become grossly distorted and assume a spindle shape. No pigment is produced. The vectors are black flies of the genus *Simulium.* A check list of species and their host has been given by Coatney (1937), while Herman (1944) has listed the North American species. The more common forms which occur are:

Leucocytozoon simondi Mathis and Leger, 1910

Leucocytozoon smithi Laveran and Lucet, 1905

Leucocytozoon caulleryi Mathis and Leger, 1909

Leucocytozoon simondi. *Hosts:* Domestic and wild ducks and geese; North America, Europe and the East. Relatively common.

Life-cycle. The endogenous developmental cycle has been described by Huff (1942) and Fallis *et al.* (1956). Sporozoites injected by the *Simulium* fly are carried by the blood stream to various cells of the body, two types of schizonts being produced. The first asexual generation takes place in the Kupffer cells of the liver. The schizonts are small, and they produce merozoites, some of which may enter blood cells to become gametocytes, while others initiate hepatic schizonts and megaloschizonts. The hepatic schizonts occur in the parenchyma liver cells, and they produce a number of cytomeres, which, by multiple fission, form a large number of small merozoites. The megaloschizonts are more numerous than the hepatic forms and apparently develop in lymphoid cells or macrophages. They are found in the brain, liver, lungs, kidney, intestinal tissue and lymphoid tissues 4–6 days after infection. As their name suggests, they are large, 60 μ–160 μ in diameter, and they contain a large number of cytomeres which in turn produce a much larger number of merozoites. With rupture of the hepatic schizonts and the megaloschizonts, merozoites are released into the blood and these appear as gametocytes in the peripheral circulation 6–7 days after infection. The majority of merozoites probably develop into gametocytes, but it is presumed that some may initiate further asexual reproduction. The identity of the host cell for the gametocytes has been debated for a number of years. One of the problems in this is that the cells containing the mature gametocytes are so distorted that their origin is difficult to determine. Huff (1942) considered the cells to be lymphocytes, or lymphocytes which have been stimulated to undergo transformation by the presence of the parasite. Other studies by Fallis *et al.* (1951) indicated that young gametocytes may occur in both lymphocytes and erythrocytes, and a similar observation was made by Cook (1954). The latter author concluded that gametocytes develop to maturity only in cells of the red blood series. An alternative opinion was expressed by Savage & Isa (1959), who suggested that young gametocytes selected monocytes and macrophages for development.

Mature gametocytes are elongate, oval bodies, usually 14 μ–15 μ in length but may reach up to 22 μ, by 4·5 μ–5·5 μ. The infected host cell is grossly distended and elongated, and it may measure up to 48 μ in length. The nucleus of the host cell is elongate and forms a long, thin, dark crescent along one side of the parasitised cell. Occasionally, round forms of the parasite occur in undistorted host cells, and there is no evidence that these differ functionally from the elongate forms. The macrogametes stain dark blue with Romanowsky stains, the nucleus is compact, and several vacuoles may occur in the darkly stained cytoplasm. The microgametocytes are slightly smaller than the macrogametes, the cytoplasm stains less deeply, usually a pale blue colour, and the nucleus is diffuse and stains pale pink.

The vectors of *L. simondi* are members of the genus *Simulium*. *Simulium venustum* has been recognised as such for some time, and *S. croxtoni*, *S. euryadminiculum* and *S. rugglesi* were added to the list by Fallis *et al.* (1956). Development in the insect vector is essentially the same as *Plasmodium* in the mosquito.

Pathogenesis. Leucocytozoon simondi is markedly pathogenic for young ducks and geese. The clinical signs of leucocytozoonosis are sudden in onset, and death may occur within a day or so. Ducklings are listless, anorexic, show rapid breathing (due to the large number of megaloschizonts in the capillaries of the lung) and may show nervous derangements prior to death. The disease in older birds is less acute and develops more slowly. Birds become emaciated and listless but seldom die in less than 4 days from the onset of the disease.

Diagnosis of *L. simondi* in ducks is based on the demonstration of the gametocytes in blood smears or, and more satisfactorily, the megaloschizonts in smears of the lung. There is no known effective treatment for

L. simondi infection, and control consists of controlling *Simulium* flies. Young ducklings should be isolated from the older birds since these may serve as carriers. Total freedom from the disease is only achieved when ducklings and goslings are raised in regions where black flies do not occur.

Leucocytozoon smithi. *Hosts:* Domestic and wild turkeys; North America, Europe. This is a markedly pathogenic species for young turkeys; heavy losses due to it have been recorded in North America. The general prevalence ranges from about 20 per cent to more than 80 per cent in domestic and wild turkeys, especially in areas where conditions are good for the breeding of *Simulium* flies.

Morphologically, this parasite resembles *L. simondi*. The mature gametocytes are elongate, approximately 20 μ–22 μ by 6 μ, and the host cell is greatly distorted and elongated and may measure up to 45 μ by 14 μ. The nucleus of the host cell is elongated, forming a dark band on one side of the parasites, and this is frequently split to form a dark band on each side of the parasite.

The endogenous developmental cycle is comparable to that of *L. simondi*, but megaloschizonts have not been observed. Hepatic schizonts (10 μ–20 μ in diameter) occur in the cells of the liver parenchyma and contain cytomeres which produce large numbers of merozoites. The prepatent period of infection is approximately 9 days. The vectors of *L. smithi* are *Simulium occidentale*, *S. nigroparvum* and *S. slossonae* in which the same developmental cycle occurs as in *L. simondi*.

Pathogenesis of L. smithi. This parasite may be extremely pathogenic for young turkeys; very heavy losses having been reported from various parts of the world, the death rate reaching up to 90 per cent in some flocks. The clinical signs consist of anorexia, emaciation, debility, while leg weakness and incoordination occur in the later stages of the disease. In fulminating outbreaks of the disease, birds usually die within 2 or 3 days after the onset of clinical signs, but if not, some undergo a chronic type of infection where there is a persistent cough and moist bronchitis, while others may appear completely recovered. In all cases recovered birds remain as carriers.

On post mortem there is jaundice, congestion of the duodenum, splenic enlargement and congestion of the lungs and kidneys.

The diagnosis of turkey leucocytozoonosis is based on similar evidence as that for *L. smithi*. For treatment Bierer (1950) has recommended sulphaquinoxaline; however, this needs confirmation as to its efficacy. Prevention and control are the same as for *L. simondi*.

Leucocytozoon caulleryi. *Hosts:* Domestic chicken, Far East and South Carolina (Levine, 1961).

The mature gametocytes of this species are round, approximately 15 μ in diameter; the host cell is not distorted as in the other species but is enlarged, measuring up to 20 μ in diameter. The host cell nucleus is compressed to one side of the cell forming a band extending about $\frac{1}{3}$ of the way around the parasite.

Disease due to this parasite has been reported in Japan by Akiba (1960). He demonstrated that *Culicoides arakawae* was probably the natural vector of *L. caulleryi* in that ookinetes, oocysts and sporozoites were demonstrable in specimens of this fly which had fed upon infected chickens. He was able also to demonstrate gametocytes in chickens 14 days after the injection of a suspension of sporozoites. An outbreak of leucocytozoonosis in chickens in Taiwan in which 20 per cent of the chickens died was reported by Liu (1958). Post-mortem changes included anaemia, haemorrhages in the lungs, liver and kidneys, enlargement of the spleen and white spots on the heart muscle. Megaloschizonts were found in the kidney, lung and heart, but hepatic schizonts were not.

Other species of *Leucocytozoon* which have been reported include *L. marchouxi* Mathis and Leger, 1910 (doves and pigeons), *L. sabrazesi* Mathis and Leger, 1910 (chicken; Far East), *L. neavei* Balfour, 1906 (guinea fowl) and *L. bonasae* Clarke, 1935 (ruffed grouse).

FAMILY: BABESIIDAE POCHE, 1913

Kudo (1966) considers this family to be one of the three of the order Haemosporidia, containing blood protozoa which lack pigment granules and are minute parasites of erythrocytes. He includes the two genera *Babesia* and *Theileria* in the family. Neitz (1956) has proposed that the genera *Babesia* and *Theileria* be assigned separately to two families, *Babesiidae* and *Theileridae*, these being families of a sub-order *Piroplasmidea* Wenyon, 1926. The two family scheme is adopted in the present text.

However, the placing of these piroplasms in the Haemosporidia, and indeed in the Sporozoa, may require reconsideration since there is little evidence that they behave as do the majority of the members of the class Sporozoa. Cheissin & Poljansky (1963) have declared that piroplasms should be included in the Plasmodroma as a separate order, the Piroplasmatida, of the class Sarcodina. They base this consideration on the fact that the piroplasms have only an asexual type of reproduction, show no alternation of generations, possess amoeboid movements and lack any developmental stages which possess kinetic elements. Though these have been reported, Rudzinska & Trager (1960) were unable to find such structures in electron micrographs of *Babesia rodhaini* of the mouse.

Organisms of the family Babesiidae are round to pyriform, amoeboid, forms occurring in the erythrocytes. They multiply by binary fission, or schizogony, in the red blood cell. The vectors are ixodid ticks, or, in avian forms, argasid ticks. Some authors differentiate three genera or three sub-genera according to the number of organisms which result from the division in the erythrocytes; thus, in *Babesia* two forms result from division, in *Nuttallia* four and in *Aegyptianella* eight to sixteen forms occur. Other authors also divide the genus *Babesia* into *Babesia* and *Babesiella*.

Genus: Babesia Starcovici, 1893

Organisms multiply in the erythrocytes by asexual division, producing two, four or more non-pigmented amoeboid parasites. When stained with Romanowsky stains they show a blue cytoplasm and a red chromatin mass usually at one pole. A string of chromatin granules may extend from the larger mass. Characteristically, they are pear-shaped forms lying at an angle with the narrow ends in apposition.

Some eighteen species of *Babesia* have been recognised, and in general they fall into 2 major groups; large forms with an average length of more than 3 microns and small forms which have an average length of less than 2·5 microns.

Life-cycle of Babesia. Multiplication of *Babesia* organisms in the vertebrate host occurs in the erythrocytes by a budding process (schizogony) to form two, four or more trophozoites. These are liberated from the erythrocyte and invade other cells, the process being repeated until a large percentage of red blood cells are parasitised. Occasionally a cell shows multiple infection with a large number of trophozoites, but it is considered that this represents a series of binary fissions or a multiple invasion of the cell. The blood forms are readily transmissible by mechanical means to another animal, and these then initiate a further cycle of asexual reproduction.

Under natural conditions the *Babesia* species are transmitted by ticks, the first demonstration of this being by Smith & Kilborne (1893) for the causal agent (*Babesia bigemina*) of Texas fever. This observation was a major landmark in the history of arthropod-borne diseases. The development of *Babesia* in ticks has occasioned much work and speculation. Dennis (1932) maintained that sexual reproduction occurred with *Babesia bigemina* in the tick *Boophilus annulatus*, but since his work the idea of a phase of sexual reproduction has been replaced by one supporting asexual reproduction.

Essentially, development and transmission of *Babesia* spp. in ticks is either by transovarian transmission or by stage to stage transmission. The former is the only mode of transmission for one host ticks, since following the attachment of larvae the rest of the tick developmental stages occur on the same animal. With two or three host ticks, stage to stage transmission becomes of importance, adult stages transmitting infection which they acquired as nymphs, or nymphs doing the same with infection acquired as larvae.

The account of the life cycle of *Babesia bigemina* in the tick *Boophilus microplus* given by Riek (1964) provides a very satisfactory account of ovarian transmission of a *Babesia* spp.

Transovarian Transmission of Babesia. The rate of development in the tick is dependent on the environmental temperature; it is much more rapid in ticks held at 28°C than those at 25°C. Riek (1964) considered that parasites in red blood cells ingested early in the engorgement of a tick either were destroyed or their development was retarded until the tick was replete. Immediately on repletion erythrocytic forms of the parasite were seen lying free in large numbers in the gut contents. Many were irregular in shape with long rays or pseudopodia and frequently were clumped together. A further stage in development consisted of a spherical body, $3\,\mu$–$5\,\mu$ in diameter, with a large vacuole surrounded by a thin layer of cytoplasm containing a single peripheral nuclear mass. Two other forms of spherical bodies were observed. The first, infrequent in appearance, showed three to four separate chromatin dots on the periphery around which the cytoplasm concentrated leaving a central vacuole. Riek considered that this form could divide into discrete elongated bodies, $4\,\mu$–$6\cdot9\,\mu$ by $1\,\mu$–$2\cdot1\,\mu$, with a central chromatin dot. A second spherical form possessed two nuclei, one elongated and extending around the periphery of the vacuolated organism and the other a round mass at the opposite pole. Riek was unable to observe division of the second spherical form into elongate bodies. He suggested that these early stages might represent part of a gametogenous cycle and syngamy with the production of a zygote. He based this opinion on several considerations, including the fact that a large number of parasite stages are taken in by the tick vector but only a minority undergo further development. These are almost exclusively oval or spherical forms. Riek suggests that the spherical form with two nuclei may result from a union of an elongated form with the spherical form with a single nuclear mass. The result of this union may be a blunt, curved, cigar-shaped body, $8\,\mu$–$10\,\mu$ long by $3\cdot5\,\mu$–$4\cdot5\,\mu$ wide. This form was found in the gut contents at the end of the first 24 hours of development. The chromatin of the cigar-shaped body was discrete and stained intensely red while the cytoplasm was intensely blue. It assumed an ovoid shape as it grew, and subsequently it became a spherical body with a vacuolated central cytoplasm with chromatin spread on the periphery. Between 24 and 48 hours after repletion, the first evidence of development in epithelial cells of gut was found, being indicated by an irregular, spindle-shaped body with a more or less centrally placed single chromatin mass. Following invasion of the epithelial cell the parasitic stage appeared to undergo multiple fission. Development proceeded rapidly, and the chromatin was distributed in the cell in a number of small dots; each dot later collected a ring of cytoplasm around it to produce a number of separate, oval or globular elements $3\cdot2\,\mu$–$6\cdot5\,\mu$ in diameter. Between 40 and 48 hours after repletion, large numbers of these spherical forms, 'fission bodies', were seen in smear preparations from the gut of ticks. The 'fission body' grew within the epithelial cell, and ultimately the cytoplasm and chromatin became separated into vacuolated bodies, these being contained within the limiting membrane of the parasite. The mature 'fission body' contained up to 200 forms which, when liberated in making smears, measured $5\,\mu$–$8\,\mu$ by $3\,\mu$–$4\,\mu$. The mature 'fission body' ruptured from the epithelial cell and liberated club-shaped bodies or 'vermicules' into the lumen of the gut. Initially, the vermicule had a homogeneous cytoplasm, and the nucleus lay to the broader end to give a cap-like appearance. Vermicules migrated through the gut wall to the haemolymph, and as they aged the anterior red staining area disappeared, the cytoplasm becoming vacuolated. At this stage they measured 9 μ–13 μ by 2 μ–2·9 μ. By 72 hours after repletion, such forms were present in the haemolymph, the ovary and other tissues of the body, while numerous fission bodies in various stages of development were still found in the epithial cells of the gut. Vermicules occurred in mature ova from 72 hours onwards. In other studies Riek (1964) found that transmission of infection to cattle by larvae, developed from eggs of infected ticks, occurred only with eggs laid after the 96th hour after repletion.

A second cycle of development was initiated about 96 hours after infection. This involved the entry of vermicules into cells of the Malpighian tubules and the haemolymph, and here they underwent further multiple fission. The cycle undertaken appeared to be essentially the same as that occurring in the epithelial cells of the gut except that these cells were not involved.

In the initial development in the egg of the tick, the vermicules were present in yoke material. For further development vermicules entered the epithelial cells of the gut of the larvae, and here the same sequence of development occurred as was seen in the Malpighian tubule cells of the parent female. Further vermicules were produced by this phase of development, and these were liberated into the gut lumen or haemolymph of the larva.

Development of the *Babesia* to the infective stage for the bovine is dependent on a moult of the tick from the larval to the nymphal stage, and Riek was unable to observe transmission of *B. bigemina* to the bovine before 8–10 days after larval attachment of the tick *Boophilus microplus*. After the moult to the nymphal stage, vermicules were found in the cells of the salivary gland, these being similar to those in the haemolymph. The vermicules assumed a spherical form, they enlarged and their chromatin became scattered in the cell and broken up into a large number of small dots, many hundreds being found in a single cell. Cytoplasm was organised around the chromatin dots to produce spherical or pyriform organisms, which Riek regarded as mature, infective forms ready for liberation from the salivary gland. Such forms, too, were comparable in appearance to the pyriform stages found in the bovine erythrocyte.

The transovarian mode of development and transmission described by Regendanz & Reichenow (1933) for *Babesia canis* of the dog in *Dermacentor reticulatus* is essentially the same as the above. Following entry of the veriform stage into the egg, it divides a few times to form some very small, round individuals, and they do not undergo further development until the larval tick has hatched and undergone a moult. Then the small forms enter the nymphal salivary glands, and by a series of binary fissions give rise to thousands of minute vermiform infective parasites. As well as occurring in the nymphal stage, this process also takes place in the adult tick.

Stage to Stage Transmission of Babesia. In a study of the stage to stage transmission of *Babesia canis* by *Rhipicephalus sanguineus*, Shortt (1936) found no evidence of sexual reproduction. Multiplication of developmental forms was seen in phagocytes which lay contiguous to the hyperdermis in the body cavity of the tick. 'Pseudocysts' of organisms occurred about 7 days after the nymph had dropped off the host, and by 11–15 days club-shaped organisms, 9 μ by 2 μ, were present in the cysts. The club-shaped forms were liberated from the host cell and migrated to the muscle sheaths of the nymphal tick where they penetrated muscle cells, rounded up and divided repeatedly to form a large number of small, ovoid forms about 1·2 μ in length. Subsequent development occurred when the recently metamorphosed adult fed on a dog; the parasites migrated to the salivary glands, entered the cells of the acini and underwent repeated binary fission to form the large numbers of small, ovoid, infective stages.

The question of sexual reproduction by *Babesia* spp. in ticks has yet to be clarified. Originally, Dennis (1932) described the formation of isogametes with fusion of these to form a motile zygote (oökinete) which passed through the intestinal wall and invaded the ovary and then the ova of the tick. Comparable developmental stages were observed by Petrov (1941) in *Ixodes ricinus* infected with *Babesia bovis*, but Muratov & Kheisin (1959) failed to find it with *Babesia bigemina* in two species of ticks, Polyanskii & Kheisin (1959) failed to find it in *Ixodes ricinus* infected with *Babesia bovis* and Shortt (1936) failed to observe it for *Babesia canis* in *Dermacentor reticulatus* or *Rhipicephalus sanguineus*.

Host Specificity of Babesia. Rosenbusch (1927) suggested that *Babesia* organisms were, in reality, parasites of ticks and did not necessarily require mammals as alternative hosts. Support for this idea came from the fact that *Babesia* infection of ticks can be maintained when ticks are fed over a long period on hosts refractory to the parasite. Thus, ticks reared for five generations on hedgehogs may still be capable of infecting dogs with *Babesia canis*. Enigk (1944a) found that equine piroplasms could be retained for several generations in ticks fed on hosts other than horses, and Markov & Abramov (1956) reported that *Babesia ovis* (of sheep) was still present fourteen generations later in ticks maintained on rabbits. However, there is increasing evidence that the babesias are not as strictly host-specific as was previously thought. Callow (Riek, 1964) has observed inapparent infections with *Babesia bigemina* in sheep, goat and horse, and the progeny of female ticks fed on such animals were infective for cattle. Enigk & Friedhoff (1962) were able to transmit *Babesia divergens* of cattle to splenectomised red deer, fallow deer, roe deer and moufflons, and *Babesia divergens* has been found in chimpanzees following the injection of heparinised blood containing this parasite (Garnham & Bray, 1959). Further weight to the lack of specificity of the babesias is given by the studies of Skravalo & Deanovic (1957), who observed a natural infection with *Babesia bovis* in a splenectomised man. The hereditary transmission of *Babesia* spp. in ticks postulated by previous workers may, in fact, be due to the acquisition of infection by the ticks from a host carrying an occult infection.

Babesia of Cattle

The five species of *Babesia* occurring in cattle are:

Babesia bigemina (Smith and Kilborne, 1893)

Babesia bovis (Babes, 1888)

Babesia divergens (M'Fadyean and Stockman, 1911)

Babesia argentina (Lignieres, 1909)

Babesia major Sergeant, Donatien, Parrot, Lestoquard and Plantureux, 1926

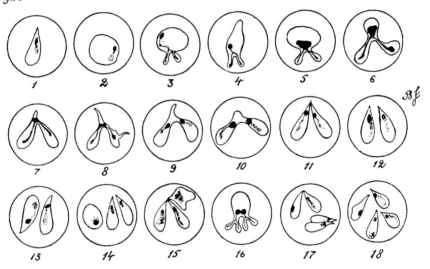

FIG. 281. *Babesia bigemina* of Cattle: Method of Multiplication in Red Blood Corpuscles (× ca. 3000). (From Wenyon, 1926)

Babesia bigemina. This organism is the cause of an important disease of cattle called cattle tick fever, red water fever, piroplasmosis and, formerly in North America, Texas fever. *Hosts:* Principally the bovine, also in zebu, water buffalo. (Levine, 1961, also gives deer (*Mazama americana reperticia*) and white-tailed deer (*Odocoelius virginianus chiriquensis*) as hosts.) Occurs throughout the tropics and subtropical areas such as Central and South America, North and South Africa, Australia and southern Europe.

Morphology: Babesia bigemina is a large piroplasm, 4 μ–5 μ in length by about 2 μ wide, round forms 2 μ–3 μ in diameter. The organisms are characteristically pear-shaped and lie in pairs forming an acute angle in the red blood corpuscle. Round, oval or irregularly shaped forms may occur depending on the stage of the development of the parasite in the red cell.

Developmental Cycle. Multiplication in the vertebrate host has been discussed previously (p. 698), and the developmental cycle in the tick has been described by Riek (1964) (p. 698).

The following ticks have been incriminated as vectors: One host ticks: *Boophilus annulatus,* North America; *Boophilus calcaratus,* North Africa; *Boophilus decoloratus,* South Africa; *Boophilus microplus,* Australia, Panama, South America: Two host ticks: *Rhipicephalus evertsi,* South Africa; *Rhipicephalus bursa,* South Africa: Three host ticks: *Haemaphysalis punctata,* Europe and Eurasia; *Rhipicephalus appendiculatus,* South Africa.

There is no conclusive evidence that *B. bigemina* can be transmitted mechanically by blood-sucking arthropods. On rare occasions it seems that intrauterine transmission may occur from mother to foetus, but this mode of infection does not seem to be of any significant importance in the general epidemiology of babesiosis.

Pathogenesis. In young animals the infection is frequently symptomless and associated with a low parasite density. There are a few reports of fatal infection in newborn calves (Smith & Kilborne, 1893), and Hall (1960) has reported the development of babesiosis in calves, born of non-immune parents, when they were inoculated with infective blood or exposed to infected ticks at 12–55 days of age. The natural resistance of the young calf to infection usually disappears at 9–12 months of age.

The incubation period after infection, or exposure to infected ticks, is 1–2 weeks, and the first evidence of the disease is a spectacular rise in body temperature to 106–108°F. The high fever lasts from 2–7, or more, days, and during this period a profound anaemia frequently develops. There is haemoglobinuria and cardiac palpitation. Initially, there is a profuse diarrhoea, and this is later followed by marked constipation. At the height of fever, up to 75 per cent of red blood cells may be destroyed, and the mortality may be very high in acute cases, death occurring 4–8 days after the onset of clinical signs. Animals which survive the acute phase go into a chronic disease syndrome which may extend over several weeks with an irregular course and intermittent temperature rises, at times reaching 104–105°F. Animals become thin and emaciated, but there is usually no marked haemoglobinuria in this stage, and finally the animal recovers.

A cerebral form of *B. bigemina* infection has been reported in cattle in Nyasaland by Zlotnik (1953). The onset of disease is sudden, the temperature reaching 106–107°F in a few hours, and death may occur within 12–36 hours after the onset of clinical signs. The parasites appear to accumulate, and probably multiply, in the cerebral capillaries since organisms are only rarely seen in blood smears.

At post mortem the lesions consist of subcutaneous and intramuscular oedema with icterus, the fat is yellow and gelatinous and the blood thin and watery. On sedimentation, the blood plasma contains haemoglobulin, and the urine in the bladder is frequently red or dark brown. The spleen is markedly enlarged with a soft, dark splenic pulp; the liver is enlarged, pale and yellowish, and the gall bladder is distended with thick, dark bile. In the cerebral form there is perivascular, perineuronal and interstitial oedema throughout the brain and spinal cord.

Immunology of B. bigemina *Infection*

An inverse age susceptibility occurs in *Babesia* infections, young animals being naturally resistant while older animals are fully susceptible. Calves in an enzootic area are free of clinical signs and have a very low parasite density. The passive transfer of maternal antibodies via the colostrum is probably responsible in part for this resistance; however, Riek (1963) suggests that additional explanations are necessary since animals of several months of age develop only a low parasitaemia when they are introduced from a clean to an infected area.

Breed of Animal. It has been suggested that some races of cattle are more resistant to *B. bigemina* than others (*Bos indicus* has been suggested to be more resistant than *Bos taurus*); however, Arnold (1948) reported no difference in the severity of *Babesia* infections when either Brahma or European breed animals were introduced into an infected area in Jamaica. Daly & Hall (1955) observed similar reactions in all breeds tested with blood-transmitted infections of *B. bigemina.*

Acquired Immunity. The immunity in babesiosis is a premunition. The immunity persists as long as the animal remains a latent carrier of the infection, and in the case of *B. bigemina* infection a period of up to 12 years has been demonstrated for this latency. If parasites disappear as the result of autosterilisation, effective therapy, or removal from the *Babesia* area, the animal becomes fully susceptible. In endemic areas, however, due to the repeated reinfection from infected ticks, it is usual for animals to retain their immunity for a considerable period. Nevertheless, there is some evidence that recovery from the disease with elimination of the organism results in a sterile immunity for a substantial time. Sergent *et al.* (1945) reported that the elimination of sources of infection for *B. bigemina* resulted in the loss of immunity 14–22 months afterwards, and Arnold (1948) found that immunity disappeared in 3–4 years in the absence of reinfection. Further discussion on this aspect is given by Riek (1963).

The spleen plays an important role in maintaining the immune state to *Babesia* infection, since immunity may be broken down by removal of the spleen. With *B. bigemina* a fatal infection may be precipitated by this procedure.

Serological studies of *B. bigemina* infection have been carried out by

Mahoney (1962). Antibodies were detectable 7–21 days after tick transmitted infection, and they persisted for more than 10 months. Antibodies may be present with no detectable parasites in the blood, but such blood can be shown to be infective by injection into splenectomised calves. At a later stage antibodies occur when blood will not create infection in susceptible animals.

Diagnosis of B. bigemina *Infection.* Diagnosis is based on the clinical signs and confirmed by the detection of parasites in the peripheral blood. Both thick and thin blood smears may be employed, being stained by one of the Romanowsky stains; however, the organisms may not always be apparent, and it may be necessary to examine a number of smears to establish their presence. In the cerebral form, examination of cerebral capillaries is necessary. In endemic areas high fever associated with haemoglobinuria and anaemia is suggestive of *Babesia* infection, and frequently animals are treated without recourse to blood examination. For wider surveys the complement fixation test of Mahoney (1962) may be of value, especially in those animals where the level of parasitaemia is low.

Treatment of B. bigemina *Infection*

Trypan blue. Dose; about 100 ml. of a 1 per cent–2 per cent solution is given intravenously in normal saline; frequently one injection is enough but two treatments may be necessary, given on successive days. Care should be taken to insure that none of the material is given subcutaneously, this producing a marked reaction in the subcutaneous tissues. Following treatment mucous membranes and muscle turn blue; recovery is relatively slow.

Acriflavine. Dose; 20 ml. of a 5 per cent aqueous solution intravenously or 5 ml. of a 5 per cent citrated solution intramuscularly.

Phenamidine (4,4-diamidinodiphenyl ether). Dose, 12 mg. per kg. subcutaneously in a 40 per cent aqueous solution. This compound eliminates all the parasites from the animal, and treated animals are no longer premune. Occasional cases of toxicity may result from its use, these being anaphylactic in type, but usually the animal recovers.

Berenil (4,4-diamidinodiazoaminobenzene aceturate). Dose, 2–3·5 mg. per kg. by deep intramuscular injection.

Pirevan (Acapron, Babesan, Piroparv, Acaprin, Piroplasmin) (quinuronium sulphate) [6:6′-di(N-methylquinolyl) urea dimethosulphate]. Dose; 1 ml. of a 5 per cent solution subcutaneously per 50 kg. body weight. Intravenous injections are contraindicated. The toxic reactions consist of vasodilation with sweating, salivation, diarrhoea, urination and sometimes collapse and death. The drug has a specific action on the parasympathetic nervous system. Pirevan has been used extensively for the treatment of babesiosis.

Diampron (3,3′-diamidinocarbanilide di-isethionate). Introduced for the treatment of *B. divergens* infection, but it is also effective against *B. bigemina* (Shone *et al.*, 1961). Dose, 10 mg. per kg. intramuscularly or subcutaneously, preferably by deep intramuscular injection.

Control of B. bigemina *Infection.* Since the natural transmission of *B. bigemina* is dependent on certain species of ticks, infection can be prevented by adequate tick control measures which keep animals free from tick infestation. This can be done by the regular dipping of cattle, this method having resulted in the elimination of *B. bigemina* from the United States. The methods and frequency of dipping are factors which must be determined for the local area and are considered on page 492.

The inverse age resistance of cattle to *B. bigemina* has been exploited for control by immunisation. Young animals are inoculated, preferrably with a mild strain of *B. bigemina*, and the subsequent infection, if necessary, is controlled by trypan blue. This method is especially useful when cattle are to be shipped to endemic areas.

Recent work has indicated that piroplasms from carrier animals may show a loss of virulence, and injection of these into calves may produce a lower level of immunity than expected. Tsur (1961) has confirmed that blood from latent carriers of *B. bigemina* may not consistently infect susceptible calves.

A further factor in such immunisation is the transmission of maternal immunity to calves. Hall (1963) has shown that passively immunised calves may be refractory to infection, and consequently artificial immunisation should be delayed until the effect of this has disappeared.

Babesia bovis. *Hosts:* Cattle, also roe deer and stag (Levine, 1961). Characteristically, this species occurs in southern Europe, and it has also been reported from Africa, Asia and the East. At one time it was considered to extend into northern Europe, including Great Britain; however, investigations by Simitch *et al.* (1955) and Davies *et al.* (1958) showed that the northern European form was *Babesia divergens*. It is also possible that *Babesia berbera* is a synonym of *B. bovis*. In view of the confusion in the literature regarding *B. bovis* and *B. divergens*, previous accounts of *B. bovis* may be inaccurate.

Morphology. A small piroplasm, 2·4 μ by 1·5 μ and slightly larger than *B. divergens*. In further contrast to *B. divergens* there are usually no divergent forms lying superficially in the red blood corpuscle, and vacuolated signet ring forms are particularly common, consisting of a centrally placed vacuole with a nuclear mass at one pole.

Developmental Cycle. The vectors of *B. bovis* include *Ixodes ricinus*, a ubiquitous tick in Europe, *Ixodes persulcatus*, which has a more northerly and easterly distribution, *Boophilus calcaratus* and *Rhipicephalus bursa* (Simitch *et al.*, 1955). However, previous information on the transmission of *B. bovis* in ticks is subject to reservations in view of the lack of specific identification of the organism.

The pathogenicity of *B. bovis* is probably similar to that of *B. divergens* and will be described along with this species.

Babesia divergens. *Hosts:* Cattle. It is essentially a northern European form, and Simitch *et al.* (1955) and Davies *et al.* (1958) have differentiated it from the more southern European and Danube Basin form, *B. bovis.* Enigk & Friedhoff (1962a) have demonstrated the transmission of *B. divergens* to splenectomised moufflon, fallow deer, red deer and roe deer. Organisms were demonstrated microscopically in these animals, and infections were subsequently transmitted back to calves. The infection persisted in red deer for 8 months, but sheep and goats were not susceptible to the infection. These authors considered that the wild game may serve as natural reservoirs for *B. divergens.*

Enigk & Friedhoff (1962b) discovered a new species of *Babesia* of the roe deer, *Babesia capreoli.* This was transmissible to other roe deer, but splenectomised cattle and sheep were refractory to the infection.

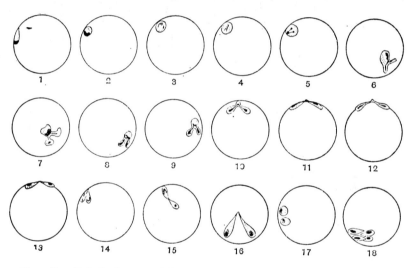

FIG. 282. *Babesia divergens* of Cattle (× ca. 3000). (From Wenyon, 1926)

Morphology. *B. divergens* is smaller than *B. bovis*, 1·5 μ by 0·4 μ, and commonly appears as paired, divergent forms lying superficially on the red blood cell. Other forms may be stout and pyriform, measuring 2 μ by 1 μ, some may be circular, and a few are vacuolated and up to 2 μ in diameter. Garnham (1962) has suggested that *Babesia pitheci* of African monkeys may be a form of *B. divergens* of cattle.

The Developmental Cycle of B. divergens. This has yet to be studied in detail. It is transmitted by *Ixodes ricinus*, and Joyner *et al.* (1963) have demonstrated transovarian transmission of *B. divergens* through larvae of *I. ricinus.* Arthur (1966) has also implicated *Dermacentor reticulatus* as a host tick.

Cases of piroplasmosis are associated with the activity of the tick. In

Great Britain where *I. ricinus* may show a bi-annual activity, cases are to be expected in late spring and autumn. Serious disease may occur in animals that have been moved into an endemic area. As with *B. bigemina*, animals up to one year of age seldom show clinical signs of the infection, though they serve as carriers for the infection and as a source of infection for ticks.

Pathogenesis. The disease entity produced by *B. divergens* or *B. bovis* is less severe than that caused by *B. bigemina*. The incubation period is 4–10 days, and the first clinical sign is a marked elevation of temperature, up to 106°F, which persists for 2–3 days. Within 48 hours of the peak of fever, haemoglobinuria is observed, followed by jaundice of the mucous membrane and palpitations of the heart. In severe infections death may occur. If an animal survives the acute syndrome, gastrointestinal upsets become evident by a thin and watery diarrhoea which is followed by a marked constipation, with the faeces being bile-stained. The animal progressively loses flesh, appetite is reduced, and death may occur if this phase is prolonged, though recovery from this clinical entity is not uncommon.

Diagnosis. This is based on the clinical signs, the history of the area and the demonstration of the parasites in blood smears. These are not readily found but are to be expected in their greatest number during the period of high fever. Recovered animals are immune, and Davies *et al.* (1958) reported that two heifers which had lost their infection with *B. divergens* remained immune to reinfection despite the lack of organisms.

Treatment. Both *B. divergens* and *B. bovis* fail to respond to trypan blue. Otherwise, the compounds used for *B. bigemina* are effective for the two small forms. Diampron has been shown to have therapeutic effect against *B. divergens* by Beveridge *et al.* (1960).

Control. This is essentially the same as for *B. bigemina* and consists of tick control and, where indicated, the immunisation of younger animals with blood from infected animals. Vaccination against *Babesia* is regularly carried out in Sweden, and Bodin & Hildar (1963) have reported that of 78,000 innoculated animals, 0·72 per cent showed clinical reactions and 0·007 per cent died. In a study of vaccinated animals at pasture, a morbidity rate of 12 per cent in nonvaccinated animals was compared with one of 0·12 per cent in vaccinated animals.

Babesia argentina. *Hosts:* Cattle. Distributed in South and Central America and Australia.

The exact relationship of this small species to the others must still await critical study. Riek (1963) states that on morphological grounds alone there is little reason to regard *B. argentina*, *B. bovis* and *B. berbera* as separate species, and in preliminary observations with a complement fixation test he found immunological similarity between *B. argentina* and *B. berbera* but a complete difference between these two and *B. divergens*. Contrary views were presented by Sergent *et al.* (1945), who considered

B. major, *B. berbera* and *B. bovis* distinct species since in cross immunity tests they failed to immunise against one another.

Morphology. In general, *B. argentina* resembles *B. bovis*, though the parasites are slightly more robust. The pyriform forms are 2 μ by 1·5 μ and usually lie in the centre of the erythrocyte, though occasionally peripheral forms are found.

Developmental Cycle. This is similar to that of the other small piroplasms of cattle, the tick vector being *Boophilus microplus*.

Pathogenesis. In Australia *B. argentina* is responsible for the majority of field outbreaks of babesiosis (Riek, 1963). It is relatively uncommon in animals under 12 months of age, and this age group is predominantly infected by *B. bigemina*. In animals over 2 years of age, however, *B. argentina* is the main infection. Under Australian conditions *B. argentina* is the more pathogenic species (Pierce, 1956), and cattle inoculated with the smaller form showed twice the mortality of those infected with *B. bigemina*.

The pathological entity is comparable to that for *B. divergens*. High fever is evident about a week to 10 days after infection, and shortly afterwards haemoglobinuria occurs. A cerebral form of disease due to *B. argentina* has been recorded by Callow & McGavin (1963). Post-mortem changes consisted of congestion of the grey and white matter of the brain and generalised dilation of capillaries by red blood cells, the majority of which were infected with *B. argentina*. In addition, perivascular, perineuronal and interstitial oedema occurred throughout the brain and cord. Clinical signs varied, consisting of convulsions, incoordination and coma. Other studies by Callow & Johnston (1963) suggested that the brain capillaries may be a predilection site for *B. argentina* in healthy animals. Of 88 artificially infected animals, 76 showed such infection, and of 458 cattle from an endemic area, 299 contained such organisms in the brain capillaries.

Recovered animals are premune to infection. Pierce (1956) has shown that the minimum time after which cattle again become susceptible is 5–6 months.

Treatment and Control. This is the same as for *B. divergens*. Control is based on the usual tick control measures.

Babesia berbera. *Hosts:* Cattle. North Africa, southern Europe.

Considerable doubts exist as to the validity of this species. Simitch *et al.* (1945) have concluded that it is synonymous with *B. bovis*, the parasite being a North African and southern European form.

Morphologically, it resembles *B. bovis*, this character suggesting the synonymy; however, Sergent *et al.* (1945) using cross immunity studies consider it a distinct species.

Transmitting ticks include *I. ricinus* and *I. persulcatus* in Europe and *B. calcaratus* and *Rh. bursa* in North Africa.

The pathogenic effects are comparable to those detailed for the other small piroplasms. For treatment the compounds previously mentioned have been used with success. Diampron has been found effective against *B. berbera* by Kemron *et al.* (1960).

Babesia major. *Hosts:* Cattle. South America, North and West Africa, southern Europe, Soviet Union.

This species resembles *B. bigemina* except that it is smaller and lies in the centre of the erythrocyte. The pyriform bodies are 2·6 μ by 1·5 μ, and the angle formed by the organisms is less than 90°. Round forms about 1·8 μ in diameter may occur.

Developmental Cycle. This is comparable to thàt of *B. bovis. Boophilus calcaratus* is the tick vector in the Soviet Union, and in Holland, Bool *et al.* (1961) suggested that *Haemaphysalis punctata* may be a vector.

Babesia major is considered less pathogenic than *B. bovis*, the temperature elevation is not so marked, and the haemoglobinuria and anaemia are mild.

For treatment the compounds mentioned above are satisfactory, though Sergent *et al.* (1945) considered the silver compound, Ichthargan, to be the only preparation which had any action on *B. major*.

Babesia of Sheep and Goats

Four species of *Babesia* have been reported from sheep and goats, consisting of one large form and three small forms:

Babesia motasi Wenyon, 1926
Babesia ovis (Babes, 1892) Starcovici, 1893
Babesia foliata Ray and Rhaghavachari, 1941
Babesia taylori (Sarwar, 1935)

Babesia motasi. *Hosts:* Sheep and goats. Southern Europe, Middle East, Soviet Union, southeast Asia, also Africa and other parts of the tropics.

This is a large form measuring 2·5 μ–4 μ by 2 μ, the pyriform stages resembling those of *B. bigemina*, the angle at which they meet being acute. They may occur singly or in pairs.

Developmental Cycle. This is similar to that of *B. bigemina*. The tick vectors include *Dermacentor silvarum, Haemaphysalis punctata* and *Rhipicephalus bursa*. Both transovarian and stage to stage transmission have been demonstrated for this parasite in *Rh. bursa*. Markov & Abramov (1957) described clavate parasites in the ovary and eggs of the tick, and Li (1958) described similar forms in other developmental stages.

Pathogenesis. The disease caused by *B. motasi* may be acute or chronic. In the former it follows a course comparable to *B. bigemina*, being characterised by high fever, haemoglobinuria and marked anaemia with prostration. Death is not uncommon. In the chronic form there are no characteristic signs and death is unusual. Recovered animals are immune to the infection but are still susceptible to *Babesia ovis*.

Diagnosis. This is based on clinical signs and the demonstration of the parasites in the peripheral blood, these being most numerous at the time of the acute fever.

Treatment. Trypan blue is effective, being given intravenously. The dose for sheep is 10–25 ml. of a 1 per cent solution in normal saline. This may be repeated 24 hours later, but a single dose is usually sufficient.

Babesia ovis. *Hosts:* Sheep and goats. Distributed throughout tropical and sub-tropical areas, also in southern Europe and the Soviet Union.

Babesia ovis is much smaller than *B. motasi*, being 1 μ–2·5 μ in length. The majority of organisms are round, occurring at the margin of the red cell. Pyriform organisms are comparatively rare, and when they occur in pairs the angle between them is obtuse, the organisms usually lying at the margin of the erythrocyte.

The developmental cycle of *B. ovis* is probably similar to that of *B. bovis*. The principal vector tick in the Soviet Union is *Rh. bursa*. This is a 2 host tick, and transovarian transmission and stage to stage transmission have been reported in it (Markov & Abramov, 1957).

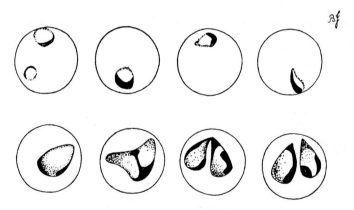

Fig. 283. *Babesia* Species of Sheep (×3000). Upper row, *Babesia ovis*. Lower row, *Babesia motasi*. (From Wenyon, 1926)

Pathogenic Effects of B. ovis. These are usually less severe than those with *B. motasi*, though an acute phase characterised by fever, jaundice, haemoglobinuria and anaemia may be seen. In the chronic form of the disease about 1 per cent of the erythrocytes are infected.

Recovered animals are immune to infection, and there is no cross immunity with *B. motasi*.

Treatment. Trypan blue is ineffective. Pirevan (quinuronium sulphate) has been used for *B. ovis* at a dose of 2 ml. of a 0·5 per cent solution per 10 kg. Simitch *et al.* (1956) used berenil at the rate of 3 mg. per kg. for *B. ovis* infection in sheep. A rapid recovery occurred in 161 out of 169 infected sheep given a single intramuscular injection.

Babesia foliata. This species has been recorded from sheep in India. It resembles *B. ovis* but lies more centrally in the erythrocyte. The vector has not yet been identified. It may be a synonym of *B. ovis*.

Babesia taylori. *Host:* Goat. India. This is a small form which may reach up to 1·5 μ—2 μ in length, but usually it is ovoid to round, about 1 μ in diameter, and appears to undergo several fissions to produce eight or even sixteen parasites per erythrocyte. The host red cell is often enlarged, and dividing forms of the organism may be seen in the plasma. The vector of this species has yet to be identified.

Pathogenicity. This is low, haemoglobinuria not being in evidence.

The control of *Babesia* spp. in sheep is similar to that in cattle and depends on tick control, the therapeutic use of drugs and immunisation of young animals with blood from older infected animals.

Babesia of Horses

Two species of *Babesia* occur in the horse:

Babesia caballi (Nuttall, 1910)

Babesia equi (Laveran, 1901)

Babesia caballi. *Hosts:* Horse, also donkey and mule. Southern Europe, Asia, Soviet Union, Africa and the Panama Zone. Recently, Sippel *et al.* (1962) reported equine babesiosis in the U.S.A., finding 97 infected horses in Florida and an additional number in Georgia. Two species of *Babesia* occur in equines in Florida, *B. caballi* representing the majority of the parasite population, but a second form typical of *Babesia equi* is also present.

Morphology. *B. caballi* is a large species resembling *B. bigemina*. Parasites commonly occur as pairs, are pyriform and measure 2·5 μ–4 μ in length; the angle formed by the organisms is acute. Round or oval forms, 1·5 μ–3 μ in diameter, may also occur.

Developmental Cycle. The tick vectors of the *Babesia* species of horses are considered in detail by Enigk (1943, 1944a, 1951). These are as follows: *Dermacentor marginatus* (southern and eastern Soviet Union, Germany), *D. reticulatus* and *D. silvarum* (European Soviet Union), *D. nitens* (Florida, Panama), *Hyalomma excavatum* and *H. dromedarii* (North Africa), *H. scupense* (Ukraine), *Rhipicephalus bursa* (Bulgaria), *Rh. sanguineus* (Greece) etc.

Pathogenesis. There is a great variation in the clinical manifestations of *B. caballi* infection. The course may be acute or chronic, mild or severe, and in some cases it may end in death. Persistent fever and anaemia with icterus commonly occur, but haemoglobinuria is rare and is not characteristic of the infection. In acute cases death may occur from 1–4 weeks after the onset of clinical signs. Disturbances of the central nervous system are common and may result in posterior paralysis. Malherbe (1956) records incoordination in foals aged 4–5 months during midsummer in South Africa. Clinical signs of this consisted of restlessness, nervousness and walking in circles with incoordination.

All breeds of horses are equally susceptible to *B. caballi* infection, though the disease is more marked in older horses, and the inverted age resistance is comparable to that seen in *B. bigemina*. Following recovery the animal is premune, and in general horses are resusceptible to piroplasmosis 1–2 years after recovery in the absence of reinfection.

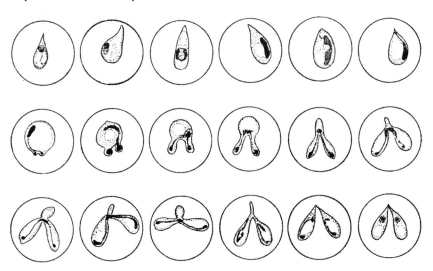

FIG. 284. *Babesia caballi* of the Horse. Various forms seen during multiplication in the red cells (× ca. 3000). (From Wenyon, 1926)

Diagnosis of B. caballi *Infection.* Diagnosis is based on the clinical signs, the presence of tick vectors, history of the area and the demonstration of the organism in the peripheral blood. Several samples may need to be examined since those taken at the onset of disease may show only a small number of parasites. The most satisfactory site to obtain the blood sample is the skin of the ear, and frequently the first drop of blood contains the greatest number of organisms. A reduction in haemoglobin amount and erythrocytes and an increase in erythrocyte sedimentation rate supply supportive evidence.

Serological tests have been used for the diagnosis of *Babesia* infection in horses. Hirato *et al.* (1945) prepared an antigen from the stromata of blood cells from an acutely infected horse and demonstrated the persistence of complement fixation antibodies for at least 100 days after infection. More recently in the United States, Ristic *et al.* (1966) have used several serological tests for diagnosis. Using a soluble antigen prepared by protamine sulphate precipitation of sonically lyzed infected erythrocytes, Ristic & Sibinovic (1964) were able to detect precipitins in the serum of horses convalescing or recovered from *Babesia* infection. The specificity of the test was shown by the absence of the reactions with sera of horses with various other infections, including viral infectious anaemia. The protamine sulphate precipitating antigen is a mucoprotein in nature (Sibinovic, 1965), and at least 1 component of the antigen can withstand boiling at 90°C for 30 minutes. This component has the characteristics of polysaccharide, and it can be adsorbed onto sheep erythrocytes so that they can be used for passive haemagglutination tests. Ristic (1966) reports a good correlation between the results of precipitation in gels and the haemagglutination tests. Soluble antigens from acute phase serum of infected animals can be prepared and adsorbed onto bentonite

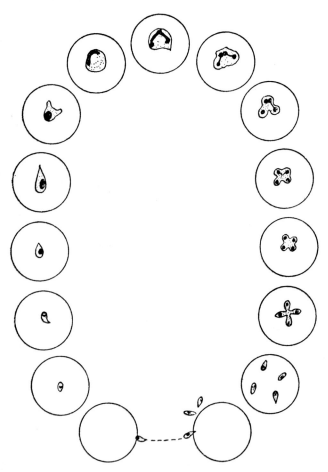

FIG. 285. *Babesia equi* of the Horse. Various forms seen during multiplication in the red cells (× ca. 3000). (From Wenyon, 1926)

particles or tanned erythrocytes and used in agglutination procedures for the detection of antibodies to *Babesia* (Ristic, 1966).

Treatment of B. caballi *Infection. Trypan blue* is effective and is given intravenously as a 1 per cent solution at the rate of 50–100 ml. according to the size of the horse. It is well tolerated and may be repeated 24 hours later.

Pirevan (Acapron, Babesan, Piroparv) is effective and superior to trypan blue. It is given subcutaneously as a 5 per cent solution at the rate of 1·2 ml. per 100 kg. body weight.

In the Soviet Union, Haemosporidin [(N, N'-di-4-dimethyl-aminophenyl) urea methylmethosulphate] is given subcutaneously as a 2 per cent solution, 5–6 ml. being given per horse. The therapeutic dose is based on the level of 0·2 mg. per kg. (Ershov, 1956).

Symptomatic treatment consists of housing animals if possible, appropriate nursing and a balanced diet. In cases of severe anaemia, blood transfusions may be indicated.

Prophylaxis of *B. caballi* infection in horses is comparable to that for *B. bigemina* in cattle.

Babesia equi. *Hosts:* Horse, mule, donkey, certain zebra. Asia, Africa, Europe, South and East Africa, South America and Soviet Union. It possibly occurs in the United States (Florida) since a form comparable to it has been recognised by Ristic (1966).

This parasite is readily distinguished from *B. caballi*. It is smaller, about 2 μ in length, and characteristically divides into four daughter organisms which frequently form a maltese cross. (Some authors prefer to refer this species to the genus *Nuttalia*.) Less usual forms in the erythrocytes are rounded or amoeboid stages.

Developmental Cycle. The tick vectors are considered by Enigk (1943, 1944). These include: *Dermacentor reticulatus* (European Soviet Union), *D. marginatus* (eastern Europe), *Hyalomma excavatum*, *H. plumbeum* (Greece, Central Asia), *H. dromedarii* (North Africa), *Rhipicephalus bursa*, *Rh. turanicus* (Soviet Union), *Rh. evertsi* (South Africa) and *Rh. sanguineus* (Central Asia, North Africa).

Pathogenicity of B. equi. In general this species is more pathogenic than *B. caballi*, but mixed infections of *B. caballi* and *B. equi* may occur. Ershov (1956) considers that simultaneous primary infections occur rarely, and he suggests an antagonism between the two, *B. equi* infection having a tendency to develop more frequently than *B. caballi*. Following infection the incubation period is 8–10 days, the first clinical sign being a marked increase in body temperature, which may reach 106°–107°F, and this coincides with the appearance of the organisms in the circulating blood. In acute cases the disease process lasts 8–10 days, and if recovery is to occur there is a fever crisis about the 10th day; thereafter the body temperature falls to normal, and the animal rapidly recovers and becomes a carrier. In peracute cases death may occur in 1–2 days after the onset of clinical signs. Anaemia and haemoglobinuria may be marked, and there is listlessness, depression and inappetence. Oedema of the dependent parts of the body and the head may occur. There may also be gastrointestinal upsets and hard faeces covered with yellowish mucus. Posterior paralysis, common in *B. caballi* infections, is not usually seen. The subacute infection develops more slowly and is more prolonged. Recovery may take several weeks or months.

The pathological changes are most readily seen in acute infections and consist of general jaundice, petechial haemorrhages, enlargement of the spleen and liver, and the kidneys are flabby and may show petechial haemorrhages. In severe cases oedema of the lungs and sometimes terminal pneumonia may be found.

Animals recovered from infection are premune, and the persistence of immunity is comparable to that with the piroplasms of cattle. The premunity may depend to some extent on the strain of organism. Abramov (1952) has observed different strains which varied in virulence, and Ershov (1956) records that a transcaucasian strain is more virulent and pathogenic than one from the temperate zones of the Soviet Union. Consequently, superimposed infection of the former on premunity induced by the latter may lead to clinical disease. There is no cross immunity between *B. equi* and *B. caballi*.

Diagnosis of B. equi *Infection.* This is made on the clinical signs and the identification of parasites in stained blood smears. Blood examination is best made during the period of fever since, subsequently, organisms become scarce in the blood. The maltese cross formation is typical of the species, and these may be readily seen if a fluorescent antibody technique is used (Ristic *et al.* 1964).

Treatment. Since *B. equi* is a small piroplasm, it is not affected by trypan blue. Acriflavine has been used as a 2 per cent solution at the rate of 10 ml. per 100 kg. body weight intravenously. This drug, under the name of tryflavine or euflavine, has been used extensively in northern Africa (Algeria) and South Africa. Pentamidine (lomidine 4,4'-diamidino 1,5-diphenoxy pentane) has been used widely by French workers in North Africa (Carmichael, 1956), and haemosporidin has been used for the infection of horses in the Soviet Union.

The control measures appropriate to *B. equi* infection are comparable to those for the other *Babesia*.

Babesia of Swine

Two species have been recorded:
Babesia trautmanni (Knuth and Du Toit, 1918)
Babesia perroncitoi (Cerruti, 1939)

Babesia trautmanni. *Hosts:* Pig; wart hog and bush pig may act as carriers (Neitz, 1956). Soviet Union, southern Europe (Italy, Bulgaria), Congo, Tanganyika.

Morphology. Organism, $2 \cdot 5 \, \mu$–$4 \, \mu$ long by $1 \cdot 5 \, \mu$–$2 \, \mu$ wide, characteristically long and narrow. Organisms frequently occur in pairs, but the cell may contain up to four organisms and sometimes five or six. Oval, amoeboid and ring forms may occur, and occasional parasites may be seen in the plasma.

The developmental cycle in the vertebrate host is probably the same as for the other species of *Babesia*. Tick vectors include *Rhipicephalus turanicus* (Soviet Union), *Boophilus decoloratus* (Tanganyika) and *Rh. sanguineus* and *Dermacentor reticulatus* (Europe) (Neitz, 1956).

Pathogenesis of B. trautmanni. Babesiosis of swine is a seasonal disease occurring during the spring and reaching a peak incidence during May and June. Piglets 2–4 months of age and adult swine are equally susceptible, and in the Soviet Union the wild boar may be infected and thereby serve as a natural reservoir for the disease (Ershov, 1956). In the acute disease there is fever with anaemia, haemoglobinuria, jaundice, oedema of the dependent parts and incoordination. Pregnant sows may abort and mortality may reach 50 per cent. The incubation period is 12–25 days.

Diagnosis is made on clinical signs, especially the haemoglobinuria and the icterus, and the demonstration of the organisms in blood smears.

Treatment. Trypan blue is effective being given intravenously as a 1 per cent solution at the rate of 10–25 ml. per animal. In Italy, Puccini *et al.* (1958) have reported that berenil is effective against *B. trautmanni* being given as a 7 per cent solution at the rate of 3·5 ml. per kg. intravenously. Lawrence & Shone (1955) found that phenamidine given subcutaneously at the rate of 1·5 ml. of a 40 per cent solution per 100 lb. body weight was effective.

Babesia perroncitoi. *Hosts:* Pig. Sardinia, Sudan.

This is a small rounded vacuolated form, 0·7 μ–2 μ in diameter. Oval to pyriform forms may occur, 1·2 μ–2·6 μ long by 0·7 μ–1·9 μ wide.

The tick vectors have yet to be established experimentally; however, Cerruti (1939) has suggested that *Rhipicephalus sanguineus* and *Dermacentor reticulatus* may be the vectors in Italy.

The pathogenesis of the infection is comparable to that caused by *B. trautmanni*. Puccini *et al.* (1958) found that berenil was effective for treatment.

Babesia of Dogs and Cats

Canine babesiosis is widespread throughout the world; four species have been described:

Babesia canis (Piana and Galli-Valerio, 1895)
Babesia gibsoni (Patton, 1910)
Babesia vogeli Reichenow, 1937
Babesia felis Davis, 1929

Of the above *Babesia canis* is the species of major importance.

Babesia canis. *Hosts:* Domestic dog. Asia, Africa, southern Europe, United States, Puerto Rico, Central and South America. Naturally infected wolves, striped jackals and black-backed jackals have been found

in Turkestan, East Africa and South Africa, respectively. The red fox
and silver fox have been artificially infected in Germany.

Morphology. This is a large piroplasm, pyriform in shape, $4\,\mu$–$5\,\mu$ in
length, pointed at one end and round at the other. Frequently there is a
vacuole in the cytoplasm. The pyriform forms may lie at an angle to
one another, but pleomorphism of shape may be seen, organisms varying
from amoeboid to ring forms. Multiple infection of erythrocytes may be
seen, up to, and sometimes more than, sixteen organisms being found in a
single red blood cell. Organisms may also be found in endothelial cells
of the lungs and liver and also in macrophages, this probably being due to
erythrophagocytosis.

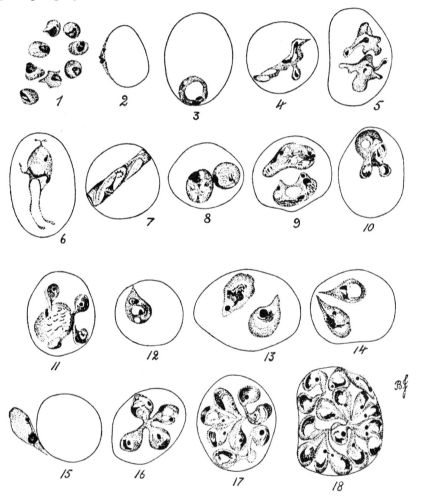

Fig. 286. *Babesia canis* in the Blood of the Dog ($\times$ ca. 2250). (From Wenyon, 1926)
1. Group of free forms, probably resulting from rupture of a cell with multiple infection;
2. Marginal form; 3–9. Various types of parasite; 10. Form producing two buds; 11.
Form producing four buds; 12–14. Pear-shaped individuals; 15. Free pear-shaped form;
16. Form producing four buds; 17, 18. Cells containing several budding parasites.

Developmental Cycle. The life cycle in *Rhipicephalus sanguineus* and *Dermacentor reticulatus* has been referred to previously. Transovarian transmission and stage to stage transmission have been reported (page 701). The principal vector of *B. canis* is *Rhipicephalus sanguineus* which occurs throughout the world; it has been specifically demonstrated as a vector in India, Germany, France, South Africa, United States and Brazil. *Dermacentor marginatus* and *D. reticulatus* have been incriminated in France, Germany and the Soviet Union. *Dermacentor venustus* (*D. andersoni*) is a possible vector in France, *Haemaphysalis leachi* in South Africa and *Hyalomma plumbeum plumbeum* in the Soviet Union.

Pathogenesis of B. canis *Infection.* Unlike other animals, the puppy may show clinical disease as severe as that seen in adult dogs.

Artificial infection of susceptible dogs with infective blood was studied by Ewing (1965). Initially, there was a transient parasitaemia which lasted 3–4 days after which the organisms disappeared from the peripheral blood for about 10 days. A second parasitaemia developed about 2 weeks after exposure, and the increase in numbers of organisms in the red blood cells resulted from binary fission within the cells; cells which harboured multiple trophozoites contained either two or exponential multiples of two.

The severity of infections with *B. canis* varies markedly according to the strain of the parasite. Ewing & Buckner (1965), in the U.S.A., found that though anaemia developed in uncomplicated infections, there was also enough active haemopoiesis to allow recovery in many cases. On the other hand, Maegraith *et al.* (1957) and Tella & Maegraith (1965) reported a strain of *B. canis* obtained from Elberfeld (Germany) in 1938, which had been maintained by subinoculation through dogs and puppies, to be highly virulent for young puppies, killing them in 4–5 days. The inoculation of 1–2 ml. of blood either intravenously or intraperitoneally resulted, almost invariably, in death a few days after the onset of clinical signs. In fully grown dogs the infection was not always fatal though severe haemolysis often developed.

Under natural conditions and in endemic areas, a wide variety of clinical manifestations of the disease may be seen. Malherbe (1956) states, 'there is almost no guise under which the disease does not masquerade at some time or another'. The common clinical signs seen in the majority of cases are as follows: An incubation period of 10–21 days is followed by a fever of 102°–105°F, malaise and listlessness. There is depression, disinclination to move, anorexia, the mucous membranes become pale, and jaundice develops in advanced or neglected cases. Haemoglobinuria is usually associated with peracute cases where the loss of red blood cells is marked. Splenic enlargement is present, the faeces are markedly yellow (except in very early or peracute cases), and usually there is a lot of bilirubin in the urine. Progressive debility is seen, and emaciation may become extreme; however, the animal frequently dies before this stage is reached. In the majority of cases organisms are readily demonstrable in smears from the peripheral blood (Malherbe, 1956).

In chronic infections there may be an irregular temperature, a capricious appetite and a marked loss of condition.

In a study of severe and fatal infections, Maegraith *et al.* (1957) found no direct relationship between the clinical condition and the degree of parasitaemia. Thus, the degree of anaemia may not be correlated with a high parasite density, and in fatal infection Tella & Maegraith (1965) found the average parasite count in puppies dying on the 5th day of infection to be 6·6 per cent in contrast to a PCV of 29·3 per cent and an RBC count of 24·6 per cent at that time. Maegraith *et al.* (1957) noted that the fall of erythrocyte numbers and haemoglobin concentration may be accompanied by intravascular haemolysis, but frequently anaemia developed without obvious haemoglobinaemia and haemoglobinuria. Maegraith *et al.* (1957) consider that very active phagocytosis of both parasitised and unparasitised RBC by macrophages in the circulating blood and in the spleen, bone marrow and liver, is largely responsible for the loss of cells in cases where haemoglobinuria is not present.

Erythropoiesis is active even in profound cases of anaemia, and reticulocytes appear at an early stage of the infection and continue to do so throughout the disease process.

The mode of death in *B. canis* infection depends on the length of illness. In rapid, fulminating infections, which cause death in 4–5 days, the animal remains conscious to the end with a strong heart action, and death is associated with acute respiratory failure, often with extensor spasm. In infections which do not kill so quickly, the animal becomes weaker and finally unconscious; it is completely relaxed, there is always a profound anaemia, the extremities are cold, respirations are shallow and rapid, the heart beat rapid and feeble, and the animal dies from circulatory failure associated with pulmonary oedema (Maegraith *et al.*, 1957).

The atypical manifestations vary from a simple catarrhal bronchitic condition to pneumonia, both of which show a remarkable response to specific therapy. Subcutaneous oedema, ascites and purpura have been described by Malherbe. In the ascites cases, characteristically there is marked abdominal distention, usually but not invariably, associated with emaciation. This is seen usually in half grown puppies or young dogs under a year of age; animals have very pale mucous membranes, the temperature may be normal or sub-normal, and blood smears may or may not show the *Babesia* organisms. In some cases organisms are undetected even after extensive examination. Such cases show a striking response to specific treatment, the peritoneal exudate being rapidy resorbed, and by 7–12 days the oedema fluid has disappeared. Purpura haemorrhagica may occur in a few cases. Petechial haemorrhages or ecchymoses occur on the iris, the mucous membranes of the mouth and lips and the skin of the abdominal wall and the inside of the thighs. Some cases may pass red urine or, occasionally, blood clots, and blood may be observed in the faeces indicating haemorrhage in the posterior bowel.

Central nervous system involvement is less common than the other manifestations. Piercey (1947) has described a case of acute cerebral canine babesiosis characterised by sudden death, and Purchase (1947) reported a case in which parasites were scarce in the peripheral blood but abundant in brain smears and in histological sections. Maegraith *et al.* (1957), in their acute experimental infections, failed to observe neurological signs other than general weakness of the limbs and coma, which developed as a terminal effect. Peripheral nerve lesions have been reported by Malherbe & Parkin (1951). These may be manifest by rheumatoid muscular pains, chiefly of the legs, causing lameness and even paraplegia. Dogs may scream with pain if their heads are touched or their mouths opened.

At post mortem there is enlargement of the liver and spleen. Centrilobular degeneration or necrosis occurs in the liver, and in a few cases this may extend almost to the periphery of the lobule. The kidneys show medullary congestion in fatal cases, and there are degenerative changes in the tubular epithelium in the cortical region. Other post-mortem changes include oedema in the pleural and the peritoneal cavities and petechial haemorrhages on various organs and the mucous membranes. The latter are also icteric and there is a profound anaemia.

The effect of combined infection with *Babesia canis* and *Ehrlichia* (*canis*) has been discussed by Ewing & Buckner (1965). They reported grave illness accompanied by severe anaemia of the normocytic, normochromic type which was due to destruction of mature erythrocytes and an impairment of erythropoiesis. These workers considered that the *Babesia* were responsible for the former and *Ehrlichia* for the latter. Dogs infected with either organism alone did not succumb to the infection. Dual infections in young dogs were often fatal, death being expected 19–45 days after exposure. It remains to be seen how commonly *Ehrlichia* is a component of the disease entity which hitherto has been attributed to *Babesia*.

Diagnosis of B. canis *Infection.* In areas where the infection is endemic, any dog with a high fever and clinical signs of anaemia and jaundice is a suspect for babesiosis. Frequently dogs are treated without a blood examination being made. Even in the absence of demonstrable organisms in the peripheral blood, there may be sufficient justification for treatment since demonstration of the organisms in blood smears may not be easy. Organisms are most readily found in the first drop of capillary blood from an ear puncture.

When atypical forms of the disease occur diagnosis may need to be based on the response to specific therapy (Malherbe, 1956), and usually this is rapid and more or less complete.

Supportive evidence for a diagnosis includes splenomegaly, an increased bleeding time, anaemia, accelerated erythrocyte sedimentation and the presence of increased amounts of bilirubin in the serum.

Treatment of B. canis *Infection*. *Trypan blue* is effective against *B. canis*. A single intravenous injection of 4–5 ml. of a 1 per cent solution is usually effective for an average sized dog (35 pounds). Care should be taken that the drug is given intravenously and not subcutaneously.

Phenamidine (4,4'-diamino diphenylether) has given excellent results at the rate of 10 ml. of a 5 per cent solution per kg. subcutaneously. A single dose is usually effective but it may be repeated 24 hours later.

Pirevan (Acapron, Babesan, Piroparv) is given subcutaneously as a 0·5 per cent solution at the rate of 0·05 ml. per kg. The drug is generally well tolerated though in some dogs minor convulsions may occur, but these are transitory. It may be repeated in 24 hours with safety.

Prevention and Control of B. canis *Infections*. This is essentially the same as that for other *Babesia*. Since *Rhipicephalus sanguineus* may occur in dog kennels, and even in human habitation, a regular programme of tick control should include periodic cleaning and fumigation of kennels.

Recovered animals are immune to *B. canis*. This is a premunition, and Kobalskii *et al.* (1963) have shown that the blood of recovered dogs may remain infective for 16 months; however, after 1·5–2 years the blood ceased to be infective for clean animals and the dogs were no longer immune.

Babesia gibsoni. *Hosts:* Domestic dog. India, Ceylon, parts of China, Turkestan, possibly parts of North Africa. In addition, the jackal (*Canis aureus*) in India, the wolf (*Canis lupus*) in Turkestan and the fox (*Vulpes vulpes dorsalis*) in Sudan are naturally infected (Neitz, 1956).

B. gibsoni is a small form, is pleomorphic and lacks the usual pyriform-shaped trophozoites. Characteristically the trophozoites are annular or oval; signet ring forms may occur and, rarely, large ovoid to circular blue forms, about half the diameter of the host cell, or elongate forms stretching across the cell, may be seen.

The developmental cycle is similar to that of *Babesia canis*. The transmitting ticks include *Haemaphysalis bispinosa* and *Rhipicephalus sanguineus* in India, both of which are three host ticks.

The disease produced by *B. gibsoni* is more chronic than that caused by *B. canis*. There are periodic exacerbations of fever and progressive anaemia and haemoglobinuria. Death may take place after several weeks, or even several months, of illness. There is a marked enlargement of the spleen and the liver, but jaundice is not a frequent clinical sign.

There is at present no satisfactory treatment for *B. gibsoni* infection. Seneviratne (1953) has reported that paludrine has been used with some degree of success for *B. gibsoni* infections in Ceylon.

Babesia vogeli. *Hosts:* Dog. North Africa and southern Asia.

Morphologically it is similar to *B. canis* but larger. It may be a synonym of *B. canis*, and the species was originally established because dogs infected with it failed to show immunity to a strain of *B. canis* transmitted by

Dermacentor. It is transmitted by *Rhipicephalus sanguineus,* and the clinical entity is comparable to that produced by *B. canis.*

Babesia felis. *Hosts:* Domestic cat. Sudan, South Africa. Also in wildcat (Sudan), Sudanese lion (Sudan), Indian leopard (*Panthera pardus fusca*) (India), American puma (*Felis concolor*) (Zoological Gardens, Cairo), American lynx (*Lynx rufus*) (Zoological Gardens, London).

This is a small species, the majority of the forms being round or oval, 1·5 μ–2 μ in diameter; pyriform stages are uncommon. Division is into four, forming a maltese cross arrangement; however, binary fission is also seen.

The development cycle is not known.

The pathogenic effects of *B. felis* consist of anaemia and icterus. Prolonged cases lead to emaciation, splenomegaly and occasionally haemoglobinuria.

The infection is effectively treated by trypan blue and acaprin.

Piroplasmosis of Poultry

Two species of the family Babesiidae occur in poultry:

Aegyptianella pullorum Carpano, 1928

Aegyptianella moshkovskii (Schurenkova, 1938) Poisson, 1953

The genus *Aegyptianella* is related to *Babesia,* but four to sixteen, or more, trophozoites are produced by division. Laird & Lari (1957) consider it unnecessary to assign a separate genus to the organisms and retain them in the genus *Babesia.*

Aegyptianella pullorum. *Hosts:* Domestic chicken, goose, also duck and turkey. (Experimentally in doves, pigeons, quail, canaries and other birds.) Sudan, North and South Africa, south-east Asia, India, south-east Europe, Soviet Union.

Morphology. The early trophozoites or initial bodies are small, 0·5 μ– 1·0 μ, round to oval and consist of a chromatin granule with a small ring of cytoplasm. Further development produces pear-shaped, oval or round forms consisting of a blue cytoplasm containing a reddish chromatin mass. A third, larger form resembles a schizont and consists of an oval or round body, 2 μ–2·5 μ by 3 μ–4 μ, with chromatin displaced to the periphery. Up to 20 merozoites may be produced.

The developmental cycle of *A. pullorum* consists of asexual multiplication by schizogony in the red cells of the fowl to produce four to sixteen or more merozoites. Transmission is through the fowl tick, *Argas persicus,* but the developmental stages in the tick have not been demonstrated. Transmission in the tick is by neither the stage to stage nor the transovarian routes. Following feeding by an adult tick on an infected fowl, 26 days or more are required before the organism is transmissible to another bird.

Pathogenesis. The disease may be acute, sub-acute or chronic. Indigenous poultry rarely suffer the acute disease, but freshly introduced stock may die within a few days of the onset of the clinical entity. The incubation period is 12–15 days after which there is fever, diarrhoea, anorexia and jaundice. At post mortem there is anaemia, enlargement of the spleen, degeneration of the liver, petechial haemorrhages on the serosae and greyish-yellow degeneration of the kidneys. The clinical condition is often complicated by fowl spirochaetosis (*Borrelia*), which is also transmitted by *A. persicus*.

Treatment. Trypan blue is ineffective. Sergent (1935) has reported that ichthargan (a silver preparation) given intravenously as a 1 per cent solution is effective.

Aegyptianella moshkovskii. *Hosts:* Chicken, possibly also turkey, pheasant, house crow and other birds. Indian sub-continent, south-east Asia, Egypt, eastern parts of the Soviet Union.

The parasite usually produces four merozoites, sometimes six. The early initial forms are 0·2 μ–0·6 μ in diameter, larger ring forms 2·1 μ by 1·4 μ and large oval or irregular forms 0·9 μ–5·3 μ in diameter. A detailed consideration of the position of this parasite in the *Babesia* group is given by Laird & Lari (1957).

The developmental cycle and the pathogenesis of this form are unknown.

FAMILY: THEILERIIDAE DU TOIT, 1918

Members of this family are round, ovoid, rod-like or irregular forms, found in lymphocytes, histiocytes and erythrocytes. They do not produce pigment and are transmitted by ixodid ticks. They occur in cattle, sheep and goats, causing the disease theileriasis.

The systematic position and classification of the theilerias has been reviewed extensively in recent years. Neitz & Jansen (1956) modified the classification by the introduction of the family Gonderidae; however, later, Neitz (1962) rejected this classification.

Theileria *Species of Cattle*

Theileria parva (Theiler, 1904)
Theileria annulata Dschunkowsky and Luhs, 1904
Theileria mutans Theiler, 1906

Theileria parva. *Hosts:* Cattle (*Bos taurus*), East, Central and South Africa; African buffalo (*Syncerus caffer*), East Africa; Indian water buffalo (*Bulbalis bubalis*), East and South Africa.

Recent studies by Barnett & Brocklesby (1966c) have shown that the species hitherto known as *Theileria lawrenci* and found in the African buffalo is, in reality, a modified strain of *Th. parva*.

Classically, *Th. parva* causes the disease East Coast fever, or bovine theileriasis, which is responsible for high mortality among susceptible and imported stock. The zebu (*Bos indicus*) in endemic areas has a high natural resistance to *Th. parva*; however, animals imported into endemic areas are highly susceptible.

Morphology. The forms in red blood cells are mainly rod-shaped, 1·5 μ–2 μ by 0·5 μ–1 μ; however, round, oval, comma- and ring-shaped forms may also occur. With Romanowsky stains they show a blue cytoplasm with a red chromatin granule at one end. Several parasites may occur in individual erythrocytes, but there is no evidence of multiplication in the red cells.

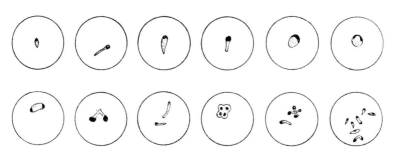

Fig. 287. *Theileria parva* of Cattle (× ca. 2500). Piroplasm forms in erythrocytes. (From Wenyon, 1926)

The actively multiplying forms of the parasite occur chiefly in the cytoplasm of lymphocytes and occasionally in the endothelial cells, especially of the lymphatic glands and the spleen. These are regarded as schizonts (Koch's Blue Bodies), being circular or irregularly shaped structures about 8 μ in diameter, but they may vary from 2 μ–12 μ or more. With Romanowsky stains they show a blue cytoplasm and a varied number of red chromatin granules. Two forms of schizonts are recognised. Those which contain large chromatin granules, 0·4 μ–2 μ in diameter (mean 1·2 μ), are referred to as macroschizonts (or agamonts) and produce macromerozoites, 2 μ–2·5 μ in diameter. The other forms contain smaller chromatin granules, 0·3 μ–0·8 μ in diameter (mean 0·5 μ), and are referred to as microschizonts (or gamonts), and produce micromerozoites. The latter invade the red blood cells and may represent sexual stages of the parasite.

Developmental Cycle of Theileria parva. Cattle are infected from infected ticks which possess large numbers of uninucleate sporozoites in their salivary glands. Injected sporozoites pass by way of the lymphatic system to the lymphoid tissues, especially the lymph nodes and spleen, and here they form schizonts. The large macroschizonts produce macromerozoites which repeat the schizogony process until large numbers of lymphoid cells are parasitised. The microschizonts produce forms (piroplasms) which invade the blood, the majority of which are rod-shaped, measuring 1·5 μ–2 μ by 0·5 μ–1 μ. Such forms do not undergo any further division until they are ingested by the vector tick.

Theileria parva has been cultivated in the macroschizont stage in tissue culture of bovine lymphocytes associated with baby hamster kidney cells (Hulliger *et al.*, 1964). The parasite propagates within the multiplying lymphoid cells and does not destroy the host cell. The nuclear particles of *Th. parva* divide at about the same rate as the host cells, and during division the theileria body is closely associated with the mitotic apparatus, being pulled apart and distributed to both daughter lymphoid cells in late mitosis. Proof that a similar mode of multiplication occurs *in vivo* is lacking but the marked lymphoid hyperplasia in the infection would imply excessive mitotic division by lymphoid cells and many of these are infected. In addition there is no evidence *in vivo* for new infection of lymphoid cells by disintegrated single theileria particles.

Hulliger *et al.* (1966) have also obtained microschizontal development *in vitro* when lymphocyte cultures were incubated at around 42°C. With this temperature of incubation, little multiplication of lymphocytes occurred but the theileria particles continued to multiply without inhibition, producing stages containing many nuclear particles. Hulliger *et al.* (1966) comment that although the significance of the high temperature requirements for microschizontal development in culture is not clear, the disease in the animal is characterised by high temperatures of up to 42·4°C during the period of microschizont development.

Under natural conditions, the distribution of *Th. parva* is limited to the distribution of the tick *Rhipicephalus appendiculatus*. This is found in Central, East and southern Africa; it is a three host tick, and stage to stage transmission of infection occurs. Several other species of ticks have been demonstrated as capable of transmitting the infection, and these include the *Rhipicephalus* species, *R. ayrei*, *R. capensis*, *R. evertsi*, *R. jeanelli*, *R. neavei*, *R. simus*, and the *Hyalomma* ticks, *H. anatolicum* (syn. *H. excavatum*), *H. dromedarii* and *H. truncatum*. Transmission of the parasite in all is on a stage to stage basis, and the organism does not survive in the ticks for more than one moult.

Throughout the years a great deal of work has been done regarding the developmental cycle of *Theileria parva* in ticks. There is still no clear understanding of this process; however, work by Riek (1966) with *Theileria mutans* may assist in the elucidation of the tick cycle for *Th. parva*. Initial work on the life cycle of *Th. parva* by Gonder (1910, 1911) and later by Cowdry & Ham (1932) suggested sexual union of parasites and the formation of a zygote, oökinete, sporoblasts and sporozoites. Such work was criticised by Reichenow (1940), who regarded the 'zygotes' as symbionts and the other stages as degenerated tissue cells. Alternatively, Reichenow (1940) maintained that the vast majority of parasites taken into the tick in a blood meal died in the intestine of the tick. A few succeeded in penetrating the gut to get into the body cavity, and they then passed directly to the salivary glands where they lay dormant until the tick dropped off the host, moulted and attached to a new host. When the next stage of the tick commenced to feed, multiplication by repeated binary fission produced several thousand minute parasites which were packed between the secretory droplets of the cells. Ultimately the cell ruptured and the parasites passed into the lumen of the salivary duct to be injected into the host at the next blood meal. Three days were required for this process in the nymphal stage and 4·5 days in adult ticks.

Recently, Martin *et al.* (1964) observed developmental stages of *Th. parva* in the gut contents, gut epithelial cells and cells of the salivary gland of infected ticks. The form in the epithelial cells of the gut was a large spherical body, but these authors were unable to detect any stages of *Th. parva* in the body cavity of the ticks, and no stages of the organism were detected in unengorged nymphs. Three distinct types of alveoli were found in the salivary glands of *R. appendiculatus*, and developmental stages of *Th. parva* were found only in the granular secretory cells. Pre-infective forms were seen in the salivary glands only after the infected nymph or adult tick had fed for 24 hours or more, and development at this stage was by multiple fission. This was rapid since cattle were infected within 48 hours of the application of infected nymphae.

Riek (1966) suggests that the stages prior to the infection of the salivary gland must either be present in very small numbers or be extremely small in size and escape detection.

Pathogenesis of Th. parva *Infection.* East Coast fever is a serious disease with high mortality in susceptible stock, being characterised by lymphoid hyperplasia, followed by exhaustion of the lymphoid tissues and leucopenia. In recently imported stock the mortality may reach 90–100 per cent. The zebu (*Bos indicus*) has a high level of natural resistance, and in enzootic areas a calfhood mortality of 5–10 per cent may be expected (Barnett, 1963). Where zebu are introduced from non-enzootic areas the mortality may be very high. There is little difference in mortality between calves and adults in highly susceptible European cattle, but where the disease is endemic young cattle are relatively more resistant than older cattle.

The incubation period following exposure is 10–25 days (mean, 13 days), and the acute form of the disease is the most common, lasting 10 to 23 days. This commences with fever, the temperature rising to 104°–107°F, which is maintained until death or recovery occurs. A few days after the onset of fever animals cease to eat, there is swelling of the superficial lymph nodes, and there may be a nasal discharge, lachrymation and swelling of the eyelids and ears. The heartbeat is rapid, diarrhoea with blood and mucus in the faeces may occur and there is marked emaciation. Lung oedema occurs in the acute form, and this is probably the immediate cause of death.

Post-mortem findings in the acute form consist of a marked enlargement of the spleen and the liver, which is also yellowish-brown in colour, friable and shows degeneration. The lymph nodes are markedly swollen and hyperemic, the kidneys show haemorrhagic or greyish-white 'infarcts', the lungs are congested and oedematous, and there may be fluid in the thorax, pericardium and underneath the kidney capsule. Ulceration of the abomasum and small and large intestines occurs, the ulcers consisting of a central necrotic area surrounded by a haemorrhagic zone.

A fatal disease of cattle, 'corridor disease', is encountered in an area called 'the corridor', a stretch of country 100 square miles in extent lying between the Hluhluwe and Umfolozi game reserves in Zululand. Corridor disease is highly pathogenic for cattle, mortality reaching 80 per cent or more, but the African buffalo is highly resistant and serves as a reservoir for the infection. Originally, corridor disease was thought to be due to *Th. lawrenci*, but an extensive survey of the Theileridae of cattle and buffalo in Africa by Barnett & Brocklesby (1966a, b, c) and Brocklesby & Barnett (1966a, b) led them to conclude that *Th. lawrenci* is a strain of *Th. parva*.

A sub-acute form of the disease frequently occurs in calves. The clinical signs are similar to the acute form but not as pronounced, and recovery from this form is more common than with the acute disease.

A mild form of the disease is seen in calves born of immune dams in endemic areas. In this form the temperature rise is mild, lasting a few days to a week, there is swelling of the superficial lymph nodes, and recovery is more common.

In East and Central Africa, the condition of 'turning sickness' has been associated with *Th. parva* and also *Theileria mutans*. Affected animals make circling movements and show abduction of the hind limbs. On post mortem there is an increase in cerebrospinal fluid, extravasations of blood in various areas of the cortex, and localised necrotic areas occur in the brain in which forms resembling the schizonts of *Theileria* are found. Barnett (1963) considers the condition to be a local or generalised breakdown in immunity. With *Th. parva* the condition sometimes occurs when animals are moved from one enzootic area to another in which there is severe reinfection challenge.

Artificial Transmission. Normally *Th. parva* is not transmissible to other animals by blood inoculation. This is in distinction to the other species of *Theileria* where blood inoculation readily creates an infection. However, it is usually fairly readily transmitted by spleen or lymph node suspensions from infected animals.

Immunology of Th. parva *Infections.* The immunity which results in a recovered animal is solid, specific, and does not depend upon premunity. The immunity is stable and in an endemic area is effective for the life of the animal. In the absence of reinfection, immunity wanes slowly though occasionally animals may lose their immunity within a few months and be susceptible to a second infection. The level of immunity is not dependent on the degree of response of the first infection, and Barnett (1963) indicated that it is not influenced by the strain of organism. There is much evidence to indicate that *Th. parva* is antigenically stable, and Barnett & Bailey (1958) found no strain differences between East African and South African forms. The immunity is not influenced by splenectomy, and Barnett (1963) considered that the increased resistance of calves to *Th. parva* is not due to immunity transferred passively via the colostrum.

Active immunisation of animals against *Th. parva* is based on the observation by Theiler (1911) that artificially induced infections have a lower mortality rate and a higher recovery rate than tick induced infections. Immunisation of cattle by the injection of spleen or lymph node suspensions was practised for a period in South Africa; however, the level of mortality (25 per cent) was high, and moreover, not all animals infected were immune, only 60-70 per cent being so on exposure to tick infection.

Following the demonstration that chlortetracyclines, when given repeatedly, can suppress the parasitaemia in clinical cases, Neitz (1953) and Barnett & Bailey (1958) developed an immunisation schedule which consisted of producing an infection with infected ticks and suppressing the disease by the intravenous administration of 10 mg./kg. of aureomycin on alternate days during the incubation period and during the first few days of the reaction. This procedure is costly, and since at present the infection can only be regularly and effectively transmitted by ticks, the large scale application of such an immunization procedure is more or less precluded.

Diagnosis. Under general field conditions, the most satisfactory diagnosis is made by the demonstration of the schizonts in material obtained from superficial lymph nodes or by spleen puncture. The forms in the erythrocytes may be difficult to see at times, and in the early part of the infection they may be very few. Differential diagnosis between *Th. parva* and other *Theileria* species is not always easy, this being based on the enzootic area, the pathology, the epidemiology and, preferably, cross immunity tests.

Treatment and Control. Despite the effectiveness of the chlortetracyclines, especially if they are given repeatedly in the early stages of the disease, there is no effective drug for field use.

Control of *Th. parva* infection is dependent on tick control and, in some areas, quarantine measures. Transmission of the infection is from stage to stage, and the aim should be to prevent infected tick larvae or nymphs from transmitting the infection to a clean animal. In some parts of East Africa animals are dipped at intervals of 3-4 days for this purpose. If an infected tick attaches to an animal which is not susceptible to the infection, it then loses its infectivity; however, in the absence of a suitable host an adult tick may remain viable and infective for as long as 18 months.

Theileria annulata. *Hosts:* Bovine, zebu, water buffalo: North Africa, Middle and Far East, Soviet Union and southern Europe.

The organism produces a highly fatal disease of cattle in North Africa and is transmitted by ticks of the genus *Hyalomma*.

Morphology. The 'piroplasm forms in the red blood cells are more or less indistinguishable from those of *Th. parva* but more commonly occur as round, oval- or ring-shaped (0.5μ–1.5μ) forms. Rod shapes, commas (1.6μ) and anaplasma-like organisms may also be found, the latter measuring 0.5μ. The erythrocytic forms undergo binary fission with the

formation of two daughter individuals. Division into four to produce a cross
may also occur. Macroschizonts and microschizonts are found in the
lymphocytes of the spleen and lymph nodes, being similar to those of *Th.
parva*. *Theileria annulata* is readily transmissible by blood passage, and
schizonts are fairly numerous in the circulating blood.

Developmental Cycle of Th. annulata. The developmental cycle in the
vertebrate host is probably comparable to that of *Th. parva*. Recent work
on the growth of *Th. annulata* in tissue culture systems has shown that the
organism may be propagated for several serial passages in 'monocytic'
cells (Tsur & Adler, 1965; Hulliger *et al.*, 1965).

The tick vectors of *Th. annulata* are all members of the genus *Hyalomma*.
These include: *H. detritum* (N. Africa, Soviet Union), *H. dromedarii*
(Central Asia), *H. excavatum* and *H. turanicum* (Asia Minor), *H. savignyi*
(syn. *H. marginatum*) (Asia Minor, India), *H. plumbeum plumbeum* and *H.
scupense* (Soviet Union).

As far as is known there is no transovarian transmission of *Th. annulata*
through the ticks, though this was claimed by Ray (1950) who stated that
it could pass through five generations of *H. savignyi*. Similar work with *H.
excavatum* (syn. *H. turkmeniense*) was described by Korienko & Shmuireva
(1944), but Delpy (1949) could find no evidence of transovarian transmission.

The developmental cycle of *Th. annulata* in the tick has received little
extensive study, though early studies by French workers indicated a sexual
cycle.

Pathogenesis of Th. annulata. In general, the disease entity is comparable
to East Coast Fever. Mortality varies considerably, being 10 per cent in
some areas and up to 90 per cent in others. For this reason there has been
a tendency to ascribe Algerian theileriasis to a mild strain, referred to as
Theileria dispar by French workers. The more pathogenic strains occur
in the Soviet Union, Israel, Iran and India.

The disease entity may be acute, sub-acute or chronic. The acute
disease occurs in all breeds and all ages of cattle as well as buffalo and
zebu, but the latter two recover more readily from the disease. The
incubation period is 9–25 days, and the disease may last as little as 3–4
days in the acute form or may be prolonged for about 20 days. A marked
rise in body temperature, reaching 104°–107°F, is followed by depression,
lachrymation, nasal discharge and swelling of the superficial lymph nodes.
Emaciation is rapid and haemoglobinuria may occur. The severity of
the disease does not necessarily correspond to the extent of the parasitaemia. An animal may be seriously ill when less than 25 per cent of
the blood cells are infected with piroplasm stages, and less severe reactions
may occur where 45 per cent of the red blood cells are infected.

The post-mortem findings consist of a markedly enlarged spleen and
liver, there are 'infarcts' in the kidneys, the lungs are usually oedematous,
and the lymph nodes may be swollen, especially in the acute form of the

disease. The mucous membranes show icterus and often petechiae, and those of the abomasum and small intestine are swollen, reddened and show characteristic ulcers 2 to 12 mm. in diameter and surrounded by a zone of inflammation. Necrotic infarcts of the brain may occur in a small number of cases (Barboni, 1932), and cutaneous lesions have been reported by Tsur-Tchernomoretz *et al.* (1960), schizonts being found in the dermis.

Immunology of Th. annulata *Infection.* Recovery from *Th. annulata* infection leads to the development of premunity, and infection can be transmitted from such animals by blood inoculation. There is no cross immunity between *Th. annulata, Th. mutans* or *Th. parva.* Practical vaccination procedures, based upon the difference in virulence of various strains, have been practised in Algeria and in Israel. Field strains of low virulence are used, but since this may not protect all calves from virulent field strains, it is often necessary to boost immunity by a virulent strain 1–2 months after the use of the mild strain. Advantages of this vaccination include the fact that the low pathogenic strain can be maintained in calves by blood or tissue inoculation and that serial passage results in the loss of the erythrocyte phase after ten to thirteen passages. Thus, vaccinated animals are not infective for ticks.

The duration of immunity to *Th. annulata* is less than that seen in *Th. parva*, and Barnett (1963) estimates that 10 per cent of animals may be completely susceptible 17 months after the first infection; however, Sturman (1959) believed protection induced by vaccination lasted 2–3 years under conditions of field exposure. Immunity to *Th. annulata* is less stable than that to *Th. parva*. Relapse and death may occur after a considerable period of premunity.

Diagnosis and Treatment of Th. annulata *Infection.* Diagnosis is based on the demonstration of parasites in the red blood cells or in smears of material obtained from lymph nodes or spleen. Differentiation between *Th. annulata* and *Th. parva* is not easy, and diagnosis is based on the evaluation of the enzootic conditions in the area. It is not uncommon for *Th. annulata* to occur along with *Babesia* or *Anaplasma*, and the disease entity may be a combination of two or all of these.

No completely satisfactory treatment exists. Richardson & Kendall (1963) state that intravenous acriflavin has been recommended, and pentamidine has been reported to have some effect.

The control of *Th. annulata* is based on tick control measures. Immunisation is practised in Algeria and Israel, and in some areas this has greatly reduced the incidence of the disease.

Theileria mutans. *Hosts:* Cattle. Africa, Asia, Australia, Soviet Union. Splitter (1950) found the organism in a splenectomised calf in the U.S.A., Kreir *et al.* (1962) have found a *Theileria* species in splenectomised deer in the U.S.A., and Hignett (1953) reported the parasite in England in cattle which had been artificially infected with *Babesia divergens.*

It is the cause of benign bovine theileriasis and it is almost always nonfatal.

Morphologically, this parasite is indistinguishable from the other species of *Theileria*. The forms in the erythrocytes are round, oval, pyriform or anaplasma-like and measure 1 μ–2 μ in diameter, two or four parasites occurring in a single red blood cell. Schizonts are not readily detectable but when they are found they occur in the lymphocytes of the spleen and lymph nodes and measure about 8 μ in diameter, but they may be up to 20 μ in diameter. They resemble the macroschizonts of the more pathogenic species.

Developmental Cycle. Little work has been done on the endogenous cycle in the mammalian host, and it is assumed to be comparable to that in the other species.

The ticks responsible for the transmission of *Th. mutans* are listed by Neitz (1956) and include *Rhipicephalus appendiculatus* and *Rh. evertsi* (South Africa), *Haemaphysalis bispinosa* (Australia) and *H. punctata* (Soviet Union). *Boophilus annulatus* and *B. microplus*, both one host ticks, have been incriminated as vectors (experimentally), but since the infection is transmitted from stage to stage the role of these ticks in natural transmission requires clarification.

The developmental stages of *Th. mutans* in the tick *H. bispinosa* were studied by Riek (1966). Parasites similar to those in the erythrocytes were found free in the gut contents of larval ticks on repletion, but 24 hours later only small numbers were found despite a parasite density of more than 10 per cent in blood. Twenty-four to 48 hours after repletion small numbers of organisms were seen inside the epithelial cells of the gut wall, but no development was detected. By 10 days, spherical bodies, up to 15 μ in diameter, with a homogeneous cytoplasm and a nucleus about 3 μ in diameter were seen in several squash preparations. In such preparations these were extracellular, but Riek considered they had been liberated from the epithelial cells when the preparation was made. The next recognisable developmental forms were found in the salivary glands of nymphs during the first 24 hours after attachment. Thereafter, development was rapid, and by 48 hours to 4 to 5 days multiple fission produced bodies, 40 μ by 30 μ, which contained large numbers of infective forms. Of the three types of alveoli which had been found in the salivary glands of *H. bispinosa*, developmental stages occurred only in the granular secretory cells, only a few alveoli were infected, and only one or two cells in these were parasitised.

Theileria Species of Sheep

Two species of theileria have been described from sheep and goats:
Theileria hirci Dschunkowsky and Urodschevich, 1924
Theileria ovis Rodhain, 1916

Theileria hirci. *Hosts:* Sheep, goats; North and East Africa, Iraq, Turkey, southern Soviet Union and Greece.

The disease may be highly fatal, mortality ranging from 50–100 per cent.

Morphology. Erythrocytic piroplasms are round to oval in the majority of cases, about 18 per cent are rod-shaped and a small percentage are anaplasma-like. Round forms measure 0·6 μ–2 μ in diameter, they may be found in pairs or in fours and multiplication takes place in the erythrocytes. Schizonts occur in the lymphocytes of the spleen and lymph nodes. They range in size from 4 μ to 10 μ (mean 8 μ) and contain up to 80 chromatin granules, 1 μ–2 μ in diameter. Both macroschizonts and microschizonts occur.

The tick vector of *Th. hirci* has yet to be established, but in enzootic areas it is likely to be *Rhipicephalus bursa* (Neitz, 1956).

Pathogenesis. The disease is highly pathogenic for sheep and goats, mortalities up to 100 per cent having been reported in endemic areas. The infection is mild in young lambs and kids, possibly due to maternal immunity. An acute form of the disease is more usual, but subacute and chronic forms have been observed. In general, it resembles East Coast Fever; there is high fever associated with listlessness, a nasal discharge, jaundice, petechial haemorrhages in submucous, subserous and subcutaneous tissues, marked enlargement of the spleen and lymph nodes, the kidneys are enlarged and pale and show infarcts, and there may be a transitory haemoglobinuria. Animals which recover are premune, and there is no cross immunity with *Theileria ovis*.

Diagnosis of the infection is based on the detection of piroplasms in blood smears or schizonts in lymph node and spleen smears.

There is no known treatment and control measures depend on tick control.

Theileria ovis. *Hosts:* Sheep, goats. Africa, Asia, India, Soviet Union, parts of Europe.

It is much more widely distributed than *Th. hirci* and causes a benign disease.

Morphologically, the organism resembles *Th. hirci*, but the blood forms are relatively scarce, as are the schizonts which occur in the lymph nodes.

The ticks responsible for transmission include *Rhipicephalus bursa* (Soviet Union), *Rh. evertsi* (South Africa), *Dermacentor sylvarum*, *Haemaphysalis sulcata* and nymphs of *Ornithodorous lahorensis* (Soviet Union) (Bitukov, 1953).

The pathogenic entity is mild, and there is seldom mortality or any distinct clinical signs.

Theileridae of Wild Ruminants

Several other species of *Theileria* have been reported from various African ruminants, and Neitz (1959) has given an account of these.

25

Theileria cervi. This organism was found in the splenectomised white-tailed deer (*Dama virginiana*) by Kreier *et al.* (1962) and was subsequently identified as *Th. cervi* by Schaeffler (1962). It cannot be transmitted to the ox or to the sheep.

Cytauxzoon taurotragi. This organism was originally described by Martin & Brocklesby (1960) and Brocklesby (1961) from a fatal infection in a yearling eland (*Taurotragus oryx pattersonianus*). Brocklesby (1962) reported schizonts in sections of liver, lung and lymph node but not in the spleen or kidney. Erythrocytic stages of the parasite were indistinguishable from those of *Th. parva*, and the schizonts in the liver were the cytauxzoon type and resembled those of *Cytauxzoon sylvicaprae* of the grey duiker and *C. strepsicerosic* of the great Kudu.

FAMILY: HAEMOGREGARINIDAE NEVEU-LEMAIRE, 1901

Organisms of this family belong to the suborder Adeleidea Léger and are similar to the *Eimeridae*, but micro- and macrogametocytes become attached to each other in pairs during development into gametes; the zygote becomes an oocyst producing numerous sporoblasts, each of which develops into a spore containing two or four sporozoites. Parasites of the above family occur in the cells of the circulatory system of vertebrates, and the genus *Hepatozoon* Miller, 1908, is the only group of interest in this book.

Genus: Hepatozoon Miller 1908

Schizogony occurs in the endothelial cells of the liver, and the gametocytes are found in leucocytes or erythrocytes according to the species of organism. Sporogony occurs in various blood-sucking arthropods.

Hepatozoon canis (James, 1905). *Hosts:* Dog, cat, jackal, hyena. Far East, Central and North Africa, Middle East, Italy.

Schizonts occur in the endothelial cells of the spleen, bone marrow and liver as round or oval bodies, more or less filling the host cell and containing thirty to forty nuclei.

Various types of schizonts have been described; one produces a small number of large merozoites (usually three) which Wenyon (1926) considered became schizonts, and another produces a large number of small merozoites which are the forms that enter leucocytes.

The blood forms, gamonts, occur in the leucocytes and are elongate, rectangular bodies measuring 8 μ–12 μ by 3 μ–6 μ (mean 6 μ by 3 μ). They are surrounded by a delicate capsule, stain pale blue with a dark reddish-purple nucleus and have a number of pink granules in the cytoplasm. In citrated blood these forms may be found free in the plasma.

Developmental Cycle. The dog is infected by the ingestion of the infected vector tick, *Rhipicephalus sanguineus*, which contains sporocysts in its body cavity. The liberated sporozoites penetrate the wall of the intestine of the dog, pass via the blood stream to the spleen, liver and bone marrow, and here they enter tissue cells and become schizonts. Several generations of schizonts occur, but ultimately merozoites enter the circulating leucocytes and become gametocytes or gamonts. These show no sexual dimorphism and undergo no further change until ingested by the tick. Gametocytes leave the host leucocyte in the alimentary canal of the tick, become associated in pairs, and the microgametocyte produces two non-flagellate microgametes, one of which fertilises the macrogamete to produce a zygote. This is motile (oökinete), and it penetrates the intestinal wall to enter the haemocoel of the tick where it grows to become an oocyst which, when mature, is about 100 μ in length. Sporoblasts (thirty to fifty) and then sporocysts are formed, each of which produces about sixteen sporozoites. On ingestion of the tick, the oocysts and sporocysts rupture to release the sporozoites.

Pathogenesis of Hepatozoon canis. The organism may be found in apparently healthy dogs, but it is associated with pathogenic effects in Africa and the Far East. The clinical signs consist of an irregular fever, anaemia, progressive emaciation with enlargement of the spleen. Lumber paralysis has been described. Death occurs in 4–8 weeks after the onset of clinical signs.

Hepatozoon canis infection is diagnosed by the demonstration of the gametocytes in stained blood smears, or the schizonts in the spleen or bone marrow.

There is no known treatment, and control is based on tick control.

Other species of *Hepatozoon:*

Hepatozoon muris (Balfour, 1905). Occurs in the brown rat (*Rattus norvegicus*) and the black rat (*Rattus rattus*) throughout the world. The schizogony cycle takes place in the parenchymal cells of the liver, the gametocytes being found in the monocytes of the blood. Development occurs in the rat mite, *Echinolaelaps echidninus*, rats being infected by ingestion of the infected mite.

Hepatozoon musculi (Porter, 1907). Is found in the white mouse in England.

Hepatozoon cuniculi (Sangiorgi, 1914). Occurs in the rabbit in Europe.

Hepatozoon griseisciuri (Clarke, 1958). Is found in the grey squirrel in the United States.

ORGANISMS OF UNCERTAIN CLASSIFICATION

The affinities of the protozoa considered in the following section are uncertain. Those that are definitely considered to be protozoa, e.g. *Toxoplasma, Sarcocystis, Besnoitia* etc., have been classified by Levine (1961) in a class Toxoplasmasida and in an order Toxoplasmorida. This order contains two families, Toxoplasmatidae and Sarcocystidae. This arrangement would appear more justified than previous ones, where, for example, the genus *Toxoplasma* was regarded as belonging to the family *Babesiidae*.

In addition to the above forms, there are some, previously regarded as protozoa, which are almost certainly non-protozoan in character and most likely rickettsiae. These include *Anaplasma, Eperythrozoon* and *Haemobartonella*. It has been customary in the past to include them in the protozoa, and though they now should be removed, they have not yet been accepted by bacteriologists and virologists as defined entities. Consequently, to avoid their being missed, a brief account of each is included in this volume.

Genus: Toxoplasma Nicolle and Manceaux, 1908

A single species, *Toxoplasma gondii* Nicolle and Manceaux, 1908, occurs.

Toxoplasma gondii. This was first observed in the African rodent, the gondi (*Ctenodactylus gondi*); but since then it has been found in a very large range of mammals and birds. Two morphological forms of the parasite occur, a proliferative form (trophozoite) and a cyst-like form (pseudocyst).

The mature proliferative trophozoite is elongate, often with a curved or crescent-like form; it measures from $4\,\mu$–$6\,\mu$ in length by $2\,\mu$–$3\,\mu$ in breadth. The vesicular nucleus, which possesses a central karyosome, is situated near the blunter end of the organism and stains red with Romanowsky stains, while the cytoplasm stains pale blue.

Electron micrographs show the trophozoite to be composed of an anterior conoid from which run five to eighteen cylindrical toxonemes. Mitochondria occur and an endosome is visible in the nucleus.

To reproduce, the organism penetrates a host cell, usually a reticuloendothelial cell, and undergoes repeated longitudinal binary division to produce eight or sixteen daughter parasites. The affected cell is grossly distended, and later the cell membrane ruptures, liberating the daughter parasites. The daughter parasites are usually smaller than the mature forms, but they enlarge in the intracellular fluid, enter new cells, and the cycle is repeated. A process of budding has been described by Goldman, *et al.* (1958).

The pseudocyst stage usually appears late in subacute or chronic infections. It is the general opinion that pseudocysts result from the active multiplication of trophozoites inside a cell, but instead of being released from the cell by rupture, a cyst wall is laid down around the stages inside the cell. Pseudocysts may measure as little as $8\,\mu$ but may reach up to $100\,\mu$ in size and contain up to 60,000 organisms. The organisms within the pseudocyst are closely packed together, are more lancet-shaped and possess a more terminal nucleus and a glycogen granule. It is undecided whether the wall of the pseudocyst consists of the remains of the host cell or whether it is primarily of parasitic origin. It is argyrophilic and elastic in its staining properties and appears quite resistant to mechanical damage (Cross, 1947).

As yet the organism has not been cultivated in artificial medium and will only proliferate in animals, in fertile eggs or in tissue culture (Cook & Jacobs, 1958).

Transmission of Toxoplasmosis. Two main methods of transmission exist; congenital or acquired. In congenital infection the organism passes across the placenta from an infected mother to the foetus; the mother usually suffers from an asymptomatic or subclinical infection, but the infection often becomes clinical in the offspring.

The natural mode of acquired transmission has yet to be determined. It is assumed that the pseudocyst form is responsible for transmission since the proliferative forms rapidly die outside the host; however, the fate of the cystic phase outside the host is not known either. The ability to survive the digestive process differs in the two forms. Thus, Jacobs (1956) found that it was easier to produce infections in mice when they were fed the carcases of mice which had suffered a chronic infection than those which had suffered an acute infection. Acutely infected mice usually only possess the proliferative stages, whereas chronically infected animals carry a large number of pseudocysts.

The oral route would appear to be the most likely way of infection, the organisms coming from a wide variety of sources such as the excretions or secretions of infected animals or directly by the consumption of infected food in an under-cooked condition. Evidence is available to suggest that persons eating meat in an under-cooked condition are more likely to contract the infection than persons that eat meat well-cooked. Probably no single mode of transmission is applicable, and several routes may be suggested. Thus, people handling meat such as butchers, slaughter-house attendants or those dealing with the carcases of animals may well acquire the infection through skin abrasions, cuts or through the conjunctival sac.

No adequate evidence exists at present to fully support arthropod transmission; however, arthropods can aquire the infection by sucking blood, and the parasite can survive in them for several days. Mice and other animals injected with material from ticks or mites collected in nature may develop toxoplasmosis (Jacobs, 1956), and toxoplasmosis is more prevalent in warm moist areas of the world than in cold or hot dry areas.

The possibility of the organism being transmitted by helminth ova has been raised by Hutchinson (1965), who was able to transmit the infection from cat to mouse with the embryonated eggs of the cat ascarid *Toxocara cati*. The form of the toxoplasma which occurs in the eggs has not been determined, but it remained viable for at least 12 months and caused infection in mice after this time.

Pathogenesis of Toxoplasmosis

General Characteristics of the Infection. Following the inoculation of the parasite into a susceptible animal, there is an incubation period which varies according to the size of the inoculum. Initially, multiplication occurs at the local site, and then there is general spread of the toxoplasms throughout the body, and invasion of various tissues and organs occurs. The parasites multiply in the proliferative form producing areas of necrosis, parasitism reaches high levels, and the animals may succumb during this period. During the height of this phase, organisms usually appear in secretions and excretions such as urine, faeces, milk, conjunctival fluid and even in the saliva. These are the proliferative forms, and they are unable to survive for any length of time outside the host. There is little spread of toxoplasmosis from one animal to another in the acute phase, even when the animals are confined in a close space (e.g. mice in the same jar). It is only under very special circumstances, where a most intimate contact is established between animals, that the proliferative form of the acute phase can result in the transmission of the disease from one animal to the other.

The subacute form of the disease is characterised by the appearance of antibodies which rapidly clear the blood and tissues of the proliferative form of the organism. The brain is cleared of organisms very late, followed by the heart, while the liver, spleen and lungs are cleared of organisms relatively quickly by the serum antibodies. Persistence of the organisms in the cyst or pseudocyst form is characteristic of the chronic infection. This phase can live for some considerable time; in dogs for up to 10 months, and in rats, mice and pigeons they have been found for as long as 3 years after infection.

A variation in strains of the organism is seen. The main criteria for differentiating strains are virulence and the characteristics of the disease produced. The most virulent strains are those which are highly pathogenic for mice and also produce severe disease in other laboratory animals. With strains of low virulence there is, in general, a lower parasitaemia, less tissue invasion and shorter persistence of the parasite. Organisms isolated from animals which have been sick or dying of the infection are usually more virulent than those that have been obtained from an animal which shows no clinical evidence of disease. In nature the organism seems very well adapted to its hosts, and the majority of infections are avirulent or at the most subclinical in character. The factors which lead to the organism adopting a more virulent behaviour are unknown.

Toxoplasmosis in the Human

Most of the cases of toxoplasmosis in children are congenital in origin, the mother usually showing a mild infection or no evidence of infection. The lesions are marked and the symptoms characteristic, namely cerebral calcification, choroidoretinitis, hydrocephalus or microcephaly and psychomotor disturbances. The child may be born either alive or dead, and if born alive may suffer serious mental retardation within a few weeks of birth. Generalised infection may be present at birth, and fever, adenopathy and enlargement of the spleen and liver occur shortly afterward. Mild cases of congenital toxoplasmosis occur, and these are more difficult to diagnose than the clinical form. Acquired toxoplasmosis (i.e. non-congenital) should be suspected when lymphadenopathy, lassitude accompanied by fever, lymphocytosis, meningoencephalitis, eye lesions of doubtful origin or myocarditis are observed. Probably hundreds or thousands of cases of human toxoplasmosis go unrecognised since only a mild illness characterised by slight fever and slight enlargement of the lymph glands is presented.

Toxoplasmosis in Dogs

Mello (1910) first described toxoplasmosis in a dog. The disease in this case was characterised by fever, anaemia, respiratory distress and haemorrhagic diarrhoea. On autopsy the animal had a sero-sanguinous exudate in body cavities, small nodules in the lungs and numerous small ulcers in the small intestine. Intracellular and extracellular parasites were seen in smears and sections. Since this time it has become clear that the clinical manifestations may vary greatly. Beverley (1957) has stated that in approximately half the cases of canine toxoplasmosis, respiratory signs are in evidence, alimentary disturbances occur in another quarter and neurological signs in the remainder. No sex difference was apparent, and all types of dogs were infected. The onset of illness is marked by an insidious development of fever with lassitude, anorexia and diarrhoea; occasionally it may be sudden with vomiting followed by fits and paralysis and other neurological manifestations (Beverley, 1957).

There is ample serological evidence to indicate that dogs are frequently infected in nature. Miller & Feldman (1953), using a dye test, found that 59 per cent of 51 dogs in New York were infected, Siim (1950) found 18·5 per cent of a group of dogs in Copenhagen had a high dye test titre and Lainson (1956) found 42·5 per cent of sera from 113 dogs in London positive by the complement fixation test.

The disease is characterised by necrosis, and the cellular infiltration is predominantly mononuclear. In the brain gliosis may develop alongside perivascular infiltrations which sometimes include plasma cells. A leptomeningitis may be present, and foci of necrosis occur in the grey matter just beneath the ependyma. Necrotic tissue may be shed into the ventricles leading to an obstructive internal hydrocephalus. It is usually the pseudocyst stage which is demonstrable in the brain (Beverley, 1957).

In the lungs necrotic nodules may be found in the parenchymatous tissue, and a pleural exudate may be present. Associated glands are swollen, and the organisms can be easily found in the cells lining the alveoli, trachea or bronchi.

The spleen and liver are usually enlarged, and organisms can be found in the liver cells, the epithelium of the biliary tubules and in the reticulo-endothelial cells of the spleen. Ulceration of the intestinal mucosa is common in canine toxoplasmosis. This tendency has also been recorded in cats, foxes and ferrets, and it may well be a factor in the transmission of the disease. The ulcers of the digestive tract are usually deep and occur in the duodenum or the rectum; organisms are found in the adjacent mucosa or lying underneath the muscle layers. Where intestinal ulceration is a feature of the infection, viable organisms have been found in the faeces.

Beverley (1957) has suggested that in many clinical cases of toxoplasmosis in dogs, some 'stress factor' has initiated the clinical entity, and Campbell (1956) in Glasgow found evidence that all the dogs with toxoplasmosis also suffered from a concomitant virus infection.

Toxoplasmosis in Cats

Few records exist as to the incidence of toxoplasmosis in cats. In a survey on the sera of cats in Hamburg, Westfal *et al.* (1950) were unable to find any evidence that cats were infected.

The lesions to be expected are enlargement and focal necrosis of the mesenteric lymph nodes, ulceration of the intestine and nodules in the lungs. The clinical syndrome is characterised by fever, dyspnoea, anorexia and blindness. Maksteneiks & Verlinde (1957) state that pseudocysts may occur in the brain and be associated with encephalomyelitis.

Toxoplasmosis in Cattle

Reports are scarce concerning toxoplasmosis in cattle. Sanger *et al.* (1953) recorded an outbreak of illness in a herd of Brown Swiss cows in which forty-five of seventy-eight calves, born over a period of a year, died at various ages. Clinical signs were dyspnoea, coughing, sneezing, a nasal discharge, trembling and shaking of the head. An elevated temperature was seen in several cases, but in others the temperature was more or less normal. At times death was sudden without any previous evidence of illness, or in other cases the disease lasted for several months. Autopsy of a 4 week old calf showed a fibrinous deposit in the peritoneal cavity, enlargement of submaxillary and bronchial lymph glands, a haemorrhagic tracheitis and pneumonia with consolidation. Toxoplasma were found in the brain, lungs and lymph nodes. Sanger *et al.* (1953) demonstrated the organism in individual animals in another herd which had suffered from signs of anorexia, weakness, ataxia and diarrhoea. Koestner & Cole (1961) have studied the neuropathology of toxoplasmosis in experimentally infected cattle and sheep, the lesions in both species being similar. In the early stages lesions consist of damage to the vascular walls producing endothelial swelling, perivascular oedema and proliferation of the adventitia cells. The process spreads to adjacent nervous tissue producing foci of necrosis which contain numerous toxoplasma organisms. Glial nodules consisting of pleomorphic microglia and oligodendroglia, astrocytes and monocytes are formed, and at this stage pseudocysts are in evidence. Healing of these lesions with scar formation occurs, and a particular feature in the chronic form is calcification of the blood vessel walls.

Toxoplasmosis in Sheep

An early report of toxoplasmosis in sheep was made by Olafson & Monlux (1942), who found the organism in sheep affected with nervous signs. Wickham & Carne (1950) recorded a single case of 'circling disease' in Australian sheep, toxoplasma being found in the brain along with congestion and perivascular cuffing.

The association of toxoplasma with ovine perinatal mortality was recorded by Harley & Marshall (1957) in New Zealand. These authors demonstrated the association of abortion with *Toxoplasma gondii*, and in Great Britain, Beverley & Watson (1961) recorded that toxoplasma infection was associated with ovine abortion in Yorkshire. Serological surveys showed toxoplasma infection to be widespread in Yorkshire flocks, and antibodies to *Toxoplasma* were found in high titres in ewes which had aborted from hitherto unknown causes. The organism was isolated from the brain or liver of aborted or still-born lambs, but there is as yet no conclusive evidence in Britain that toxoplasma plays the same role in ovine abortion as it does in New Zealand. However, the evidence suggests that the situation might be such. New Zealand toxoplasmosis is probably the most widespread and most important cause of infectious ovine perinatal mortality (Hartley & Marshall, 1957). Toxoplasmosis, other than the disease causing abortion, has not been previously recognised in New Zealand, and Hartley & Marshall suggested that the New Zealand strain of *Toxoplasma* was less virulent than, for example, American (RH) strain, and they postulated that the organism has become adapted to the pregnant ovine uterus.

Hartley *et al.* (1954) and Hartley & Marshall (1957) have detailed the clinical aspects of toxoplasma abortion in sheep. Death of the foetus may occur antepartum, at the end of an apparently normal parturition or within a few hours of birth. Mummification, mild to marked uterine decomposition, subcutaneous oedema of the foetus and an excess of fluid in the body cavities are seen. However, these changes are not specific for toxoplasmosis and are generally indicative of abortion and uterine infection, and essentially there is no diagnostic lesion which can be specifically attributed to toxoplasma infection.

Histological examination of the foetal membranes, particularly of those where the infection is still active, shows oedema of the mesenchyme of the foetal villi with a moderately diffuse invasion of mononuclear cells. Focal areas of epithelial swelling and necrosis, with desquamation, are evident, and where large areas of the trophoblast are shed necrotic nodules may result. Cotyledons show intra- and extracellular toxoplasms.

The neuropathological lesions in experimental toxoplasmosis in sheep are similar to those found in cattle (Koestner & Cole, 1961) and occur in 75 per cent of cases. The principal lesion is a focal necrosis in the acute form, while in the more chronic form glial nodules are much in evidence, and toxoplasma cysts are found associated with these.

Toxoplasmosis in Pigs

Toxoplasmosis in pigs was first recorded by Farrell *et al.* (1952). Since then pigs in America, Norway and Japan have been found infected, and Harding *et al.* (1961) reported the infection in British pigs. Newly born animals and those up to 3 weeks of age tend to be affected, and usually the disease is manifest by excessive losses of young pigs at farrowing time. The clinical signs include fever, shivering, weakness, coughing, incoordination, relaxation of abdominal muscles and diarrhoea. Pulmonary signs may be a common feature of acute toxoplasmosis in the young pig, and frequently this is associated with subclinical pneumonia in the herd.

Cole *et al.* (1953) state that the most common post-mortem signs are pneumonia, focal necrosis of the liver, hydrothorax, ascites, lymphadenitis and enteritis.

As with toxoplasmosis in other animals, the mode of transmission from pig to pig or mother to offspring is not known. Cole *et al.* (1953) have demonstrated by mouse inoculation that milk from lactating sows, which reacted to intradermal and serological tests, contained the organism, and they suggested that the milk may be a source of infection for the young pig.

Toxoplasmosis in Birds

A large number of records have been made concerning the prevalence of toxoplasma infection in birds. However, many of these records have been made upon the histological appearance of an organism resembling toxoplasma, and no direct serological or mouse inoculation evidence exists to support many of the reports.

In domestic poultry, a disease ascribed to toxoplasmosis has been reported by Ericksen & Harbor (1953) in Norway. Fowls were found dead without any evidence of previous illness, and others showed signs of anorexia, emaciation and pallor for periods of up to a month. Diarrhoea and blindness were features in some of the poultry. Histologically, there was a pericarditis, focal or diffuse myocarditis, focal encephalitis, a necrotic hepatitis and ulcers of the gastro-intestinal tract. Toxoplasma were found in various organs.

Jacobs *et al.* (1952) carried out a survey of the prevalence of toxoplasma in pigeons in Washington. A prevalence of 12·5 per cent was found, and strains isolated from them were morphologically and serologically identical with the virulent RH (human) strain.

Toxoplasmosis in Other Animals

Christiansen (1948) and Christiansen & Siim (1951) recorded outbreaks of toxoplasmosis in hares in the winter months in Denmark. In nearly all the cases the infections were of the acute, fatal type and showed general systemic infections. A marked increase in the size of the spleen was evident, and the livers were enlarged, pale and contained scattered submiliary foci. The mesenteric lymph nodes were swollen, there was oedema of the lungs and a sero-sanguinous fluid in the body cavities. Toxoplasma were present in large numbers in most of the organs, being particularly associated with the changes in the lungs, liver and spleen.

Toxoplasmosis in wild rabbits was studied by Beverley *et al.* (1954), who found in Great Britain that 34 per cent showed serological evidence of infection. Lainson (1955) demonstrated that the organism may be found in the brain of rabbits, even in those which had been bred under conditions which excluded them from contact with the wild rabbit. Strains recovered from such rabbits failed to produce disease in mice.

The prevalence of toxoplasma in rats has not been widely investigated. Perrin *et al.* (1943) found 8·7 per cent of savannah rats infected with toxoplasma in the brain, and Eyles (1952) found a prevalence of 3·2 per cent in rats in the Memphis area. Spontaneous disease in the rat, due to toxoplasmosis, is rare, and it is also difficult to induce disease artificially in rats, even with large doses of the organism.

Public Health Significance of Toxoplasmosis

Numerous reports attest the widespread prevalence of toxoplasmosis in domestic and wild animals and in man. Despite the 'sea of toxoplasma infection around us' (Jacobs, 1956), the mode of the transmission is still in doubt. There have been some suggestions that human infections are associated with infections of pets such as dogs and cats or with the consumption of the flesh of infected animals. The latter, however, does not offer a satisfactory explanation of how herbivors such as cattle, sheep, goats, rabbits and hares are infected.

Westphal & Bauer (1952) have stressed that toxoplasmosis is 'not normally a disease', rather it appears to be a condition of symbiosis between the host and the animal, and only rarely is the balance tipped in favour of the parasite. Beverley *et al.* (1954), in a study of toxoplasmosis in the Sheffield area of Great Britain, ranked various occupational groups according to their susceptibility to toxoplasmosis. The general prevalence of toxoplasmosis, judged by serological tests, was 25 per cent of the adult population. The prevalence increased up to the age of 20, after which it remained steady. There was no significant difference between the prevalence in men or in women, but significantly higher antibody titres were found in the sera of veterinarians and abattoir workers. A still higher prevalence was noted in individuals who handled rabbits, and highest of all was the group who were concerned with the trapping of rabbits.

Diagnosis of Toxoplasmosis

Diagnosis of toxoplasmosis on clinical grounds is usually difficult, and recourse must be made to the demonstration of either the organism or antibodies against it. The most convincing diagnosis is the isolation of the parasite by inoculation of suspect material into mice. Mice are probably the most useful animals for this since they are highly susceptible and rarely suffer from spontaneous infection. A highly virulent strain produces an acute and generalised fatal infection 1–14 days after the intraperitoneal route of injection, and a few days earlier if the intracerebral route has been used. Ascites develops after intraperitoneal injection, and abundant proliferative stages can be found in films prepared from peritoneal or pleural fluids or in smears from the cut surfaces of lung, liver, spleen and brain.

With strains of lower virulence a transient disease is produced in a few mice about the 3rd week after inoculation, but mostly the disease is asymptomatic. Infected mice can be detected by serological tests about 6 weeks after inoculation and the infection confirmed by examination of the brain for pseudocysts. This is done by emulsifying the brain in saline and examining a drop of this under the low power of a microscope. The number of cysts found in a smear may vary from one to 100 or more depending on the virulence.

Where diagnosis is uncertain it is sometimes desirable to carry out blind passage of material from the first set of mice to a second or further set of mice. Several passages may be necessary before the organism appears in a form virulent enough to cause acute peritonitis. Alternatively, cortisone can be given to enable strains of low virulence to produce the acute fatal type of infection.

Various strains of *Toxoplasma* exist. Some are highly virulent, as illustrated by the RH (human) strain, which will cause an acute fulminating and fatal disease in mice (the RH strain of toxoplasma has been serially passaged in mice since its original isolation from a human case of encephalitis); but on the other hand apparently completely avirulent toxoplasms appear. The rabbit strain of Lainson (1955) can be passaged in rabbits for a year with no apparent increase in pathogenicity, and it has been passaged rapidly, on fourteen occasions, in mice without alteration of the virulence. However, the introduction of this strain into multimammate rats (*Mastomys* = *Rattus coucha*) resulted in a highly pathogenic strain which would produce fatal infections in animals. Similarly, the passage of organisms through canaries will result in a marked elevation of virulence. The increased virulence is fully maintained when the organism is put back into ordinary laboratory mice and guinea pigs (Lainson, 1957).

Serological Tests. Fulton (1963) has reviewed the serological procedures available for the diagnosis of toxoplasmosis. Of many tests available the complement fixation test (Sabin, 1949; Warren & Sabin, 1942), the dye test (Sabin & Feldman, 1948; Beverley & Beattie, 1952), the skin test (Frenkel, 1948), the inhibition of fluorescence (Goldman, 1957) and the haemagglutination test (Jacobs & Lunde, 1957) are in more general use.

Dye Test. The dye test depends on the principle that antibody and an accessory factor (a complement-like serum factor) modify living *Toxoplasma* so that these fail to stain with methylene blue at pH 11. Proliferative forms of *Toxoplasma* which have not been modified by antibody stain readily, and the test is quantitated by finding the highest dilution of serum which will modify 50 per cent of the toxoplasms in a standard suspension. Beverley (1960) has emphasised that constant practice is necessary in order to perform and interpret the dye test, and it is best carried out in a large laboratory which is routinely doing serological surveys. Because of the exacting value of the test and, at times, the difficulty in obtaining sera containing accessory factor, many diagnostic laboratories have stopped using it.

In man a dye test titre of 1 in 16 is regarded as suspect, 1 in 32 as probable and 1 in 64 as strong presumptive evidence of toxoplasma infection. In artificial infections it is possible to produce extraordinarily high titres. In man antibody levels rise to a maximum a few weeks to a few months after primary clinical infection, and they then fall slowly over a period of years. It is possible that a positive dye test persists in an infected person for the rest of his life.

Complement Fixation Test. This has been widely used as a diagnostic test. The titres, though lower, generally follow those delineated by the dye test. Complement-fixing antibodies usually appear later and disappear sooner than those detected by the other tests, and in most cases antibodies disappear following the disappearance of clinical signs. The antigens which have been used include preparations from infected chorio-allantoic membranes of the chick embryo (Cathie, 1957) and lysed organisms from mouse peritoneal exudates (Thalhammer, 1956).

Skin Test. The antigen for this is prepared by rapidly freezing and thawing toxoplasms obtained from a mouse peritoneal exudate. The reaction is of the delayed hypersensitivity type. There is, generally, good agreement between the positive skin test and dye test positive sera, though no relationship exists between the area of the erythema in the skin test and the serum antibody titres. Its main use is in population surveys.

Haemagglutination Test. Jacobs & Lunde (1957) developed a passive haemagglutination test which has gained wide acceptance and now serves as a routine serological test in many laboratories. Various modifications of it have increased its usefulness; thus formalinised cells provide a stable supply of standardised cells, and human group O cells avoid heterophile reactions which may occur with sheep cells.

Indirect Fluorescent Antibody Test (I.F.A.). Goldman (1957) described this test, which is based on the inhibition of the specific staining of the *Toxoplasma* organism with fluorescent antibody by antibody in the test serum. This test has yet to achieve widespread use, but it has been shown to be sensitive, specific and reproducible and, together with the haemagglutination technique, may ultimately prove to be the most practical method for the diagnosis of toxoplasmosis.

Treatment. No completely satisfactory treatment for toxoplasmosis is known. Daraprim (pyrimethamine) (2,4-diamino-5-*p*-chlorophenyl-6-ethyl-pyrimidine) has been found effective in monkeys and humans at adequate blood levels and is effective against the proliferative forms of the organisms. It is of little value against the cyst forms.

Pyrimethamine, with triple sulpha drugs, has given good results in many cases, especially in ocular cases of toxoplasmosis. There is synergy between the sulphonamides and the diamino pyrimidines, this producing sequential blocks in the metabolic pathways involving para-amino benzoic acid, folic acid and folinic acid (Eyles, 1956).

Genus: Encephalitozoon Levaditi, Nicolau and Schoen, 1923

The genera *Toxoplasma* and *Encephalitozoon* are very similar, and Biocca (1949) has suggested that they may be synonymous. One species is recognised, *Encephalitozoon cuniculi* Levaditi, Nicolau and Schoen, 1923, originally found in the brain and kidney of a rabbit affected with motor paralysis. It has been demonstrated subsequently in mice, guinea pigs, rats and occasionally the dog.

Encephalitozoon cuniculi. The organisms are smaller than *Toxoplasma*, being straight or slightly curved, uninucleate rods with rounded ends, one end being a little larger than the other. Extracellular forms are $2 \cdot 4 \mu - 3 \cdot 4 \mu$ by $1 \cdot 8 \mu - 2 \cdot 8 \mu$, and intracellular forms are $1 \cdot 5 \mu - 3 \mu$ by $1 \cdot 4 \mu - 2 \cdot 8 \mu$. Parasites may be found in compact pseudocyst accumulations containing 100 or more trophozoites in nerve cells, macrophages or other tissue cells.

The differentiation between *Toxoplasma* and *Encephalitozoon* is based on immunological and morphological characteristics. No cross immunity exists between the two, the cytoplasm of *Encephalitozoon* stains uniformly light blue with Giemsa stain, whereas that of *Toxoplasma* is granulated. *Encephalitozoon* is Gram-positive and *Toxoplasma* Gram-negative; *Encephalitozoon* stains poorly with haematoxylin and eosin, whereas *Toxoplasma* stains well; and with iron haematoxylin *Encephalitozoon* stains black and *Toxoplasma* does not. *Encephalitozoon* may be rapidly frozen and stored at $-70°C$, whereas *Toxoplasma* fails to survive this; *Toxoplasma* grows readily in tissue culture of monkey kidney monolayers, but *Encephalitozoon* fails to do so; *Toxoplasma* is usually fatal to mice, especially on serial passage, but *Encephalitozoon* is not and its virulence is not enhanced by serial passage.

The developmental cycle of *Encephalitozoon* is unknown, but the organisms can be transmitted to mice, rats and rabbits by intracerebral and intraperitoneal inoculation of material from brain, liver, spleen or peritoneal exudate. It has also been transmitted *via* the urine, and it is likely that congenital infection also occurs.

Pathogenesis of E. cuniculi. In many instances the infection is not apparent and, at the most, is indicated by a mild temperature increase. In the rabbit the infection is usually chronic, and motor paralysis may occur with death. Lesions occur in the brain, and fatal or acute cases show necrotic areas with lymphocytic cuffing about the blood vessels of the cerebrum. Granulomatous lesions occur in the kidneys and other organs, and necrotic lesions have been described in the heart and kidneys.

Disease due to *E. cuniculi* has been reported in dogs by Plowright (1952) and Plowright & Yeoman (1952). Fox hound puppies were affected with posterior weakness and incoordination, the animals fatigued quickly, and there was loss of condition and ocular changes. The animals died from 6 weeks to 15 months of age. In both outbreaks the clinical signs resembled those of rabies. Animals became vicious, attempted to bite people, and some puppies had epileptiform fits or uncontrolled spasms. The major lesions consisted of encephalitis and nephritis, the lesions being similar so those seen in the rabbit.

Diagnosis of *Encephalitozoon* infection is based on the demonstration of the lesions and organisms in sections. Differentiation from *Toxoplasma* is necessary, and this is done on serological evidence and on staining reactions.

No treatment is known.

Genus: Sarcocystis Lankester, 1882

A large number of species of *Sarcocystis* have been described from the striated muscles of herbivors, birds and man. The validity of the speciation is open to question since species have been differentiated on host basis, on their size and wall structure. Some forms show little host specificity and the morphology may vary in different hosts.

Spindler & Zimmerman (1945) reported the isolation of an *Aspergillus*-like organism from the sarcocystis of pigs, and later Spindler (1947) described hyphae-like structures in *Sarcocystis* from sheep and geese. This led to the speculation that *Sarcocystis* was fungal in nature; however, the studies of Ludvik (1958, 1960, 1963) leave little doubt that *Sarcocystis* is a protozoan with relationships to *Toxoplasma* and the M organism.

Morphology of Sarcocystis

The organisms (Miescher's tubes) are usually readily visible as spindles or cylindrical shaped structures lying in the muscle bundles. They vary greatly in size, from microscopic dimensions to several centimetres in length. Essentially, the organism is enclosed in a cyst wall, from the inside of which septa run into the body of the parasite dividing it into a number of chambers. When mature, it is filled with banana shaped spores or trophozoites $10\,\mu$–$12\,\mu$ by $4\,\mu$–$9\,\mu$ (Rainey's corpuscles). Detailed examinations of the structure of *Sarcocystis* and the trophozoites have been carried out by Ludvik (1958, 1960, 1963). The cyst wall is a unicellular syncitium with many nuclei surrounded by cell organelles, and the surface is provided with hollow projections which enable the parasite to come into close contact with the host tissue. The cyst is divided into a large number of chambers, the walls being formed by the projection of an inner, granular layer of the cyst wall which show connections with the superficial hollow projections. The trophozoite is covered by a double layered pellicle and in the anterior third there is a fibrillar zone with a well developed anterior hollow conoid, $0\cdot3\,\mu$–$0\cdot4\,\mu$ long. Covering the conoid and within the pellicle is a polar ring, $0\cdot4\,\mu$–$0\cdot5\,\mu$ in diameter, and from this twenty-two to twenty-six fibrils run back along the whole length of the body under the double layered pellicle. The anterior third of the body is filled with a large number (up to 350) of parallel fibrils or channels, 50 mμ in diameter, the sarconemes, which arise from the conoid and end abruptly at about the third of the cell. A large number of spherical central granules, $0\cdot4\,\mu$–$0\cdot5\,\mu$ in diameter, occur in the middle of the body; these impregnate well with osmium and stain with Heidenhein's hematoxylin but not with Giemsa. A large number of small granules, some of which contain RNA and some volutin, also occur here. The nucleus is in the posterior third of the body. It is finally granulated and surrounded by a double nuclear membrane and contains a small number of chromatin granules and an endosome which stains well with silver. A large number of granules and vacuoles occur around the nucleus, some containing glycogen, and lying amongst them are 1 to 3 elongated mitochondria with a typical tubular interior structure.

Developmental Cycle of Sarcocystis. It is generally believed that infection is by ingestion, animals acquiring muscle cysts at some stage in the faeces of animals. Resistant forms of the parasite have been described in the intestines of mice, and passage through the intestine may be a necessary part of the developmental cycle. Spindler *et al.* (1946) failed to infect pigs directly with *Sarcocystis* material from pig muscle, but pigs became infected when they ate their own faeces. Similarly, the passage of infected pork through the digestive tract of dogs, cats, mice and chickens produced a form which was infective for swine. There is no evidence for an intermediate host or an insect vector.

It is assumed that the infective stage or trophozoite passes through the intestinal wall and is carried by the blood stream to various striated muscles of the body. The earliest stage, detectable 6 or more weeks after infection, consists of a single-celled amoeboid parasite, the nucleus of which undergoes a series of binary fissions to produce a number of rounded nucleated cells (sporoblasts), the whole being enclosed in a cyst

PLATE XXVIII

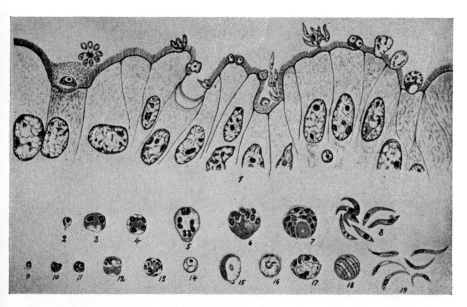

Cryptosporidium parvum from the small intestine of mice (× approx. 2000). (From Wenyon, 1926)

1. Various stages of parasite on the surface of the epithelium. 2–8. Schizogony cycle. 9–13. Development of microgametocyte and formation of microgametes. 14, 15. Development of macrogametocyte. 16–18. Development of oocyst and formation of sporozoites. 19. Escape of sporozoites from oocysts

PLATE XXIX

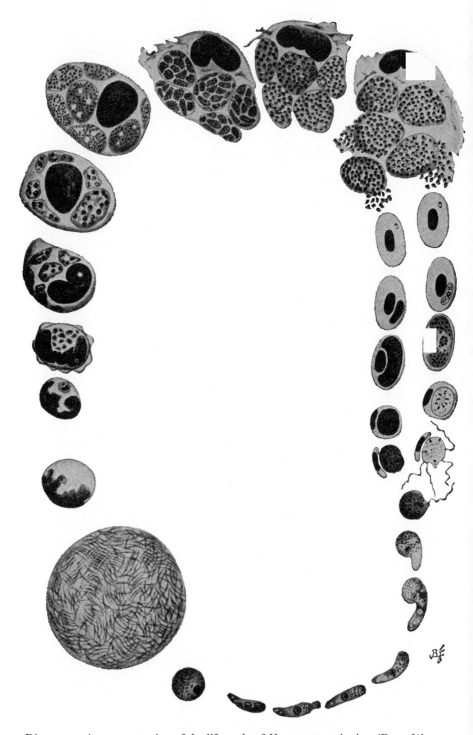

Diagrammatic representation of the life cycle of *Haemoproteus columbae*. (From Wenyon, 1926)

PLATE XXX

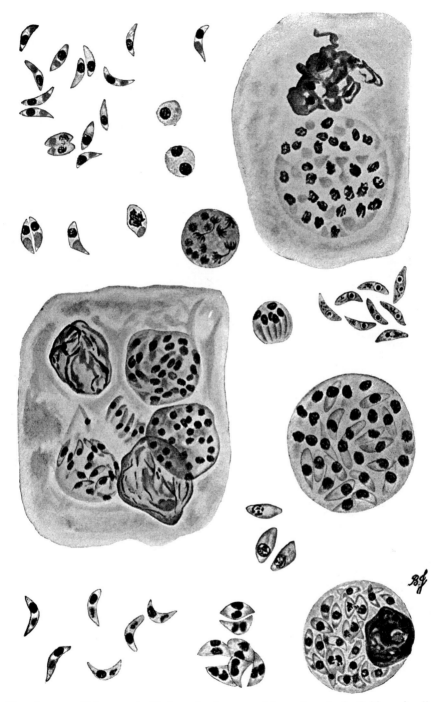

Toxoplasma gondii (× 1750). Various developmental forms from body fluids and cells.
(From Wenyon, 1926)

PLATE XXXI

A. *Encephalitozoon cuniculi* in atrophying nerve cell and scattered through the brain substance (× 1200). (From Wenyon, 1926)

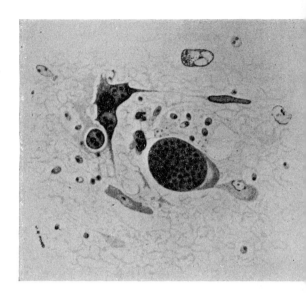

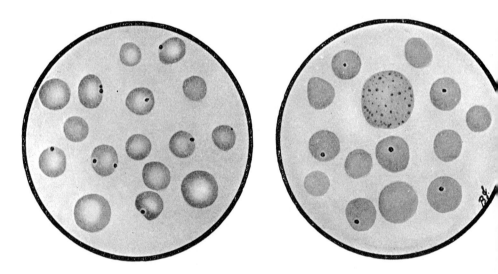

B. Anaplasmosis of cattle (× approx. 2000). (From Wenyon, 1926). At left, *Anaplasma marginale.* At right, *Anaplasma centrale;* an enlarged red blood corpuscle showing basophilic spots is also shown

wall (Scott, 1943). Repeated binary fission results in ellipsoidal and later banana-shaped forms (trophozoites), and as these increase in number, the cyst enlarges in size, and ingrowths of the cyst wall divide the organism into chambers or compartments. The process continues and as the cyst grows new trophoblasts are produced at the periphery of the cyst and trophozoites accumulate inside the cyst.

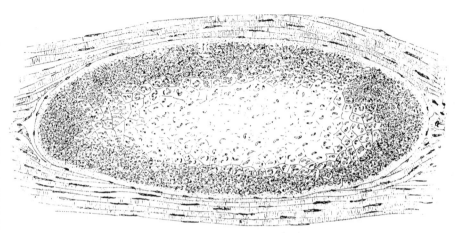

Fig. 288. Diagrammatic Representation of Longitudinal Section of a Sarcocyst in the Muscles of the Ox. (× ca. 500). (From Wenyon, 1926)

Pathogenesis of Sarcocystis. In the living animal, *Sarcocystis* spp. are not considered to be of any serious pathogenic significance. Meat intended for human consumption may be condemned if it is infected with the parasite. Spindler *et al.* (1946) have reported that pigs with more than forty cysts per g. of diaphragm muscle were unthrifty and showed signs of muscular stiffness.

Sarcocystis tenella Railliet, 1886. *Hosts:* Sheep, goats. Commonly in the oesophagus, also in the diaphragm and the heart. Readily visible, ellipsoidal, up to 1 cm. in length. Common.

Sarcocystis fusiformis Railliet, 1897. *Hosts:* Ox. Striated and heart muscles. Up to 1 cm. in length. World wide in distribution. Common.

Sarcocystis miescheriana (Kühn, 1865) Lankester, 1882. *Hosts:* Pig. Tongue and heart muscle. World wide in distribution. Common. Cyst generally just visible to the naked eye, may reach up to 4 mm. in length.

Sarcocystis bertrami Doflein, 1901. *Hosts:* Horses, asses, mules. Heart, diaphragm and other muscles. World wide and common. Resembles *S. miescheriana.*

Sarcocystis lindemanni (Rivolta, 1878). *Hosts:* Man. Heart, larynx, tongue and extremities. World wide in distribution; rare. Cysts up to 5 cm. in length, usually very much smaller.

Sarcocystis muris Blanchard, 1885. *Hosts:* Mice, rats. Heart muscles and other striated muscles. World wide in distribution. Cysts up to several cm. in length, appearing as white tubules in the muscle fibers.

Genus: Besnoitia Henry, 1913

The status of this genus has been under discussion in recent years (Jellison, 1956). Previously, the name *Globidium* has been used, but it is now clear that the intestinal globidia represent macroschizont development of one or more species of *Eimeria* (Pellerdy, 1963). Pols (1960) considers that the genus *Besnoitia* has affinities with *Toxoplasma* but is differentiated from it by occurring temporarily in monocytes and permanently in histocytes, whereas *Toxoplasma* occurs chiefly in cells of the reticulo-endothelial system such as macrophages, monocytes and endothelial cells.

Cutaneous besnoitiasis is a serious skin condition of cattle and horses, especially in South Africa. It is characterised by painful swellings, thickening of the skin, loss of hair and necrosis.

Morphology. The *Besnoitia* pseudocyst may reach up to 600 μ in diameter. It is usually spherical, and when mature it is packed with crescentic trophozoites, each 2 μ–7 μ in length. Animals may be infected artificially by the intraperitoneal, intravenous or subcutaneous injection of blood from an infected animal.

The morphology of the developmental stages has been followed by Pols (1960) in artificially infected rabbits. Trophozoites appear 16–18 days after inoculation and occur extracellularly or in monocytes in the blood stream or in smears from the lung or testes. The early forms are mainly crescentic, 5 μ–9 μ by 2 μ–5 μ, with a blue granular cytoplasm and a more or less central nucleus. Invasion of histocytes occurs, a vacuole is produced, and here the forms multiply by binary fission. As the *Besnoitia* grow the host cell nucleus divides to form a multinucleate cell, and as the cyst becomes larger the cytoplasm of the host cell is flattened to form the inner coat of the pseudocyst. As the parasite becomes larger, collagen is laid down around the host cell membrane to form the hyaline capsule of the pseudocyst.

The natural mode of transmission is probably by ingestion, and Hofmeyr (1945) has suggested that in South Africa contaminating watering troughs may be the source of infection. More recently, Bigalke (1960) has reported that the *Besnoitia besnoiti* may be transmitted mechanically by *Glossina palpalis*.

Besnoitia besnoiti (Marotel, 1912) Henry, 1913. *Hosts:* Cattle, rabbit experimentally. The parasite is endemic in South Africa and also occurs in the Congo, Sudan, Angola, southern France and Portugal.

The parasite is found in the dermis, subcutaneous tissues and fascia and in the laryngeal, nasal and other mucosae.

Pathogenesis of B. besnoiti. The mortality of infection is usually below 10 per cent, though animals may lose condition markedly, pregnant animals may abort, bulls may become sterile and the hides are of little value for leather making purposes. Animals of all ages, from 6 months upwards, may be infected, and after an incubation period of 6–10 days there is a temperature rise which lasts 2–10 days. Cyst formation in the skin occurs 1–4 weeks after the start of the temperature rise. The febrile stage of the infection is accompanied by photophobia, enlargement of the lymph nodes and oedematous swellings on the limbs and the lower parts of the body. These are tender and warm, the animals are reluctant to move and are anorexic, respiration is rapid, diarrhoea may be present and abortion may occur at this stage. The initial stage may be mild with little obvious clinical alteration, and such animals usually recover. However, the acute febrile stage may progress to the second, or depilatory, stage in which the skin becomes markedly thickened; it loses its elasticity, and it may crack open and ooze a serous sanguinous fluid. The hair falls out over the swollen parts, and the skin is left very much wrinkled. Animals may start to feed again, but the loss of condition is very marked. Death may occur during the second stage, but if the animal survives the third, or seborrhoea sicca, stage supervenes. The animals remain emaciated for several months, there is a further loss of hair over the areas which were oedematous, and a markedly thickened and folded hide results. This skin is also scurfy, and the whole appearance is one of extensive mange. The hairless condition may remain for several months if not the life of the animal, though in milder cases a certain amount of regrowth of hair may occur giving checkered markings on the animal. There is no satisfactory treatment for the condition.

Besnoitia bennetti Babudieri, 1932. *Hosts:* Horse, ass. Africa, Sudan, southern France. Two cases have been found in imported burros in the United States. The species is less common than *B. besnoiti* of cattle. The parasite was originally described in both horses and cattle in the Sudan, but Pols (1960) has clearly separated the parasites of the horse and those of the cow.

The morphology is essentially the same as for *B. besnoiti*, and the life cycle is presumed to be the same.

Pathogenesis. The pathogenesis of *B. bennetti* was described by Bennett (1933). The disease has a chronic course, animals being ill for 7–8 months. There is marked weakness, a general thickening of the skin, loss of hair and a scurfy appearance. Occasionally the disease may run a more acute course ending in death.

Other species of *Besnoitia* include:

Besnoitia tarandi (Hadwen, 1922). Of the reindeer and caribou in Alaska.

Besnoitia jellisoni Frenkel, 1955. Of the wild mouse (*Peromyscus maniculatus*) in the U.S.A. (Idaho).

Genus: Anaplasma Theiler, 1910

There is little doubt that *Anaplasma* can no longer be regarded as a protozoan, and there is every evidence of its rickettsial nature. Nevertheless, it is frequently dealt with in courses on protozoology, at conferences on parasitology and in textbooks on parasitology and for the convenience of persons who may inadvertently turn to a textbook on veterinary parasitology for information, the following general outline is presented.

Anaplasma appears as small, spherical bodies, red to dark red in colour when stained with Romanowsky stains, inside the red blood cells of cattle, deer, sheep and goats. They are 0·2 μ–0·5 μ in diameter, with no cytoplasm, but a faint halo may appear around them. Sometimes two organisms may lie close to each other, giving the appearance of binary fission; occasionally multiple invasion of a cell may occur.

Anaplasma marginale Theiler, 1910. This organism is widely distributed throughout the tropical and subtropical areas of the world. It is common in Africa, the Middle East, southern Europe and the Far East; and in the United States it is stated that the disease is a major problem in 18 states, costing 34 to 35 million dollars annually. Deer may be infected experimentally, and the carrier state may occur in wild deer in the United States, in antelope in South Africa and the elk in the Soviet Union. It is transmitted by ticks of various species, and mechanical transmission by tabanid flies and mosquitoes is important in some areas.

Morphology of A. marginale. Recent work on the morphology of *Anaplasma* has indicated its rickettsia-like character. Espana & Espana (1963) distinguished two morphological types, a normal, rounded form and a filamented form, both of which occurred in the majority of infected animals, but in some cases only the rounded form of organism was seen. Further work by Kreier & Ristic (1963a, b, c) distinguished three morphological types from various parts of the United States, and these authors have suggested that the three forms are distinct organisms for which they propose the names *Anaplasma marginale* for a rounded, marginal body type, *Paranaplasma caudata* for a tailed form and *Paranaplasma discoides* for a bipolar disc type.

Electron microscopic studies of bovine erythrocytes infected with *Anaplasma* have shown that the organism is structurally similar to the inclusion bodies produced by members of the psittacosis lymphogranuloma group of organisms. The inclusion body consists of two to eight smaller sub-units (initial bodies) (Ristic & Watrach, 1961), which are round or oval, 300 mμ to 400 mμ in diameter and enclosed in a double membrane.

The invasion and the multiplication of *Anaplasma* in red cells was studied by Ristic (1963). Initial bodies enter mature erythrocytes by penetration of the erythrocyte membrane. Reproduction of the initial body is by binary fission, and this occurs by an elongation of the initial body and a constriction of its double membrane. A further marked constriction occurs, and electron-dense material is present in each of two daughter organisms formed, these being still connected by a narrow strand of plasma. Ultimately, the two separate but remain close to one another.

Transmission of Anaplasma. On a world-wide basis, it is probable that ticks are the primary vectors of anaplasmosis; however, tabanid flies, deerflies, mosquitoes and stable flies have all been demonstrated to act as vectors. Piercy (1956) has listed nineteen species of seven genera of ticks, including *Argas, Boophilus, Dermacentor, Hyalomma, Ixodes, Ornithodorus* and *Rhipicephalus*, which are concerned in transmission.

Transmission by biting flies has been considered in detail by Piercy (1956), and this method of transmission appears to be common in the southern United States. Transmission by mosquitoes is thought to be of lesser importance and is possibly responsible for active transmission under natural conditions in a few instances.

Mechanical transmission of anaplasmosis is well known, and major and minor operations in cattle husbandry such as dehorning, castration, vaccination, blood sampling etc. may be responsible for the transmission of anaplasmosis both in and out of season.

Clinical Manifestations of Anaplasmosis. Anaplasmosis is essentially a disease of adult cattle, and in general severe clinical infections do not occur until an animal is about 18 months of age. Younger animals are susceptible to the infection but exhibit little detectable reaction, though they can be made clinical cases by splenectomy. In mature cows the incubation period is from 15–36 days with an average of 26 days. There is an increase in body temperature, and in mature animals the infection may be fatal during the fever period. Organisms appear in the red blood cells several days before the fever; at first only a few are found, but by the time fever is initiated, 30–48 per cent of cells may be parasitised; and as the fever progresses, the number of parasitised red cells increases. Anorexia develops and animals show severe anaemia which is especially noticeable at the time of, or shortly after, the fever crisis.

Mortality, especially in susceptible imported cattle, may be as high as 80 per cent, but in an enzootic area the seasonal death rate may be of the order of 10 per cent.

In more chronic cases there is a severe anaemia, and recovery is slow, the animal being susceptible to numerous other conditions which may affect it; in Africa, for example, malnutrition, virus diseases etc. may terminate the life of the animal.

Anaplasma centrale Theiler, 1911. This organism is morphologically similar to and possibly a variant of *A. marginale*. As its name suggests, it is centrally placed in the erythrocyte. *A. centrale* infections are comparable to those of *A. marginale* except that they are milder.

Anaplasma ovis. This organism is referred to in the literature, but there is some doubt as to the validity of the species. *Anaplasma* *marginale* may be maintained by sub-passage through sheep and goats in which it is usually nonpathogenic, and during passage the virulence of the organism for cattle is reduced or lost. This organism resembles *A. marginale*, and it may, under natural conditions, be a form which has become adapted to sheep. Infections in sheep have been reported from North America, North and South Africa, Israel and the Soviet Union.

Genus: Eperythrozoon Schilling, 1928

The exact systematic position of the eperythrozoa has yet to be determined. Organisms of this genus are minute forms occurring on the surface of erythrocytes and in the plasma; they are usually minute rings or coccoid-shaped granular bodies, $0.5\,\mu$–$2\,\mu$–$3\,\mu$ in diameter, and stain reddish-purple with Romanowsky stains. Electron microscope studies by Ristic (1963) showed them to be oblong, rod-shaped structures surrounded by a double membrane with a cytoplasm containing an accumulation of high electron density substances near each end. Partial cross serological staining by the fluorescent antibody technique was demonstrated between *Anaplasma* and *Eperythrozoon*.

Several species of *Eperythrozoon* have been recorded from various parts of the world. *Eperythrozoon wenyoni* occurs in cattle, being widespread in various parts of the world, including North America; *Eperythrozoon ovis* has been reported in sheep in South Africa; *Eperythrozoon parvum* and *Eperythrozoon suis* occur in swine; and *Eperythrozoon felis* has been described from the cat, though this may represent a misidentification of *Haemobartonella*. *Eperythrozoon coccoides* is found in mice.

The developmental cycle of the eperythrozoa is not fully known. It is believed the parasites multiply in the blood and have an affinity with erythrocytes. The infection is readily transmissible by blood inoculation, but the natural mode of transmission has not been fully investigated. Jansen (1952) has demonstrated that lice may be responsible in the transmission of these organisms.

Eperythrozoonosis of Swine

Of the two species in pigs (*E. suis* and *E. parvum*), *E. suis* is the larger form, occurring as rings $2\,\mu$ to $3\,\mu$ in diameter. It is also the more pathogenic, severe infections causing ictero-anaemia (Splitter, 1950), which is an anaplasmosis-like disease of swine. The smaller form, *E. parvum*, is $0.5\,\mu$–$0.8\,\mu$ in diameter, and it is generally nonpathogenic, though clinical signs may be seen in splenectomised pigs.

The pathogenicity of *E. suis* has been described by Splitter (1950). Following an incubation period of about 9 days, the organisms appear in the blood, and this coincides with the elevation of temperature, which may reach $107°F$. Severe infections cause anaemia, anorexia, and jaundice. The highest morbidity and mortality occur in suckling pigs, and in acute infections pigs may die in less than five days. In older animals, such as weanlings, death may be delayed, or the animal may recover. Though the infection is widespread, it is, in general, not responsible for significant losses.

The pathological changes consist of anaemia, jaundice (yellow belly), the liver is brownish in colour and the bile yellowish-green and viscid. The spleen is enlarged and hyperplastic, and there is hyperplasia of the bone marrow. Blood smears show large numbers of organisms on the red blood cells and in the plasma.

Diagnosis of eperythrozoonosis in pigs is based on the clinical signs and the demonstration of organisms in blood smears.

The organisms are susceptible to the tetracycline antibiotics, and oxy-tetracycline (terramycin) given at the rate of 25–50 mg. per lb. orally, or intramuscularly or intravenously at the rate of 2 mg. per lb. daily, is effective.

Eperythrozoon wenyoni. Cattle infected with this organism usually show little or no clinical manifestation. Occasionally, in severe infections, acute fever occurs, to be followed by emaciation and some jaundice. At this time parasites are very common in the blood.

Eperythrozoon ovis. This infection, though not widespread, occurs as an occasional pathogen of sheep in South Africa. The organisms are small pleomorphic forms, assuming ovals, rods or rings, on and between, the red blood cell. The infection is usually benign in nature, but occasionally it produces an anaemia with icterus, an irregular fever, progressive emaciation and poor condition.

Genus: Haemobartonella

This genus includes a number of forms which have affinities with the rickettsiae, and it is now fairly certain that they are not protozoa. Electron microscopy shows them to consist of round, oval bodies, usually in pairs and containing a mass of undifferentiated internal structure (Ristic, 1963). Cross serological reactions with *Haemobartonella* are seen with *Anaplasma* and *Eperythrozoon*.

Haemobartonella canis occurs in the dog and on occasion may be responsible for producing anaemia, emaciation and anorexia. Young puppies are the most susceptible to the disease. *Haemobartonella felis* has received substantial attention recently, and it is considered to be the cause of feline infectious anaemia.

Haemobartonellae are similar to the eperythrozoa, appearing as bacilliform, coccoid, ring or other pleomorphic forms on and between the red cells of the infected animal. Small colonies of organisms may occur in the red blood cell; such forms indicate multiplication. They stain intensely with Romanowsky stains, so much so that at first appearance the blood smear appears to be very poorly stained.

Pathogenesis of Haemobartonella *Infection.* It is likely that a large number of infections are undetected due to their benign and inapparent nature.

Splenectomy may cause clinical parasitaemia with anaemia, emaciation and perhaps death. In the cat acute, sub-acute and chronic forms of the infection may occur. In the acute form there is intermittent fever with a progressive anaemia, this corresponding to the level of organisms in the circulating blood. The infection is most common in young cats; if not diagnosed and treated, it results in an extended illness with anaemia and perhaps death. The tetracycline antibiotics are effective given orally for 18–21 days at the rate of 100 mg. 3 times a day for chloramphenicol (Chloromycetin), or 50 mg. per kg. daily orally or 5 mg. per kg. daily intravenously or intramuscularly for terramycin.

No information is available on the mode of transmission of the haemo-bartonellae of cats and dogs, though *H. muris* of rats may be transmitted by the spiny rat louse, *Polyplax spinulosa*. It is possible, therefore, that blood sucking arthropods are responsible for transmission of the other species.

CLASS: CILIATA Perty, 1852

Organisms of this class possess cilia for locomotion. They are highly organised forms possessing two nuclei, a macronucleus which is large and massive and responsible for the cytoplasmic activities of the organism, and a micronucleus, which is vesicular and is concerned with the reproductive process. Reproduction is asexual by transverse binary fission or, in the sexual phase, by conjugation.

A large number of ciliates exist, the majority of which are free living, inhabiting water of all kinds. The whole group has been reviewed by Corliss (1961).

The genus of immediate importance is *Balantidium*, which is a parasite of the large intestine of man, pig, monkey and possibly other animals. In addition to this pathogen, however, a large number of ciliates occur in the rumen of ruminants and the large intestine of equines. These are not parasitic in the sense that they produce disease, rather they are concerned in digestive processes; but their exact role in this has yet to be determined. No attempt will be made to discuss these forms, and further information on them may be obtained from Lubinsky (1957) and Levine (1961).

Genus: Balantidium Claparède and Lachmann, 1858

Organisms of this genus are oval to ellipsoidal in outline; there is a distinct macronucleus and a small micronucleus. The cilia are arranged in longitudinal rows over the whole of the body; a mouth, or peristome, is situated near the anterior end of the organism, and there is a weakly developed cytopharynx.

A large number of species of *Balantidium* have been described, the description of them being based largely on the host in which they have been found and on the size of the body and the macronucleus. The synonymy of the genus has not been investigated in detail, but it is likely that many of the forms are synonyms.

Balantidium coli (Malmsten, 1857) Stein, 1862. The vegetative forms averages 50 μ–60 μ in length, but larger forms are not uncommon, and some may measure up to 150 μ in length. The body surface is covered with slightly oblique longitudinal rows of cilia, the peristome is subterminal and at the narrower end, the macronucleus is kidney-shaped, and the micronucleus lies in the notch of the macronucleus. One contractile vacuole occurs near the posterior end of the body, another near the centre, and the cytoplasm contains numerous food vacuoles. The organism is actively motile and moves quickly over the microscopic field.

Cysts are produced, these being ovoid to spherical, and measure 40 μ–60 μ. They are faintly yellowish-green in colour, and the organism can be recognised within the cyst by the macronucleus.

Reproduction is by transverse binary fission, but conjugation may also take place. Transmission to other hosts is by the cysts.

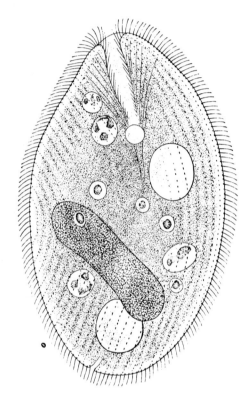

FIG. 289. *Balantidium coli* from the Human Intestine (×1200). (From Wenyon, 1926)

Balantidium coli is widespread in swine, and it is likely that it will be found in any pig if an adequate examination is made. The prevalence of the infection in man is much lower, and prevalences of 0·6 per cent to 1 per cent have been recorded. The organism also occurs in other higher primates, and it may be a troublesome infection in zoological gardens. Occasional infections of other animals with *B. coli* have been reported; thus, Bailey & Williams (1949) reported a clinical infection in a dog in the U.S.A.

Pathogenesis of B. coli. The pig appears to be the primary host, and in it *B. coli* is generally regarded as a commensal, since under normal conditions it is found in the lumen of the large intestine and is associated with no change in the mucosa. Occasionally, and for undetermined reasons, it may invade the mucosa and cause superficial and even deep ulcerations, these being associated with a mild to severe enteritis. Almejew (1963) has reported acute and at times fatal infections in pigs characterised by dysentery with haemorrhage. Organisms were found as deep as the muscular layer of the caecum and colon, being associated with lymphocytic and leucocytic infiltrations. Almejew suggested that *B. coli* had a plasmolytic effect and produced damage to the nuclei of the epithelial cells of the mucosa. Tempelis & Lysenko (1957) have shown that *B. coli* produces hyaluronidase, and this may assist the organism to enter the tissues.

In man *B. coli* produces superficial to deep ulcers associated with dysentery. The early lesions of *B. coli* infection resemble those produced by *Entamoeba histolytica*, but they do not show the same tendency to enlarge and spread. Only rarely does *B. coli* invade other tissues, such as the liver.

Human infection is a zoonosis and is usually acquired from swine through the contamination of food stuffs, fingers etc. with pig faeces. Normally, the cysts are the source of infection, and these remain viable for days or weeks in moist pig faeces. Under conditions of gross contamination, trophozoites may initiate human infection, but these are very much less resistant than the cysts, and they die within 15–30 minutes at temperatures above 40°C, though in a moist environment they may survive 1–3 days at room temperature. *Balantidium* infection in the higher primates in zoological gardens is normally maintained by the animals themselves.

Diagnosis of *B. coli* infection is based on the clinical signs, post-mortem evidence of an ulcerative condition of the large intestine and the presence of very large numbers of *B. coli*. Because of the common occurrence of the organism in apparently normal animals, it is unwise to ascribe intestinal upsets to its presence without additional evidence of its invasive properties.

Treatment. Acute infections may be treated with the tetracycline antibiotics, and in man carbarsone and tetracyclines have been used. Carbarsone is also of value in captive primates, a dose of 250 mg. being given daily for 10 days.

REFERENCES

TRYPANOSOMA

ASHCROFT, M. T. (1959). The Tinde experiment: a further study of the long term cyclical transmission of *Trypanosoma rhodesiense*. *Ann. trop. Med. Parasit.*, **53**, 137–146

BARBER, H. J. & BERG, S. S. (1962). Structure and activity of antiprotozoal drugs. In *Drugs, Parasites and Hosts* (Ed. by L. G. Goodwin & R. H. Nimmo-Smith). London: Churchill

BISHOP, A. (1959). Drug resistance in protozoa. *Biol. Rev.*, **34**, 445–500

BISHOP, A. (1962). Chemotherapy and drug resistance in protozoal infections. In *Drugs, Parasites and Hosts* (Ed. by L. G. Goodwin & R. H. Nimmo-Smith). London: Churchill

BROOM, J. C. & BROWN, H. C. (1940). Studies on trypanosomiasis. IV. Notes on the serological characters of *Trypanosoma brucei* after cyclical development in *Glossina morsitans*. *Trans. R. Soc. trop. Med. Hyg.*, **34**, 53–64

BROWN, K. N. & WILLIAMSON, L. (1962). Antigens of Brucei trypanosomes. *Nature, Lond.*, **194**, 1253–1255

BROWN, K. N. (1963). The antigenic character of the *'Brucei'* trypanosomes. In *Immunity to Protozoa* (Ed. by P. C. C. Garnham, A. E. Pierce & E. Roitt). Oxford: Blackwell Scientific Publications

BUXTON, P. A. (1955). *The Natural History of Tsetse Flies.* Mem. No. 10, London School Hyg. & trop. Med. London: H. K. Lewis

CARMICHAEL, J. A. (1939). Turning sickness of cattle and *Trypanosoma theileri. Parasitology*, **31**, 498–500

CHANDLER, R. L. (1958). Studies on the tolerance of N'dama cattle to trypanosomiasis. *J. comp. Path.*, **68**, 253–260

CUNNINGHAM, M. P. & VICKERMAN, K. (1961). An improved agglutination reaction for use in analysis of African trypanosomes. *Trans. R. Soc. trop. Med. Hyg.*, **55**, 12

DAVEY, D. G. (1950). Experiments with antrycide in the Sudan and East Africa. *Trans. R. Soc. trop. Med. Hyg.*, **43**, 583–616

DESOWITZ, R. S. (1956). Observations on the metabolism of *Trypanosoma vivax. Exp. Parasit.*, **5**, 250–259

DESOWITZ, R. S. (1959). Studies on immunity and host-parasite relationships. I. The immunological response of resistant and susceptible breeds of cattle to trypanosomal challenge. *Ann. trop. Med. Parasit.*, **53**, 293–313

DESOWITZ, R. S. & WATSON, H. J. C. (1953). Studies on *Trypanosoma vivax*. IV. The maintenance of a strain in white rats without sheep-serum supplement. *Ann. trop. Med. Parasit.*, **47**, 62–67

DESOWITZ, R. S. (1963). Adaptation of trypanosomes to abnormal hosts. *Ann. N. Y. Acad. Sci.*, **113**, 74–87

DIKMANS, G., MANTHEI, C. A. & FRANK, A. H. (1957). Demonstration of *Trypanosoma theileri* in the stomach of an aborted bovine fetus. *Cornell Vet.*, **47**, 344–353

FAIRBAIRN, H. & BURTT, E. (1946). The infectivity to man of a strain of *Trypanosoma rhodesiense* transmitted cyclically to *Glossina mositans* through sheep and antelope: Evidence that man requires a minimum infective dose of metacyclic trypanosomes. *Ann. trop. Med. Parasit.*, **40**, 207–213

FAIRBAIRN, H. (1953). Studies on *Trypansoma vivax*. IX. Morphological differences in strains and their relation to pathogenicity. *Ann. trop. Med. Parasit.*, **47**, 394–405

FAUST, E. C. (1949). The etiologic agent of Chagas' disease in the United States. *Boln. Of. sanit. Pan-Am.*, **28**, 455–461

FIENNES, R. N. T. W. (1952). The cattle trypanosomiases. A cryptic focus of parasites in association with a secondary stage of disease. *Br. vet. J.*, **108**, 298–305

GOBLE, F. C. (1958). A comparison of strains of *Trypanosoma cruzi* indigenous to the United States with certain strains from South America. *Proc. 6th Int. Congr. trop. Med. Malaria*, **3**, 158–166

GOMEZ, R. J. (1956). Estudio do la tripanosomiasis natural del canino (*Canis fam*) en Venezuela. *Rec. Med. Vet. Parasit. Caracas*, **15**, 63–105

GOODWIN, L. G. & ROLLO, I. M. (1955). The chemotherapy of malaria, piroplasmosis, trypanosomiasis and leishmaniasis. In *Biochemistry and Physiology of Protozoa*. Vol. 2 (Ed. by S. H. Hutner & A. Lwoff). New York & London: Academic Press

GOODWIN, L. G. (1964). The chemotherapy of trypanosomiasis. In *Biochemistry and Physiology of Protozoa*. Vol. 3. (Ed. by S. H. Hutner). New York & London: Academic Press

GRANT, P. T. & FULTON, J. D. (1957). The catabolism of glucose by strains of *Trypanosoma rhodesiense. Biochem. J.*, **66**, 242–250

GRAY, A. R. (1963). Serum transaminase levels in cattle and sheep infected with *Trypanosoma vivax. Exp. Parasit.*, **14**, 374–381

GRAY, A. R. (1960). Precipitating antibody in trypanosomiasis of cattle and other animals. *Nature, Lond.*, **186**, 1058–1059

HOARE, C. A. (1949). *Handbook of Medical Protozoology.* London: Baillière, Tindall & Cox

HOARE, C. A. (1954). The loss of the kinetoplast in trypanosomes with special reference to *Trypanosoma evansi. J. Protozool.*, **1**, 28–33

HOARE, C. A. (1959). Morphological taxonomic studies on mammalian trypanosomes. IX. Revision of *Trypanosoma dimorphon. Parasitology*, **49**, 210–231

HOARE, C. A. (1964). Morphological and taxonomic studies on mammalian trypanosomes. X. Revision of the systematics. *J. Protozool.*, **11**, 200–207

HOOF, L. (1947). Observations on trypanosomiasis in the Belgian Congo. *Trans. R. Soc. trop. Med. Hyg.*, **40**, 728–761

HORNBY, H. E. (1953). *African trypanosomiasis in Eastern Africa*, pp. 39 ff. H.M. Stationery Office

KNIERIM, F. (1959). Tecnica de la reaccion de fijacion del complemento segun el methodo del 50% de hemolisis de Bozicevich etc. *Boln. chil. Parasit.*, **13**, 75–78

LEACH, T. M. (1961). Observations on the treatment of *Trypanosoma evansi* infection in camels. *J. comp. Path, Ther.*, **71**, 109–117

LEACH, T. M. & EL KARIB, E. A. A. (1960). Prophylaxis against repeated artificial challenge with *Trypanosoma congolense*. A comparative trial of antrycide prosalt and prothidium bromide. *J. comp. Path. Ther.*, **70**, 385–395

LEVINE, N. D., WATRACH, A. M., KANTOR, S. & HARDENBROCH, H. J. (1956). A case of bovine trypanosomiasis due to *Trypanosoma theileri* in Illinois. *J. Parasit.*, **42**, 553

LINCICOME, D. R. (1957). Growth of *Trypanosoma lewisi* in the heterologous mouse host. *Am. J. trop. Med. Hyg.*, **6**, 392

MULLIGAN, H. W. (1951). Tolerance of indigenous West African cattle to trypanosomiasis. *Bull. Bur. perm. Interafr. Tsétsé*, No. **164**, p. 4

NOBLE, E. R. (1955). The morphology and life cycles of trypanosomes. *Q. Rev. Biol.*, **30**, 1–28

OMEROD, W. E. (1963). The initial stages of infection with *Trypanosoma lewisi*; control of parasitaemia by the host. In *Immunity to Protozoa* (Ed. by P. C. C. Garnham, A. E. Pierce & I. Roitt). Oxford: Blackwell Scientific Publications.

OLSEN, P. F., SHOEMAKER, J. P., TURNER, H. F. & HAYS, K. L. (1964). Incidence of *Trypanosoma cruzi* (Chagas) in wild vectors and reservoirs in East Central Alabama. *J. Parasit.*, **50**, 599–603

PELL, E. & CHARDOME, M. (1954). *Trypanosoma suis* Ochmann, 1905—Trypanosome monomorphe pathogène de mammifères évoluant dans les glandes salivaires de *Glossina brevipalpis*, Newst., Mosso (Urundi). *Annls Soc. Belge Méd. trop.*, **34**, 277–295

PIZZI, T. & TALIAFERRO, W. H. (1960). A comparative study of protein and nucleic acid synthesis in different species of trypanosomes. *J. infect. Dis.*, **107**, 100–107

RISTIC, M. & TRAGER, W. (1958). Cultivation at 37°C of a trypanosome (*Trypanosoma theileri*) from cows with depressed milk production. *J. Protozool.*, **5**, 146–148

ROBSON, J. T. (1961). Prophylaxis against trypanosomiasis in Zebu cattle. *Vet. Rec.*, **73**, 641–645

SOLTYS, M. A. (1959). Immunity in trypanosomiasis III. Sensitivity of antibody resistant strains to chemotherapeutic drugs. *Parasitology*, **49**, 143–152

SPLITTER, E. J. & SOULSBY, E. J. L. (1967). Isolation and cultivation of *Trypanosoma theileri* in tissue culture media. *Exp. Parasit.* (In Press)

STEINERT, M. (1963). Structures et fonction du kinetonucleus des trypanosomes. In *Progress in Protozoology* (Ed. by J. Luduck, J. Lom & J. Vavra), p. 397. New York and London: Academic Press

STEWART, J. L. (1951). The West African shorthorn cattle. Their value to Africa as trypanosomiasis-resistant animals. *Vet. Rec.*, **63**, 454–457

TALIAFERRO, W. H. (1923). A reaction product in infections with *Trypanosoma lewisi* which inhibits the reproduction of the trypanosomes. *J. exp. Med.*, **39**, 171–190

TALIAFERRO, W. H. (1932). Trypanocidal and reproduction-inhibiting antibodies to *Trypanosoma lewisi* in rats and rabbits. *Am. J. Hyg.*, **16**, 32–84

TALIAFERRO, W. H. (1948). The inhibition of reproduction of parasites by immune factors. *Bact. Rev.*, **12**, 1–17

TALIAFERRO, W. H. (1963). Cellular and humoral factors in immunity to protozoa. In *Immunity to Protozoa* (Ed. by P. C. C. Garnham, A. E. Pierce & I. Roitt). Oxford: Blackwell Scientific Publications

WATSON, E. A. (1915). Durine and the complement fixation test. *Parasitology*, **8**, 156–182

WEITZ, B. (1960). A soluble protective antigen of *Trypanosoma brucei*. *Nature, Lond.*, **185**, 788

WEITZ, B. (1962). Immunity in trypanosomiasis. In *Drugs, Parasites and Hosts* (Ed. by L. G. Goodwin & R. H. Nimmo-Smith). London: Churchill

WEITZ, B. (1963). Immunological relationships between African trypanosomes and their hosts. *Ann. N. Y. Acad. Sci.*, **113**, 400–408

WENYON, C. M. (1926). *Protozoology*. 2 Vols. London: Baillière, Tindall & Cox

WHITESIDE, E. F. (1962). Interactions between drugs, trypanosomes and cattle in the field. In *Drugs, Parasites and Hosts*. (Ed. by L. G. Goodwin & R. H. Nimmo-Smith). London: Churchill

WHITESIDE, E. F. (1960). Recent work in Kenya on the control of drug-resistant cattle trypanosomiasis. *Proc. VIIth Sci. Comm. Tryp. Res., Jos.*, 141–154

WIJERS, D. J. B. & WILLETT, K. C. (1960). Factors that may influence the infection rate of *Glossina palpalis* with *Trypanosoma gambiense*. II. The number and morphology of the trypanosomes present in the blood of the host at the time of the infected feed. *Ann. trop. Med. Parasit.*, **54**, 341–350

WILDE, J. K. H. & ROBSON, J. T. (1953). The effect against *Trypanosoma congolense* in Zebu cattle of three phenanthridine compounds. *Vet. Rec.*, **65**, 49–51

WILLETT, K. (1950). Trypanosomiasis research. *An. Rep. East Africa High Com., Nairobi*, pp. 33–35

WILLETT, K. (1961). West African Institute for Trypanosomiasis Research, Annual Report, 1961

WILLIAMSON, J. & BROWN, K. N. (1964). The chemical composition of trypanosomes. III. Antigenic constituents of brucei trypanosomes. *Exp. Parasit.*, **15**, 44–68

WOODY, N. C. & WOODY, H. B. (1955). American trypanosomiasis (Chagas disease); first indigenous case in the United States. *J. Am. med. Ass.*, **195**, 676–677

LEISHMANIA

ADLER, S. (1963). Immune phenomena in leishmaniasis. In *Immunity to Protozoa* (Ed. by P. C. C. Garnham, A. E. Pierce & I. Roitt). Oxford: Blackwell Scientific Publications

ADLER, S. (1964). Leishmania. In *Adv. Parasit.* **2**, 35–96 (Ed. by B. Dawes). London & New York: Academic Press

ANSARI, N. & MOFIDI, CH. (1950). Contribution à l'étude des 'formes humides' de Leishmaniose cutanée. *Bull. Soc. Path. exot.*, **43**, 601–607

BERBERIAN, D. A. (1939). Vaccination and immunity against oriental sore. *Trans. R. Soc. trop. Med. Hyg.*, **33**, 87–94

BERBERIAN, D. A. (1944). Cutaneous leishmaniasis (oriental sore). I. Time required for development of immunity after vaccination. *Archs. Derm. Syph.*, **49**, 433–435

BIAGI, F. F. (1953). Algunos comentarios sobre gicos: *Leishmania tropica mexicana*, nueva subespecie. *Med. Rev. Mex.*, **33**, 401–406

CHOPRA, R. N., GUPTA, J. C. & BASU, N. K. (1927). Further observations on the serum test for Kala-azar with organic antimony compounds. A simple blood test for Kala-azar. *Indian med. Gaz.*, **62**, 434–437

FLOCH, H. (1954). *Leishmania tropica guyanensis* n. Sp., the agent of tegumentary leishmaniasis in the Guianas and Central America. *Bull. Soc. Path. exot.*, **47**, 784–787

GOODWIN, L. G. & ROLLO, I. M. (1955). The chemotherapy of malaria, proplasmosis, trypanosomiasis, and leishmaniasis. In *Biochemistry and Physiology of Protozoa* (Ed. by S. H. Hutner & A. Lwoff). New York & London: Academic Press

HOARE, C. A. (1949). *Handbook of Medical Protozoology*. London: Baillière, Tindall & Cox

KOZHEVNIKOV, P. V. (1959). On cross immunity between rural and urban skin leishmaniasis. *Med. Parasit. Moscow*, **28**, 695–699

LEVINE, N. D. (1963). *Protozoan Parasites of Domestic Animals and of Man*. Minneapolis: Burgess Publ.

MANSON BAHR, P. E. C. (1963). Active immunization in leishmaniasis. In *Immunity to Protozoa* (Ed. by P. C. C. Garnham, A. E. Pierce & I. Roitt). Oxford: Blackwell Scientific Publications

NAPIER, L. E. (1927). The infectivity of the flagellate form of *Leishmania donovani*. *Indian J. med. Res.*, **15**, 481–483

NUSSENZWEIG, V. (1959). Diagnostico serologico da leishmaniose visceral humana e canina. *Proc. 6th int. Congr. trop. Mea. Malaria. Lisbon*, **3**, 779–790

PELLIGRENO, J. (1951). Nota preliminar sobre a reação intradérmica feita com a fração Polissacaridea isolada de formas de cultura da *Leishmania braziliensis* em Casos de Leishmaniose Teguimentar Americana. *Hospital (Rio de Janiero)*, **39**, 859

PESSOA, S. B. (1961). Classification of leishmanioses and of species of the genus leishmania. *Arches Hig. Saù de públ.*, **26**, 41–50

STAUBER, L. (1963). Immunity to Leishmania. *Ann. N. Y. Acad. Sci.*, **113**, 409–417

THORSON, R. E., BAILEY, W. S., SHERRILL, W., HOERLEIN, A. B. & SIEBOLD, H. R. (1955). A report in a case of imported visceral leishmaniasis of a dog in the United States. *Am. J. trop. Med. Hyg.*, **4**, 18–22

ZUCKERMAN, A. (1962). Some observations on immunity to *Leishmania tropica*. *Sci. Rept. 1st Super. Sanita*, **2**, 95–102

TRICHOMONAS FOETUS

BARTLETT, D. E. (1948). Further observations on experimental treatments of *Trichomonas foetus* infection in bulls. *Am. J. vet. Res.*, **9**, 351–359

DIAMOND, L. S. (1957). The establishment of various trichomonads of animals and man in axenic cultures. *J. Parasit.*, **43**, 488–490

FEINBERG, J. G. (1952). A capillary agglutination test for *Trichomonas foetus*. *J. path. Bact.*, **64**, 645–647

FEINBERG, J. G. & MORGAN, M. T. J. (1953). The isolation of a specific substance, and a glycogen-like polysaccharide from *Trichomonas foetus*. *Br. J. exp. Path.*, **34**, 104–118

FITZGERALD, P. R., JOHNSON, A. E. & HAMMOND, D. M. (1963). Treatment of genital trichomoniasis in bulls. *J. Am. vet. med. Ass.*, **143**, 259–262

FITZGERALD, P. R., JOHNSON, A. E., THORNE, J. L. & HAMMOND, D. M. (1958). Experimental infections of the bovine genital system with trichomonads from the digestive tracts of swine. *Am. J. vet. Res.*, **19**, 775–779

GRASSÉ, P. P. (1952). *Traité de Zoologie*. I. Fasc. 1. Paris: Masson

HAMMOND, D. M. & BARTLETT, D. E. (1945). Pattern of fluctuations in numbers of *Trichomonas foetus* occurring in the bovine vagina during initial infections. I. Correlation with time of exposure and with subsequent estrual cycles. *Am. J. vet. Res.*, **6**, 84–90

HAMMOND, D. M., FITZGERALD, P. R., BINNS, W. & MINER, M. L. (1953). The efficacy of bovoflavin salve in the experimental treatment of trichomoniasis in bulls. *Cornell Vet.*, **43**, 121–127

JOHNSON, A. E. (1964). Incidence and diagnosis of trichomoniasis in western beef bulls. *J. Am. vet. med. Ass.*, **145**, 1007–1010

KERR, W. R. (1944). The intradermal test in bovine trichomoniasis. *Vet. Rec.*, **56**, 303–307

KERR, W. R. (1964). Immobilization and agglutination of *Trichomonas foetus*. In *Immunological Methods* (Ed. by J. F. Ackroyd). Oxford: Blackwell Scientific Publications

KERR, W. R. & ROBERTSON, M. (1941). An investigation into the infection of cows with *Trichomonas foetus* by means of the agglutination reaction. *Vet. J.*, **97**, 351–365

KERR, W. R. & ROBERTSON, M. (1943). A study of the antibody response of cattle to *Trichomonas foetus*. *J. comp. Path.*, **53**, 280–297

KERR, W. R. & ROBERTSON, M. (1945). A note on the appearance of serological varieties among *T. foetus* strains isolated from infected cattle. *Vet. Rec.*, **57**, 221–222

KERR, W. R. & ROBERTSON, M. (1953). Active and passive sensitization of the uterus of the cow *in vivo* against *Trichomonas foetus* antigen and the evidence for the local production of antibody in that site. *J. Hyg. Camb.*, **51**, 405–415

KERR, W. R. & ROBERTSON, M. (1954). Passively and actively acquired antibodies for *Trichomonas foetus* in very young calves. *J. Hyg. Camb.*, **52**, 253–263

KUDO, R. R. (1954). *Protozoology*. 4th Ed. Springfield, Illinois: Thomas

LARSEN, L. (1953). The internal pudendal (pudic) nerve block for anesthesia of the penis and relaxation of the retractor penis muscle. *J. Amer. med. Ass.*, **123**, 18–27

LEVINE, N. D. (1961). *Protozoan Parasites of Domestic Animals and of Man*. Minneapolis, Minnesota: Burgess

LEVINE, N. D., ANDERSON, F. L., LOSCH, M. J., NOTZOLD, R. A. & MEHRER, K. N. (1962). Survival of *Trichomonas foetus* stored at −28 and −95°C after freezing in the presence of glycerol. *J. Protozool.*, **9**, 347–350

LEVINE, N. D., MIZELL, M. & HOULAHAN, D. A. (1958). Factors affecting the protective action of glycerol on *Trichomonas foetus* at freezing temperatures. *Exp. Parasit.*, **7**, 236–248

MORGAN, B. B. (1948). Studies on the precipitin and skin reactions of *Trichomonas foetus* (Protozoa) in cattle. *J. Cell. Comp. Physiol.*, **32**, 235–246

MORGAN, B. B. & HAWKINS, P. A. (1952). *Veterinary Protozoology*. 2nd Ed. Minneapolis, Minn.: Burgess

PIERCE, A. E. (1949a). The mucous agglutination test for the diagnosis of bovine trichomoniasis. *Vet. Rec.*, **61**, 347–349

PIERCE, A. E. (1949b). The agglutination reaction of bovine serum in the diagnosis of trichomoniasis. *Br. vet. J.*, **105**, 286–294

PIERCE, A. E. (1953). Specific antibodies at mucous surfaces. *Proc. R. Soc. Med.*, **46**, 31–33

PIERCE, A. E. (1959). Specific antibodies at mucous surfaces. *Vet. Rev. Annot.*, **5**, 17–36

ROBERTSON, M. (1960). The antigens of *Trichomonas foetus* isolated from cows and pigs. *J. Hyg. Camb.*, **58**, 207–213

ROBERTSON, M. (1963). Antibody response in cattle to infection with *Trichomonas foetus*. In *Immunity to Protozoa* (Ed. by P. C. C. Garnham, A. E. Pierce & I. Roitt). Oxford: Blackwell Scientific Publications

SCHOOP, G. & OEHLIKERS, H. (1939). Die Züchtung der Rindertrichomonaden in eiweissarmem Nährboden. *Dt. tierärztl. Wschr.*, **47**, 401–403

SCHOOP, G. & STOLZ, A. (1939). Trichomoniasis bei Rehen. *Dt. tierärztl. Wschr.*, **47**, 113–114

SHORB, M. S. (1964). The physiology of trichomonads. In *Biochemistry and Physiology of Protozoa* (Ed. by S. H. Hutner). New York: Academic Press

SWITZER, W. P. (1951). Atrophic rhinitis and trichomonads. *Vet. Med.*, **46**, 478–481

OTHER TRICHOMONADS, CHILOMASTIX, COCHLOSOMA, HEXAMITA, GIARDIA, ETC.

ABRAHAM, R. & HONIGBERG, B. M. (1965). Cytochemistry of chick liver cell cultures infected with *Trichomonas gallinae*. *J. Parasit.*, **51**, 823

ALLEN, E. A. (1936). A pentatrichomonas associated with certain cases of enterohepatitis or 'blackhead' of poultry. *Trans. Am. microsc. Soc.*, **55**, 315–322

ALLEN, E. A. (1940). A redescription of *Trichomonas gallinarum* Martin and Robertson, 1911, from the chicken and turkey. *Proc. helminth. Soc. Wash.*, **7**, 65–68

ALLEN, E. A. (1941). Microscopic differentiation of lesions of histomoniasis and trichomonas in turkeys. *Am. J. vet. Res.*, **2**, 214–217

ANDERSON, F. L., LEVINE, N. D. & HAMMOND, D. M. (1962). The morphology of *Trichomonas ovis* from the cecum of domestic sheep. *J. Parasit.*, **48**, 589–595

BEMRICK, U. J. (1961). A note on the incidence of three species of Giardia in Minnesota. *J. Parasit.*, **47**, 87–89

BRIGGS, J. E. (1959). Nitrofurans in Feeds. *14th Kansas Formula Feed Conf. Kansas State College*, 4–6 Jan., 1959, pp. 15–21

CAMPBELL, J. G. (1945). An infectious enteritis of young turkeys associated with *Cochlosoma* sp. *Vet. J.*, **101**, 255–259

CRAIGE, J. E. (1948). Differential diagnosis and specific therapy of dysenteries in dogs. *J. Am. vet. med. Ass.*, **113**, 343–347

CRAIGE, J. E. (1949). Intestinal disturbances in dogs: Differential diagnosis and specific therapy. *J. Am. vet. med. Ass.*, **114**, 425–428

DELAPPE, I. P. (1957). Effect of inoculating the chicken and the turkey with a strain of *Trichomonas gallinarum*. *Exp. Parasit.*, **6**, 412–417

DIAMOND, L. S. (1957). The establishment of various trichomonads of animals and man in axenic cultures. *J. Parasit.*, **43**, 488–490

FAUST, E. C. & RUSSELL, P. F. (1964). *Craig and Faust's Clinical Parasitology*. 7th Ed. Philadelphia: Lea & Febiger

FELICE, F. P. (1952). Studies on the cytology and life history of a giardia from the laboratory rat. *Univ. Calif. Publ. Zool.*, **57**, 53–143

FLICK, E. W. (1954). Experimental analysis of some factors influencing variation in the flagellar number of *Trichomonas hominis* from man and other primates, and their relationship to nomenclature. *Exp. Parasit.*, **3**, 105–121

FOGG, D. E. (1957). *Merck Poultry Nutrition and Health Symposium*. St. Louis, 5 Aug., 1957, pp. 16–18

FROST, J. K. & HONIGBERG, B. M. (1962). Comparative pathogenicity of *Trichomonas vaginalis* and *Trichomonas gallinae* to mice. II. Histopathology of subcutaneous lesions. *J. Parasit.*, **48**, 898–918

FROST, J. K., HONIGBERG, B. M. & MCLURE, M. T. (1961). Intracellular *Trichomonas vaginalis* and *Trichomonas gallinae* in natural and experimental infections. *J. Parasit.*, **47**, 302–303

HAGEN, K. W. (1950). Treatment of giardia in the chinchilla. *Calif. Vet.*, **3**, 11

HAIBA, M. H. (1956). Further study on the susceptibility of murines to human giardiasis. *Z. Parasitenk.*, **17**, 339–345

HAYES, B. S. & KITCHER, E. (1960). Evaluation of techniques for the demonstration of *Trichomonas vaginalis*. *J. Parasit.*, **46**, 45

HINSHAW, W. R. (1959). In *Diseases of Poultry*, 4th Ed. (Ed. by H. E. Biester & L. H. Schwarte). Ames: Iowa State Univ. Press

HINSHAW, W. R. & MCNEIL, E. (1941). Carriers of *Hexamita meleagridis*. *Am. J. vet. Res.*, **2**, 453–458

HIBLER, C. P., HAMMOND, D. M., CASKEY, F. H., JOHNSON, A. E. & FITZGERALD, P. R. (1960). The morphology and incidence of the trichomonads of swine, *Trichomonas suis* (Gruby & Delaford) *Trichomonas rotunda* n. sp. and *Trichomonas buttreyi* n. sp. *J. Protozool.*, **7**, 159–171

HOARE, C. A. (1955). Life cycle of *Hexamita meleagridis*. *Vet. Rec.*, **67**, 324

HONIGBERG, B. M. (1961). Comparative pathogenicity of *Trichomonas vaginalis* and *Trichomonas gallinae* to mice. I. Gross pathology, quantitative evaluation of virulence, and some factors affecting pathogenicity. *J. Parasit.*, **47**, 545–571

HONIGBERG, B. M., BECKER, D., LIVINGSTON, M. C. & MCLURE, M. T. (1964). The behavior, and pathogenicity of two strains of *Trichomonas gallinae* in cell cultures. *J. Protozool.*, **11**, 447–465

HUGHES, W. F. & ZANDER, D. V. (1954). Isolation and culture of *Hexamita* free of bacteria. *Poultry Sci.*, **33**, 810–815

GRASSÉ, P. P. (1952). *Traité de Zoologie*. I Fasc. 1. Paris: Masson

KOTT, H. and ADLER, S. (1961). A serological study of *Trichomonas* sp. parasitic in man. *Trans. R. Soc. trop. Med. Hyg.*, **55**, 333–344

LEVINE, N. D. (1961). *Protozoan Parasites of Domestic Animals and of Man*. Minn, Minn.: Burgess

MANGRUM, J. F., FERGUSON, T. M., COUCH, J. R., WILLS, F. K. & DELAPLANE, J. P. (1955). The effectiveness of furazolidone in the control of hexamitiasis in turkey poults. *Poultry Sci.*, **34**, 836–840

MARTIN, C. L. & ROBERTSON, M. (1911). Further observations on the caecal parasites of fowls, with some reference to the rectal fauna of other vertebrates. Report *J. micro Sci.*, **57**, 53–81

MCDOWELL, S. (1953). A morphological and taxonomic study of the caecal protozoa of the common fowl, *Gallus gallus*. *J. Morphol.*, **92**, 337–399

MCENTEGART, M. G., CHADWICK, C. S. & NAIRN, R. C. (1958). Fluorescent antisera in the detection of serological varieties of *Trichomonas vaginalis*. *Br. J. vener. Dis.*, **34**, 1–3

MCLOUGHLIN, D. K. (1957). Age of host and route of administration as factors influencing the susceptibility of turkeys to *Trichomonas gallinarum*. *J. Parasit.*, **43**, 321

MCNEIL, E. & HIRSHAW, W. R. (1941). Experimental infection of chicks with *Hexamita meleagridis*. *Cornell Vet.*, **31**, 345–350

MESA, C. P., STABLER, R. M. & BERTHRONG, M. (1961). Histopathological changes in the pigeon infected with *Trichomonas gallinae*. *Avian Dis.*, **5**, 48–60

MIESSNER, H. & HANSEN, K. (1936). Trichomoniasis der Tauben. *Dt. tierärztl. Wschr.*, **44**, 323–330

MUELLER, J. F. (1959). Is chilomastix a pathogen? *J. Parasit.*, **45**, 170

NOLLER, W. & BUTTGEREIT, F. (1923). Über ein neues parasitisches Protozoon der Haustaube (*Octomitus columbae* nov. spec.) *Zbl. Bakt. Orig.*, **75**, 239–240

PIZZI, T. (1957). Pathogenic role of *Giardia lamblia*. *Boln. chil. Parasit.*, **12**, 10–12

RICHARDSON, U. F. & KENDALL, S. B. (1963). *Veterinary Protozoology*. Edinburgh & London: Oliver & Boyd

SHELTON, G. C. (1954). Giardiasis in the chinchilla. II. Incidence of the disease and results of experimental infections. *Am. J. vet. Res.*, **15**, 75–78

SLAVIN, D. & WILSON, J. E. (1954). *Hexamita meleagridis*. *Nature, Lond.*, **172**, 1179–1181

SLAVIN, D. & WILSON, J. E. (1960). A fuller conception of the life cycle of *Hexamita meleagridis*. *Poultry Sci.*, **39**, 1559–1576

STABLER, R. M. (1951). Effect of *Trichomonas gallinae* from diseased mourning doves on clean domestic pigeons. *J. Parasit.*, **37**, 437–478

STABLER, R. M. (1953). Effect of *Trichomonas gallinae* (Protozoa: Mastigophora) on nestling passerine birds. *J. Colo.-Wyo. Acad. Sci.*, **4**, 58

STABLER, R. M. (1954). *Trichomonas gallinae*: A review. *Exp. Parasit.*, **3**, 368–402

STABLER, R. M. (1957). The effect of furazolidone on pigeon trichomoniasis due to *Trichomonas gallinae*. *J. Parasit.*, **43**, 280–282

STABLER, R. M. & HERMAN, C. M. (1951). Upper digestive tract trichomoniasis in mourning doves and other birds. *Trans. N. Am. Wild Life Conf.*, **16**, 145–163
STABLER, R. M. & MELLENTIN, R. W. (1953). Effect of 2-amino-5-nitrothiazole (enheptin), and other drugs on *Trichomonas gallinae* infection in the domestic pigeon. *J. Parasit.*, **39**, 637–642
WALKER, R. V. L. (1948). Enterohepatitis (blackhead) in turkeys. I. Pentatrichomonas associated with enterohepatitis and its propagation in developing chick embryos. *Can. J. comp. Med.*, **12**, 43–46
WILSON, J. E. & SLAVIN, D. (1955). Hexamitiasis of turkeys. *Vet. Rec.*, **67**, 236–242

HISTOMONAS

BRADLEY, R. E., JOHNSON, J. & REID, W. M. (1964). Apparent obligate relationship between *Histomonas meleagridis* and *Escherichia coli* in producing disease. *J. Parasit.*, **50**, (Suppl.) 51
CONNELL, R. (1950). Enterohepatitis (blackhead) in turkeys. VI. Abnormalities, possibly caused by a stage of *Histomonas meleagridis* occurring in second stage larvae of blackhead-transmitting *Heterakis gallinae*. *Canad. J. comp. Med.*, **14**, 331–337
CRAIG, F. R., BLOW, W. L. & BARBER, C. W. (1959). *N. Carolina State College Prog. Rept.*, March 25, 1959
DOLL, J. P. & FRANKER, C. K. (1963). Experimental histomoniasis in gnotobiotic turkeys. I. Infection and histopathology of the bacteria-free host. *J. Parasit.*, **49**, 411–414
DRBOHLAV, J. J. (1924). The cultivation of the protozoon of blackhead. *J. med. Res.*, **44**, 677–678
FARMER, R. K., HUGHES, D. L. & WHITING, G. (1951). Infectious enterohepatitis (blackhead) in turkeys: A study of the pathology of the artificially induced disease. *J. comp. Path. Ther.*, **61**, 251–262
FARMER, R. K. & STEPHENSON, J. (1949). Infectious enterohepatitis (blackhead) in turkeys: A comparative study of methods of infection. *J. comp. Path. Ther.*, **59**, 119–126
FARR, M. M. (1956). Survival of the protozoan parasite, *Histomonas meleagridis*, in feces of infected birds. *Cornell Vet.*, **46**, 178–187
FARR, M. M. (1961). Further observations on survival of the protozoan parasite, *Histomonas meleagridis*, and eggs of poultry nematodes in feces of infected birds. *Cornell Vet.*, **51**, 3–13
FOGG, D. E. (1957). *Merck Poultry Nutrition and Health Symposium*. St. Louis, Mo. 5 August, 1957, p. 16–28
FRANKER, C. K. & DOLL, J. P. (1964). Experimental histomoniasis in gnotobiotic turkeys. II. Effects of some caecal bacteria on pathogenesis. *J. Parasit.*, **50**, 636–640
GRAYBILL, H. W. & SMITH, T. (1920). Production of fatal blackhead in turkeys by feeding embryonated eggs of *Heterakis papillosa*. *J. exp. Med.*, **31**, 647–655
HARRISON, A. P., HANSEN, P. A., DEVOLT, H. M., HOLST, A. P. & TROMBA, F. G. (1954). Studies on the pathogenesis of infectious enterohepatitis (blackhead) of turkeys. *Poultry Sci.*, **33**, 84–93
HORTON-SMITH, C. & LONG, P. L. (1956). Further observations on the chemotherapy of histomoniasis (blackhead) in turkeys. *J. comp. Path. Ther.*, **66**, 378–388
KENDALL, S. B. (1957). Some factors influence resistance to histomoniasis in turkeys. *Br. vet. J.*, **113**, 435–439
KENDALL, S. B. (1959). The occurrence of *Histomonas meleagridis* in *Heterakis gallinae*. *Parasitology*, **49**, 169–172
LESSER, E. (1960). Cultivation of *Histomonas meleagridis* in a modified tissue culture medium. *J. Parasit.*, **46**, 686
LUCAS, J. M. S. (1961). 1,2-dimethyl-5-nitromidazole, 8595 R. P. Part. I. Prophylactic activity against experimental histomoniasis in turkeys. *Vet. Rec.*, **73**, 465–467
LUND, E. E. (1957). The immunizing action of a nonpathogenic strain of histomonas against blackhead in turkeys. *J. Protozool*, **4**, (Suppl.) 6
LUND, E. E. (1959). Immunizing action of a nonpathogenic strain of histomonas against blackhead in turkeys. *J. Protozool.*, **6**, 182–185
LUND, E. E. (1963). *Histomonas wenrichi* n. sp. (Mastigophora: Mastigamoebidae), a nonpathogenic parasite of gallinaceous birds. *J. Protozool.*, **10**, 401–404
LUND, E. E. & BURTNER, R. H. (1957). Infectivity of *Heterakis gallinae* eggs with *Histomonas meleagridis*. *Exp. Parasit.*, **6**, 189–193
MALEWITZ, T. D., RUNNELS, R. A. & CALHOUN, M. L. (1958). The pathology of experimentally produced histomoniasis in turkeys. *Am. J. vet. Res.*, **19**, 181–185
TYZZER, E. E. (1919). Developmental phases of the protozoon of 'blackhead' in turkeys. *J. med. Res.*, **40**, 1–30
TYZZER, E. E. (1926). *Heterakis vesicularis* Frölich 1791: A vector of an infectious disease. *Proc. Soc. ept. Biol. Med.*, **23**, 708–709
TYZZER, E. E. (1933). Loss of virulence in the protozoon of 'blackhead' a fatal disease of Turkeys, and the immunizing properties of attenuated strains. *Science*, **78**, 522–523
TYZZER, E. E. (1934). Studies on histomoniasis or 'blackhead' infection, in the chicken and the turkey. *Proc. Am. Acad. Arts Sci.*, **69**, 189–264
TYZZER, E. E. (1936). A study of immunity produced by infection with attenuated culture strains of *Histomonas meleagridis*. *J. comp. Path. Ther.*, **49**, 285–303

26

TYZZER, E. E. & COLLIER, J. (1925). Induced and natural transmission of blackhead in the absence of heterakis. *J. infect. Dis.*, **37**, 265–267

WEHR, E. E., FARR, M. M. & McLOUGHLIN, D. K. (1958). Chemotherapy of blackhead in poultry. *J. Am. vet. med. Ass.*, **132**, 439–445

ENTAMOEBA

ANDREWS, J. M. (1932). Cysts of the dysentery-producing *Endamoeba histolytica* in a Baltimore dog. *Am. J. trop. Med.*, **12**, 401–404

BRUMPT, E. (1925). Etude sommaire de l'*Entamoeba dispar* n. sp. Amibe a Kyster Quadrinuclées parasite de l'homme. *Bull. Acad. Med., Paris*, **94**, 943–952

DERRICK, E. H. (1948). A fatal case of generalized amoebiasis due to a protozoon closely resembling, if not identical with, *Iodamoeba bütschlii*. *Trans. R. Soc. trop. Med. Hyg.*, **42**, 191–198

EYLES, D. E., JONES, F. E., JUMPER, J. R. & DRINNON, V. P. (1954). Amebic Infection in Dogs. *J. Parasit.*, **40**, 163–166

FAUST, E. C. & RUSSELL, P. F. (1964). *Craig and Faust's Clinical Parasitology*. Philadelphia: Lea & Febiger

FREMMING, B. D., VOGEL, F. S., BENSON, R. E. & YOUNG, R. J. (1955). A fatal case of amebiasis with liver abscesses and ulcerative colitis in a chimpanzee. *J. Am. vet. med. Ass.*, **126**, 406–407

GOLDMAN, M. (1954). Use of fluorescein-tagged antibody to identify cultures of *Endamoeba histolytica* and *Endamoeba coli*. *Am. J. Hyg.*, **59**, 318–325

GOLDMAN, M. (1960). Antigenic analysis of *Entamoeba histolytica* by means of fluorescent antibody. I. Instrumentation for microfluorimetry of stained amebae. *Exp. Parasit.*, **9**, 25–36

GOLDMAN, M., CARVER, R. K. & GLEASON, N. N. (1960). Antigen analysis of *Entamoeba histolytica* by means of fluorescent antibody. II. *E. histolytica* and *E. hartmanni*. *Exp. Parasit.*, **10**, 366–388

HOARE, C. A. (1950). *Handbook of Medical Protozoology*. London: Baillière, Tindall & Cox

HOARE, C. A. (1959). Amoebic infections in animals. *Vet. Rev. Annot.*, **5**, 91–102

KESSEL, J. F. (1928). Intestinal protozoa of the domestic pig. *Am. J. trop. Med.*, **8**, 481–501

LEVINE, N. D. (1961). *Protozoan Parasites of Domestic Animals and of Man*. pp. iii–412. Minneapolis: Burgess

MADDISON, S. E. (1965). Characterization of *Entamoeba histolytica* antigen–antibody reaction by gel diffusion. *Exp. Parasit.*, **16**, 224–235

MADDISON, S. E. & ELSDON-DEW, R. (1961). Non-specific antibodies in amebiasis. *Exp. Parasit.*, **11**, 90–92

MAEGRAITH, B. G. (1963). Pathogenesis and pathogenic mechanisms in protozoal diseases with special reference to amoebiasis and malaria. In *Immunity to Protozoa* (Ed. by P. C. C. Garnham, A. E. Pierce & I. Roitt). Oxford: Blackwell Scientific Publications

NOBLE, E. R. & NOBLE, G. A. (1961). *Parasitology. The Biology of Animal Parasites*. London: Kimpton

NOBLE, G. A. & NOBLE, E. R. (1952). Entamoebae in farm mammals. *J. Parasit.*, **38**, 571–595

PIPKIN, A. C. (1949). Experimental studies on the role of filth flies in the transmission of *Endamoeba histolytica*. *Am. J. Hyg.*, **49**, 255–275

PHILLIPS, B. P., WOLFE, P. A., REES, C. W., GORDON, H. A., WRIGHT, W. H. & REYNIERS, J. A. (1955). Studies on the ameba-bacteria relationship in amebiasis. Comparative results of the intracecal inoculation of germ-free, monocontaminated and conventional guinea pigs with *Entamoeba histolytica*. *Am. J. trop. Med. Hyg.*, **4**, 675–692

THIERY, G. and MOREL, P. (1956). Amibiase pulmonaire chez un zebu. *Rev. Elev.*, **9**, 343–350

THORSON, R. E., SEIBOLD, H. R. & BAILEY, W. S. (1956). Systemic amebiasis with distemper in a dog. *J. Am. vet. med. Ass.*, **129**, 335–337

WALKIERS, J. (1930). Un cas d'amibiase intestinale chez un bovidé. *Annl. Soc. belge Méd. trop.*, **10**, 379–380

COCCIDIA OF CATTLE, SHEEP AND PIGS

ALICATA, J. E. (1930). Globidium in the abomasum of American sheep. *J. Parasit.*, **16**, 162–163

ALICATA, J. E. & WILLETT, E. L. (1946). Observation on the prophylactic and curative value of sulphaguanidine in swine coccidiosis. *Am. J. vet. Res.*, **7**, 74–100

ANDERSON, F. L., LOWDER, L. J. & HAMMOND, D. M. (1965). Antibody production in experimental *Eimeria bovis* infection in calves. *Exp. Parasit.*, **16**, 23–25

ARTHUR, G. H. (1944). Coccidiosis of calves treated with sulphaguanidine. *Vet. Rec.*, **56**, 250

BAKER, D. W. (1938). Observations on *Eimeria bukidnonensis* in New York State cattle. *J. Parasit.*, **24**, (Suppl.) 15–16

BAKER, D. W. (1939). Species of eimerian coccidia found in New York State cattle. *Rept. N. Y. State vet. Coll.*, 1937–1938, pp. 160–166

BALOZET, L. (1932). Etude experimental d'eimeria nina-kohl-Yakimovi, V. L. Yakimoff et Rastegaieva, 1930. *Bull. Soc. Path. exot.*, **25**, 715–720

BECKER, E. R. (1956). Measurements of the unsporulated oocysts of *Eimeria acervulina*, *E. maxima*, *E. tenella*, amd *E. mitis*; coccidian parasites of the common fowl. *Iowa State Coll. J. Sci.*, **31**, 85

BECKLUND, W. W. (1957). An epizootic of coccidiosis in western feeder lambs in Georgia. *N. Am. Vet.*, **38**, 262–264

BIESTER, H. E. & MURRAY, C. (1934). Studies on infectious enteritis of swine. *J. Am. vet. med. Ass.*, **85**, 207–219

BISWAL, G. (1948). Coccidiosis in Buffalo Calves. *Indian vet. J.*, **25**, 36–38

BOCH, J. & WIESENHÜTTER, E. (1963). Beitrag zur Klärung der Pathogenität der Schweine-kokeidien. *Tierärztl. Umschau*, **18**, 223–225

BOUGHTON, D. C. (1943). Sulfaguanidine therapy in experimental bovine coccidiosis. *Am. J. vet. Res.*, **4**, 66–72

BOUGHTON, D. C. (1945). Bovine Coccidiosis: From carrier to clinical cases. *N. Am. Vet.*, **26**, 147–153

BRACKETT, S. & BLIZNICK, A. (1952). The reproductive potential of five species of coccidia of the chicken as demonstrated by oocyst production. *J. Parasit.*, **28**, 133–139

BRUCE, E. A. (1921). Bovine coccidiosis in British Columbia with a description of the parasite, *Eimeria canadensis*, sp. n. *J. Am. vet. med. Ass.*, **58**, 638–662

CHALLEY, J. R. & BURNS, W. C. (1959). The invasion of the cecal mucosa by *Eimeria tenella* sporozoites and their transport by macrophages. *J. Protozool.*, **6**, 238–241

CHATTON, E. (1910). La kyste de Gilruth dans la muqueuse stomacale des ovides. *Archs. Zool. exp. gén.*, **5**, 114

CHEISSIN, E. M. (1940). Rabbit coccidiosis. III. *Eimeria magna* and its developmental cycle. *Uchennye Tapiski Inst. Imena Gertsena*, **30**, 65–91

CHEISSIN, E. M. (1959). Cytochemical investigations of different stages of the life cycle of coccidia of the rabbit. *Proc. 15th Int. Cong. Zool. London*, 16–23, 713–716

CHRISTENSEN, J. F. (1938a). Species differentiation in the coccidia from the domestic sheep. *J. Parasit.*, **24**, 453–467

CHRISTENSEN, J. F. (1938b). Occurrence of the coccidian *Eimeria bukidnonensis* in American cattle. *Proc. helminth. Soc. Wash.*, **5**, 24

CHRISTENSEN, J. F. (1940). The source and availability of infective oocysts in an outbreak of Coccidiosis in lambs in Nebraska feedlots. *Am. J. vet. Res.*, **1**, 27–35

CHRISTENSEN, J. F. (1941). Experimental production of coccidiosis in silage-fed feeder lambs with observations on oocyst discharge. *N. Am. Vet.*, **22**, 608–610

CHRISTENSEN, J. F. (1941a). The oocysts of coccidia from domestic cattle in Alabama. *J. Parasit.*, **27**, 203–220

CHRISTENSEN, J. F. & PORTER, D. A. (1939). A new species of coccidium from cattle with observations on its life history. *Proc. Helminth. Soc. Wash.*, **6**, 45–48

CLARKSON, M. J. (1959). The life history and pathogenicity of *Eimeria meleagrimitis*, Tyzzer 1929, in the turkey poult. *Parasitology*, **49**, 70–82

CORDERO DEL CAMPILLO, M. (1960). Neuvos casos de coccidiosis bovina en leon: Denuncia de *Eimeria bovis* (Zublin, 1908) Fiebiger, 1912, *E. auburnensis* Christensen y Porter, 1939, y *E. ellipsoidalis* Becker y Frye, 1929. *Revtr. ibér. Parasit.*, **20**, 189–198

DAVIS, L. R., HERLICH, H. & ROHRBACHER, G. H. (1957). Observations on an outbreak of coccidiosis in a flock of western lambs in Alabama. *J. Protozool.*, **4**, (Suppl.) 10

DAVIS, L. R., HERLICH, H. & BOWMAN, G. W. (1959). Studies on experimental concurrent infections of dairy calves with coccidia and nematodes. I. *Eimeria* spp. and the small intestinal worm *Cooperia punctata*. *Am. J. vet. Res.*, **20**, 281–286

DAVIS, L. R., HERLICH, H. & BOWMAN, G. W. (1960a). Studies on experimental concurrent infections of dairy calves with coccidia and nematodes. III. *Eimeria* spp. and the thread worm, *Strongyloides papillosus*. *Am. J. vet. Res.*, **21**, 181–187

DAVIS, L. R., HERLICH, H. & BOWMAN, G. W. (1960b). Studies on experimental concurrent infections of dairy calves with coccidia and nematodes. IV. *Eimeria* spp. and the small hair-worm, *Trichostrongylus colubriformis*. *Am. J. vet. Res.*, **21**, 188–194

DAVIS, L. R., BOUGHTON, D. C. & BOWMAN, G. W. (1955). Biology and pathogenicity of *Eimeria alabamensis* Christensen, 1941, an intranuclear coccidium of cattle. *Am. J. vet. Res.*, **16**, 274–281

DAVIS, L. R. & BOWMAN, G. W. (1952). Coccidiosis in cattle. *Proc. U. S. Livestock Sanit. Ass.*, *58th Ann. Meeting*, pp. 39–50

DAVIS, L. R. & BOWMAN, G. W. (1954). The use of sulfamethazine in experimental coccidiosis of dairy calves. *Cornell Vet.* **44**, 71–79

DAVIS, L. R. & BOWMAN, G. W. (1957). The endogenous development of *Eimeria zürnii*, a pathogenic coccidium of cattle. *Am. J. vet. Res.*, **18**, 569–574

DAVIES, L. R., BOWMAN, G. W. & BOUGHTON, D. C. (1957). The endogenous development of *Eimeria alabamensis* Christensen, 1941, an intranuclear coccidium of cattle. *J. Protozool.*, **4**, 219–225

DAVIS, L. R. & BOWMAN, G. W. (1962). Schizonts and microgametocytes of *Eimeria auburnensis* Christensen and Porter, 1939, in calves. *J. Protozool.*, **9**, 424–427

VAN DOORNINCK, W. M. & BECKER, E. F. (1957). Transport of sporozoites of *Eimeria necatrix* in macrophages. *J. Parasit.*, **43**, 40–43

DUNLAP, J. S., HAWKINS, P. A. & NELSON, R. H. (1949). Studies on sheep parasites. IX. The development of naturally-acquired coccidial infection in lambs. *Ann. N.Y. Acad. Sci.*, **52**, 505–511

EDGAR, S. A. (1955). Sporulation of oocysts at specific temperatures and notes on the prepatent period of several species of avian coccidia. *J. Parasit.*, **41**, 214–216

EDGSON, F. A. (1948). Mepacrine hydrochloride in the treatment of bovine coccidiosis. *Vet. Rec.*, **60**, 517–518

FAVATI, V. & GUERIERI, E. (1961). Ovine coccidiosis in Tuscany, Italy. *Annal. Fac. Med. Vet. Univ. Pisa*, **14**, 305–313

FOSTER, A. O. (1949). The economic losses due to coccidiosis. *Ann. N. Y. Acad. Sci.*, **52**, 434–442

FOSTER, A. O., CHRISTENSEN, J. F. & HABERMANN, R. T. (1941). Treatment of coccidial infections of lambs with sulfaguanidine. *Proc. Helminth. Soc. Wash.*, **8**, 33–38

GILRUTH, J. A. (1910). Notes on a protozoon parasite found in the mucous membrane of the abomasum of a sheep. *Bull. Soc. Path. exot.*, **3**, 297–299

HAMMOND, D. M. (1964). Coccidiosis of cattle. Some unsolved problems. 130th Faculty Honor Lecture. *The Fac. Ass. Utah State University, Logan*, Utah, 1961

HAMMOND, D. M., ANDERSON, F. L. & MINER, M. L. (1963). The site of the immune reaction against *Eimeria bovis* in calves. *J. Parasit.*, **49**, 415–424

HAMMOND, D. M., ANDERSON, F. L. & MINER, M. L. (1964). Response of immunized and non-immunized calves to cecal inoculation of first generation merozoites of *E. bovis*. *J. Parasit.*, **50**, 209–213

HAMMOND, D. M., BOWMAN, G. W., DAVIS, L. R. & SIMMS, B. T. (1946). The endogenous phase of the life cycle of Eimeria. *J. Parasit.*, **32**, 409–427

HAMMOND, D. M., CLARK, G. W., MINER, M. L., TROST, W. A. & JOHNSON, A. E. (1959). Treatment of experimental bovine coccidiosis with multiple small doses and single large doses of sulfamethazine and sulfabromomethazine. *Am. J. vet. Res.*, **20**, 708–713

HAMMOND, D. M., CLARK, W. N. & MINER, M. L. (1961). Endogenous phase of the life cycle of *Eimeria auburnensis* in calves. *J. Parasit.*, **47**, 591–596

HAMMOND, D. M., FERGUSON, D. L. & MINER, M. L. (1960). Results of experiments with nitrofurazone and sulfamethazine for controlling coccidosis in calves. *Cornell Vet.*, **50**, 351–362

HAMMOND, D. M., MINER, M. L. & ANDERSON, F. L. (1960a). The timing of the merozoite stage in the life cycle of *Eimeria bovis*. *J. Protozool.*, **7**, (Suppl.) 11

HAMMOND, D. M., SAYIN, F. & MINER, M. L. (1963b). Developmental cycle and pathogenicity of *Eimeria ellipsoidalis* in calves. *Berl. Münch. tierärztl. Wschr.*, **76**, 331–333

HAMMOND, D. M., SENGER, C. M., THORNE, J. L., SHUTE, J. L., FITZGERALD, P. R. & JOHNSON, A. E. (1958). Experience with nicarbazin in coccidiosis (*Eimeria bovis*) in cattle. *Cornell Vet.*, **48**, 260–263

HAMMOND, D. M., SHUPE, J. L., JOHNSON, A. E., FITZGERALD, P. R. & THORNE, J. L. (1956). Sulfaquinoxaline and sulfamerazine in the treatment of experimental infections with *Eimeria bovis* in calves. *Am. J. vet. Res.*, **17**, 463–470

HASCHE, M. R. & TODD, A. C. (1959). *Eimeria brasiliensis* Torres and Ramos, 1939, in Wisconsin. *J. Parasit.*, **45**, 202

HENNING, M. W. (1956). *Animal Diseases in South Africa*. 3rd Ed. South Africa: Central News Agency

HOARE, C. A. (1933). Studies on some new ophidian and avian coccidia from Uganda, with a revision of the classification of the Eimeriidea. *Parasitology*, **25**, 359–388

HORTON-SMITH, C. (1958). Coccidiosis in domestic animals. *Vet. Rec.*, **70**, 256–262

HORTON-SMITH, C. & LONG, P. L. (1963). Coccidia and coccidiosis in the domestic fowl and turkey. *Adv. Parasit.*, **1**, 67–107

HUIZINGA, H. and WINGER, R. N. (1942). *Eimeria wyomingensis*, a new coccidium from cattle. *Trans. Am. Microsc. Soc.*, **61**, 131–133

IKEDA, M. (1960). Factors necessary for *E. tenella* infection of the chicken. VI. Excystation of oocysts *in vitro*. *Jap. J. vet. Sci.*, **22**, 27–41

ITAGAKI, K. and TSUBOKURA, M. (1958). Studies on the infectious process of coccidium in fowl. Further investigations on the liberation of sporozoites. *Jap. J. vet. Sci.*, **20**, 105–109

JACOB, E. (1943). Zur Unterscheidung der Kokzidienarten bei Schafen, Ziegen und Rehen. *Berl. Münch. tierärztl. Wschr.* (31–32) Aug. 6, 258–260

KOTLAN, S., PELLERDY, L. & VERSENYR, L. (1951). Experimentelle Studien über die Kokzidiose der Schafe. I. Die endogene Entwicklung von *Eimeria parva*. *Acat. Vet. Budapest*, **1**, 317–331

KUDO, R. R. (1954). *Protozoology*. Springfield, Ill.: Thomas

LANDERS, E. J. (1952). A new species of coccidia from domestic sheep. *J. Parasit.*, **38**, 569–570

LANDERS, E. J. (1953). The effect of low temperatures upon the viability of unsporulated oocysts of ovine coccidia. *J. Parasit.*, **39**, 547–552

LANDERS, E. J. (1960). Studies on excystation of coccidial oocysts. *J. Parasit.*, **46**, 195–200

LAPAGE, G. (1940). The study of coccidiosis (*Eimeria caviae*) in the guinea pig. *Vet. J.*, **96**, 144–190

LEE, R. P. (1954). The occurrence of the coccidian *Eimeria bukidnonensis* Tubangui, 1931, in Nigerian cattle. *J. Parasit.*, **40**, 464–466

LEE, R. P. & ARMOUR, J. (1958). A note on *Eimeria braziliensis* Torres and Ramos, 1939, and its relationship to *Eimeria böhmi* Supperer, 1952. *J. Parasit.*, **44**, 302–304

LEVINE, N. D. (1961). *Protozoan Parasites of Domestic Animals and of Man*. Minneapolis, Minn.: Burgess Publishing

LEVINE, N. D., IVENS, V. & FRITZ, T. E. (1962). *Eimeria christenseni* sp. n. and other coccidia (protozoa: Eimeriidae) of the goat. *J. Parasit.*, **48**, 255–269

LEVINE, P. P. (1940). The initiation of avian coccidial infection with merozoites. *J. Parasit.*, 26, 337–343
LEVINE, P. P. (1942). Excystation of coccidial oocysts of the chicken. *J. Parasit.*, 28, 426–428
LONG, P. L. (1959). A study of *Eimeria maxima* Tyzzer, 1929, a coccidium of the fowl (*Gallus gallus*). *Ann. trop. Med. Parasit.*, 53, 325–333
LOTZE, J. C. (1952). The pathogenicity of the coccidian parasite, *Eimeria arloingi*, in domestic sheep. *Cornell Vet.*, 42, 510–517
LOTZE, J. C. (1953). Life history of the coccidian parasite, *Eimeria arloingi* in domestic sheep. *Am. J. vet. Res.*, 14, 86–95
LOTZE, J. C. (1954). The pathogenicity of the coccidian parasite *Eimeria ninakohlyakimovae*, Yakimov and Rastegaeva, 1930, in domestic sheep. *Proc. Am. vet. med. Ass.*, 1953, pp. 141–146
LOTZE, J. C. (1959). The effect of experimental infections of the coccidium *Eimeria faurei* on wool. *J. Parasit.*, 45, (Suppl.) 40
MARQUARDT, W. C. (1959). The morphology and sporulation of the oocyst of *Eimeria brasiliensis*, Torres and Ildefonso Ramos 1939, of cattle. *Am. J. vet. Res.*, 20, 742–746
MARQUARDT, W. C., SENGER, C. M. & SEGHETTI, L. (1960). The effect of physical and clinical agents on the oocyst of *Eimeria zurnii* (protozoa, coccidia). *J. Protozool.*, 7, 186–189
MASKE, H. (1893). Gregarinen im Labmagen des Schafes. Vorläufige Mittheilung. *Z. Fleisch-u. Milchhyg.*, 4, 28–29
McCULLOUGH, S. F. (1952). M.Sc. Thesis, Queen's University, Belfast, Ireland
MONNÉ, L. & HÖNIG, G. (1954). On the properties of the shells of the coccidian oocysts. *Arch. Zool. Stockholm*, 7, 251–256
PATTILLO, W. H. (1959). Invasion of the cecal mucosa of the chicken by sporozoites of *Eimeria tenella*. *J. Parasit.*, 45, 253–258
PATILLO, W. H. & BECKER, E. R. (1955). Cytochemistry of *Eimeria brunetti* and *E. acervulina* of the chicken. *J. Morphol.*, 96, 61–95
PEARDON, D. L., BILKOVICH, F. R. & TODD, A. C. (1963). Trials of candidate bovine coccidiostats. *Am. J. vet. Res.*, 24, 743–748
PELLERDY, L. P. (1965). *Coccidia and Coccidiosis*. Budapest: Akademiai Kiado
RAO, S. R. & HIREGAUDAR, L. S. (1954). Coccidial fauna of cattle in Bombay State with particular reference to a recent outbreak at Aery Milk Colony, together with a description of two species, *Eimeria bombayensis* and *Eimeria khurodensis*. *Bombay vet. Coll. Mag.*, 4, 24–28
REICHENOW, E. (1940). Über das Kokzid des Equiden *Globidium leuckarti*. *Z. InfektKrankh. parasit. Krankh. Hyg. Haustiere*, 56, 126–134
RICHARDSON, U. F. (1939). The incidence of coccidiosis of sheep in Scotland. *Vet. J.*, 95, 349–351. *J. Parasit.*, 29, 10–32
RUTHERFORD, R. L. (1943). The life cycle of four intestinal coccidia of the domestic rabbit. *J. Parasit.*, 29, 10–32
SALISBURY, R. M. & WHITTEN, L. K. (1953). Coccidiosis in sheep. A review. *N. Z. vet. J.*, 1, 69–72
SARWAR, M. M. (1951). Occurrence of *Globidium gilruthi*, a protozoon parasite of sheep and goats from the Indo-Pakistan sub-continent. *Parasitology*, 41, 282
SCHAUDINN, F. (1900). Untersuchungen über den Generationswechsel bei Coccidien. *Zool. Jb. Jena Abt. Anat.*, 13, 197–292
SCHOLTYSECK, E. (1953). Beitrag zur Kenntnis des Entwicklungsganges des Hühnercoccids *Eimeria tenella*. *Arch. Protistenk.*, 98, 415–465
SENGER, C. M., HAMMOND, D. M., THORNE, J. L., JOHNSON, A. E. & WELLS, M. (1959). Resistance of calves to reinfection with *Eimeria bovis*. *J. Protozool.*, 6, 51–58
SHUMARD, R. F. (1957). Ovine coccidiosis-incidence, possible endotoxin, and treatment. *J. Am. vet. med. Ass.*, 131, 559–561
SHUMARD, R. F. (1959a). Experimentally induced ovine coccidiosis. I. Use of nitrofurazone in the feed. *Vet. Med.*, 54, 421–425
SHUMARD, R. F. (1959b). Experimentally induced ovine coccidiosis. II. Use of water soluble nitrofurazone as a therapeutic. *Vet. Med.*, 54, 477–479
SHUMARD, R. F. & EVELETH, D. F. (1955). A preliminary report on a toxic substance produced by *Eimeria* spp. in a lamb. *Agric. Res. Serv. Bull. USDA*, p. 6
SMETANA, H. (1933). Coccidiosis of the liver in rabbits. II. Experimental study on the excystation of oocysts of *Eimeria stiedae*. *Archs Path.*, 15, 175–192
SMITH, W. N., DAVIS, L. R. & BOWMAN, G. W. (1960). The pathogenicity of *Eimeria ahsata*, a coccidium of sheep. *J. Protozool.*, 7, (Suppl.) 8.
SOLIMAN, K. N. (1960). Globidium infections in the Sudan with special reference to *Globidium gilruthi*. *J. Parasit.*, 46, 29–32
SUPPERER, R. (1952). Die Coccidien des Rindes in Oesterreich. *Ost. Zool.*, 3, 591–601
SVANBAEV, S. K. (1957). Sur la question de la faune et de la morphologie des coccidia des moutons et des chèvres de l'ouest du Kazakhstan. *Trudy. Inst. Zool.*, Alma-Ata, 7, 252–257
TARLATZIS, C., PANETSOS, A. & DRAGONAS, P. (1955). Furacin in the treatment of ovine and caprine coccidiosis. *J. Am. vet. med. Ass.*, 126, 391–392
TARLATZIS, E., PANETSOS, A. & DRAGONAS, P. (1957). Further experience with furacin in treatment of ovine and caprine coccidiosis. *J. Am. vet. med. Ass.*, 131, 474

TORRES, S. & RAMOS, J. I. (1939). Eimerias dos bovinos em Pernambuco, E. *ildefonsoi* e E. *braziliensis* spcs. ns. *Archos Inst. Pesq. agron.*, *Pernambuco*, **2**, 79–96

TABANGUI, M. A. (1931). *Eimeria bukidnonensis*, a new coccidium from cattle and other coccidial parasites of domesticated animals. *Philipp. J. Sci.*, **44**, 253–271

WHITTEN, L. K. (1953). A preliminary field experiment on the treatment of coccidiosis in lambs. *N. Z. vet. J.*, **1**, 78–80

WIESENHÜTTER, E. (1962a). Ein Beitrag zur Kenntnis der endogen Entwicklung von *Eimeria spinosa* des Schweines. *Berl. Münch tierärztl. Wschr.*, **75**, 72–173

WIESENHÜTTER, E. (1962b). Experimentelle Studien über die Entwicklung von *Eimeria debliecki* und *Eimeria spinosa* des Schweines. Inaug. Diss., Berlin

WILSON, I. D. (1931). A study of bovine coccidiosis. *Va. Agric. exp. Stn. Tech. Bull.*, p. 42

WILSON, I. D. & MORLEY, L. C. (1933). A study of bovine coccidiosis. II. *J. Am. vet. med. Ass.*, **82**, 826–850

YAKIMOFF, W. L. (1931). The coccidia of the Zebu. *Bull. Soc. Path. exot.*, **24**, 644–645

YAKIMOFF, W. L., GOUSSEFF, W. F. & RASTEGAIEFF, E. F. (1933). Die Coccidiose der wilden kleinen Wiederkäuer. *Z. ParasitKde.*, **5**, 85–93

COCCIDIA OF POULTRY, DOGS, CATS, RABBITS ETC.

ALLEN, E. A. (1936). *Tyzzeria perniciosa* gen. et sp. Nov., a new coccidium from the small intestine of the pekin duck, *Anas domesticus* L. *Arch. Protistk.*, **87**, 262–267

ALTMEN, J. E. (1951). Treatment of canine coccidiosis (*Isospora bigemina*) with Aureomycin. *J. Am. vet. med. Ass.*, **119**, 207–209

ANDREWS, J. M. (1926). A factor in host-parasite specificity of coccidiosis. *Anat. Rec.*, **34**, 154

ANDREWS, J. S. & SPINDLER, L. A. (1952). *Eimeria spinosa* recovered from swine raised in Maryland and Georgia. *Proc. Helminth. Soc. Wash.*, **19**, 64

ARUNDEL, J. H. (1960). Chemotherapy of caecal coccidiosis in chickens: 3:5 Dinitro-o-toluamide. *Austral. vet. J.*, **36**, 49–53

BALL, S. J. (1959). Chemotherapy of caecal coccidiosis in chickens: the activity of Nicarbazin. *Vet. Rec.*, **71**, 86–91

BECKER, E. R. (1934). *Coccidia and Coccidiosis of Domesticated, Game and Laboratory Animals and of Man*. Ames, Iowa: Iowa State College Press

BECKER, E. R. (1956). Catalogue of Eimeriidae in genera occurring in vertebrates and not requiring intermediate hosts. *Iowa State Coll. J. Sci.*, **31**, 85–139

BECKER, E. R., ZIMMERMAN, W. J. & PATTILLO, W. (1955). A biometrical study of the oocysts of *Eimeria brunetti*, a parasite of the common fowl. *J. Protozool.*, **2**, 145–150

BOCH, J., PEZENBURG, E. & ROSENFELD, V. (1961). Ein Beitrag zur Kenntnis der Kokzidien der Schweine. *Berl. Münch. tierärztl Wschr.*, **74**, 449–451

BOLES, J. I. & BECKER, E. R. (1954). The development of *Eimeria brunetti* Levine, in the digestive tract of chickens. *Iowa State Coll. J. Sci.*, **29**, 1–26

BOYLER, C. I. & BROWN, J. A. (1953). The comparative coccidiostatic activity of some drugs against turkey coccidia. Proc. 90th Mtg. Am. vet. med. Ass., 20–30 July, 1953, pp. 328–336

BRACKETT, S. & BLIZNICK, A. (1950). The occurrence and economic importance of coccidiosis in chickens. *Bull. Lederle Lab.*, 78

BRUMPT, L. C. (1943). Le traitement des coccidioses des animaux domestiques par quinacrine ou atebrine. *Annls Parasit. hum. comp.*, **19**, 95–115

BURNS, W. C. & CHALLEY, J. R. (1959). Resistance of birds to challenge with *Eimeria tenella*. *Exp. Parasit.*, **8**, 515–526

CATCOTT, E. J. (1946). The incidence of intestinal protozoa in the dog. *J. Am. vet. med. Assoc.*, **107**, 34–36

CHAMPION, L. R. (1954). The inheritance of resistance to caecal coccidiosis in the domestic fowl. *Poultry Sci.* **33**, 670–681

CHEISSIN, E. M. (1946). Duration and life cycle in rabbit coccidia. *C.R. Acad. Sci. USSR*, **52**, 557–570

CHEISSIN, E. M. (1947). A new species of rabbit coccidia (*Eimeria coecicola* N. sp.). *C.R. Acad. Sci. USSR*, **55**, 177–179

CLARKSON, M. J. (1956). Experimental infection of turkey poults with *Eimeria adenoeides* (Moore and Brown, 1951) isolated from a natural case in Great Britain. *Nature, Lond.*, **178**, 196–197

CLARKSON, M. J. (1958). Life history and pathogenicity of *Eimeria adenoeides*, Moore and Brown, 1951 in the turkey poult. *Parasitology*, **48**, 70–88

CLARKSON, M. J. & GENTLES, M. A. (1958). Coccidiosis in turkeys. *Vet. Rec.*, **70**, 211–214

CLARKSON, M. J. (1959a). The life history and pathogenicity of *Eimeria meleagrimitis* Tyzzer 1929 in the turkey poult. *Parasitology*, **49**, 70–82

CLARKSON, M. J. (1959b). The life history and pathogenicity of *Eimeria meleagridis* Tyzzer, 1927 in the turkey poult. *Parasitology*, **49**, 519–528

CRITCHER, S. (1950). Renal coccidiosis in Pea Island Canada geese. *Wildl. in N. Carolina*, **14**, 14–15

CUCKLER, A. C. & OTT, W. H. (1947). The effect of Sulfaquinoxaline on the developmental stages of *Eimeria tenella*. *J. Parasit.*, **33**, Suppl. 10–11

CUCKLER, A. C. & MALANGA, C. M. (1955). Studies on drug resistance in coccidia. *J. Parasit.*, **41**, 302–311

CUCKLER, A. C., MALANGA, C. M., BASSO, A. J. & O'NEILL, R. C. (1955). The antiparasitic activity of substituted carbanilide complexes. *Science*, **122**, 244–245

DAVIES, S. F. M. & KENDALL, S. B. (1954a). The effect of sodium sulphaquinoxaline and sodium sulphamezathene in interrupted schedules of treatment on the development of *Eimeria tenella*. *J. comp. Path. Ther.*, **64**, 87–93

DAVIES, S. F. M. & KENDALL, S. B. (1954). The practical application of sulphamezathine therapy for caecal coccidiosis. *Vet. Rec.*, **66**, 19

DAVIES, S. F. M. (1956). Intestinal coccidiosis in chickens caused by *Eimeria necatrix*. *Vet. Rec.*, **68**, 853–857

DAVIES, S. F. M. (1957). An outbreak of duck coccidiosis in Britain. *Vet. Rec.*, **69**, 1051–1052

DAVIES, S. F. M., JOYNER, L. P. & KENDALL, S. B. (1963). *Coccidiosis*. Edinburgh & London: Oliver & Boyd

DAVIES, S. F. M. (1963). *Eimeria brunetti*, an additional cause of intestinal coccidiosis in the domestic fowl in Britain. *Vet. Rec.*, **75**, 1–4

DEOM, J. & MORTELMANS, J. (1954). Observations sur la coccidiose du porc à *Eimeria debliecki* en Congo Belge. *Annls Soc. belge Méd. trop.*, **34**, 43

DUBERMAN, D. (1960). Treatment of canine coccidiosis using nitrofurazone and sulphonamides. *J. Am. vet. med. Ass.*, **136**, 29–30

EDGAR, S. A. & SIEBOLD, C. T. (1964). A new coccidium of chickens. *Eimeria mivati* sp. N. (Protozoa: Eimeriidae) with details of its life history. *J. Parasit.*, **50**, 193–204

EDGAR, S. A., FLANAGAN, C. & HWANG, J. (1956). Breeding and immunizing chickens for resistance to coccidiosis. I. Immunization phase. *66th & 67th Ann. Rep. Agric. expl. Stn, Alabama Polytech. Inst.*, 1955–1956, pp. 46–47

EDGAR, S. A. (1958). Control of coccidiosis of chickens and turkeys by immunization. *Poultry Sci.* **37**, 1200

GARDINER, J. L. (1955). The severity of cecal coccidiosis infection in chickens as related to the age of the host and the number of oocysts ingested. *Poultry Sci.*, **34**, 415–420

GASSNER, E. X. (1940). Studies in canine coccidiosis. *J. Am. vet. med. Ass.*, **96**, 225–229

HANSON, H. C., LEVINE, N. D. & IVENS, V. (1957). Coccidia (Protozoa: Eimeriidae) of North American wild geese and swans. *Canad. J. Zool.*, **35**, 715–733

HARWOOD, P. D. & STEMZ, D. (1949). Nitrofurazone in the medication of avian coccidiosis. *J. Parasit.*, **35**, 175–182

HARWOOD, P. D., STUNZ, D. I. & WOLFGANG, R. W. (1957). The effect of furazolidone administered in the feed upon coccidiosis (*Eimeria necatrix*). *J. Parasit.*, **43**, Suppl. 17

HAUSER, K. W. (1959). Erfahrungen bei der Bekämpfung der Kokzidiose der Tauben. *Berl. Münch. tierärztl. Wschr.*, **72**, 481–483

HAWKINS, P. A. (1952). Coccidiosis in turkeys. *Mich. State Coll. Technol. Bull.*, **226**, 1–87

HEIN, H. (1963). Vaccination against infection with *Eimeria tenella* in broiler chickens. *Proc. 17th vet. Congr. Hannover*, **1**, 1443–1452

HEMMERT-HALSWICK, A. (1943). Infektion mit *Globidium leuckarti* beim Pferd. *Z. VetKde.*, **55**, 192–199

HERMAN, C. M., JANKIEWICZ, H. A. & SAARNI, R. W. (1942). Coccidiosis in California quail. *Condor*, **44**, 168

HITCHCOCK, D. J. (1955). The life-cycle of *Isospora felis* in the kitten. *J. Parasit.*, **41**, 383–393

HORTON-SMITH, C. (1947). Treatment of hepatic coccidiosis in rabbits. *Vet. J.*, **103**, 207

HORTON-SMITH, C. & LONG, P. L. (1959). The effects of different anticoccidial agents on the intestinal coccidioses of the fowl. *J. comp. Path.*, **69**, 192–207

HORTON-SMITH, C. & LONG, P. L. (1961). The effect of sulphonamide medication on the life cycle of *Eimeria meleagrimitis* in turkeys. *Exp. Parasit.*, **11**, 93–101

HORTON-SMITH, C., BEATTIE, J. & LONG, P. L. (1961). Resistance to *Eimeria tenella* and its transference from one caecum to the other in individual fowls. *Immunology*, **4**, 111–121

HORTON-SMITH, C., LONG, P. L., PIERCE, A. E. & ROSE, M. E. (1963). Immunity to coccidia in domestic animals. In *Immunity to Protozoa* (Ed. by P. C. C. Garnham. A. E. Pierce & I. Roitt). Oxford: Blackwell Scientific Publications

HYMAS, T. A. & STEVENSON, G. T. (1960). A study of the action of zoalene on *Eimeria tenella* and *Eimeria necatrix* when administered in the diet or in the drinking water. *Poultry Sci.*, **39**, 1261–1262

JACKSON, A. R. B. (1962). Excystation of *Eimeria arloingi* (Marotel, 1905): stimuli from the host sheep. *Nature*, **194**, 847–849

JOYNER, L. P. (1957). Induced drug-fastness to nitrofurazone in a laboratory strain of *Eimeria tenella*. *Vet. Rec.*, **69**, 1415–1418

JOYNER, L. P. (1958). Experimental *Eimeria mitis* infections in chickens. *Parasitology*, **48**, 101–112

KENDALL, S. B. & McCULLOUGH, F. S. (1952). Relationships between sulphamezathine therapy and the acquisition of immunity to *Eimeria tenella*. *J. comp. Path.*, **62**, 116–124

KLIMES, B. (1963). Coccidia of the domestic goose (*Anser anser dom.*). *Zbl. vet. Med.*, **10**, 427–448

KOTLAN, A. (1933). Zur Kenntnis der Kokzidiose der Wassergeflügels. Die Kokzidiose der Hausgans. *Zblt. Bakt. Abt. I. Orig.*, **129**, 11–21

KUTZER, E. (1960). Über die Kokzidien des Schweines in Österreich. *Z. ParasitKde.*, **19**, 541–547

LAARMAN, J. J. (1963). *Isospora hominis* (Railliet and Lucet, 1891) in the Netherlands. In *Progress in Protozoology* (Ed. by J. Ludvik, J. Lom & J. Vavra). New York & London: Academic Press

LEE, C. D. (1934). The pathology of coccidiosis in the dog. *J. Amer. vet. med. Ass.*, **85**, 760–781

LEVINE, N. D., (1952). *Eimeria magnalabia* and *Tyzzeria* spp. (Protozoa: Eimeriidae) from the common Canada goose. *Cornell Vet.*, **42**, 247–252

LEVINE, N. D. & IVENS, V. (1965). *Isospora* species in the dog. *J. Parasit.*, **51**, 859–864

LEVINE, P. P. (1938). *Eimeria hagani* N. sp. (Protozoa: Eimeriidae) a new coccidium of the chicken. *Cornell Vet.*, **28**, 263–266

LEVINE, P. P. (1939). The effect of sulfanilamide on the course of experimental avian coccidiosis. *Cornell Vet.*, **29**, 309

LEVINE, P. P. (1942). A new coccidium pathogenic for chickens, *Eimeria brunetti* N. sp. (Protozoa: Eimeriidae). *Cornell Vet.*, **32**, 430–439

LICKFELD, K. G. (1959). Untersuchungen über das Katzencoccid *Isospora felis* Wenyon, 1923. *Arch. Protistenk.*, **103**, 427–456

LONG, P. L. (1959). A study of *Eimeria maxima* Tyzzer, 1929. A coccidium of the fowl (*Gallus gallus*). *Ann. trop. Med. Parasit.*, **53**, 325–333

LONG, P. L. (1963). The effect of a combination of sulphaquinoxaline and Amprolium against different species of *Eimeria* in chickens. *Vet. Rec.*, **75**, 645–650

LUND, E. E. (1949). Considerations on the practical control of intestinal coccidiosis of domestic rabbits. *Ann. N.Y. Acad. Sci.*, **52**, 611–620

LUND, E. E. (1954). The effect of sulphaquinoxaline on the course of *Eimeria stiedae* infections in the domestic rabbit. *Exp. Parasit.*, **3**, 497–503

MADSEN, H. (1941). The occurrence of helminths and coccidia in partridges and pheasants in Denmark. *J. Parasit.*, **27**, 29–34

MCDERMOTT, J. J. & STAUBER, L. A. (1954). Preparation and agglutination of merozoite suspensions of the chicken coccidium *Eimeria tenella*. *J. Parasit.*, **40**, (Suppl.) 23

MCGEE, H. L. (1950). Coccidiosis in the dog. Clinical Observation. *J. Am. vet. med. Ass.*, **117**, 227–228

MCGREGOR, J. K. (1952). Renal coccidiosis in geese. *J. Am. vet. med. Ass.*, **121**, 452–453

MCLOUGHLIN, D. K. & WEHR, E. E. (1960). Stages in the life of *Eimeria tenella* affected by Nicarbazin. *Poultry Si.*, **39**, 534–538

MOORE, E. N. & BROWN, J. A. (1951). A new coccidium pathogenic for turkeys, *Eimeria adenoeides* N. sp. (Protozoa: Eimeriidae), *Cornell Vet.*, **41**, 124–125

MOORE, E. N. and BROWN, J. A. (1952). A new coccidium of turkeys, *Eimeria innocua* N. sp. (Protozoa: Eimeriidae). *Cornell Vet.*, **42**, 395–402

MOORE, E. N. (1954). Species of coccidia affecting turkeys, *Proc. 91st ann. Meet. Am. vet. med. Ass.*, pp. 300–304

MOORE, E. N., BROWN, J. A. & CARTER, R. D. (1954). A new coccidium of turkeys: *Eimeria subrotunda* N. sp. (Protozoa: Eimeriidae). *Poultry Sci.*, **33**, 925–929

MOREHOUSE, N. F. & MCGUIRE, W. C. (1958). The pathogenicity of *Eimeria acervulina*. *Poultry Sci.*, **37**, 665–672

MORINI, E. G. (1950). Coccidiosis in pigeons. *Rev. Med. Vet. B. Aires*, **32**, 207

NEMESERI, L. (1960). Beiträge zur Ätiologie der Coccidiose der Hunde. I. *Isospora canis* sp. Nov. *Acta vet. hung.*, **10**, 95–99

NEWBERNE, P. M. & BUCK, W. B. (1956). Studies on drug toxicity in chicks. *Poultry Sci.*, **35**, 1259–1264

NIESCHULZ, O. (1925). Über die Entwicklung des Taubencoccids *Eimeria pfeifferi* (Labbé, 1896). *Arch. Protistenk.*, **51**, 479–494

PARKIN, B. S. (1943). Treatment of canine coccidiosis. *J. S. Afr. vet. med. Ass.*, **14**, 73–76

PELLERDY, L. (1949). Studies on coccidia occurring in the domestic pig, with the description of a new *Eimeria* species (*Eimeria polita* sp. N.) of that host. *Acta vet. hung.*, **1**, 101–109

PELLERDY, L. S. (1953). Beiträge zur Kenntnis der Darmkokzidiose des Kaninchens. Die endogene Entwicklung von *Eimeria piriformis*. *Acta vet. hung.*, **3**, 365–377

PELLERDY, L. S. (1954). Beiträge zur Spezifizität der Coccidien des Hasen und Kaninchens. *Acta vet. hung.*, **4**, 481–487

PELLERDY, L. P. & BABOS, S. (1953). Untersuchungen über die endogene Entwicklung sowie pathologische Bedeutung von *Eimeria media*. *Acta vet. hung.*, **3**, 173–178

PELLERDY, L. P. (1956). On the status of the *Eimeria* species of *Lepus europaeus* and related species. *Acta vet. hung.*, **6**, 451–467

PELLERDY, L. P. (1960). Adatok a maxima-coccidiosis ismeretehez es hazai elofordulasahoz magy. *Allatorv. Lap.*, **15**, 307–309

PELLERDY, L. P. (1965). *Coccidia and Coccidiosis*. Budapest: Akademiai Kiado

PETERSON, E. H. (1949). Sulfonamides in the control of experimental coccidiosis in the turkey. *Vet. Med.*, **44**, 126–128

PETERSON, E. H. (1960). A study of anti-coccidial drugs against experimental infections with *Eimeria tenella* and *necatrix*. *Poultry Sci.*, **39**, 739–745

PETERSON, E. H. & MUNRO, S. S. (1949). The chemotherapy of coccidiosis due to *Eimeria acervulina*. *Ann. N. Y. Acad. Sci.*, **52**, 597–582

PIERCE, A. E., LONG, P. L. & HORTON-SMITH, C. (1962). Immunity to *Eimeria tenella* in young fowls (*Gallus domesticus*). *Immunology*, **5**, 129–152

PIERCE, A. E., LONG, P. L. & HORTON-SMITH, C. (1963). Attempts to induce a passive immunity to *Eimeria tenella* in young fowls (*Gallus domesticus*). *Immunology*, **6**, 37–47

RAY, H. N. (1945). On a new coccidium *Wenyonella gallinae* N. Sp. from the gut of the domestic fowl, *Gallus gallus domesticus*. *Linn. Curr. Sci.*, **14**, 275

ROSE, M. E. (1963). Some aspects of immunity to *Eimeria* infections. *Ann. N. Y. Acad. Sci.*, **113**, 383–399

ROSE, M. E. & LONG, P. L. (1962). Immunity to four species of *Eimeria* in the fowl. *Immunology*, **4**, 346–353

ROSENBERG, M. M., ALICATA, J. E. & PALAFOX, A. L. (1954). Further evidence of hereditary resistance and susceptibility to cecal coccidiosis in chickens. *Poultry Sci.*, **33**, 972–980

RUTHERFORD, R. L. (1943). The life cycle of four intestinal coccidia of the domestic rabbit. *J. Parasit.*, **29**, 10–32

SADEK, S. E., HANSON, L. E. & ALBERTS, J. (1955). Suspected drug induced anemias in the chicken. *J. Am. vet. med. Ass.*, **127**, 201–203

SCHOLTYSECK, E. (1955). *Eimeria anatis* N. sp. ein neues Coccid aus der Stockente (*Anas platyrhynchos*). *Arch. Protistenk.*, **100**, 431–434

SCHOLTYSECK, E. (1959). Zur Pathologie der *Eimeria maxima*—Coccidiose. *Zbl. Bakt. Abt. I. Orig.*, **175**, 305–317

SCHOLTYSECK, E. (1963). Vergleichende Untersuchungen über die Kernverhältnisse und das Wachstum bei Coccidiomorphen unter besonderer Berücksichtigung von *Eimeria maxima*. *Z. ParasitKde.*, **22**, 428–474

SKAMSER, L. M. (1947). Coccidiosis in Poults. *Turkey Wld.*, 3

SLAVIN, D. (1955). *Cryposporidium meleagridis* sp. Nov. *J. comp. Path. Ther.*, **65**, 262–266

SMETANA, H. (1933a). Coccidiosis of the liver of Rabbits. I. Experimental study on the excystation of oocysts of *Eimeria stiedae*. *Arch. Path.*, **15**, 175–192

SMETANA, H. (1933b). Coccidiosis of the liver of rabbits. II. Experimental study of the mode of infection of the liver of sporozoites of *Eimeria stiedae*. *Arch. Path.*, **15**, 330–339

SMETANA, H. (1933c). Coccidiosis of the liver of rabbits. III. Experimental study of the histogenesis of coccidiosis of the liver. *Arch. Path.*, **15**, 516–536

SMITH, M. J. & EDMONDS, R. S. (1959). Use of nitrofurazone in canine coccidiosis. *Mod. vet. Pract.*, **40**, 31–32

STUART, E. E., BRUINS, H. W. & KEENUM, R. D. (1963). The immunogenicity of a commercial coccidiosis vaccine in conjunction with Trithiadol and Zoalene. *Avian Dis.*, **7**, 12–18

STUBBS, E. L. (1957). Case report—renal coccidiosis in geese. *Avian Dis.*, **1**, 349

SWANSON, L. E. & KATES, K. C. (1940). Coccidiosis in a litter of pigs. *Proc. Helminth. Soc. Wash.*, **7**, 29–30

TOMIMURA, T. (1957). Experimental studies on coccidiosis in dogs and cats. I. The morphology of oocysts and sporogony of *Isospora felis* and its artificial infection in cats. *Riseichugaku Zasshi*, **6**, 12–14

TYZZER, E. E. (1929). Coccidiosis in gallinaceous birds. *Am. J. Hyg.*, **10**, 269–382

TYZZER, E. E. (1932). Criteria and methods in the investigation of avian coccidiosis. *J. Amer. vet. med. Ass.*, **80**, 474

VETTERLING, J. M. (1965). Coccidia (Protozoa: Emeriidae) of swine. *J. Parasit.*, **51**, 897–912

WALETSKY, E., NEAL, R. & HABEL, I. (1954). A field strain of *Eimeria tenella* resistant to sulfonamides. *J. Parasit.*, **40**, (Suppl.) 24

WALETSKY, E., HUGHES, C. O. & BRANDT, M. C. (1949). The anticoccidial activity of nitrophenide. *Ann. N. Y. Acad. Sci.*, **52**, 543

WARREN, E. W. & BALL, S. J. (1963). The effect of sulphoquinoxaline and amprolium in the life cycle of *Eimeria adenoeides* Moore and Brown, 1951, in turkey poults. *Parasitology*, **53**, 653–662

WAXLER, S. H. (1941). Immunization against cecal coccidiosis in chickens by the use of X-ray attenuated oocysts. *J. Am. vet. med. Ass.*, **99**, 481–485.

WENYON, C. M. (1923). Coccidiosis of cats and dogs and the status of the Isospora of man. *Ann. trop. Med. Parasit.*, **17**, 231–288

WENYON, C. M. & SHEATHER, A. L. (1925). *Isospora* infections of dogs. *Trans. R. Soc. trop. Med. Hyg.*, **19**, 10

WENYON, C. M. (1926b). Coccidia of the genus *Isospora* in cats, dogs and man. *Parasitology*, **18**, 253–266

ZAPFE, H. (1921). Zur Kenntnis der Kokzidiose des Hundes. *Inaug. Diss. Berlin*

ZULINSKI, T. (1957). Two cases of coccidiosis of the kidneys caused by *Eimeria* sp. in horses. *Med. Vet. Varsovie*, **13**, 579

HAEMOSPORIDEA (PLASMODIUM)

AL-DABAGH, M. A. (1961). Symptomatic partial paralysis in chicks infected with *Plasmodium juxtanucleare*. *J. comp. Path.*, **71**, 217–221

BISHOP, A. (1955). Problems concerned with gametogenesis in haemosporidea with particular reference to the genus *Plasmodium*. *Parasitology*, **45**, 163–185

BISHOP, A. (1962). Chemotherapy and drug resistance in protozoal infections. In *Drugs, Parasites and Hosts.* Biological Council Symposium (Ed. by L. G. GOODWIN & R. H. SMITH). London: Churchill

BOYE, H. K., GETZ, M. E., COATNEY, G. R., ELDER, H. A. & EYLES, D. E. (1961). Simian malaria in man. *Am. J. trop. Med. Hyg.*, **10**, 311

BRAY, R. S. (1957). Studies on the exoerythrocytic cycle in the genus Plasmodium. *Lond. School Hyg. trop. Med.*, **12**, 192

COATNEY, G. R. & ROUNDABUSH, R. L. (1949). In *Malariology* (Ed. by M. F. BOYD). Philadelphia: Saunders

EYLES, D. E., COATNEY, G. R. & GETZ, M. E. (1960). Vivax-type malaria parasite of Macaques transmissible to man. *Science*, **131**, 1812–1813

FAUST, E. C. & RUSSELL, P. F. (1964). *Craig and Faust's Clinical Parasitology.* 7th Ed. Philadelphia: Lea & Febiger

HEWITT, R. I. (1940). Bird Malaria. *Am. J. Hyg. Monogr. Series No.* **15**, *Johns Hopkins Press, Baltimore*

HUFF, C. G. (1963). Experimental research, on avian malaria. In *Advances in Parasitology* (Ed. by B. Dawes). Vol. 1, pp 1-65. London: Academic Press

HUFF, C. G. & COULSTON, F. (1944). The development of *Plasmodium gallinaceum* from sporozoite to erythrocytic trophozoite. *J. infect. Dis.*, **75**, 231–239

JEFFERY, G. M. (1961). Inoculation of human malaria into a simian host, *Macaca mulatta.* *J. Parasit.*, **47**, 90

KUDO, R. R. (1954). *Protozoology.* Springfield, Ill.: Thomas

LEVINE, N. D. (1961). *Protozoan Parasites of Domestic Animals and of Man.* Minneapolis: Burgess Publishing

LEVINE, N. D. & HANSON, H. C. (1953). Blood parasites of the Canada goose, *Branta canadensis interior. J. Wildl. Man.*, **17**, 185–196

LEVINE, N. D. & KANTOR, S. (1959). Check-list of blood parasites of birds of the order Columbiformes. *Wildl. Dis.*, **1**, 1–38

MANWELL, R. D. (1963). Factors making for host-specificity, with special emphasis on the blood protozoa. *Ann. N. Y. Acad. Sci.*, **113**, 332–342

PURCHASE, H. S. (1942). Turkey malaria. *Parasitology*, **34**, 278–283

ROLLO, I. M. (1964). The chemotherapy of malaria. In *Biochemistry and Physiology of Protozoa*, Vol. III (Ed. by S. H. HUNTER). New York: Academic Press

RUSSELL, P. F., WEST, L. S., MANWELL, R. D. & MACDONALD, G. (1963). *Practical Malariology*, 2nd Ed. London: Oxford Press

HAEMOSPORIDEA (BABESIIDAE)

ABRAMOV, I. V. (1952). Summary of the 36th Plenary Session of the USSR Leningrad Academy. Veterinary Section, on Protozoan Diseases. *Veterinariya Moscow* **9**, 55–57. (*Abs. Vet. Bull* (1953) **23**, 140)

ARNOLD, R. M. (1948). Resistance to tick-borne disease. *Vet. Rec.*, **60**, 426

ARTHUR, D. A. (1966). The ecology of ticks with reference to the transmission of protozoa. In *The Biology of Parasites* (Ed. by E. J. L. SOULSBY). New York: Academic Press

BEVERIDGE, C. G. L., THWAITE, J. W. & SHEPHERD, G. (1960). A field trial of Amicarbalide—a new Babesicide. *Vet. Rec.*, **72**, 383–386

BODIN, S. & HILDAR, G. (1963). Immunization of Swedish cattle against piroplasmosis. *Proc. 9th Nordic Vet. Congr. Copenhagen*, **1**, 328–333

BOOL, P. H., GOEDBLOED, E. & KEIDEL, H. J. W. (1961). The bovine babesia species in the Netherlands: *Babesia divergens* and *Babesia major. Tijdschr. Diergeneesk*, **86**, 28–37

CALLOW, L. L. & JOHNSTON, L. A. Y. (1963). *Babesia* spp. in the brains of clinically normal cattle and their detection by a brain smear technique. *Austral. vet. J.*, **39**, 25–31

CALLOW, L. L. & McGAVIN, M. D. (1963). Cerebral babesiosis due to *Babesia argentina. Austral. vet. J.*, **39**, 15–20

CARMICHAEL, J. (1956). Treatment and control of babesiosis. *Ann. N. Y. Acad. Sci.*, **64**, 147–151

CERRUTI, C. G. (1939). Recherches sur les piroplasmoses du porc. *Ann. Parasit.*, **17**, 114–136

CHEISSIN, E. M. & POLJANSKY, G. I. (1963). On the position of piroplasms in the system of Protozoa. In *Progress in Protozoology* (Ed. by J. LUDVIK, J. LOM & J. VAVRA). Prague: Czechoslovak Academy Sciences. New York: Academic Press

DALY, G. D. & HALL, W. T. K. (1955). A note on the susceptibility of British and some Zebutype cattle to tick fever (Babesiosis). *Austral. vet. J.*, **31**, 152

DAVIĘS, S. F. M., JOYNER, L. P. & KENDALL, S. B. (1958). Studies on *Babesia divergens* (McFadyean and Stockman, 1911). *Ann. trop. Med. Parasit.*, **52**, 206–215

DENNIS, E. W. (1932). The life-cycle of *Babesia bigemina* (Smith and Kilborne) of Texas cattlefever in the tick *Margaropus annulatus* (Say) with notes on embryology of *Margaropus. Univ. Calif. (Berkeley) Publ. Zool.*, **36**, 263–298

ENIGK, K. (1943). Die Überträger der Pferdepiroplasmose, ihre Verbreitung und Biologie. *Arch. wiss. prakt. Tierheilk*, **78**, 209–240

ENIGK, K. (1944a) Weitere Üntersuchungen zur Überträgerfrage der Pferdepiroplasmose. *Arch. wiss. prakt. Tierheilk.*, **79**, 58–80

ENIGK, K. (1944b). Das Vorkommen der Hundepiroplasmose in den besetzten Ostgebieten. *Dt. tropenmed. Z.*, **48**, 88–93

ENIGK, K. (1951). Der Einfluss des Klimas auf das Auftreten der Pferdepiroplasmosen. A. *Tropenmed. Parasit.*, **2**, 401–410

ENIGK, K. & FRIEDHOFF, K. (1962a). Zur Wirtsspezifität von *Babesia divergens* (Piroplasmidea). *Z. ParasitKde.*, **21**, 238–256

ENIGK, K. & FRIEDHOFF, K. (1962b). *Babesia capreoli* n. sp. beim Reh (*Capreolus capreolus* L). *Z. Tropenmed. Parasit.*, **13**, 8–20

ERSHOV, V. S. (1956). *Parasitology and Parasitic Diseases of Livestock*. Moscow: State Publishing House for Agricultural Literature. Engl. Ed.: National Science Foundation, Washington, D.C. and Department of Agriculture, U.S.A.

EWING, S. A. (1965). Method of reproduction of *Babesia canis* in erythrocytes. *Am. J. vet. Res.*, **26**, 727–733

EWING, S. A. & BUCKNER, R. G. (1965). Manifestations of babesiosis, ehrlichiosis and combined infections in the dog. *Am. J. vet. Res.*, **26**, 815–828

GARNHAM, P. C. C. (1962). Discussion in *Aspects of Disease Transmission by Ticks*. Symposium No. 6. Zool. Soc. Lond. (Ed. by D. R. ARTHUR). pp. 257–258

GARNHAM, P. C. C. & BRAY, R. S. (1959). The susceptibility to piroplasms. *J. Protozool.*, **6**, 352–355

HALL, W. T. K. (1960). The immunity of calves to *Babesia argentina* infection. *Austral. vet. J.*, **36**, 361–366

HALL, W. T. K. (1963). The immunity of calves to tick-transmitted *Babesia argentina* infection. *Austral. Vet. J.*, **39**, 386–389

HIRATO, K., NINOMIYA, Y., UWANO, Y. & KUTII, T. (1945). Studies on the complement-fixation reaction for equine piroplasmosis. *Jap. J. vet. Sci.*, **7**, 197–205

KEMRON, A., PIPANO, E., HADANI, A. & NEUMAN, M. (1960). Trials with a diamidine compound (M & B 5062A) in the treatment of *Babesiella berbera* in cattle. *Refuah. Vet.*, **17**, 216–226

KOLABSKII, N. A., GAIDUKOV, A. K. & TARVERDYAN, T. N. (1963). Duration of immunity and carriage of piroplasms in animals recovered from piroplasmosis. *Trudy Vsesoyuz Inst. eksp. Vet.*, **28**, 170–176. (Abstr. *Vet. Bull.*, **33**, 674)

KUDO, R. R. (1954). *Protozoology*. 4th Edit. Springfield, Ill. Thomas

KUDO, R. R. (1966). *Protozoology*. 5th Edit. Springfield, Ill. Thomas

LAIRD, M. & LARI, F. A. (1957). The avian blood parasite *Babesia moshkovskii* (Schurenkova, 1938) with a record from *Corvus splendens* Vieillot in Pakistan. *Canad. J. Zool.*, **35**, 783–795

LAWRENCE, D. A. & SHONE, D. K. (1955). Porcine piroplasmosis. *Babesia trautmanni* infection in Southern Rhodesia. *J. S. Afr. vet. med. Ass.*, **26**, 89–93

LEVINE, N. D. (1961). *Protozoan Parasites of Domestic Animals and of Man*. Minneapolis, Minn.: Burgess Publishing

LI, P. N. (1958). Developmental forms of *Babesiella ovis* in the larvae and nymphae of *Rhipicephalus bursa*. *Nauch. Trud. Ukrainsk. Inst. Exp. Vet.*, **24**, 283–287

MAEGRAITH, B. G., GILLES, H. M. & DEKAVUL, K. (1957). Pathological processes in *Babesia canis* Infections. *Z. Tropenmed. Parasit.*, **8**, 485–514

MAHONEY, D. F. (1962). Bovine babesiosis: Diagnosis of infection by a complement fixation test. *Austral. vet. J.*, **38**, 48–52

MALHERBE, W. D. (1956). The manifestations and diagnosis of babesia infections. *Ann. N.Y. Acad. Sci.*, **64**, 128–146

MALHERBE, W. D. & PARKIN, B. S. (1951). A typical symptomatology in *Babesia canis* infection. *J. S. Afr. vet. med. Ass.*, **22**, 25–36

MARKOV, A. A. & ABRAMOV, I. V. (1957). Peculiarities of circulation of *Babesiella ovis* (Babes, 1892) in the tick *Rhipicephalus bursa* Can. et Fanz. 1877. *Veterinariya Moscow*, **34**, 27–30

MURATOV, E. A. & CHEISSIN, E. M. (1959). Development of *Piroplasma bigeminum* in the tick *Boophilus calcaratus*. *Zool. Zh.*, **38**, 970–986

NEITZ, W. O. (1956). Classification, transmission and biology of piroplasms of domestic animals. *Ann. N.Y. Acad. Sci.*, **64**, 56–111

PETROV, V. G. (1941). Development of *Babesiella bovis* in the tick *Ixodes ricinus* L. and a method of investigating the ability of ticks to transmit viruses. *Vestnik. Sel. skokhoz. Nauk. Vet.*, **3**, 136

PIERCE, A. E. (1956). Protozoan diseases transmitted by the cattle tick. *Austral. vet. J.*, **32**, 210–215

PIERCEY, S. E. (1947). Hyper-acute canine babesia (tick fever). *Vet. Rec.*, **59**, 612–613

POLYANSKII, Y. I. & CHEISSIN, E. M. (1959). Some data on development of *Babesiella bovis* in tick-vectors. *Trudy. Karel. Filiala. Akad. Nauk. SSSR*, **14**, 5–13

PUCCINI, V., MUZIO, F. & GIANUBILO, G. (1958). Efficacia del 'Berenil' nella cura della Piroplasmosi suina da *Piroplasma trautmanni* e da *Babesiella perroncitoi*. *Vet. ital.*, **9**, 611–616

PURCHASE, H. S. (1947). Cerebral babesiosis in dogs. *Vet. Rec.*, **59**, 269–270

REGENDANZ, P. & REICHENOW, E. (1933). Die Entwicklung der Piroplasmen. *Z. Bakt. Parasit., Abt. I. Orig.*, **135**, 108–119

REIK, R. F. (1963). Immunity to babesiosis. In *Immunity to Protozoa* (Ed. by P. C. C. GARNHAM, A. E. PIERCE & I. ROITT). Oxford: Blackwell Scientific Publications

REIK, R. F. (1964). The life cycle of *Babesia bigemma* (Smith and Kilborne, 1893) in the tick vector *Boophilus microplus* (Canastrini). *Austral. J. agric. Res.*, **15**, 802–821

RISTIC, M. (1966). The vertebrate developmental cycle of *Babesia* and *Theileria*. In *Biology of Parasites* (Ed. by E. J. L. SOULSBY). New York: Academic Press

RISTIC, M., OPPERMANN, J., SIBINOVIC, S. & PHILLIPS, T. N. (1964). Equine piroplasmosis: A mixed strain of *Piroplasma caballi* and *Piroplasma equi* isolated in Florida and studied by the fluorescent-antibody technique. *Am. J. vet. Res.*, **25**, 15–23

RISTIC, M. & SIBINOVIC, K. H. (1964). Equine babesiosis. Diagnosis by a precipitation in gel and by a one-step fluorescent antibody inhibition test. *Am. J. vet. Res.*, **25**, 1519–1526

ROSENBUSCH, F. (1927). Study of Tristeza (Piroplasmosis): Development of *Piroplasma bigeminum* in the tick (*Boophilus microplus* Can. Lah.). *Rev. Univ. Buenos Aires*, **5**, 863–867

RUDZINSKA, M. A. & TRAGER, W. (1960). The fine structure of *Babesia rodhaini*. *J. Protozool.*, **7** (suppl.) 11

SIBINOVIC, K. H. (1965). Serological Activity and Biologic Properties of a Soluble Antigen of *Babesia caballi*. M. S. Thesis Vet. Sci. University of Illinois. Urbana

SENEVIRATNE, P. (1953). Piroplasmosis of dogs in Ceylon. Preliminary notes on the chemotherapeutic treatment of *B. gibsoni* Infections with paludrine hydrochloride. *Ceylon vet. J.*, **1**, 95–98

SERGENT, E. (1935). Report of the Pasteur Institute for 1934. *Arch. Inst. Pasteur Algér.*, **13** 418–450

SERGENT, E., DONATIEN, A., PARROT, L. & LESTOGUARD, F. (1945). *Etudes sur les piroplasmosis bovines.* Algér: Inst. Pasteur

SHONE, D. K., WELLS, G. E. & WALTER, F. J. A. (1961). The activity of Amicarbalide against *Babesia bigemina*. *Vet. Rec.*, **73**, 736

SHORTT, H. E. (1936). Life-history and morphology of *Babesia canis* in the dog-tick *Rhipicephalus sanguineus*. *Ind. J. med. Res.*, **23**, 885–920

SIMITCH, C. P., NEVENIC, V. & SIBALIC, S. (1956). Le traitement de la piroplasmose ovine et la piroplasmose bovine par 'berenil'. *Acta vet. Belgrad*, **6**, 3–13

SIMITCH, T., TETROVIC, Z. & RAKOVEC, R. (1955). Les espèces de babesiella du boeuf d'Europe. *Archs. Inst. Pasteur Algér*, **33**, 310–314

SIPPEL, W. L., COOPERRIDER, D. E., GAINER, J. H., ALLEN, R. W., MOUW, J. E. B. & TEIGLAND, M. B. (1962). Equine piroplasmosis in the United States. *J. Am. vet. med. Ass.*, **141**, 694–698

SKRABALO, Z. & DEANOVIC, Z. (1957). Piroplasmosis in man. *Documenta Med. geogr. trop.*, **9**, 11–16

SMITH, T. & KILBORNE, F. L. (1893). Investigations into the nature, causation and prevention of Texas or southern cattle fever. *U.S. Dept. Agric. Bur. Ann. Ind. Bull.*, **1**, 1–301

TELLA, A. & MAEGRAITH, B. G. (1965). Physiopathological changes in primary acute blood transmitted malaria and *Babesia* infections. I. Observations on parasites and blood cells in rhesus monkeys, mice, rats and puppies. *Ann. trop. Med. Parasit.*, **59**, 135–146

TSUR TCHERNOMARETZ, I. (1961). Immunization trials against bovine babesiasis. I. Vaccination with blood from latent carriers. *Refuah. Vet.*, **18**, 63–67 (Hebrew Text); 103–110 (English Text).

ZLOTNIK, I. (1953). Cerebral piroplasmosis in cattle. *Vet. Rec.*, **65**, 642–643

HAEMOSPORIDAE (THEILERIDAE)

BARBONI, E. (1942). Multiple brain haemorrhage in cattle with *T. annulata* infection. *Nuova Vet.* **21**, 11–15

BARNETT, S. F. (1963). The biological races of the bovine *Theileria* and their host parasite relationship. In *Immunity to Protozoa* (Ed. by P. C. C. GARNHAM, A. E. PIERCE & I. ROITT). Oxford: Blackwell Scientific Publications

BARNETT, S. F. & BAILEY, K. P. (1958). Immunization against East Coast fever with Aurofac. *East Afr. vet. Res. Organ. Rept.* 1956–1957. p. 47. Nairobi: Government Printer

BARNETT, S. F. & BROCKLESBY, D. E. (1966a). A mild form of East Coast fever (*Theileria parva*) with persistence of infection. *Br. vet. J.*, **112**, 361–370

BARNETT, S. F. & BROCKLESBY, D. W. (1966b). Susceptibility of the African buffalo (*Syncerus caffer*) to infection with *Theileria parva* (Theiler, 1904). *Br. vet. J.*, **112**, 379–386

BARNETT, S. F. & BROCKLESBY, D. W. (1966c). The passage of *Theileria lawrencie* (Kenya) through cattle. *Br. vet. J.*, **112**, 396–409

BITIUKOV, P. A. (1953). Experiments on the transmission of ovine theileriasis and anaplasmosis by the ticks *Ornithodorus lahorensis* and *Haemaphysalis sulcata*. *Trudy Akad. Nauk. Kazahkstan. S. S. R. Inst. Zool.*, **1**, 30–36

BROCKLESBY, D. W. (1962). *Cytauxzoon taurotragi* Martin and Brocklesby, 1960, a piroplasm of the eland (*Taurotragus oryx pattersonianus* Lydekker, 1906). *Res. vet. Sci.*, **3**, 334–344

BROCKLESBY, D. W. & BARNETT, S. F. (1966a). A review of the literature concerning *Theileridae* of the African buffalo (*Syncerus caffer*). *Br. vet. J.*, **112**, 371–378

BROCKLESBY, D. W. & BARNETT, S. F. (1966b). The isolation of *Theileria lawrencei* (Kenya) from a wild buffalo (*Syncerus caffer*) and its passage through captive buffaloes. *Br. vet. J.*, **112**, 387–395

COWDRY, E. V. and HAM, A. W. (1932). Studies on East Coast fever. I. Life cycle of the parasite in ticks. *Parasitology*, **24**, 1–49

DELPY, L. P. J. (1949). Studies in Iran on *Theileria annulata* Dschunkowsky and Luhs, and its natural and experimental transmission. *Bull. Soc. Path. exot.*, **42**, 285–294

GONDER, R. (1910). The life cycle of *Theileria parva:* The cause of East Coast fever of cattle in South Africa. *J. comp. Path.*, **23**, 328–335

GONDER, R. (1911). Die Entwicklung von *Theileria parva*, dem Erreger des Küstenfiebers der Rinder in Afrika. 2. Teil. *Arch. Protistenk.*, **22**, 170–178

HIGNETT, P. G. (1953). *Theileria mutans* detected in British cattle. *Vet. Rec.*, **65**, 893–894

HULLIGER, L., BROWN, C. G. D. & WILDE, J. K. H. (1966). Transition of developmental stages of *Theileria parva* in vitro at high temperature. *Nature (Lond.)*, **211**, 328–329

HULLIGER, L., BROWN, C. G. D. & WILDE, J. K. H. (1965). Theileriosis (*T. parva*) immune mechanism investigated *in vitro*. In *Progress in Protozoology* II. p. 37. International Congress Protozoology. Internat. Conf. Series No. 91. Amsterdam: Exerpta Med. Foundation

HULLIGER, L., WILDE, J. K. H., BROWN, C. G. D. & TURNER, L. (1964). Mode of multiplication of *Theileria* in cultures of bovine lymphocytic cells. *Nature (Lond.)*, **203**, 728–730

KORNIENKO, Z. P. & SHMUIREVA, M. K. (1944). On the possibility of the transmission of Theileria to its own progeny by *Hyalomma turkmeniense* (Olenev, 1931). *Veterinariya, Moscow*, **21**, 24–25

KREIER, J. P., RISTIC, M. & WATRACH, A. M. (1962). *Theileria* sp. in a deer in the United States. *Am. J. vet. Res.*, **23**, 657–662

MARTIN, H. M., BARNETT, S. F. & VIDLER, B. O. (1964). Cyclic development and longevity of *Theileria parva* in the tick *Rhipicephalus appendiculatus*. *Exp. Parasit.*, **15**, 527–533

MARTIN, H. M. & BROCKLESBY, D. W. (1960). A new parasite of the eland. *Vet. Rec.*, **72**, 331–332

NEITZ, W. O. (1953). Aureomycin in *Th. parva* infection. *Nature. Lond.*, **171**, 34–35

NEITZ, W. O. (1956). Classification, transmission and biology of piroplasms of domestic animals. *Ann. N.Y. Acad. Sci.*, **64**, 56–111

NEITZ, W. O. (1959). Theilerioses. *Adv. vet. Sci.*, **5**, 241–247

NEITZ, W. O. (1962). Second meeting FAO/OIE Expert Panel on tick-borne diseases of livestock. p. 34. Cairo 1962

NEITZ, W. O. & JANSEN, B. C. (1956). A discussion on the classification of the Theileridae. *Onderstepoort J. vet. Res.*, **27**, 7–18

RAY, H. (1950). Hereditary transmission of *Theileria annulata* infection in the tick *Hyalomma aegyptium* Neum. *Trans. R. Soc. trop. Med. Hyg.*, **44**, 93–104

REICHENOW, E. (1940). Der Entwicklungsgang des Küstenfieber-regers im Rinde und in der übertragenden Zecke. *Arch. Protistenk*, **94**, 1–56

REIK, R. F. (1966). The Development of *Babesia* spp. and *Theileria* spp. in ticks with special reference to those occurring in cattle. In *The Biology of Parasites* (Ed. by E. J. L. SOULSBY). New York: Academic Press

RICHARDSON, U. F. & KENDALL, S. B. (1963). *Veterinary Protozoology*. 3rd Ed. Edinburgh: Oliver & Boyd

SCHAEFFLER, W. L. (1962). *Theileria cervi* infection in white-tailed deer (*Dama virginiana*) in the United States. Ph.D.Diss. (Diss. Abstr., **23**, 389–391) University of Illinois, Urbana

SPLITTER, E. J. (1950). *Theileria mutans* associated with bovine anaplasmosis in the United States. *J. Amer. med. Ass.*, **117**, 134–135

STURMAN, M. (1959). Tick fever in Israel. *Symposium for Veterinariana*. Rehovah

THEILER, A. (1911). Progress report on the possibility of vaccinating cattle against East Coast fever. *1st Rept. Dir. Vet. Res. Pretoria* 1911. 47–207. Dept. Agric. South Africa

TSUR-TCHERNOMORETZ, I. & ADLER, S. (1965). Growth of lymphoid cells and *Theileria annulata* schizonts from bovine blood during the reaction period. In *Progress in Protozoology* II. Internat. Congr. Protozool. Internat. Conf. Series No. 91, pp. 37–38. Amsterdam: Excerpta Medica Foundation

TSUR-TCHERNOMORETZ, I., DAVIDSON, M. & WEISSENBERG, I. (1960). Two cases of bovine Theileriasis (*Th. annulata*) with cutaneous lesions. *Refuah. Vet.*, **17**, 100–199

HAEMOSPORIDEA (HAEMOPROTEUS, LEUCOCYTOZOON)

AKIBA, S. K. (1960). Studies on the Leucocytozoon found in the chicken in Japan. II. On the transmission of *L. caulleryi* by *Culicoides arakawae*. *Jap. J. vet. Sci.*, **22**, 309–317

ARAGÃO, H. B. (1908). Über den Entwicklungsgang und die Übertragung von *Haemoproteus columbae*. *Arch. Protistenk.*, **12**, 154–167

BAKER, J. R. (1957). A new vector of *Haemoproteus columbae* in England. *J. Protozool.*, **4**, 204–208

BENNETT, G. F. & FALLIS, A. M. (1960). Blood parasites of birds in Algonquin Park, Canada, and a discussion of their transmission. *Canad. J. Zool.*, **38**, 261–273

BIERER, B. W. (1950). Leucocytozoon infection in turkeys. *Vet. Med.*, **45**, 87–88

CHERNIN, E. (1952). The epizootiology of *Leucocytozoon simondi* infections in domestic ducks in northern Michigan. *Am. J. Hyg.*, **56**, 39–57

COATNEY, G. R. (1935). The effect of atebrin and plasmochin on the Haemoproteus infection of the pigeon, *Am. J. Hyg.*, **21**, 249–259

COATNEY, G. R. (1936). A check-list and host-index of the genus Haemoproteus. *J. Parasitol.*, **22**, 88–105

COATNEY, G. R. (1937). A catalog and host-index of the genus Leucocytozoon, *J. Parasit.*, **23**, 202–212

COOK, A. R. (1954). The gametocyte development of *Leucocytozoon simondi*. *Proc. Helminth. Soc. Wash.*, **21**, 1–9

COWAN, Z. B. (1957). Reactions against the megaloschizonts of *Leucocytozoon simondi* Mathis and Leger in ducks. *J. infect. Dis.*, **100**, 82–87

FALLIS, A. M., DAVIES, D. M. & VICKERS, M. A. (1951). Life history of *Leucocytozoon simondi* Mathis and Leger in natural and experimental infections and blood changes produced in the avian host. *Canad. J. Zool.*, **29**, 305–328

FALLIS, A. M. & WOOD, D. M. (1957). Biting midges (Diptera: Ceratopogonidae) as intermediate host for *Haemoproteus* of ducks. *Canad. J. Zool.*, **35**, 425–435

FALLIS, A. M. & BENNETT, G. F. (1958). Transmission of *Leucocytozoon bonasae* Clarke to furred grouse (*Bonasa umbellus L.*) by the black flies *Simulium latipes* Mg. and *Simulium aureum* Fries. *Canad. J. Zool.*, **36**, 533–539

FALLIS, A. M. & BENNETT, G. F. (1960). Description of *Haemoproteus canachites* n. sp. (Sporozoa: Haemoproteidae) and sporogony in Culicoides (Diptera: Ceratopogonidae). *Canad. J. Zool.*, **38**, 455–464

HERMAN, C. M. (1944). The blood protozoa of North American birds. *Bird-Banding*, **15**, 89–112

HERMAN, C. M. (1954). Haemoproteus infections in waterfowl. *Proc. Helminth. Soc. Wash.*, **21**, 37–42

HUFF, C. G. (1942), Schizogony and gametocyte development in *Leucocytozoon simondi* and comparisons with Plasmodium and Haemoproteus. *J. infect. Dis.*, **71**, 18–32

HUFF, C. G. (1963). Experimental research in avian malaria. In *Advances in Parasitology* (Ed. by BEN DAWES), Vol. 1., pp. 1–65. New York & London: Academic Press

LEVINE, N. D. (1954). Leucocytozoon in the avian order Columbriformes with a description of *L. marchouxi* Mathis and Leger 1910 from the mourning dove. *J. Protozool.*, **1**, 140–143

LEVINE, N. D. (1961). *Protozoan Parasites of Domestic Animals and of Man.* Minneapolis, Minn.: Burgess Publishing

LIU, S. K. (1958). The pathology of Leucocytozoon disease in chicks. *Mem. Coll. Agric. Nat. Taiwan Univ.*, **5**, 74–80

RAWLEY, J. (1953). Observations on the maturation of gametocytes of *Leucocytozoon simondi*. *Proc. Helminth. Soc. Wash.*, **20**, 127–128

SAVAGE, A. & ISA, J. M. (1959). Note on the blood of ducks with Leucocytozoon disease. *Canad. J. Zool.*, **37**, 1123–1126

TARSHIS, I. B. (1955). Transmission of *Haemoproteus lophortyz* O'Roke of the California quail by hippoboscid flies of the species *Stilbometropa impressa* (Bigot) and *Lynchia hirsuta* Ferris. *Exp. Parasit.*, **4**, 464–492

TOXOPLASMA

BEVERLEY, J. K. A. & BEATTIE, C. D. (1952). Standardization of the dye test for toxoplasmosis. *J. clin. Path.*, **5**, 350–353

BEVERLEY, J. K. A., BEATTIE, C. P. & ROSEMAN, C. (1954). Human toxoplasma infection. *J. Hyg. Cambridge*, **52**, 37–46

BEVERLEY, J. K. A. (1957). Toxoplasmosis. *Vet. Rec.*, **69**, 591–492

BEVERLEY, J. K. A. (1960). Toxoplasmosis. In *Recent Advances in Clinical Pathology*. Series III. London: Churchill

BEVERLEY, J. K. A. & WATSON, W. A. (1961). Ovine abortion and toxoplasmosis in Yorkshire. *Vet. Rec.*, **73**, 6–10

CAMPBELL, R. S. F. (1956). Canine toxoplasmosis. *Vet. Rec.*, **68**, 591–592

CATHIE, I. A. B. (1957). An appraisal of the diagnostic value of the serologic tests for toxoplasmosis. *Trans. R. Soc. trop. Med. Hyg.*, **51**, 104–110

CHRISTIANSEN, M. (1948). Toxoplasmose Nos Hare i Damark. *Medlemsbl. Danske Dyrlaegeforen*, **31**, 93–104

CHRISTIANSEN, M. & SIIM, J. C. (1951). Toxoplasmosis in hares in Denmark. Serological identity of human and hare strains of Toxoplasma. *Lancet*, **260**, 1201–1203

COOK, M. K. & JACOBS, L. (1958). In vitro investigations on the action of pyrimethamine against *Toxoplasma gondii*. *J. Parasit.*, **44**, 280–288

CROSS, J. B. (1947). A cytologic study of Toxoplasma with special reference to its effect on the host's cell. *J. infect. Diss.*, **80**, 2780296

ERICKSEN, S. & HARBOE, A. (1953). Toxoplasmosis in chickens. I. An epidemic outbreak of toxoplasmosis in a chicken flock in south-eastern Norway. *Acta Path. microbiol. scand.*, **33**, 56–71

EYLES, D. E. (1952). Incidence of *Trypanosoma lewisi* and *Hepatozoon muris* in the Norway rat. *J. Parasit.*, **38**, 222–225

EYLES, D. E. (1956). Newer knowledge of the chemotherapy of toxoplasmosis. *Ann. N.Y. Acad. Sci.*, **64**, 252–267

FARRELL, R. L. (1952). Toxoplasmosis. I. Toxoplasma isolated from swine. *Am. J. vet. Res.*, **13**, 181–185

FRENKEL, J. K. (1948). Dermal hypersensitivity to Toxoplasma antigens (toxoplasmins). *Proc. Soc. exp. Biol. Med.*, **68**, 634–639

FULTON, J. D. (1963) Serological tests in Toxoplasmosis. In *Immunity to Protozoa* (Ed. by P. C. C. GARNHAM, A. E. PIERCE & I. ROITT). Oxford: Blackwell Scientific Publications

GOLDMAN, M. (1957) Staining *Toxoplasma gondii* with fluorescein-labelled antibody. I. The reaction in smears of peritoneal exudate. *J. exp. Med.*, **105**, 549–556

GOLDMAN, M., CALVER, R. K. & SOLZER, A. J. (1958). Reproduction of *Toxoplasma gondii* by internal budding. *J. Parasit.*, **44**, 161–171

HARDING, J. D. J., BEVERLEY, J. K. A., SHAW, I. G., EDWARDS, B. L. & BENNETT, G. H. (1961). Toxoplasma in English pigs. *Vet. Rec.*, **73**, 3–6

HARTLEY, W. J., JEBSON, J. L. & McFARLANE, D. (1954). New Zealand type II abortion in ewes. *Austral. vet. J.*, **30** (7), 216–218

HARTLEY, W. J. & MARSHALL, S. C. (1957). Toxoplasmosis as a cause of ovine perinatal mortality. *N.Z. vet. J.*, **5**, 119–124

HUTCHINSON, W. M. (1965). Experimental transmission of *Toxoplasma gondii*. *Nature*, **206**, 961–962

JACOBS, L. & LUNDE, M. N. (1957). Hemagglutination test for toxoplasmosis. *Science*. **125**, 1035

JACOBS, L., MELTON, M. L. & JONES, F. E. (1952). The prevalence of toxoplasmosis in wild pigeons. *J. Parasit.*, **38**, 457–461

JACOBS, L. (1956). Propagation, morphology and biology of toxoplasmosis. *Ann. N.Y. Acad. Sci.*, **64**, 154–179

KOESTNER, A. & COLE, C. R. (1961). Neuropathology of ovine and bovine toxoplasmosis. *Am. J. vet. Res.*, **22**, 53–66

LAINSON, R. (1955). Toxoplasmosis in England. II. Variation factors in the pathogenesis of Toxoplasma infections; the sudden increase in virulence of a strain after passage in multimammate rats and canaries. *Ann. trop. Med. Parasit.*, **49**, 397–416

LAINSON, R. (1957). Symposium on toxoplasmosis. III. The demonstration of Toxoplasma in animals, with particular reference to members of the Mustelidae. *Trans. R. Soc. trop. Med. Hyg.*, **51**, 111–117

LAINSON, R. (1956). Toxoplasmosis in England. III. Toxoplasmosis infections in dogs: the incidence of complement-fixing antibodies among dogs in London. *Ann. trop. Med. Parasit.*, **50**, 172–186

LEVINE, N. D. (1961). *Protozoan Parasites of Domestic Animals and of Man.* Minneapolis: Burgess Publishing

MAKSTENIEKS, O. & VERLINDE, J. D. (1957). Toxoplasmosis in the Netherlands. Clinical interpretation of parasitological and serological examination and epidemiological relationships between toxoplasmosis in man and animals. *Documenta Med. geogr. trop.*, **9**, 213–224

MILLER, L. T. & FELDMAN, H. A. (1953). Incidence of antibodies for Toxoplasma among various animal species. *J. infect. Dis.*, **92**, 118–120

MELLO, U. (1910). Un cas de toxoplasmose du chien observé à Turin. *Bull. Soc. Path. exot.*, **3**, 359–363

OLAFSON, P. & MONLUX, W. S. (1942). Toxoplasma infection in animals. *Cornell Vet.*, **32**, 176–190

OTTEN, E., WESTPHAL, A. & KAJAHN, E. (1950). Über das Vorkommen von Toxoplasmose beim Hunde; statistische Erhebungen. *Mh. prakt. Tierheilk.*, **2**, 305–308

PERRIN, T., BRIGHAM, C. & KAJAHN, E. (1943). Toxoplasmosis in wild rats. *J. infect. Dis.*, **72**, 91–96

SABIN, A. B. (1949). Complement fixation test in toxoplasmosis and persistence of the antibody in human beings. *Pediatrics, Am. Acad. Pediat.*, **4**, 443–453

SABIN, A. B. & FELDMAN, H. A. (1948). Dyes as microchemical indicators of a new immunity phenomenon affecting a protozoan parasite (Toxoplasma). *Science*, **108**, 660–663

SANGER, V. L., CHAMBERLAIN, D. M., CHAMBERLAIN, R. W., COLE, C. R. & FARREL, R. S. (1953). Toxoplasmosis. V. Isolation of Toxoplasma from Cattle. *J. Am. vet. med. Ass.*, **123**, 87–91

SIIM, J. C., BIERING, SORENSEN, V. & MØLLER, T. (1963). Toxoplasmosis in domestic animals. *Adv. Vet. Sci.*, **8**, 335–429

THALHAMMER, O. (1956). Über ein neues haltbares Antigen für KBR und Hauttest auf Toxoplasmose. *Mschr. Kinderheilk.*, **104**, 110–112

WARREN, J. & SABIN, A. B. (1942). The complement fixation reaction in toxoplasmic infection. *Proc. Soc. exp. Biol. Med.*, **51**, 11–14

WESTPHAL, A. & BAUER, F. (1952). Weitere Untersuchungen und Betrachtungen zur Toxoplasmose-Komplementbindungsreaktion nach Westphal. *Z. Tropenmed. Parasit.*, **3**, 326–339

WICKHAM, N. & CARNE, H. R. (1950). Toxoplasmosis in domestic animals in Australia. *Austral. vet. J.*, **26**, 1–3

ENCEPHALITOZOON

BIOCCA, E. (1949). Osservazioni sulla posizione sistematica del Toxoplasma. *Riv. Parasit. Roma.*, **10**, 73–92

PLOWRIGHT, W. (1952). An encephalitis-nephritis syndrome in the dog probably due to congenital Encephalitozoon infection. *J. comp. Path. Ther.*, **62**, 83–92

PLOWRIGHT, W. & YEOMAN, G. (1952). Probable Encephalitozoon infection of the dog. *Vet. Rec.*, **64**, 381–383

SARCOCYSTIS

LUDVIK, J. (1958). Elektronenoptische Befunde zur Morphologie der Sarcosporidien (*Sarcocystis tenella* Railliet, 1886). *Zbl. Bakt., I. Abt., Orig.*, **172**, 330–350
LUDVIK, J. (1960). The electron microscopy of *Sarcocystis miescheriana* Kuhn, 1865. *J. Protozool.*, **7**, 128–135
LUDVIK, J. (1963). Electron microscopic study of some parasitic protozoa. *Progress in Protozoology* (Ed. by J. LUDVIK, J. LOM & J. VÁVRA). New York: Academic Press
SCOTT, J. W. (1943). Life history of Sarcosporidia, with particular reference to *Sarcocystis tenella*. *Bull.* 259, *Univ. Wyoming Agric. exp. Station*
SPINDLER, L. A. & ZIMMERMAN, H. E. (1945). The biological status of Sarcocystis. *J. Parasit.*, **31**, 13
SPINDLER, L. A., ZIMMERMANN, H. E. & JAQUETTE, D. S. (1946). Transmission of Sarcocystis to swine. *Proc. helminth. Soc. Wash.*, **13**, 1–11
SPINDLER, L. A. (1947). A note on the fungoid nature of certain internal structures of Miescher's sacs (Sarcocystis) from a naturally infected duck. *Proc. helminth. Soc. Wash.*, **14**, 28–30

BESNOITIA

BENNETT, S. C. J. (1933). Globidium infections in the Sudan. *J. comp. Path. Ther.*, **46**, 1–14
BIGALKE, R. D. (1960). Preliminary observations on the mechanical transmission of cyst organisms of *Besnoitia besnoiti* (Marotel, 1912) from a chronically infected bull to rabbits by *Glossina brevipalpis* Newstead, 1910. *J. S. Afr. vet. med. Ass.*, **31**, 37–44
HOFMEYR, C. F. B. (1945). Globidiosis in cattle. *J. S. Afr. vet. med. Ass.*, **16**, 102–109
JELLISON, W. L. (1956). On the nomenclature of *Besnoitia besnoiti*, a protozoan parasite. *Ann. N.Y. Acad. Sci.*, **64**, 268–270
PELLERDY, L. P. (1963). *Coccidia and Coccidiosis*. Budapest: Akademiai Kiado.
POLS, J. W. (1960). Studies on bovine besnoitiosis with special reference to the aetiology. *Onderstepoort J. vet. Res.*, **28**, 265–356

ANAPLASMA

ESPANA, E. & ESPANA, C. (1963). *Anaplasma marginale*. II. Further studies of morphologic features with phase contrast and light microscopy. *Am. J. vet. Res.*, **24**, 713–722
KREIER, J. P. & RISTIC, M. (1963a). Anaplasmosis. X. Morphologic characteristics of the parasites present in the blood of calves infected with the Oregon strain of *Anaplasma marginale*. *Amer. J. vet. Res.*, **24**, 672–676
KREIER, J. P. & RISTIC, M. (1963b). Anaplasmosis. XI. Immunoserologic characteristics of the parasites present in the blood of calves infected with the Oregon strain of *Anaplasma marginale*. *Am. J. vet. Res.*, **24**, 688–696
KREIER, J. P. & RISTIC, M. (1963c). Anaplasmosis. XII. The growth and survival in deer and sheep of the parasites present in the blood of calves infected with the Oregon strain of *Anaplasma marginale*. *Am. J. vet. Res.*, **24**, 697–702
PIERCY, P. L. (1956). Transmission of Anaplasmosis. *Ann. N.Y. Acad. Sci.*, **64**, 40–48
RISTIC, M. & WATRACH, A. (1961). Studies in Anaplasmosis. II. Electron-microscopy of *Anaplasma marginale* in deer. *Am. J. vet. Res.*, **22**, 109–116
RISTIC, M. (1963). Morphology, antigenicity, growth and multiplication of *Anaplasma marginale*. *17th World Vet. Congr. Hannover*, 1963, **1**, 815–819

EPERYTHROZOON

JANSEN, B. C. (1952). The occurrence of *Eperythrozoon parvum* Splitter, 1950 in South African swine. *Onderstepoort J. vet. Res.*, **25**, 5–6
RISTIC, M. (1963). Electron microscopy and serological staining of Anaplasma, Eperythrozoon, Haemobartonella and Theileria. In *Progress in Protozoology* (Ed. by J. LUDVIK, J. LOM & J. VAVRA). Prague: Czechoslovakia Acad. Sci. and New York: Academic Press
SPLITTER, E. J. (1950). Ictero-anaemia of Swine. Proc. 54th Ann. Meeting U.S. Livestock Sanit. Ass. Phoenix 1950. pp. 279–386

BALANTIDIUM

ALMEJEW, C. (1963). Propagation of balantidium in the porcine intestine. *Mh. Vet. Med.*, **18**, 250
BAILEY, W. S. & WILLIAMS, A. G. (1949). Balantidium infection in the dog. *J. Am. vet. med. Ass.*, **114**, 238
CORLISS, J. O. (1961). *The Ciliated Protozoa*. New York: Pergamon Press
LEVINE, N. D. (1961). *Protozoan Parasites of Domestic Animals and of Man*. Minneapolis, Minn.: Burgess Publishing

LUBINSKY, G. (1957). Studies on the evolution of the Ophryoscolecidae (Ciliata: Oligotricha). I. A new species of Entodinium with 'caudatium', 'lobosospino-sum', and 'dubardi' forms, and some evolutionary trends in the genus Entodinium. II. On the origin of the higher Ophryoscolecidae. III. Phylogeny of the Ophyroscolecidae based on their comparative morphology. *Canad. J. Zool.*, **35**, 111–159

TEMPELIS, C. H. & LIPENKO, M. G. (1957). The production of Hyaluronidase by *Balantidium coli. Exp. Parasit.*, **6**, 31–36

TECHNIQUE

Technique

THE COLLECTION AND PRESERVATION OF HELMINTHS

THE collection of parasites from an animal should be carried out as systematically and completely as possible. For this purpose it is wise to follow a definite scheme and examine each organ as it is examined at autopsy, beginning with the outside of the body, then the subcutaneous tissues, the body cavities and so forth.

Filarioid worms found under the skin and in the body cavities and blood vessels are very liable to burst and are best placed immediately in a 10 per cent solution of formalin, without washing in saline, unless they are soiled with blood.

Large nematodes should be collected and washed by shaking in 0·9 per cent saline and immediately dropped into 70 per cent hot alcohol or 5 per cent formal saline, which causes them to be fixed in an extended state. They can be stored in the fixative.

It is difficult to remove nematode larvae or small adult nematodes situated in tissues, but they will often leave the tissues if these are placed into a dish of warm physiological saline. The worms should be removed and fixed as soon as they are free.

Cestodes must be collected with the heads, as these are of great importance for identification. The worms are placed into a dish of warm water at about 40°C, and if their heads are attached to the intestinal wall, a piece of the latter is cut out and also placed in the dish. The worms will die fully extended usually in about an hour, and the heads will be free or may have to be dissected out. The worms are fixed, for permanent preparations, in 5 per cent formal saline, in cold 70 per cent alcohol with 5 per cent glycerin, or equal parts of 70 per cent alcohol, glycerin and distilled water, or Zenker's fluid, drawing large forms a few times over the hand or the edge of the vessel and small ones rapidly through the fluid, in order to get them fully extended. When fixing in Zenker's fluid the worms must be removed after 24 hours and thoroughly washed in running water.

The segments can be stained alive in a freshly made mixture of 97 parts of a saturated solution of carmine in 45 per cent acetic acid and 3 parts of a saturated solution of ferric acetate in glacial acetic acid, staining for 5–30 minutes and then mounting in lactophenol.

Trematodes are treated like cestodes, but if greater extension is required, they should be placed between glass slides pressed together by rubber bands. Trematodes may be cleaned by shaking them in a 1 per cent salt solution or in cold or lukewarm water. Much of their anatomy may be seen before they are fixed. Fix by pouring off the salt solution and adding 10 per cent formalin, replacing this with 3 per cent formalin when the flukes are fixed. Flukes may be fixed in Bouin's, Müller's or Helly's fixative, the corrosive sublimate in the

785

latter two fixatives, being removed with iodine in 70 per cent alcohol in the usual way.

Acanthocephala should be pressed between glass slides, in order to get the proboscis extended, and so fixed in 70 per cent alcohol.

Small worms of all kinds are usually of great importance and should not be missed. After the large worms have been removed the intestine is cut into convenient lengths, and each is vigorously shaken in a dish of warm water, collecting the worms that are liberated.

Faeces containing eggs are fixed by mixing them with an equal quantity of hot 10 per cent formalin. Cold formalin can be used, but the eggs of ascarids may continue to develop in the fixative. The material should be transferred gradually to 70 per cent alcohol if it is to be kept for an indefinite period.

THE COLLECTION AND PRESERVATION OF ARTHROPOD PARASITES

Specimens for dry mounting, such as adult *Diptera*, are killed in a cyanide killing bottle, made by placing into a wide-mouthed bottle a freshly mixed paste of potassium cyanide and plaster of Paris, which is covered with a few layers of blotting paper. Strips of paper are placed into the bottle to prevent the insects from clinging together and damaging their appendages. They are set out on a mounting board in the ordinary way and then pinned down in boxes, the floors of which are covered with a mixture of wax and naphthalin. Some material should also be collected in 70 per cent alcohol for making mounts of important parts.

Dipterous larvae, lice, fleas, mites, etc, are fixed and stored in 70 per cent alcohol or 10 per cent formalin. Care must be exercised not to miss the small parasites, and it may be necessary to make deep skin scrapings of affected areas in order to find them. Fleas should be put in small tubes containing 70–80 per cent alcohol, which will preserve them indefinitely. A drop of glycerin may be added if they are to be preserved for a long time. Formalin should not be used for fleas.

Ticks can be preserved in their natural colours by dropping them alive into a carefully made solution of chloroform in 10 per cent formalin. The formalin should be made up with distilled water. Chloroform is added in slight excess; the mixture is shaken and left for a few minutes to settle, and then the solution is poured off into a bottle with a well-fitting glass stopper. The live ticks are dropped in and the bottle is left well closed for about a month.

THE MAKING OF PERMANENT PREPARATIONS

Canada balsam is an excellent mounting medium, but requires careful preparation of the material by passing it through increasing concentrations of alcohol to draw out all water, during which shrinkage, especially of nematodes, is difficult to avoid. Glycerin gelatin is simpler, but also frequently causes shrinkage. It is very useful for eggs and small nematodes that tend to become too transparent in other media.

For all unstained material, such as nematodes, tapeworm heads, Acanthocephala and arthropods, a suitable medium is the following mixture: gum arabic 60, glycerin 40, chloral hydrate 100, distilled water 100, and thymol 1. The specimens are transferred from 70 per cent alcohol into 50 per cent glycerin and then mounted in the gum arabic medium. For small insects and mites Berlese's fluid is useful. It is made by dissolving 15 g. gum arabic in 20 ml. distilled water and adding 10 ml. glucose syrup and 5 ml. acetic acid, the whole being then saturated with chloral hydrate (up to 100 g.). This should set in 1–2 weeks and the slide may then be ringed. Keilin's medium is valuable for dipterous larvae and small insects. Its formula is: gum acacia 30 g.; cocaine hydrochloride 0·5 g.; glycerin 20 ml.; distilled water 50 ml. Mites may also be mounted in a jelly made of 20 parts gelatin, 100 parts glycerin, 120 parts carbolic acid and 2 parts distilled water, the slide being ringed after mounting.

Arthropod material, such as heads of flies, whole fleas etc., must first be boiled in 10 per cent potassium hydroxide solution to remove the soft internal parts, and it may be necessary to puncture the body for this purpose. The material is then washed in water and transferred to 70 per cent alcohol etc.

While nematodes are usually examined in lactophenol, into which they can be placed from 70 per cent alcohol, cestodes and trematodes have to be stained so that the internal organs can be seen, and the preparation is mounted in balsam in the ordinary way. Various stains are employed, *e.g.* Delafield's haematoxylin, Ehrlich's acid haematoxylin, paracarmine, acid alum carmine, lithium carmine and haemalum with 2 per cent acetic acid. It is usually advisable to dilute the stain considerably with distilled water and to stain for a prolonged period, rather than to use the concentrated stain. The specimens should be slightly overstained and differentiated in a 0·1 per cent acid alcohol or alum solution.

CLINICAL DIAGNOSTIC METHODS

1. EXAMINATION OF THE OUTSIDE OF THE BODY

The body is searched for external parasites or their eggs (bots, oxyurids), not only on the surface but also in the ears and in the conjunctival sac (eye-worms), and the skin should be palpated to determine the presence of sub-cutaneous larvae. If mange-like lesions are present, the hair round the affected area should be clipped and scrapings made with a scalpel, the blade being held at such an angle that the material scraped away falls onto a piece of card or paper or a microscope slide held underneath. A little oil on the blade used will cause the material to adhere to the blade, so that it is not lost. Scraping should continue until a little blood appears, especially when sarcoptic mange is suspected. The lesion should then be dressed and the material examined for the presence of mites or of fragments of them. Some material may be examined directly, either in water or saline or in clove oil. If it is too dense for direct examination, it should be brought just to the boil in 10 per cent caustic soda or caustic potash to break it up. It may then be examined in the hydroxide used, but it is better to centrifuge it lightly and examine the sediment. It may be possible to find mites in the external auditory canal by rotating a cotton-wool swab in this canal. A little oil on the swab will help to capture the mites. Examination with an electrically-illuminated auriscope may be useful.

2. EXAMINATION OF ALL EXCRETIONS

Excretions of the body may be carriers of parasite eggs or larvae. The nasal discharge and the sputum may, therefore, aid in the diagnosis of parasites in the air-passages, the vomit may bear evidence of parasites in the stomach, and the urine may contain eggs which can be concentrated by centrifuging. The faeces are by far the most important, as the eggs or larvae of all gastro-intestinal parasites and many others leave the body in this vehicle. It should be remembered, however, that no eggs may be found if the worms are still immature or if only males are present. In some cases abnormally shaped eggs may be found.

Faeces are examined in the first place for ripe segments of tapeworms and the student should be familiar with their appearance, otherwise he may be at a loss to recognise these bodies. If a tapeworm infection is suspected, a purgative may be given to cause the expulsion of segments in case they are not readily found.

Birds that have caeca, as the fowl e.g., pass two kinds of faeces, those from the small intestine being relatively coarse and loose with particles of varying colour, while those from the caeca are of a fine, pasty nature with a homogeneous brown or brownish-green colour. The eggs of small-intestinal worms will be found in both types of faeces, while those of caecal worms are found only in the caecal faeces.

Egg Counts. For the counting of the number of eggs in faeces there are various methods. The following are a few simple ones:

(a) *The Direct Smear.* A small quantity of faeces is placed on a slide, mixed with a drop of water, spread out and examined directly. At least three slides from different parts of the faecal sample should be examined. This method is suitable for a very rapid examination, but will usually fail to detect low-grade infections.

(b) *Concentration Methods.* The purpose of these methods is to detect light infections as well as others, and to save time by concentrating the eggs in a small volume and by eliminating the trouble caused by large faecal particles. Advantage is taken of the low specific gravity of most helminth eggs to separate them from the faeces, as described below. Many different methods have been suggested, but it is considered that, for the purposes of the veterinary student or practitioner, the selection of a few simple methods for regular use is more important than an exposition of all known methods.

In the *Willis technique* about 1 ml. of the mixed specimen is diluted with 10–20 ml. of concentrated salt solution in a suitable narrow cylinder, which is filled to the top with the liquid. A clean slide or cover glass is slid sideways over the top of the cylinder so that it is in contact with the liquid, care being taken that there are no air bubbles between the slide or cover glass and the salt solution. After about 30–45 minutes the slide or cover glass is quickly removed and examined under a low power of the microscope. This method is not suitable for eggs of trematodes and most cestodes, but shows the majority of nematode eggs in the sample. Sugar solution ($\frac{3}{4}$ lb. to 1 pint of water) may be used instead of salt solution, one advantage of it being that it is sticky so that the eggs are less likely to be washed off the slide or cover glass when it is removed.

By *centrifugal flotation* methods more time is saved and greater accuracy obtained. A fair sample, if possible 15–30 ml. of stirred faeces, is well mixed with about 500 ml. water and strained through a sieve of 1 mm. mesh, or better a set of sieves with mesh ranging from 3 mm. to 0·25 mm. The mixture is left to sediment for 10–15 minutes, and the supernatant fluid then poured off until the sediment is about to flow out. If the supernatant fluid still contains debris, sedimentation should be repeated until it is clear. The sediment is then shaken up and a sample is poured into a centrifuge tube and mixed with an equal volume of glycerin. After centrifuging at about 1000 revolutions for 1–2 minutes, the eggs will be floating at the top. They are removed by touching the surface with the end of a squarely cut glass rod and transferred to a slide for examination. Instead of glycerin, a concentrated solution of sugar ($\frac{3}{4}$ lb. sugar to 1 pint of water), or a saturated salt solution can be used. Zinc sulphate and other substances of high specific gravity are also used, but some of them bring up so much debris with the eggs that the eggs may be obscured. Methods of this type may not show eggs of trematodes, but these can be found if a heavy waterglass solution is used instead of glycerin. If schistosome eggs are expected, the faeces sample should first be fixed in formalin or spirit before mixing with water, to prevent the eggs from hatching.

The faeces may also contain larvae—for instance, those of lungworms. Such larvae will be found by the flotation methods used for detecting the presence of eggs. A simpler method for sheep faeces is to place a few pellets in a Petri dish containing a small quantity of water, when the larvae will rapidly leave the pellets and can be found in the water. In the case of soft faeces the material is spread out in a Petri dish and several small holes are made by means of a glass rod going down to the bottom. The holes are filled with water and the larvae migrate into them from the surrounding faeces.

The eggs of some worms can be recognized by their shape and size, and the student should become familiar with eggs that may be found in the faeces of the different species of domestic animals, as well as with different objects that occur in faeces and may be mistaken for eggs or larvae, as, for instance, pollen grains, plant cells or hairs, fungus spores and cysts of Protozoa. The eggs commonly found are shown in Plates XXXII–XXXVIII and the infective larvae of some nematodes of sheep on p. 807.

(c) *Egg-counting Techniques.* To obtain more accurate information with regard to the severity of an infection, egg-counting methods, by means of which the number of eggs per gramme of faeces can be determined, have been devised. All these methods, however, involve so many unavoidable sources of error that the results given by them must be regarded as being approximate only.

Stoll's Dilution Method for counting nematode eggs uses 3 g. of faeces weighed into a test-tube graduated to 45 ml. The tube is then filled to the 45 ml. mark with decinormal caustic soda solution and 10 or 12 glass beads are added. The tube is then closed with a rubber stopper and is shaken to give a homogeneous suspension of the faecal material. If much froth appears the tube can be left till it disappears. As soon as possible after shaking, 0·15 ml. of the well mixed suspension is drawn off with a pipette graduated to show this amount, and placed on a slide. The total number of eggs in the 0·15 ml. sample is then counted and this number, multiplied by 100, gives the number of eggs in 1 gramme of faeces. Coarse material, such as horse faeces, can be sieved to remove fibres which may block the pipette. For field work a heavy flask graduated at 56 and 60 ml. may be used. The flask is filled to the 56 ml. mark with decinormal caustic soda solution and faeces are added till the fluid reaches the 60 ml. mark. The 0·15 ml. is withdrawn and the number of eggs in it is multiplied by 100 to give the number of eggs per gramme of faeces. This method gives reliable counts of trematode as well as nematode eggs.

In the *McMaster egg-counting technique* the eggs are floated up in a counting chamber which dispenses with the need for a graduated pipette. The counting chamber is made of two glass slides, separated by three or four narrow, transversely placed strips of glass 1·5 mm. thick, so that two or three spaces of 1·5 mm. depth are obtained between the two slides. On the upper slide an area of 1 cm.² is ruled over each space. The volume underneath this ruled area will therefore be 0·15 ml. From the faeces 2 g. are weighed off and soaked in 30 ml. water until they are sufficiently soft. To this is added 30 ml. saturated salt solution and some steel ball bearings. After thorough shaking a sample is withdrawn by means of a wide (8 mm.) pipette and run into the counting chamber, filling all the spaces. The eggs rise to the top, so that they are all in focus against the upper slide. The number of eggs within each ruled area, multiplied by 200, represents the number per gramme in the original sample. Several counts are made and the mean taken. A simplified method is to weigh 2 g. faeces into a mortar, grind up in 10 ml. water and add 50 ml. saturated salt solution, taking enough of this, while it is being stirred, to fill the counting chambers. When large numbers of samples are being counted electrically-operated stirrers may be used.

Trematode Eggs. These are often heavier than the eggs of other helminths and the methods just described may fail to detect them all. This may be especially important when only a few eggs are present, as, for example, in light infections, or when anthelmintics have been administered.

For counting the eggs of *Fasciola hepatica* the following methods are available:

For Sheep Faeces. 10 g. of the faeces are weighed into an Erlenmeyer flask, calibrated to the 300 ml. mark and partially filled with 0·4 N sodium hydroxide solution. The flask is stoppered and allowed to stand overnight. Next morning it is vigorously shaken to break up the faeces and it is then filled to the 300 ml. mark with 0·4 sodium hydroxide solution and is again shaken. Immediately after this shaking 7·5 ml. of the mixture in the flask is transferred to a 15 ml. centrifuge tube and is centrifuged. The supernatant fluid is then drawn off and replaced by saturated NaCl solution with a specific gravity of 1·2. This also is centrifuged and the supernatant fluid is drawn off. Centrifugation is continued with repeated changes of sodium chloride solution until the supernatant fluid is clear. The final sediment is then passed through an 80-mesh screen into a counting chamber made by marking a 70 mm. diameter Petri dish with parallel lines 3 mm. apart. The eggs in this are then counted under a dissecting microscope. Since the 7·5 ml. sample contains 0·25 g. of faeces, the number of eggs counted is multiplied by 4 to give the number of eggs per gramme.

For Cattle Faeces a similar method is used, except that 30 g. of cattle faeces are taken and 5 ml. samples are taken for centrifugation. Since these contain 0·5 g. of faeces, the number of eggs counted in the final sediment is multiplied by 2 to give the number of eggs per gramme.

Factors Influencing Egg Counts. It is obvious that all egg counts will be influenced by the consistency of the faeces, wet faeces being much heavier than a drier specimen, and further by the total amount of faeces passed per day, because in dry faeces the eggs are concentrated in a smaller output of faeces. The first source of error may be corrected by taking 2 g. of normal, formed faeces, 2·5 g. of soft faeces, 3 g. of a medium soft stool not formed into pellets, 5 g. of a pultaceous stool, and 7 g. of a watery stool. Because egg counts vary widely both in individual animals and at different times of the day and for other reasons, one egg count is not of much value. Several should be done on different days, and the average of these taken. The interpretations of the results obtained requires considerable experience. The following figures may be taken as a guide, but clinical signs and other circumstances should also be taken into account:

Nematodes. (*i*) Equines; 500 eggs per gramme, mild infection; 800–1000 moderate; 1500–2000 severe. (*ii*) Lambs; much depends on the species of worm present, but 2000–6000 eggs per gramme indicates a severe infestation, and treatment is advisable when 1000 eggs per gramme or more are found; (iii) cattle; 300–600 eggs per gramme indicates the advisability of treatment. *Trematodes.* The presence of 100–200 eggs of *Fasciola hepatica* per gramme of faeces of cattle, or 300–600 eggs per gramme of faeces of sheep, indicate an infection likely to be pathogenic.

More satisfactory results are obtained if the count per gramme is multiplied by the total weight of the faeces passed in 24 hours, so that the total egg output per day is obtained. If this is done for 3 consecutive days, the average obtained is a very fair measure of the infection, and can be used for accurate experimental work—for instance, the testing of anthelmintics. It is important, however, to remember that the egg production of the female worms of different species is influenced by various factors. These include the immunity of the host, the age of the parasites, the consistency of the faeces, diet etc.

(d) *Faeces Cultures.* Because a specific diagnosis cannot always be made from the eggs, it may be necessary to cultivate the larvae from those eggs that hatch in the free state. For this purpose the faeces are broken up and placed in a glass jar, which is closed and kept at a temperature of about 26°C for a suitable time, usually 7 days. The faeces must be neither too dry nor too wet; the consistency of normal sheep and horse faeces is the correct one. If they are too dry, the faeces are moistened with water; if too wet, sterilised and dried sheep faeces are added or a good grade of animal charcoal can be used instead. After incubation the jar is placed in a dull light and many species of larvae will migrate up the walls of the jar, from which they can be removed by means of a needle or soft brush for examination in a drop of water on a slide. It is advisable to kill the larvae by heating carefully over a small flame until movement ceases and the worms lie fully extended.

Larvae that do not migrate can be separated by means of the Baermann technique as follows: a glass funnel 20 cm. wide at the top and closed at the bottom with a clamped piece of rubber tubing is fixed in a stand and a circular piece of wire gauze, about 9 cm. in diameter, is placed in the funnel and on it a larger piece of linen. The incubated faeces are spread 2 cm. deep on the linen, and water at 40°C is poured down the side of the funnel until it covers the faeces. The apparatus is left for a few hours, when the larvae will be found in a few ml. of water drawn off at the bottom. This method was devised for the separation of larvae from soil and is very useful for that purpose as well.

Another culture method which gives good results, for instance with dog faeces, is to mix equal parts of faeces and charcoal, placing the mixture in a Petri dish and in the lid of the dish a piece of moist blotting paper. The larvae will later be found on the paper.

Counts of Immature and Mature Worms. These may be required for the estimation of the effects of anthelmintics, or to estimate, for other reasons, the number of helminths present in the alimentary tract. In general the procedure is to ligature off the various parts of the alimentary canal and to pass their contents through a series of graded screens to remove solid debris. The worms can then be picked out of the clarified fluid remaining and can be identified and counted. If necessary the contents of portions of the alimentary canal can be preserved in formalin and dealt with when time is available. The mucosa of the alimentary tract may be digested with acid pepsin (10 g. pepsin, 30 ml. HCl, 1000 ml. of water) at 37°C for several hours. The material is then sieved through a mesh of 200 apertures to the linear inch, which retains the immature worms. These are preserved in 5 per cent formal saline.

3. BLOOD EXAMINATION FOR LARVAE

The larvae of most filarial worms are found in the blood, and the diagnosis of filariasis has to be made by finding them. Several methods may be employed:

(a) A drop of fresh blood is placed on a slide, covered with a cover-slip and examined immediately. The microfilariae will be seen moving about. This method can be carried out as a preliminary, but is not suitable for a specific determination. A few slides examined in this way will show whether larvae are present and, since the larvae of some species occur in the blood at night and others during the day, it is necessary to carry out the examination at the correct time.

(b) If the larvae are abundant, a thin smear can be made; if they are rare, a thick film is made and this gives better results in the majority of cases. The films are completely air-dried as quickly as possible and the thick film is then placed into a vessel of distilled water in a slanting position and facing downwards, until it has been completely dehaemoglobinised. It is then air-dried again, fixed in methyl alcohol for ten minutes and then stained (see also details of special techniques for *Dirofilaria*).

(c) When the microfilariae are rare, several ml. of blood are placed in a centrifuge tube and 5 per cent acetic acid is added to produce haemolysis. When this is complete, the mixture is centrifuged and the larvae are removed from the bottom by means of a pipette.

DIAGNOSTIC METHODS IN PROTOZOOLOGY

FAECES OR INTESTINAL CONTENTS

Where motile organisms are to be searched for (*e.g. Hexamita, Trichomonas* etc.), material should be examined as soon as possible since the organisms lose their motility in cold material. The preparation should be kept warm until examination and a simple smear is made, mixing the specimen with warm saline. Direct examination is useful for the detection of motile organisms, and the use of a phase contrast or dark field microscope greatly facilitates this.

With less delicate forms (e.g. cysts of *Entamoeba, Balantidium, Coccidia*, etc.), concentration can be employed, the faeces being passed through a screen to remove course debris and then repeatedly sedimented or concentrated by the flotation technique described for helminth eggs. The sample from the concentration may be stained to facilitate examination. Thus, an aqueous solution of eosin (1 per cent) stains faecal debris a bright red, but living protozoa and cysts fail to stain and are recognized as colourless bodies in the sample. An aqueous solution of iodine (1 per cent) is useful to facilitate detection of protozoal cysts.

Where it is necessary to sporulate oocysts for accurate identification, these may be obtained by concentration techniques (e.g. the top layer of a salt or sugar flotation is washed in water and the oocysts collected by sedimentation or light centrifugation), or, if oocysts are numerous in a faecal sample, the sample may be used in an unconcentrated form. For sporulation the material is mixed with an excess of 2 per cent potassium dichromate solution and poured into Petri dishes; the depth of fluid should not exceed half an inch. The dishes are then incubated at room temperature or 27°C for the appropriate time.

Intestinal contents or faeces may need to be stained for more accurate identification of intestinal protozoa. Cover glass preparations are the most suitable, and these should be coated with albumen fixative to facilitate adherence of faeces etc. to the glass. A thin layer of faeces or intestinal contents is spread on the cover glass, and this is fixed before it is allowed to dry. The most satisfactory fixative is Schaudinn's fluid (saturated solution of mercuric chloride, two parts; absolute alcohol, 1 part; glacial acetate acid, few drops), and cover glasses should be gently dropped into this or floated on it, smear down, and left for about 10 to 15 minutes. Fixed smears are then washed in 70 per cent alcohol and can be stored in this. It is useful to add a little iodine (to give a port wine colour) to remove excess mercuric chloride. Smears are most satisfactorily stained with Heidenheim's iron haematoxylin. For best results, overnight staining should be used (e.g. stain overnight in a mixture of one part 3 per cent iron alum in distilled water to 9 parts 50 per cent alcohol: wash in 70 per cent alcohol: stain overnight in 1 part haematoxylin and 9 parts 70 per cent alcohol: differentiate in dilute iron alum: wash in 70 per cent alcohol: dehydrate, mount); however, for rapid diagnostic purposes 2 per cent iron alum in distilled water for one hour, 0·1 per cent aqueous haematoxylin for 2 hours and destaining with either saturated aqueous picric acid or iron alum can be used to produce an adequate preparation.

Other staining methods include Mayer's acid haemalum and Mallory's phosphomolybdic-acid haematoxylin. A quick diagnosis may often be made if the smear is fixed in absolute methanol and stained with Giemsa, though this stain is not recommended for faecal smears when the finer structures of intestinal protozoa are to be examined.

BLOOD OR TISSUE FLUIDS

Wet blood smears can be examined for living trypanosomes, the search for organisms being greatly facilitated by phase contrast or dark field illumination.

Blood smears should be stained by one of the Romanowsky stains (methylene blue–eosin combination). Where organisms are plentiful, a thin blood smear is satisfactory and allows a more satisfactory examination. Slides should be absolutely clean, and the blood smear should be spread evenly and thinly. Thick blood smears allow more blood cells to be examined but require more care in interpretation. Thick blood smears cannot be used with avian or camel blood because of the nucleated erythrocytes. Thick blood smears need to be dehaemoglobinized before staining, and this may be done by placing them in distilled water until the colour has disappeared. Thin smears or dehaemoglobinized smears are fixed in absolute methanol and may then be stained by Leishman, Giemsa, Wright's or Field's stain. Wright's stain is the most useful for quick staining, but added detail is produced if smears are stained overnight in dilute Giemsa. For best results it is important to adjust the pH of the stain to pH 7·2 for mammalian blood and pH 6·7 for avian blood.

TISSUES

Usually, the most satisfactory method of examination of tissues is for sections to be cut and stained with haematoxylin and eosin, Giemsa or other appropriate stain. Frozen sections provide a rapid means of examination. A diagnosis may often be made by mixing a scraping, or a small sample, of the tissue with a little saline and examining the preparation in the fresh state (e.g. schizonts of coccidia, toxoplasma, pseudocysts, sarcosporidia etc.). Such preparations may also be stained to achieve a more critical examination.

CULTURAL TECHNIQUES

A variety of these exist for the isolation of protozoa (e.g. for trichomonads, amoebae, leishmaniae etc.). References to these may be found in the appropriate section dealing with the parasite and information is also available in Levine (1961) and Richardson & Kendall (1963).

IMMUNODIAGNOSTIC TECHNIQUES

Several serological and other techniques (e.g. complement fixation, haemagglutination, fluorescent antibody, skin tests) are in use for the detection of various protozoal infections (e.g. trichomoniasis, leishmaniasis, toxoplasmosis etc.). Further details of these may be obtained from the references quoted in the appropriate section dealing with the parasite.

REFERENCES

LEVINE, N. D. (1961). *Protozoan Parasites of Domestic Animals and of Man.* Minneapolis, Minn.: Burgess Publishing
RICHARDSON, U. F. & KENDALL, S. B. (1963). *Veterinary Protozoology.* Edinburgh and London: Oliver & Boyd

Host Parasite List

THIS list includes only the parasites mentioned in this volume and it is therefore not complete. Occasional parasites and temporary parasites, such as the blood sucking Diptera, are not included. Ticks are listed only under those hosts which are the most important or to which they transmit diseases. *In all cases the main text should be consulted to ascertain the full extent of the host range of a parasite.*

MAN

DIGESTIVE TRACT

Trematodes
  Opisthorchis sinensis
  Fasciolopsis buski
  Echinostoma revolutum
  Heterophyes heterophyes
  Metagonimus yokogawi
  Nanophyetus schikhobalowi
  Gastrodiscoides hominis

Cestodes
  Diphyllobothrium latum
  Mesocestoides spp.
  Dipylidium caninum
  Taenia solium
  Taenia saginata
  Hymenolepis nana

Nematodes
  Ascaris lumbricoides
  Strongyloides stercoralis
  Trichinella spiralis
  Trichuris trichiura
  Ancylostoma caninum
  Ancylostoma braziliense
  Ancylostoma duodenale
  Necator americanus
  Trichostrongylus colubriformis
  Trichostrongylus vitrinus
  Trichostrongylus probolurus
  Trichostrongylus axei
  Mecistocirrus digitatus

Protozoa
  Chilomastix mesnili
  Giardia lamblia
  Trichomonas hominis
  Entamoeba coli
  Entamoeba histolytica
  Endolimax nana
  Iodamoeba bütschlii
  Balantidium coli

LIVER

Trematodes
  Dicrocoelium dendriticum

Opisthorchis tenuicollis
Pseudamphistomum truncatum
Fasciola hepatica
Schistosoma spp.

Cestodes
  Hydatid cyst

Nematodes
  Toxocara spp. (larvae)

CIRCULATORY SYSTEM

Trematodes
  Schistosoma mansoni
  Schistosoma japonicum
  Schistosoma haematobium
  Schistosoma bovis
  Schistosoma mattheei

Nematodes
  Dirofilaria immitis
  Dipetalonema perstans
  Dipetalonema streptocerca
  Mansonella ozzardi
  Brugia malayi
  Wuchereria bancrofti
  Toxocara spp. (larvae)

Protozoa
  Trypanosoma gambiense
  Trypanosoma rhodesiense
  Trypanosoma cruzi
  Toxoplasma gondii (rarely)
  Babesia spp.
  Plasmodium vivax
  Plasmodium falciparum
  Plasmodium ovale
  Plasmodium malariae
  Leishmania donovani

RESPIRATORY SYSTEM

Trematodes
  Paragonimus westermanii

Cestodes
  Hydatid cyst

Nematodes
 Metastrongylus apri
Protozoa
 Toxoplasma gondii

URINARY SYSTEM
Nematodes
 Dioctophyma renale

SKIN AND SUBCUTANEOUS TISSUE
Cestodes
 Sparganum mansoni
Nematodes
 Dracunculus medinensis
 Gnathostoma spinigerum
Arthropods
 Limnatis africana
 Gastrophilis intestinalis (larva)
 Hypoderma bovis (larva)
 Hypoderma lineata (larva)
 Dermatobia hominis (larva)
 Callitroga hominivorax (larva)
 Cordylobia anthropophaga (larva)
 Pulex irritans
 Ceratophyllus gallinae
 Pediculus humanus
 Phthirus pubis
 Argas persicus
 Otobius megnini
 Ornithodoros moubata
 Haemaphysalis leporispalustris

Ixodes spp.
Dermacentor spp.
Sarcoptes scabiei
Ornithonyssus bacoti
Ornithonyssus sylviarum
Ornithonyssus bursa
Trombicula spp.
Demodex folliculorum

MUSCLES, TENDONS, ETC
Cestodes
 Cysticercus cellulosae
Nematodes
 Trichinella spiralis
Protozoa
 Sarcocystis lindemanni

EYE
Nematodes
 Thelazia callipaeda
 Toxocara spp. (larvae)
Arthropods
 Oestrus ovis (larvae)
Protozoa
 Toxoplasma gondii

CENTRAL NERVOUS SYSTEM
Cestodes
 Cysticercus cellulosae
 Hydatid cyst

HORSE, MULE AND DONKEY

DIGESTIVE TRACT
Trematodes
 Gastrodiscus aegyptiacus
 Gastrodiscus secundus
 Pseudodiscus collinsi

Cestodes
 Anoplocephala magna
 Anoplocephala perfoliata
 Paranoplocephala mamillana

Nematodes
 Parascaris equorum
 Habronema muscae
 Habronema microstoma
 Habronema megastoma
 Gongylonema pulchrum
 Strongyloides westeri
 Strongylus equinus
 Strongylus edentatus
 Strongylus vulgaris
 Triodontophorus spp.
 Oesophagodontus robustus
 Craterostomum spp.
 Gyalocephalus capitatus
 Poteriostomum spp.
 Trichonema spp.
 Trichostrongylus axei
 Probstmayria vivipara
 Oxyuris equi

Arthropods
 Gastrophilus intestinalis (larva)
 Gastrophilus inermis (larva)

Gastrophilus nasalis (larva)
Gastrophilus pecorum (larva)
Gastrophilus haemorrhoidalis (larva)

Protozoa
 Tritrichomonas equi
 Trichomonas equibuccalis
 Giardia equi
 Entamoeba equi
 Entamoeba equibuccalis
 Entamoeba gedoelsti
 Eimeria leuckarti
 Eimeria solipedum
 Eimeria uniungulati

LIVER
Trematodes
 Dicrocoelium dendriticum
 Fasciola gigantica
 Fasciola hepatica
 Fascioloides magna

Cestodes
 Cysticercus tenuicollis
 Hydatid cyst

CIRCULATORY SYSTEM
Trematodes
 Schistosoma bovis
 Schistosoma indicum

EGGS OF WORM PARASITES

PLATE XXXII

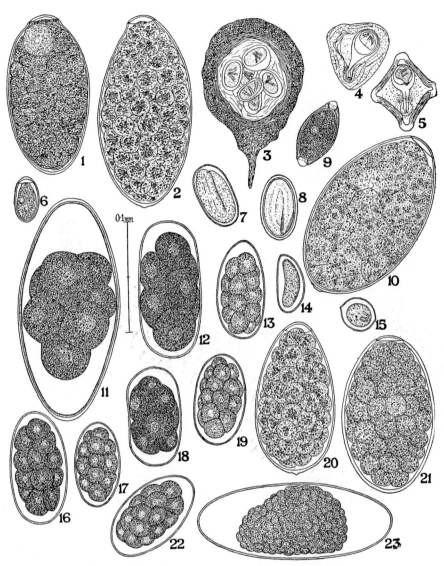

EGGS OF WORM PARASITES OF THE SHEEP. (ORIGINAL)

1, *Fasciola hepatica;* 2, *Paramphistomum cervi;* 3, *Thysaniezia giardi;* 4, *Moniezia expansa;* 5, *Moniezia benedeni;* 6, *Dicrocoelium dendriticum;* 7, *Strongyloides papillosus;* 8, *Gongylonema pulchrum;* 9, *Trichuris globulosa;* 10, *Fasciola gigantica;* 11, *Nematodirus spathiger;* 12, *Gaigeria pachyscelis;* 13, *Trichostrongylus* spp.; 14, *Skrjabinema ovis;* 15, *Avitellina centripunctata;* 16, *Chabertia ovina;* 17, *Haemonchus contortus;* 18, *Bunostomum trigonocephalum;* 19, *Oesophagostomum columbianum;* 20, *Cotylophoron cotylophorum;* 21, *Fascioloides magna;* 22, *Ostertagia circumcincta;* 23, *Marshallagia marshalli.*

PLATE XXXIII

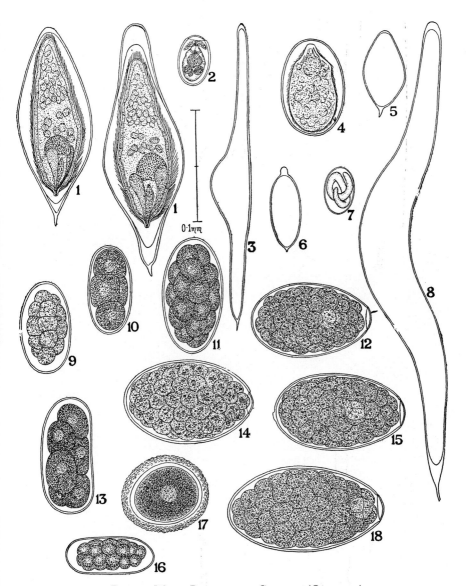

EGGS OF WORM PARASITES OF CATTLE. (ORIGINAL)

1, *Schistosoma bovis*; 2, *Eurytrema pancreaticum*; 3, *Schistosoma spindalis*; 4, *Schistosoma japonicum*; 5, *Schistosoma indicum*; 6, *Ornithobilharzia turkestanicum*; 7, *Thelazia rhodesii*; 8, *Schistosoma nasalis*; 9, *Oesophagostomum radiatum*; 10, *Syngamus laryngeus*; 11, *Mecistocirrus digitatus*; 12, *Fischoederius cobboldi*; 13, *Bunostomum phlebotomum*; 14, *Carmyerius spatiosus*; 15, *Gastrothylax crumenifer*; 16, *Cooperia pectinita*; 17, *Ascaris vitulorum*; 18, *Fischoederius elongatus*.

PLATE XXXIV

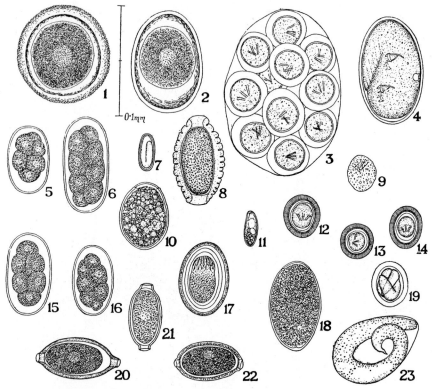

0.1mm

EGGS OF WORM PARASITES OF THE DOG AND FOX. (ORIGINAL)

1, *Toxocara canis*; 2, *Toxascaris leonina*; 3, *Dipylidium caninum*; 4, *Linguatula serrata*; 5, *Ancylostoma caninum*; 6, *Ancylostoma braziliense*; 7 *Spirocerca lupi*; 8, *Dioctophyma renale*; 9, *Mesocestoides lineatus*; 10, *Diphyllobothrium latum*; 11, *Euryhelmis squamula*; 12, *Echinococcus granulosus*; 13, *Taenia hydatigena*; 14, *Taenia ovis*; 15, *Uncinaria stenocephala*; 16, *Necator americanus*; 17, *Oncicola canis*; 18, *Troglotrema salmincolo*; 19, *Physaloptera canis*; 20, *Trichuris vulpis*; 21, *Capillaria plica*; 22, *Capillaria aerophila*; 23, *Filaroides osleri*.

PLATE XXXV

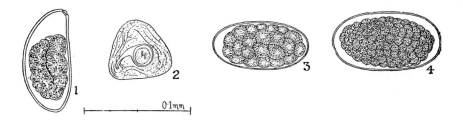

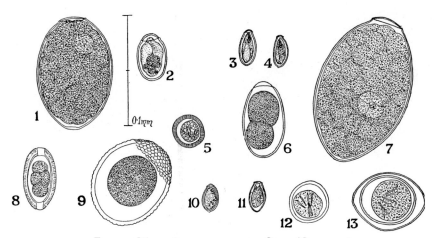

EGGS OF WORM PARASITES OF THE CAT. (ORIGINAL)

1, *Echinochasmus perfoliatus;* 2, *Platynosomum concinnum;* 3, *Opisthorchis sinensis;* 4, *Opisthorchis tenuicollis;* 5, *Taenia taeniaeformis;* 6, *Gnathostoma spinigerum;* 7, *Euparyphium melis;* 8, *Capillaria hepatica;* 9, *Toxocara mystax;* 10, *Heterophyes heterophyes;* 11, *Metagonimus yokogawai;* 12, *Diplopylidium zschokkei;* 13, *Joyeuxiella furhmanni.*

PLATE XXXVI

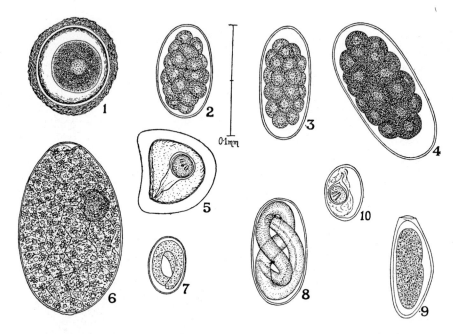

EGGS OF WORM PARASITES OF EQUINES. (ORIGINAL)

1, *Ascaris equorum;* 2, *Strongylus* spp.; 3, *Trichomena* spp.; 4, *Triodontophorus tenuicollis;* 5, *Anoplocephala* spp.; 6, *Gastrodiscus aegyptiacus;* 7, *Strongyloides westeri;* 8, *Dictyocaulus arnfieldi;* 9, *Oxyuris equi;* 10, *Paranoplocephala mamillana.*

PLATE XXXVII

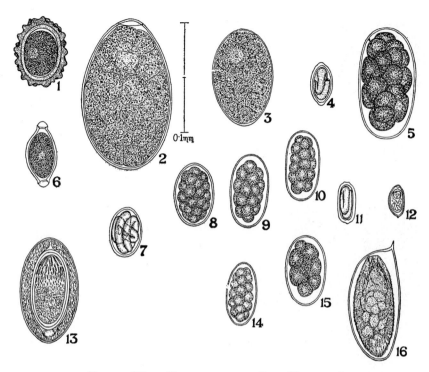

EGGS OF WORM PARASITES OF THE PIG. (ORIGINAL)

1, *Ascaris lumbricoides;* 2, *Fasciolopsis buski;* 3, *Paragonimus westermanii;* 4, *Ascarops strongylina;* 5, *Stephanurus dentatus;* 6, *Trichuris trichiura;* 7, *Metastrongylus apri;* 8, *Bourgelatia diducta;* 9, *Oesophagostomum dentatum;* 10, *Hyostrongylus rubidus;* 11, *Physocephalus sexalatus;* 12, *Brachylaemus suis;* 13, *Macracanthorhynchus hirudinaceus;* 14, *Globocephalus connorfilii;* 15, *Necator* sp.; 16, *Schistosoma suis.*

PLATE XXXVIII

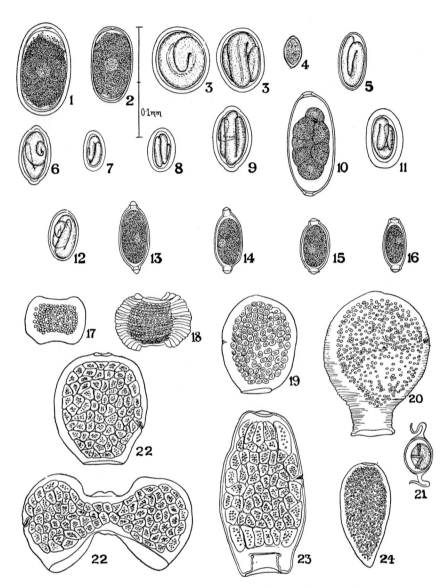

0·1mm

EGGS OF WORM PARASITES OF THE FOWL. (ORIGINAL)

1, *Ascaridia galli;* 2, *Heterakis galliae;* 3, *Subulura brumpti;* 4, *Prosthogonimus* sp.; 5, *Strongyloides avium;* 6, *Tetrameres americana;* 7, *Acuaria spiralis;* 8, *Acuaria hamulosa;* 9, *Gongylonema ingluvicola;* 10, *Syngamus trachea;* 11, *Hartertia gallinarum;* 12, *Oxyspirura mansoni;* 13, *Capillaria annulata;* 14, *Capillaria retusa;* 15, *Capillaria columbae;* 16, *Capillaria longicollis.* Ripe segments of tapeworms (not drawn to scale); 17, *Amaebotaenia sphenoides;* 18, *Hymenolepis carioca;* 19, *Raillietina cesticillus;* 20, *Choanotaenia infundibulum;* 21, single egg of *C. infundibulum;* 22, *Raillietina echinobothrida;* 23, *Raillietina tetragona;* 24, *Davainea proglottina.*

Schistosoma japonicum
Ornithobilharzia turkestanicum

Nematodes
 Elaeophora böhmi
 Strongylus vulgaris (larvae)

Protozoa
 Babesia caballi
 Babesia equi
 Trypanosoma brucei
 Trypanosoma congolense
 Trypanosoma dimorphon
 Trypanosoma equinum
 Trypanosoma equiperdum
 Trypanosoma evansi
 Trypanosoma vivax

UROGENITAL SYSTEM

Nematodes
 Dioctophyma renale

Protozoa
 Trypanosoma equiperdum

RESPIRATORY SYSTEM

Trematodes
 Schistosoma nasalis

Cestodes
 Hydatid cyst

Nematodes
 Dictyocaulus arnfieldi
 Habronema spp. (larvae)

SKIN AND SUBCUTANEOUS TISSUES

Nematodes
 Dracuncutus medinensis
 Habronema spp. (larvae)
 Parafilaria multipapillosa

Arthropods
 Hypoderma bovis (larva)
 Hypoderma lineata (larva)
 Callitroga hominivorax (larva)
 Chrysomyia bezziana (larva)
 Hippobosca equina
 Hippobosca maculata
 Hippobosca rufipes
 Damalinia equi
 Haematopinus asini
 Otobius megnini
 Ixodes ricinus
 Ixodes canisuga
 Ixodes pacificus
 Ixodes cookei

Ixodes scapularis
Boophilus annulatus
Boophilus decoloratus
Boophilus microplus
Margaropus winthemi
Rhipicephalus appendiculatus
Rhipicephalus evertsi
Rhipicephalus bursa
Dermacentor albipictus
Dermacentor nigrolineatus
Dermacentor venustus
Dermacentor nitens
Dermacentor occidentalis
Dermacentor reticulatus
Amblyomma hebraeum
Amblyomma americanus
Amblyomma cajennense
Amblyomma imitator
Amblyomma maculatum
Sarcoptes scabiei
Psoroptes communis equi
Chorioptes equi
Trombicula spp.

Protozoa
 Besnoitia bennetti

MUSCLES, TENDONS ETC

Nematodes
 Onchocerca cervicalis
 Onchocerca reticulata

Protozoa
 Sarcocystis bertrami

EYE

Nematodes
 Thelazia lacrymalis
 Setaria equina (microfilariae)

CENTRAL NERVOUS SYSTEM

Cestodes
 Hydatid cyst
 Coenurus cerebralis

Nematodes
 Setaria digitata

SEROUS CAVITIES

Cestodes
 Cysticercus tenuicollis

Nematodes
 Setaria equina

SHEEP, GOAT AND DEER

DIGESTIVE TRACT

Trematodes
 Cymbiforma indica
 Skrjabinotrema ovis
 Paramphistomum cervi
 Paramphistomum ichikawai
 Paramphistomum microbothaium
 Paramphistomum orthocoelium
 Cotylophoron cotylophorum
 Calicophoron calicophorum
 Ceylonocotyle streptocoelium
 Gastrothylax crumenifer
 Platynosomum ariestis

Cestodes
 Moniezia expansa
 Moniezia benedeni
 Avitellina spp.
 Stilesia globipunctata
 Thysanosoma actinioides
 Thysaniezia giardi

Nematodes
 Gongylonema pulchrum
 Gongylonema verrucosum
 Gongylonema mönnigi
 Gaigeria pachyscelis

27

Haemonchus similis
Haemonchus contortus
Haemonchus placei
Mecistocirrus digitatus
Marshallagia marshalli
Trichostrongylus axei
Trichostrongylus colubriformis
Trichostrongylus falculatus
Trichostrongylus vitrinus
Trichostrongylus capricola
Trichostrongylus probolurus
Trichostrongylus rugatus
Trichostrongylus longispicularis
Trichostrongylus drepanoformis
Ostertagia ostertagi
Ostertagia circumcincta
Ostertagia trifurcata
Ostertagia lyrata
Ostertagia mentulata
Ostertagia occidentalis
Teladorsagia davtiani
Cooperia curticei
Cooperia punctata
Cooperia pectinata
Cooperia oncophora
Nematodirus spathiger
Nematodirus battus
Nematodirus helvetianus
Nematodirus abnormalis
Nematodirus rufaevastitatis
Oesophagostomum columbianum
Oesophagostomum venulosum
Chabertia ovina
Bunostomum trigonocephalum
Skrjabinema ovis
Skrjabinema alata
Strongyloides papillosus
Trichuris ovis
Trichuris globulosa
Capillaria longipes

Protozoa
  Trichomonas ovis
  Giardia caprae
  Entamoeba ovis
  Eimeria ahsata
  Eimeria arkhari
  Eimeria arloingi
  Eimeria christenseni
  Eimeria crandallis
  Eimeria faurei
  Eimeria gilruthi
  Eimeria granulosa
  Eimeria intricata
  Eimeria ninakohlyakimovae
  Eimeria pallida
  Eimeria parva
  Eimeria punctata

LIVER

Trematodes
  Dicrocoelium dendriticum
  Eurytrema pancreaticum
  Fasciola hepatica
  Fasciola gigantica
  Fascioloides magna
  Cymbiforma indica
  Parafasciolopsis fasciolaemorpha

Cestodes
  Stilesia hepatica

Thysanosoma actinioides
Cysticercus tenuicollis
Hydatid cyst

CIRCULATORY SYSTEM

Trematodes
  Schistosoma mattheei
  Schistosoma bovis
  Schistosoma spindalis
  Schistosoma indicum
  Ornithobilharzia turkestanicum

Nematodes
  Elaeophora schneideri
  Parelaphostrongylus odocoilei

Protozoa
  Trypanosoma brucei
  Trypanosoma congolense
  Trypanosoma dimorphon
  Trypanosoma evansi
  Babesia motasi
  Babesia ovis
  Babesia foliata
  Babesia taylori
  Trypanosoma melophagium
  Trypanosoma uniforme
  Trypanosoma vivax
  Theileria hirci
  Theileria ovis
  Theileria cervi
  Anaplasma ovis
  Eperythrozoon ovis
  Toxoplasma gondii

RESPIRATORY TRACT

Trematodes
  Schistosoma nasalis
  Paragonimus westermannii
  Paragonimus kellicotti

Cestodes
  Hydatid cyst

Nematodes
  Syngamus nasicola
  Dictyocaulus filaria
  Protostrongylus rufescens
  Cystocaulus nigrescens
  Muellerius capillaris
  Bicaulus schulzi
  Bicaulus sagittatus
  Neostrongylus linearis

Arthropods
  Oestrus ovis (larvae)

Protozoa
  Toxoplasma gondii

SKIN AND SUBCUTANEOUS TISSUE

Nematodes
  Elaeophora schneideri (microfilariae)
  Wehrdikmansia cervipedis
  Wehrdikmansia rugosicauda
  Wehrdikmansia flexuosa

Arthropods
  Hypoderma aeratum
  Hypoderma crossi
  Hypoderma diana
  Hypoderma silenus
  Oedemagena tarandi

Dermatobia hominis (larva)
Lucilia sericata (larva)
Lucilia cuprina (larva)
Calliphora albifrontalis (larva)
Calliphora augur (larva)
Calliphora erythrocephala (larva)
Calliphora fallax (larva)
Calliphora stygia (larva)
Calliphora vomitoria (larva)
Microcalliphora varipes (larva)
Callitroga hominivorax (larva)
Chrysomyia chloropyga (larva)
Chrysomyia albiceps (larva)
Chrysomyia rufifacies (larva)
Chrysomyia micropogon (larva)
Melophagus ovinus
Damalinia ovis
Linognathus ovillus
Linognathus africanus
Linognathus pedalis
Otobius megnini
Ornithodoros moubata
Ixodes ricinus
Ixodes pilosus
Ixodes rubicundus
Ixodes pacificus
Ixodes persulcatus
Ixodes scapularis
Haemaphysalis cinnabarina punctata
Haemaphysalis leporispalustris
Boophilus decoloratus
Rhipicephalus appendiculatus
Rhipicephalus evertsi
Rhipicephalus sanguineus
Dermacentor venustus
Dermacentor variabilis
Dermacentor nitens
Dermacentor occidentalis

Amblyomma hebraeum
Amblyomma variegatum
Amblyomma americanum
Amblyomma cajennense
Amblyomma maculatum
Sarcoptes scabiei
Chorioptes ovis
Psoroptes communis ovis
Psorergates ovis
Trombicula spp.

MUSCLES AND TENDONS

Cestodes
Cysticercus ovis

Nematodes
Elaphostrongylus cervi

Protozoa
Sarcocystis tenella

EYE

Nematodes
Thelazia rhodesii
Thelazia californiensis

CENTRAL NERVOUS SYSTEM

Cestodes
Coenurus cerebralis

Nematodes
Elaphostrongylus panticola
Elaphostrongylus rangiferi
Odocoileostrongylus tenuis
Setaria digitata (immature)

Protozoa
Toxoplasma gondii

BOVINE (Including Zebu)

DIGESTIVE TRACT

Trematodes
Paramphistomum cervi
Paramphistomum scotiae
Paramphistomum hiberniae
Paramphistomum ichikawi
Paramphistomum gotoi
Paramphistomum liorchis
Paramphistomum microbothridoides
Paramphistomum orthocoelium
Calicophoron calicophorum
Cotylophoron cotylophorum
Gastrothylax crumenifer
Fischoederius cobboldi
Fischoederius elongatus
Carmyerius spatiosus
Carmyerius gregarius
Ceylonocotyle streptocoelium
Cymbiforma indica

Cestodes
Moniezia expansa
Moniezia benedeni
Avitellina spp.
Thysanosoma actinioides
Thysaniezia giardi

Nematodes
Gongylonema pulchrum
Gongylonema verrucosum
Mecistocirrus digitatus
Haemonchus contortus
Haemonchus placei
Haemonchus similis
Trichostrongylus axei
Trichostrongylus colubriformis
Trichostrongylus longispicularis
Ostertagia ostertagi
Ostertagia lyrata
Cooperia punctata
Cooperia pectinata
Cooperia oncophora
Cooperia mcmasteri
Nematodirus battus
Nematodirus filicollis
Nematodirus helvetianus
Nematodirus spathiger
Neoascaris vitulorum
Agriostomum vryburgi
Bunostomum phlebotomum
Strongyloides papillosus
Trichuris ovis
Trichuris globulosa
Oesophagostomum radiatum
Chabertia ovina
Macracanthorhychus hirudinaceus

Protozoa
  Giardia bovis
  Entamoeba bovis
  Tritrichomonas enteris
  Eimeria alabamensis
  Eimeria auburnensis
  Eimeria bovis
  Eimeria braziliensis
  Eimeria bukidnonensis
  Eimeria canadensis
  Eimeria cylindrica
  Eimeria ellipsoidalis
  Eimeria mundaragi
  Eimeria pellita
  Eimeria subspherica
  Eimeria wyomingensis
  Eimeria zürnii

LIVER

Trematodes
  Dicrocoelium dendriticum
  Dicrocoelium hospes
  Eurytrema pancreaticum
  Eurytrema coelomaticum
  Fasciola hepatica
  Fasciola gigantica
  Fascioloides magna
  Gigantocotyle explanatum

Cestodes
  Hydatid cyst
  Cysticercus tenuicollis
  Stilesia hepatica
  Thysanosoma actinioides

CIRCULATORY SYSTEM

Trematodes
  Schistosoma japonicum
  Schistosoma bovis
  Schistosoma mattheei
  Schistosoma spindalis
  Schistosoma indicum
  Ornithobilharzia turkestanicum
  Ornithobilharzia bomfordi

Nematodes
  Elaeophora poeli
  Dipetalonema evansi (Camel)
  Onchocerca armillata

Protozoa
  Trypanosoma brucei
  Trypanosoma congolense
  Trypanosoma dimorphon
  Trypanosoma evansi
  Trypanosoma theileri
  Trypanosoma uniforme
  Trypanosoma vivax
  Babesia argentina
  Babesia berbera
  Babesia bigemina
  Babesia bovis
  Babesia divergens
  Babesia major
  Theileria annulata
  Theileria mutans
  Theileria lawrenci
  Theileria parva
  Toxoplasma gondii
  Anaplasma marginale
  Anaplasma centrale
  Eperythrozoon wenyoni

UROGENITAL SYSTEM

Nematodes
  Stephanurus dentatus
  Dioctophyma renale
Protozoa
  Tritrichomonas foetus

RESPIRATORY SYSTEM

Trematodes
  Fasciola hepatica
  Schistosoma nasalis

Cestodes
  Hydatid cyst

Nematodes
  Dictyocaulus viviparus
  Syngamus laryngeus
  Syngamus nasicola

Protozoa
  Toxoplasma gondii

SKIN AND SUBCUTANEOUS TISSUE

Nematodes
  Stephanofilaria dedoesi
  Stephanofilaria stilesi
  Stephanofilaria kaeli
  Stephanofilaria assamensis
  Parafilaria bovicola
  Dracunculus medinensis

Arthropods
  Hypoderma bovis (larva)
  Hypoderma lineata (larva)
  Dermatobia hominis (larva)
  Chrysomyia bezziana (larva)
  Callitroga hominovorax (larva)
  Lyperosia exigua
  Lyperosia irritans
  Lyperosia minuta
  Haematobia irritans
  Haematobia stimulans
  Hippobosca equina
  Hippobosca maculata
  Hippobosca rufipes
  Damalinia bovis
  Haematopinus eurysternus
  Linognathus vituli
  Solenopotes capillatus
  Otobius megnini
  Ixodes ricinus
  Ixodes pilosus
  Ixodes rubicundus
  Ixodes cookei
  Ixodes pacificus
  Ixodes persulcatus
  Ixodes scapularis
  Boophilus annulatus
  Boophilus decoloratus
  Boophilus microplus
  Boophilus calcaratus
  Margaropus winthem
  Hyalomma mauritanicum
  Rhipicephalus appendiculatus
  Rhipicephalus capensis
  Rhipicephalus sanguinens
  Rhipicephalus simus
  Rhipicephalus evertsi
  Haemaphysalis cinnabarina punctata
  Dermacentor albipictus

Dermacentor nitens
Dermacentor occidentalis
Dermacentor variabilis
Dermacentor venustus
Amblyomma americanum
Amblyomma cajennense
Amblyomma imitator
Amblyomma hebraeum
Amblyomma variegatum
Sarcoptes scabiei
Psoroptes communis bovis
Psoroptes natalensis
Chorioptes bovis
Psorergates bos
Trombicula spp.
Demodex bovis
Raillietia auris

Protozoa
Besnoitia besnoiti

MUSCLES AND TENDONS

Cestodes
Cysticercus bovis

DIGESTIVE TRACT

Trematodes
Fasciolopsis buski
Echinochasmus perfoliatus
Gastrodiscoides hominis
Gastrodiscus aegyptiacus
Brachylaemus suis
Metagonimus yokogawai

Cestodes
Diphyllobothrium latum

Nematodes
Ascaris suum
Ascarops strongylina
Ascarops dentata
Physocephalus sexalatus
Simondsia paradoxa
Gongylonema pulchrum
Gnathostoma hispidum
Strongyloides westeri
Strongyloides ransomi
Trichinella spiralis
Trichuris suis
Bourgelatia diducta
Oesophagostomum dendatum
Oesophagostomum brevicaudum
Oesophagostomum longicaudum
Oesophagostomum georgianum
Ancylostoma duodenale
Necator suillus
Globocephalus urosubulatus
Globocephalus longimucronatus
Trichostrongylus colubriformis
Trichostrongylus axei
Hyostrongylus rubidus
Ollulanus tricuspis
Mecistocirrus digitatus
Macracanthorhynchus hirudinaceus

Arthropods
Gastrophilus haemorrhoidalis (larva)
Gastrophilus intestinalis (larva)

Nematodes
Onchocerca gibsoni
Onchocerca gutturosa

Protozoa
Sarcocystis fusiformis

EYE

Nematodes
Thelazia rhodesii
Thelazia gulosa
Thelazia alfortensis
Thelazia skrjabini
Setaria spp. (immature)

CENTRAL NERVOUS SYSTEM

Cestodes
Coenurus cerebralis

Protozoa
Toxoplasma gondii

SEROUS CAVITIES

Nematodes
Setaria labiato-papillosa
Setaria digitata

PIG

Protozoa
Chilomastix mesnili
Giardia lamblia
Tritrichomonas buttreyi
Tritrichomonas suis
Tritrichomonas rotunda
Entamoeba suis
Iodamoeba bütschlii
Eimeria debleicki
Eimeria perminuta
Eimeria polita
Eimeria scabra
Eimeria scrofae
Eimeria spinosa
Isospora suis
Isospora almaataensis
Balantidium coli

LIVER

Trematodes
Dicrocoelium dendriticum
Opisthorchis tenuicollis
Opisthorchis sinensis
Fasciola hepatica
Eurytrema pancreatum (pancreas)

Cestodes
Cysticercus tenuicollis
Hydatid cyst

Nematodes
Ascaris suum (Aberrant)

CIRCULATORY SYSTEM

Trematodes
Schistosoma japonicum
Schistosoma suis

Protozoa
Trypanosoma brucei
Trypanosoma congolense
Trypanosoma cruzi

Trypanosoma dimorphon
Trypanosoma evansi
Trypanosoma simiae
Trypanosoma suis
Babesia perroncitoi
Babesia trantmanni
Toxoplasma gondii
Eperythrozoon parvum
Eperythrozoon suis

UROGENITAL SYSTEM
Nematodes
Stephanurus dentatus
Dioctophyma renale

RESPIRATORY SYSTEM
Trematodes
Paragonimus westermannii
Paragonimus kellicotti

Cestodes
Hydatid cyst

Nematodes
Metastrongylus apri
Metastrongylus pudendotectus
Metastrongylus salmi

SKIN AND SUBCUTANEOUS TISSUES
Nematodes
Suifilaria suis
Arthropods
Callitroga hominivorax
Cuterebra spp.
Haematopinus suis
Boophilus decoloratus
Amblyomma americanum
Amblyomma maculatum
Dermacentor nitens
Dermacentor variabilis
Dermacentor venustus
Ixodes scapularis
Sarcoptes scabiei
Demodex phylloides

MUSCLES AND TENDONS
Cestodes
Cysticercus cellulosae
Sparagana
Nematodes
Trichinella spiralis
Protozoa
Sarcocystis miescheriana

SEROUS CAVITIES
Nematodes
Setaria congolensis

DOG, CAT AND FOX

DIGESTIVE TRACT
Trematodes
Alaria alata
Alaria canis
Alaria americana
Alaria michiganensis
Alaria mustelae
Apophallus mühlingi
Cryptocotyle lingua
Cryptocotyle concava
Cryptocotyle jejuna
Echinochasmus perfoliatus
Euparyphium melis
Euparyphium ilocanum
Euryhelmis squam,ıla
Metagonimus yokogawai
Heterophyes heterophyes
Rossicotrema donicum
Nanophyetus salmincola

Cestodes
Spirometra mansoni
Spirometra mansonoides
Spirometra erinacei
Diphyllobothrium latum
Mesocestoides lineatus
Dipylidium caninum
Taenia hydatigena
Taenia pisiformis
Taenia ovis
Taenia krabbei
Taenia multiceps
Taenia gaigeri
Taenia serialis
Echinococcus granulosus
Hydatigera taeniaeformis

Joyeuxiella spp.
Diplopylidium spp.
Nematodes
Toxascaris leonina
Toxocara canis
Toxocara cati
Strongyloides stercoralis
Strongyloides cati
Ancylostoma caninum
Ancylostoma tubaeforme
Ancylostoma braziliense
Uncinaria stenocephala
Necator americanus
Trichinella spiralis
Trichuris vulpis
Physaloptera praeputialis
Physaloptera canis
Physaloptera felidis
Gnathostoma spinigerum
Ollulanus tricuspis
Spirocerca lupi
Spirocerca artica
Onicola canis
Soboliphyme baturini

Protozoa
Giardia canis
Giardia felis
Trichomonas canistomae
Trichomonas felistomae
Entamoeba histolytica
Eimeria canis
Eimeria felina
Eimeria cati
Isospora canis
Isospora bigeminia

Isospora rivolta
Isospora felis
Toxoplasma gondii

LIVER

Trematodes
  Dicrocoelium dendriticum
  Opisthorchis tenuicollis
  Opisthorchis sinensis
  Pseudamphistomum truncatum
  Fasciola hepatica
  Fasciolopsis buski
  Platynosomum fastosum
  Eurytrema procyonis
  Metorchis albidus
  Metorchis conjunctus
  Parametorchis complexus

Protozoa
  Hepatozoon canis
  Leishmania donovani

CIRCULATORY SYSTEM

Trematodes
  Schistosoma japonicum
  Schistosoma rhodhaini
  Schistosoma spindale
  Ornithobilharzia turkestanicum

Nematodes
  Dirofilaria immitis
  Brugia patei
  Brugia pahangi
  Gurltia paralysans

Protozoa
  Trypanosoma brucei
  Trypanosoma congolense
  Trypanosoma cruzi
  Trypanosoma dimorphon
  Trypanosoma evansi
  Trypanosoma rangeli
  Leishmania donovani
  Babesia canis
  Babesia felis
  Babesia gibsoni
  Babesia vogeli
  Eperythrozoon felis
  Haemobartonella canis
  Haemobartonella felis

UROGENITAL SYSTEM

Nematodes
  Dioctophyma renale
  Capillaria plica

RESPIRATORY SYSTEM

Trematodes
  Paragonimus westermanni
  Paragonimus kellicotti
  Troglotrema acutum

Nematodes
  Aelurostrongylus abstrusus
  Angiostrongylus vasorum
  Filaroides osleri
  Filaroides milski
  Anafilaroides rostratus
  Broncostrongylus subcrenatus
  Vogeloides massinoi
  Metathelazia spp.
  Skrjabingylus nasicola

Capillaria aerophila
Crenosoma vulpis

Arthropods
  Pneumonyssus caninum
  Linguatula serrata

Protozoa
  Toxoplasma gondii

SKIN AND SUBCUTANEOUS TISSUE

Nematodes
  Rhabditis strongyloides
  Dirofilaria repens
  Dipetalonema reconditum
  Dipetalonema grassi
  Dracunculus medinensis
  Dracunculus insignis

Arthropods
  Dermatobia hominis (larva)
  Cordylobia arthropophaga (larva)
  Trichodectes canis
  Felicola subrostratus
  Heterodoxus spiniger
  Heterodoxus longitarsus
  Linognathus setosus
  Ctenocephalides canis
  Ctenocephalides felis felis
  Echidnophaga gallinacea
  Otobius megnini
  Amblyomma americanum
  Amblyomma cajennense
  Amblyomma maculatum
  Ixodes ricinus
  Ixodes holocyclus
  Ixodes hexagonus
  Ixodes canisuga
  Ixodes cookei
  Ixodes kingi
  Ixodes muris
  Ixodes pacificus
  Ixodes rubicundus
  Ixodes persulcatus
  Ixodes scapularis
  Boophilus decoloratus
  Rhipicephalus simus
  Rhipicephalus sanguineus
  Rhipicephalus bursa
  Haemaphysalis leachi
  Haemaphysalis bispinosum
  Haemaphysalis leporispalustris
  Dermacentor variabilis
  Dermacentor reticulatus
  Dermacentor venustus
  Sarcoptes scabiei
  Otodectes cynotis
  Demodex canis
  Cheyletiella parasitivorax
  Trombicula spp.
  Ornithonyssus bacoti

MUSCLES, TENDONS ETC

Nematodes
  Trichinella spiralis

EYE

Nematodes
  Thelazia californiensis
  Thelazia callipaeda

CENTRAL NERVOUS SYSTEM

Protozoa
Toxoplasma gondii
Encephalitozoon cuniculi

SEROUS CAVITIES

Nematodes
Dipetalonema dracunculoides

FOWL

DIGESTIVE TRACT

Trematodes
Echinostoma revolutum
Echinoparyphium recurvatum
Hypoderaeum conoideum
Plagiorchis arcuatus
Notocotylus attenuatus
Catatropis verrucosa
Brachylaemus commutatus
Prosthogonimus pellucidus

Cestodes
Davainea proglottina
Raillietina tetragona
Raillietina echinobothrida
Raillietina cesticillus
Cotugnia digonopora
Amoebotaenia sphenoides
Choanotaenia infundibulum
Metroliasthes lucida
Hymenolepis carioca
Fimbriaria fasciolaris

Nematodes
Heterakis gallinarum
Heterakis brevispiculum
Heterakis putaustralis
Heterakis indica
Ascaridia galli
Subulura brumpti
Subulura differens
Strongyloides avium
Capillaria caudinflata
Capillaria obsignata
Capillaria contorta
Capillaria anatis
Trichostrongylus tenuis
Hartertia gallinarum
Gongylonema ingluvicola
Gongylonema crami
Acuaria hamulosa
Acuaria spiralis
Tetrameres americana
Tetrameres fissispina
Physaloptera truncata
Polymorphus boschadis

Protozoa
Histomonas meleagridis
Chilomastix gallinarum
Trichomonas gallinae
Trichomonas gallinarum
Tritrichomonas eberthi
Eimeria acervulina
Eimeria brunetti
Eimeria hagani
Eimeria maxima
Eimeria mivati
Eimeria mitis
Eimeria necatrix
Eimeria praecox
Eimeria tenella
Wenyonella gallinae
Cryptosporidium tyzzeri

LIVER

Protozoa
Histomonas meleagridis

CIRCULATORY SYSTEM

Protozoa
Leucocytozoon caulleryi
Plasmodium gallinaceum
Plasmodium juxtanucleare
Aegyptianella pullorum
Aegyptianella moshkovskii

UROGENITAL SYSTEM

Trematodes
Prosthogonimus pellucidus
Prosthogonimus ovatus
Prosthogonimus macrorchis

RESPIRATORY SYSTEM

Trematodes
Typhlocoelum cymbium

Nematodes
Syngamus trachea

Arthropods
Cytodites nudus

SKIN AND SUBCUTANEOUS TISSUE

Trematodes
Collyriclum faba

Cestodes
Dithyridium variabile

Arthropods
Callitroga hominivorax
Menopon gallinae
Menacanthus stramineus
Cuclotogaster heterographus
Lipeurus caponis
Goniocotes gallinae
Goniodes gigas
Goniodes dissimilis
Ceratophyllus gallinae
Echidnophaga gallinacea
Argas persicus
Amblyomma americanum
Haemaphysalis cinnabarina
Haemaphysalis leporispalustris
Amblyomma hebraeum
Cnemidocoptes gallinae
Cnemidocoptes mutans
Epidermoptes bilobatus
Epidermoptes bifurcata
Mégninia cubitalis
Pterolichus obtusus
Laminosioptes cysticola
Dermanyssus gallinae
Ornithonyssus bursa
Ornithonyssus bacoti
Ornithonyssus sylviarum

Neoschöngastia americana
Trombicula spp.

MUSCLES AND TENDONS

Protozoa
Sarcocystis rileyi

EYE

Nematodes
Oxyspirura mansoni
Oxyspirura parvovum

TURKEY

DIGESTIVE TRACT

Trematodes
Brachylaemus commutatus
Plagiorchis megalorchis

Cestodes
Raillietina cesticillus
Choanotaenia infundibulum
Metroliasthes lucida

Nematodes
Heterakis gallinarum
Ascaridia galli
Subulura brumpti
Strongyloides avium
Capillaria obsignata
Capillaria contorta
Trichostrongylus tenuis
Acuaria hamulosa
Acuaria spiralis
Tetrameres americana
Tetrameres fissispina

Protozoa
Chilomastix gallinarum
Hexamita meleagridis
Histomenas meleagridis
Histomenas wenrichi
Trichomonas gallinae
Trichomonas gallinarum
Cryptosporidium meleagridis
Eimeria adenoeides
Eimeria dispersa
Eimeria gallopavonis
Eimeria innocua
Eimeria meleagridis
Eimeria meleagrimitis
Eimeria subrotunda

LIVER

Protozoa
Histomonas meleagridis
Trichomanas gallinarum

CIRCULATORY SYSTEM

Protozoa
Haemoproteus meleagridis
Leucocytozoon smithi
Plasmodium durae
Aegyptianella pullorum

RESPIRATORY SYSTEM

Nematodes
Syngamus trachea

Arthropods
Cytodites nudus

SKIN AND SUBCUTANEOUS TISSUE

Trematodes
Collyriclum faba

Cestodes
Dithyridium variabile

Arthropods
Menacanthus stramineus
Chelopistes meleagridis
Argas persicus
Cnemidocoptes mutans
Freyana chanayi
Dermanyssus gallinae
Ornithonyssus bursa

DUCK AND GOOSE

DIGESTIVE TRACT

Trematodes
Opisthorchis simulans
Echinostoma revolutum
Echinoparyphium paraulum
Echinoparyphium recurvatum
Hypoderaeum conoideum
Prosthogonimus pellucidus
Notocotylus attenuatus
Catatropis verrucosa
Typhlocoelum cymbium
Typhlocoelum obovale
Hyptiasmus tumidus
Apatemon gracilis
Parastrigea robustus
Cotylurus cornutus

Cestodes
Cotugnia fastigata
Hymenolepis lanceolata
Fimbriaria fasciolaris

Nematodes
Porrocaecum crassum
Heterakis gallinarum
Heterakis dispar
Ascaridia galli
Capillaria contorta
Amidostomum anseris
Trichostrongylus tenuis
Acuaria uncinata
Tetrameres fissispina
Tetrameres crami
Hystrichis tricolor
Polymorphus boschadis
Filicollis anatis

Protozoa
Trichomonas anatis
Trichomonas anseris
Cochlosoma anatis
Eimeria anatis
Eimeria anseris

Eimeria nocens
Eimeria parvula
Eimeria stigmosa
Tyzzeria anseris
Tyzzeria perniciosa

CIRCULATORY SYSTEM

Trematodes
Bilharziella polonica

Protozoa
Haemoproteus nettionis
Leucocytozoon simondi
Aegyptianella pullorum

UROGENITAL SYSTEM

Trematodes
Prosthogonimus pellucidus
Prosthogonimus macrorchis
Prosthogonimus ovatus

Protozoa
Eimeria truncata

RESPIRATORY SYSTEM

Trematodes
Typhlocoelum cymbium

Nematodes
Cyathostoma bronchialis

Protozoa
Toxoplasma gondii

SKIN AND SUBCUTANEOUS TISSUE

Trematodes
Collyriclum faba

Nematodes
Avioserpens taiwana

Arthropods
Trinoton anseris
Menopon gallinae
Argas persicus

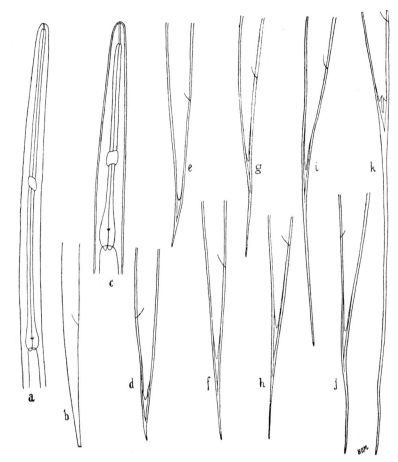

a, Strongyloides papillosus, oesophageal region; *b*, hind end of same; *c, Trichostrongylus*, oesophageal region; *d*, hind end of same; *e, Ostertagia*, hind end; *f, Cooperia*, hind end; *g, Haemonchus*, hind end; *h, Bunostomum*, hind end; *i, Oesophagostomum*, hind end; *j, Chabertia*, hind end; *k, Nematodirus*, hind end. (All drawn to same scale)

	Total length	Oeso-phagus	Tail of larva	Tail of sheath
Strongyloides papillosus (filariform larva)	0·6	0·23	0·09	Sheath absent
Trichostrongylus instabilis	0·69	0·165	0·06	0·094
Ostertagia spp.	0·84	0·16	0·075	0·112
Cooperia spp.	0·78	0·16	0·067	0·124
Haemonchus contortus	0·69	0·136	0·06	0·142
Bunostomum trigonocephalum	0·57	0·16	0·06	0·140
Chabertia ovina	0·73	0·165	0·064	0·165
Oesophagostomum columbianum	0·79	0·16	0·07	0·214
Nematodirus spathiger	1·1	0·225	0·056	0·326

INDEX